a LANGE medical book

1989

Medical Microbiology & Immunology

Examination and Board Review

Warren Levinson, MD, PhD
Professor of Microbiology
Department of Microbiology and Immunology
University of California, San Francisco

Ernest Jawetz, MD, PhD
Professor of Microbiology and Medicine Emeritus
Department of Microbiology and Immunology
University of California, San Francisco

APPLETON & LANGE
Norwalk, Connecticut/San Mateo, California

0-8385-6235-3

Notice: Our knowledge in clinical sciences is constantly changing. As new information becomes available, changes in treatment and in the use of drugs become necessary. The authors and the publisher of this volume have taken care to make certain that the doses of drugs and schedules of treatment are correct and compatible with the standards generally accepted at the time of publication. The reader is advised to consult carefully the instruction and information material included in the package insert of each drug or therapeutic agent before administration. This advice is especially important when using new or infrequently used drugs.

90 91 92 93 / 10 9 8 7 6 5 4 3 2

Prentice Hall International (UK) Limited, *London*
Prentice Hall of Australia Pty. Limited, *Sydney*
Prentice Hall Canada, Inc., *Toronto*
Prentice Hall Hispanoamericana, S.A., *Mexico*
Prentice Hall of India Private Limited, *New Delhi*
Prentice Hall of Japan, Inc., *Tokyo*
Simon & Schuster Asia Pte. Ltd., *Singapore*
Editora Prentice Hall do Brasil Ltda., *Rio de Janeiro*
Prentice Hall, *Englewood Cliffs, New Jersey*

ISBN 0-8385-6235-3
ISSN 1042-8070

PRINTED IN THE UNITED STATES OF AMERICA

Cover Design: Steven M. Byrum

Table of Contents

Preface

This book is a concise review of the medically important aspects of microbiology. It covers both the basic and clinical aspects of bacteriology, virology, mycology, parasitology, and immunology. Its 2 major aims are (1) to assist those who are preparing for the National Boards and (2) to provide students who are presently taking medical microbiology courses with a rapid and flexible source of information.

These aims are achieved by utilizing several different formats, which should make the book useful to students with varying study objectives and learning styles:

(1) A narrative text for complete information.
(2) Summaries of important microorganisms for rapid review of essentials.
(3) Review questions at the end of each chapter.
(4) Practice questions in National Board style, with answers provided after each group of questions.
(5) Clinical case discussions to illustrate the relevance of the material to patient problems.

In addition, the following specific features should be emphasized:

(1) The information is presented succinctly, with stress on making it clear, interesting, and up to date.
(2) There is strong emphasis in the text on the clinical application of microbiology and immunology to infectious diseases.
(3) In the clinical bacteriology and virology sections, the organisms are separated into major and minor pathogens. This allows the student to focus on the clinically most important microorganisms.
(4) Key information is summarized in useful review tables.
(5) The more than 650 National Board practice questions have been constructed to cover the important aspects of each of the sub-disciplines on the board examination—Bacteriology, Virology, Mycology, Parasitology and Immunology.
(6) Brief summaries of medically important microorganisms are presented together in a separate section to facilitate access to the information and to encourage comparisons of one organism with another.
(7) Ten clinical cases are presented as unknowns for the reader to analyze in a realistic, problem-solving way. These cases illustrate the importance of basic science information in clinical decision-making.

After teaching both medical microbiology and clinical infectious disease for many years, we believe that students appreciate a book that presents the essential information in a readable, interesting and varied format. We hope you find this book meets those criteria.

Warren Levinson, MD, PhD
Ernest Jawetz, MD, PhD

San Francisco
June, 1989

Acknowledgments

We gratefully acknowledge the thoughtful comments of Dr Bertie Argyris and Dr Candice McCoy, who reviewed the immunology section, and Dr Donald Heyneman, who reviewed the parasitology section. The excellent secretarial skills of Grace Stauffer and Bertha Cooke are greatly appreciated. We are indebted to our editor, Yvonne Strong, who ensured that the highest standards of grammar and style were met.

W. L. gratefully acknowledges the invaluable assistance of his wife, Barbara, in making this book become a reality.

W. L. dedicates this book to his father and mother who instilled a love of scholarship, the joy of teaching, and the value of being organized.

Part I: Basic Bacteriology

Bacteria Compared With Other Microorganisms

1

AGENTS The agents of human infectious diseases belong to 5 major groups of organisms: bacteria, fungi, protozoa, helminths, and viruses. The first 3 groups are members of the kingdom of **protists,** one of the primary biologic subdivisions along with animals and plants (Table 1–1). The protists are distinguished from animals and plants by being either unicellular or relatively simple multicellular organisms. The helminths are complex multicellular organisms that are classified as metazoa within the animal kingdom. Taken together, the helminths and the protozoa are commonly called parasites. Viruses are quite distinct from the other organisms, as they are not cells but can replicate only within cells.

Table 1–1. Biologic relationships of pathogenic microorganisms.

Kingdom	Pathogenic Microorganisms	Type of Cells
Animal	Helminths	Eukaryotic
Plant	None	Eukaryotic
Protist	Protozoa Fungi Bacteria	Eukaryotic Eukaryotic Prokaryotic
	Viruses	Noncellular

IMPORTANT FEATURES Many of the essential characteristics of these organisms are described in Table 1–2. One salient feature is that bacteria, fungi, protozoa, and helminths are cellular, whereas viruses are not. This distinction is based primarily on 3 criteria.

(1) Structure. Cells have a nucleus or nucleoid (see below) containing DNA; this is surrounded by cytoplasm, within which proteins are synthesized and energy is generated. Viruses have an inner core of genetic material (either DNA or RNA) but no cytoplasm, and so they depend on host cells to provide the machinery for protein synthesis and energy generation.

(2) Method of replication. Cells replicate by binary fission, during which one parent cell divides to make 2 progeny cells while retaining its cellular structure. In contrast, viruses disassemble, produce many copies of their nucleic acid and protein, and then reassemble into multiple progeny viruses. Furthermore, viruses must replicate within host cells, because, as mentioned above, they lack protein-synthesizing and energy-generating systems. With the exception of rickettsiae and chlamydiae, which are bacteria that also require living host cells for growth, bacteria can replicate extracellularly.

(3) Nature of the nucleic acid. Cells contain both DNA and RNA, whereas viruses contain either DNA or RNA but not both.

EUKARYOTES & PROKARYOTES Cells have evolved into 2 fundamentally different types, **eukaryotic** and **prokaryotic,** which can be distinguished on the basis of their structure and the complexity of their organization. Fungi and protozoa are eukaryotic, whereas bacteria are prokaryotic.

Table 1–2. Comparison of medically important organisms.

Characteristic	Viruses	Bacteria	Fungi	Protozoa and Helminths
Cells	No	Yes	Yes	Yes
Approximate diameter (μm)[1]	0.02–0.2	1–5	3–10 (yeasts)	15–25 (trophozoites)
Nucleic acid	Either DNA or RNA	Both DNA and RNA	Both DNA and RNA	Both DNA and RNA
Type of nucleus	None	Prokaryotic	Eukaryotic	Eukaryotic
Ribosomes	Absent	70S	80S	80S
Mitochondria	Absent	Absent	Present	Present
Nature of outer surface	Protein capsid and lipoprotein envelope	Rigid wall containing peptidoglycan	Rigid wall containing chitin	Flexible membrane
Motility	None	Some	None	Most
Method of replication	Not binary fission	Binary fission	Binary fission or budding[2]	Binary fission[3]

[1]For comparison, a human red blood cell has a diameter of 7 μm.
[2]In general, molds divide by binary fission, whereas yeasts divide by budding.
[3]Helminth cells divide by binary fission, but the organism reproduces itself by complex, sexual life cycles.

(1) The eukaryotic cell has a true nucleus with multiple chromosomes surrounded by a nuclear membrane and uses a mitotic apparatus to ensure equal allocation of the chromosomes to progeny cells.

(2) The **nucleoid** of a prokaryotic cell consists of a single circular molecule of loosely organized DNA lacking a nuclear membrane and mitotic apparatus (Table 1–3).

In addition to the different types of nuclei, the 2 classes of cells are distinguished by several other criteria.

(1) Eukaryotic cells contain **organelles**, such as mitochondria and lysosomes, and larger (80S) ribosomes, whereas prokaryotes contain no organelles and smaller (70S) ribosomes.

(2) Most prokaryotes have a rigid external cell wall that contains **peptidoglycan**, a polymer of amino acids and sugars, as its unique structural component. Eukaryotes, on the other hand, do not contain peptidoglycan. Either they are bound by a flexible cell membrane or, in the case of fungi, they have a rigid cell wall with chitin, a homopolymer of N-acetylglucosamine, typically forming the framework.

(3) The eukaryotic cell membrane contains **sterols**, whereas no prokaryote, except the wall-less *Mycoplasma,* has sterols in its membranes.

Another criterion by which these organisms can be contrasted is **motility**. Most protozoa and some bacteria can move, whereas fungi and viruses are nonmotile. The protozoa are a heterogeneous group that possess 3 different organs of locomotion: flagella, cilia, and pseudopods. The motile bacteria move only by means of flagella.

Table 1–3. Characteristics of prokaryotic and eukaryotic cells.

Characteristic	Prokaryotic Bacterial Cells	Eukaryotic Human Cells
DNA within a nuclear membrane	No	Yes
Mitotic division	No	Yes
DNA associated with histones	No	Yes
Chromosome number	One	More than one
Membrane-bound organelles such as mitochondria and lysosomes	No	Yes
Size of ribosome	70S	80S
Cell wall containing peptidoglycan	Yes	No

Review Questions

1. What are the differences between bacteria and viruses?
2. Are bacteria prokaryotic or eukaryotic? What are the differences between prokaryotic and eukaryotic cells?
3. What are the similarities and the differences among bacteria, fungi, and protozoa?

Structure of Bacterial Cells

2

SHAPE & SIZE Bacteria have 3 basic shapes: **cocci, bacilli,** and **spirochetes** (Fig. 2–1). Some bacteria are variable in shape and are said to be **pleomorphic** (many-shaped). The shape of a bacterium is determined by its rigid cell wall. The microscopic appearance of a bacterium is one of the most important criteria used in its identification.

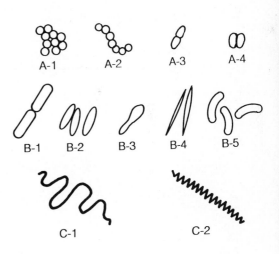

Figure 2–1. Bacterial morphology. **A:** Cocci: in clusters, eg, *Staphylococcus* (A-1); chains, eg, *Streptococcus* (A-2); in pairs with pointed ends, eg, *Streptococcus pneumoniae* (A-3); in pairs, eg, *Neisseria* (A-4). **B:** Rods: with square ends, eg, *Bacillus* (B-1); with rounded ends, eg, *Salmonella* (B-2); club-shaped, eg, *Corynebacterium* (B-3); fusiform, eg, *Fusobacterium* (B-4); comma-shaped, eg, *Vibrio* (B-5). **C:** Spirochetes: relaxed coil, eg, *Borrelia* (C-1); tightly coiled, eg, *Treponema* (C-2). (Modified and reproduced, with permission, from Joklik WK et al: *Zinsser Microbiology,* 19th ed. Appleton & Lange, 1988.)

In addition to their characteristic shapes, the arrangement of bacteria is important. For example, certain cocci occur in pairs (**diplococci**), some in chains (**streptococci**), and others in grapelike clusters (**staphylococci**). These arrangements are determined by the orientation and degree of attachment of the bacteria at the time of cell division.

Bacteria range in size from about 0.2 to 5 μm (Fig 2–2). The smallest bacteria are about the same size as the largest viruses (poxviruses) and are the smallest organisms capable of existing outside the host. The longest bacterial rods approach the size of some yeasts and human red blood cells (7 μm).

STRUCTURE The structure of a typical bacterium is illustrated in Fig 2–3, and the important features of each component are presented in Table 2–1.

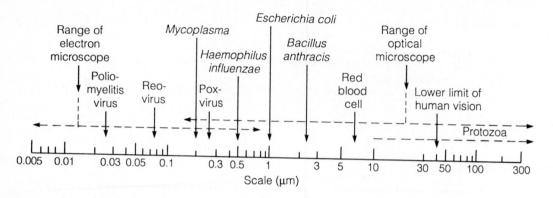

Figure 2-2. Sizes of representative bacteria, viruses, protozoa, and human red cells. (Modified and reproduced, with permission, from Joklik WK et al: *Zinsser Microbiology,* 19th ed. Appleton & Lange, 1988.)

Cell Wall

The cell wall is the outermost component common to all bacteria (except *Mycoplasma* species, which are bounded by a cell membrane, not a cell wall). Some bacteria have surface features external to the cell wall, such as a capsule, flagella, and pili, which are less common components and are discussed below.

The cell wall is a multilayered structure located external to the cytoplasmic membrane. It is composed of an inner layer of **peptidoglycan** (see p 5) surrounded by an outer layer that varies in thickness and chemical composition depending upon bacterial type (Fig 2-4). The peptidoglycan provides structural support and maintains the characteristic shape of the cell.

A. Cell Walls of Gram-Positive and Gram-Negative Bacteria: The structure, chemical composition, and thickness of the cell wall differ in gram-positive and gram-negative bacteria (box and Table 2-2).

(1) The peptidoglycan layer is much thicker in gram-positive than in gram-negative bacteria. Some gram-positive bacteria also have a layer of teichoic acid on the outside of the peptidoglycan, whereas gram-negative bacteria have no teichoic acid.

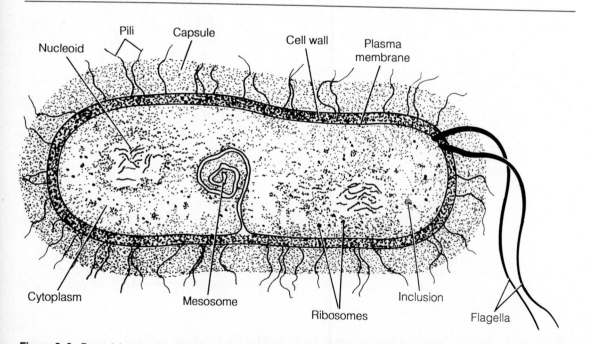

Figure 2-3. Bacterial structure. (Modified and reproduced, with permission, from Tortora G, Funk B, Case C: *Microbiology: An Introduction,* 2nd ed. Benjamin/Cummings, 1986.)

Table 2–1. Bacterial structures.

Structure	Chemical Composition	Function
Essential components		
Cell wall		
Peptidoglycan	Sugar backbone with peptide side chains that are cross-linked	Gives rigid support, protects against osmotic pressure; is the site of action of penicillins and cephalosporins and is degraded by lysozyme.
Outer membrane (gram-positive organisms)	Teichoic acid	Major surface antigen but rarely used in laboratory diagnosis.
Outer membrane (gram-negative organisms)	Lipid A	Toxic moiety of endotoxin.
	Lipopolysaccharide	Major surface antigen used frequently in laboratory diagnosis.
Cytoplasmic membrane	Lipoprotein bilayer without sterols	Site of oxidative and transport enzymes.
Ribosome	RNA and protein in 50S and 30S subunits	Protein synthesis; site of action of aminoglycosides, erythromycin, tetracyclines, and chloramphenicol.
Nucleoid	DNA	Genetic material.
Mesosome	Invagination of plasma membrane	Participates in cell division and secretion.
Periplasm	Space between plasma membrane and outer membrane	Contains many hydrolytic enzymes, including β-lactamases.
Nonessential components		
Capsule	Polysaccharide[1]	Protects against phagocytosis.
Pilus or fimbria	Glycoprotein	Adherence to cell surfaces; attachment to bacteria during conjugation.
Flagellum	Protein	Motility.
Spore	Keratinlike coat, dipicolinic acid	Resistance to dehydration, heat, and chemicals.
Plasmid	DNA	Contains a variety of genes for antibiotic resistance, enzymes, and toxins.
Granule	Glycogen, lipids, polyphosphates	Storage sites of food.

[1]Except in *Bacillus anthracis,* in which it is a polypeptide of D-glutamic acid.

(2) In contrast, the gram-negative organisms have a complex outer layer consisting of lipopolysaccharide, lipoprotein, and phospholipid. Lying between the outer-membrane layer and the cytoplasmic membrane in gram-negative bacteria is the **periplasmic space**, which is the site, in some species, of enzymes (eg, β-lactamases) that degrade penicillins and other β-lactam drugs.

Table 2–2. Comparison of cell walls of gram-positive and gram-negative bacteria.

Component	Gram-Positive Cells	Gram-Negative Cells
Peptidoglycan	Thicker; multilayer	Thinner; single layer
Teichoic acids	Yes	No
Lipopolysaccharide (endotoxin)	No	Yes
Lipoprotein and phospholipid	No	Yes

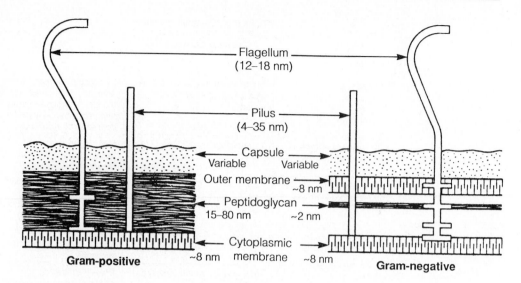

Figure 2–4. Cell walls of gram-positive and gram-negative bacteria. (Reproduced, with permission, from Ingraham JL, Maalφe O, Neidhardt FC: *Growth of the Bacterial Cell.* Sinauer Associates, 1983.)

The cell wall has several other important properties:

(1) in gram-negative organisms, it contains **endotoxin**, a lipopolysaccharide (see p 8);

(2) its polysaccharides and proteins are antigens that are useful in laboratory identification; and

(3) its porin proteins play a role in regulating the passage of molecules into the cell.

B. Cell Walls of Acid-Fast Bacteria: Mycobacteria, eg, *Mycobacterium tuberculosis,* have an unusual cell wall, resulting in their inability to be Gram-stained. These bacteria are said to be "**acid-fast**," since they resist decolorization with acid-alcohol after being stained

---

Gram Stain: This staining procedure, developed in 1884 by the Danish physician Christian Gram, is the most important procedure in microbiology. It separates most bacteria into 2 groups: the gram-positive bacteria, which stain blue, and the gram-negative bacteria, which stain red. The Gram stain involves the following 4-step procedure.

(1) The crystal violet dye stains all cells blue.

(2) The iodine solution (a mordant) is added to form a crystal violet-iodine complex; all cells continue to appear blue.

(3) The organic solvent, such as acetone or ethanol, extracts the blue dye complex from the lipid-rich, thin-walled gram-negative bacteria to a greater degree than from the lipid-poor, thick-walled gram-positive bacteria. The gram-negative organisms appear colorless; the gram-positive bacteria remain blue.

(4) The red dye safranin stains the decolorized gram- negative cells red; the gram positive bacteria remain blue.

The Gram stain is useful in 2 ways:

(1) in the identification of many bacteria, and

(2) in influencing the choice of antibiotic, since, in general, gram-positive bacteria are more susceptible to penicillin G than are gram-negative bacteria.

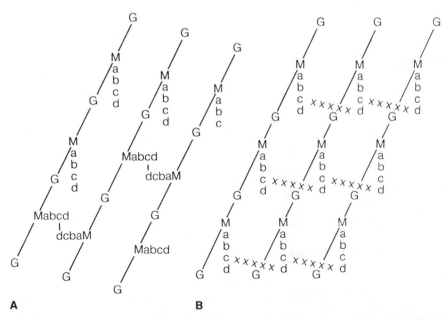

Figure 2–5. Peptidoglycan structure: *A:* Escherichia coli. *B: Staphylococcus aureus.* M, muramic acid; G, glucosamine; a, L-alanine; b, D-glutamic acid; c, diaminopimelic acid (*A*) or L-lysine (*B*); d, D-alanine; x, pentaglycine bridge. (Modified and reproduced, with permission, from Joklik WK et al: *Zinsser Microbiology,* 19th ed. Appleton & Lange, 1988).

with carbolfuchsin. This property is related to the high concentration in the cell wall of lipids called mycolic acids.

In view of their importance, 3 components of the cell wall, ie, peptidoglycan, lipopolysaccharide, and teichoic acid, will be discussed in detail.

C. Peptidoglycan: Peptidoglycan is a complex, interwoven network that surrounds the entire cell. It is found only in bacterial cell walls. It provides rigid support for the cell, is important in maintaining the characteristic shape of the cell, and allows the cell to withstand media of low osmotic pressure, such as water. A representative segment of the peptidoglycan layer is shown in Fig 2–5. The term "peptidoglycan" is derived from the peptides and the sugars (glycan) that make up the molecule. Synonyms for peptidoglycan are murein and mucopeptide.

Fig 2–5 illustrates the carbohydrate backbone, which is composed of alternating N-acetylmuramic acid and N-acetylglucosamine molecules. Attached to each of the muramic acid molecules is a tetrapeptide consisting of both D- and L-amino acids, the precise composition of which differs from one bacterium to another. Two of these amino acids are worthy of special mention: diaminopimelic acid, which is unique to bacterial cell walls, and D-alanine, which is involved in the cross-links between the tetrapeptides and in the action of penicillin. Note that this tetrapeptide contains the rare D-isomers of amino acids; most proteins contain the L-isomer. The other important component in this network is the peptide cross-link between the 2 tetrapeptides. The cross-links vary among species; in *Staphylococcus aureus,* for example, 5 glycines link the terminal D-alanine to the penultimate L-lysine.

Since peptidoglycan is present in bacteria but not in human cells, it is a good target for antibacterial drugs. Several of these drugs, such as the penicillins and cephalosporins, inhibit its synthesis (see Chapter 10).

The enzyme **lysozyme**, which is present in human tears, mucus, and saliva, can cleave the peptidoglycan backbone by breaking its glycosyl bonds, thereby contributing to the natural resistance of the host to microbial infection. Lysozyme-treated bacteria may swell and rupture owing to the entrance of water into the cells, which have a high internal osmotic pressure. However, if the lysozyme-treated cells are in a solution with the same osmotic pressure as that of the bacterial interior, they will survive as spherical forms, called protoplasts, surrounded only by a cytoplasmic membrane.

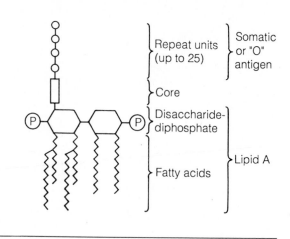

Figure 2–6. Lipopolysaccharide (LPS) structure. (Modified and reproduced, with permission, from Jawetz E et al: *Review of Medical Microbiology*, 18th ed. Appleton & Lange, 1989.)

D. Lipopolysaccharide (LPS): The LPS of the outer layer of the cell wall of gram-negative bacteria is **endotoxin.** It is responsible for many of the features of disease, such as fever and shock, caused by these organisms. It is called endotoxin because it is an integral part of the cell wall, in contrast to exotoxins, which are freely released from the bacteria. The pathologic effects of endotoxin are the same irrespective of the organism from which it is derived.

The LPS is composed of 3 distinct units (Fig 2–6):

(1) a phospholipid called lipid A, which is responsible for the toxic effects;

(2) a core polysaccharide of 5 sugars linked through ketodeoxyoctulonate to the lipid A; and

(3) an outer polysaccharide consisting of up to 25 repeating units of 3–5 sugars. This outer polymer is the important somatic or O antigen of several gram-negative bacteria that is used to identify certain organisms in the clinical laboratory.

E. Teichoic Acid: These polymers of glycerol phosphate or ribitol phosphate are located in the outer layer of the gram-positive cell wall. Some polymers of glycerol teichoic acid penetrate the peptidoglycan layer and are covalently linked to the lipid in the cytoplasmic membrane, in which case they are called **lipoteichoic acid;** others anchor to the muramic acid of the peptidoglycan. Teichoic acids are antigenic and induce antibodies that are species-specific. The physiologic role of teichoic acids is uncertain.

Cytoplasmic Membrane Just inside the peptidoglycan layer of the cell wall lies the cytoplasmic membrane, which is composed of a phospholipid bilayer similar in microscopic appearance to that in eukaryotic cells. They are chemically similar, but eukaryotic membranes contain sterols, whereas prokaryotes do not. The only prokaryotes that have sterols in their membranes are members of the genus *Mycoplasma*. The membrane has 4 important functions:

(1) active transport of molecules into the cell,

(2) energy generation by oxidative phosphorylation,

(3) synthesis of precursors of the cell wall, and

(4) secretion of enzymes and toxins.

Mesosome This invagination of the cytoplasmic membrane is important during cell division, when it functions as the origin of the transverse septum that divides the cell in half and as the binding site of the DNA which will become the genetic material of each daughter cell.

Cytoplasm The cytoplasm has 2 distinct areas when visualized in the electron microscope:

(1) an amorphous matrix that contains ribosomes, nutrient granules, metabolites, and ions; and

(2) an inner, nucleoid region composed of DNA.

A. Ribosomes: Bacterial ribosomes are the site of protein synthesis as in eukaryotic cells, but they differ in size and chemical composition. Bacterial ribosomes are 70S in size, with 50S and 30S subunits, whereas eukaryotic ribosomes are 80S in size, with 60S and 40S subunits. The differences in both the ribosomal RNAs and proteins constitute the basis of the selective action of several antibiotics that inhibit bacterial, but not human, protein synthesis (see Chapter 10).

B. Granules: The cytoplasm contains several different types of granules that serve as storage areas for nutrients and stain characteristically with certain dyes. For example, volutin is a reserve of high energy stored in the form of polymerized metaphosphate. It appears as a "metachromatic" granule, since it stains red with methylene blue dye instead of blue as one would expect.

C. Nucleoid: The nucleoid is the area of the cytoplasm in which DNA is located. The DNA of prokaryotes is a single, circular molecule that has a molecular weight of approximately 2×10^9 and contains about 2000 genes. The nucleoid contains no nuclear membrane, no mitotic apparatus, and no histones, so there is little resemblance to the eukaryotic nucleus.

D. Plasmids: Plasmids are extrachromosomal, double-stranded, circular DNA molecules that are capable of replicating independently of the bacterial chromosome. Although plasmids are usually extrachromosomal, they can be integrated into the bacterial chromosome.

(1) Transmissible plasmids can be transferred from cell to cell by conjugation (see Chapter 4 for a discussion of conjugation). They are large (MW 40–100 million), since they contain about a dozen genes responsible for synthesis of the sex pilus and for the enzymes required for transfer. They are usually present in a few (one to 3) copies per cell.

(2) Nontransmissible plasmids are small (MW 3–20 million), since they do not contain the transfer genes; they are frequently present in many (10–60) copies per cell.

Plasmids occur in both gram-positive and gram-negative bacteria, and several different types of plasmids can exist in one cell. Treatment with some compounds, such as acridine dyes, can "cure" bacteria of their plasmids in vitro.

The genes for the following functions and structures of medical importance are carried by plasmids:

(1) antibiotic resistance, which is mediated by a variety of enzymes;

(2) resistance to heavy metals such as mercury (the active component of some antiseptics, such as Merthiolate and Mercurochrome) and silver, which is mediated by a reductase enzyme;

(3) resistance to ultraviolet light, which is mediated by DNA repair enzymes;

(4) pili (fimbriae), which mediate the adherence of bacteria to epithelial cells; and

(5) exotoxins, including several enterotoxins.

Other plasmid-encoded products of interest are

(1) bacteriocins, which are toxins or enzymes that are produced by certain bacteria and are lethal for other bacteria;

(2) nitrogen fixation enzymes in *Rhizobium* in the root nodules of legumes;

(3) tumors caused by *Agrobacterium* in plants;

(4) several antibiotics produced by *Streptomyces*; and

(5) a variety of degradative enzymes that are produced by *Pseudomonas* and are capable of cleaning up environmental hazards such as oil spills and toxic chemical-waste sites.

E. Transposons: Transposons are pieces of DNA that move readily from one site to another, either within or between the DNAs of bacteria, plasmids, and bacteriophages. In view of their unusual ability to move, they are nicknamed "jumping genes." They can code for drug resistance enzymes, toxins, or a variety of metabolic enzymes, and they can either cause mutations in the gene into which they insert or alter the expression of nearby genes.

Transposons typically have 4 identifiable domains. On each end is a short DNA sequence of **inverted repeats,** which are involved in the integration of the transposon into the recipient DNA. The second domain is the gene for the transposase, which is the enzyme that mediates the excision and integration processes. The third region is the gene for the repressor that regulates the synthesis both of the transposase and of the gene product of the fourth domain, which, in many cases, is an enzyme mediating antibiotic resistance (Fig 2–7).

In contrast to plasmids or bacterial viruses, transposons are not capable of independent replication; they replicate as part of the recipient DNA. More than one transposon can be located in the DNA; for example, a plasmid can contain several transposons carrying drug resistance genes. **Insertion sequences** are a type of transposon that have fewer bases (800–1500 base pairs), since they do not code for their own integration enzymes. They can cause mutations at their site of integration and can be found in multiple copies at the ends of larger transposon units.

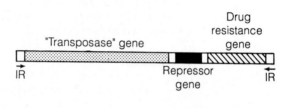

Figure 2–7. Transposon genes. IR, inverted repeat. (Modified and reproduced, with permission, from Fincham JR: *Genetics.* Jones and Bartlett, 1983.)

Specialized Structures Outside the Cell Wall

A. Capsule: The capsule is a gelatinous layer covering the entire bacterium. It is composed of polysaccharide, except in the anthrax bacillus, which has a capsule of polymerized D-glutamic acid. The sugar components of the polysaccharide vary from one species of bacteria to another and frequently determine the serologic type within a species. For example, there are 80 different serologic types of *Streptococcus pneumoniae,* which are distinguished by the antigenic differences of the sugars in the polysaccharide capsule.

The capsule is important for 4 reasons:

(1) It is a determinant of virulence of many bacteria, since it limits the ability of phagocytes to engulf the bacteria. Variants of encapsulated bacteria that have lost the ability to produce a capsule are usually nonpathogenic.

(2) Specific identification of an organism can be made by using antiserum against the capsular polysaccharide. In the presence of the homologous antibody, the capsule will swell greatly. This swelling phenomenon, which is used in the clinical laboratory to identify certain organisms, is called the **quellung reaction.**

(3) Capsular polysaccharides are used as the antigens in certain vaccines, since they are capable of eliciting protective antibodies. For example, the purified polysaccharides of 23 types of *S pneumoniae* are present in the current vaccine.

(4) The capsule may play a role in the adherence of bacteria to human tissues, which is an important initial step in causing infection.

In certain organisms, eg, *Streptococcus mutans,* a loose network of polysaccharide strands (the glycocalyx) mediates adherence to the tooth surface. This plays a role in the formation of plaque, the precursor of dental caries.

B. Flagella: Flagella are long, whiplike appendages that propel the bacteria toward food and other attractants, a process called **chemotaxis.** The ability of flagella to impart movement is a function of their structure (Fig 2–8). The base is anchored to the cell membrane and cell wall by a series of rings. Extending from this is a curved, hooklike area that rotates, thereby turning the long filament, which acts as a propeller. The filament is composed of many subunits of a single protein, flagellin, arranged in several intertwined chains. The energy for

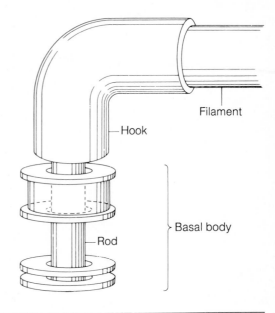

Figure 2–8. Structure of flagella. (Modified and reproduced, with permission, from De Pamphilis ML, Adler J: Fine structure and isolation of the hook-basal body complex of flagella from *Escherichia coli* and *Bacillus subtilis.* *J Bacteriol* 1971; 105: 384.)

movement, the **proton motive** force, is provided by adenosine triphosphate (ATP), derived from the passage of ions across the membrane.

Flagellated bacteria have a characteristic number and location of flagella: some bacteria have one, and others have many; in some the flagella are located at one end, and in others they are all over the outer surface. Only certain bacteria have flagella; many rods do, but most cocci do not and are therefore nonmotile. Spirochetes move by using a flagellumlike structure called the **axial filament**, which wraps around the spiral-shaped cell to produce an undulating motion.

Flagella are important for 2 reasons:

(1) They are the means by which bacteria move toward nutrients or away from harmful substances. This property (chemotaxis) is a function of sensors on the outer surface of the cell that detect differences in the concentration of the medium.

(2) Some species of bacteria, eg, *Salmonella* species, are identified in the clinical laboratory by the use of specific antibodies against flagellar proteins.

C. Pili (Fimbriae): Pili are hairlike filaments that extend from the cell surface. They are shorter and straighter than flagella and are composed of subunits of a protein, pilin, arranged in helical strands. They are found mainly on gram-negative organisms.

Pili have 2 important roles:

(1) They mediate the attachment of bacteria to specific receptors on the human cell surface, which is a necessary step in the initiation of infection for some organisms. Mutants of *Neisseria gonorrhoeae* that do not form pili are nonpathogens.

(2) A specialized kind of pilus, the sex pilus, forms the attachment between the male (donor) and the female (recipient) bacteria during conjugation (see Chapter 4).

Spores   These highly resistant structures are formed in response to adverse conditions by 2 genera of medically important gram-positive rods: the genus *Bacillus*, which includes the agent of anthrax, and the genus *Clostridium*, which includes the agents of tetanus and botulism. Spore formation (sporulation) occurs when nutrients, such as sources of carbon and nitrogen, are depleted (Fig 2–9). The spore forms inside the cell and contains bacterial DNA, a small amount of cytoplasm, cell membrane, peptidoglycan, very little water, and, most importantly, a thick, keratinlike coat that is responsible for the remarkable resistance of the spore to heat, dehydration, radiation, and chemicals. This resistance may be mediated by dipicolinic acid, a chelator of calcium ion found only in spores.

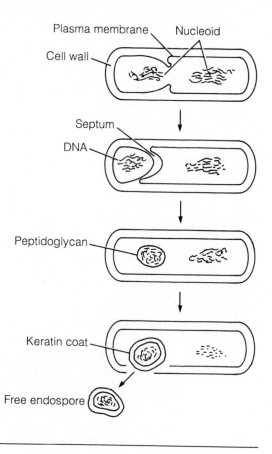

Figure 2–9. Bacterial spores. (Modified and reproduced, with permission, from Tortora G, Funk B, Case C: *Microbiology: An Introduction,* 2nd ed. Benjamin/Cummings, 1986.)

Once formed, the spore has no metabolic activity and can remain dormant for many years. Upon exposure to water and the appropriate nutrients, specific enzymes degrade the coat; water and nutrients enter; and germination into a metabolizing, reproducing bacterial cell occurs. Note that this differentiation process is *not* a means of reproduction, since one cell produces one spore that germinates into one cell.

The medical importance of spores lies in their extraordinary resistance to heat and chemicals. As a result of their resistance to heat, sterilization cannot be achieved by boiling. Steam-heating under pressure (autoclaving) at 121° C, usually for 30 minutes, is required to ensure the sterility of products for medical use. Spores are sometimes not seen in clinical specimens recovered from patients infected by spore-forming organisms, since the supply of nutrients is adequate.

Review Questions

1. What is the structure of the bacterial cell wall? What is its function?
2. Where is the periplasmic space, and what is its importance?
3. What are the differences between gram-positive and gram-negative cell walls?
4. What attribute of the cell wall of *Mycobacterium tuberculosis* makes it acid-fast?
5. Describe the Gram stain procedure and the function of each step.
6. What is the structure of peptidoglycan? What is its function?
7. If certain bacteria are treated with lysozyme, a protoplast may result. What is the mode of action of lysozyme? What is a protoplast?
8. What is the importance of the lipopolysaccharide in the cell wall of gram-negative bacteria?
9. What are the similarities and differences between the cytoplasmic membranes of bacteria and eukaryotic cells?

10. What is the function of mesosomes?
11. How do bacterial ribosomes differ from eukaryotic ones?
12. How does the bacterial nucleoid differ from the nucleus of a eukaryotic cell?
13. What are plasmids, and what is their function?
14. What are transposons, and how do they differ from plasmids?
15. What is the function of (1) bacterial capsules, (2) bacterial flagella, and (3) pili?
16. What is the medical importance of bacterial spores? Describe the circumstances under which they form.

Growth

3

GROWTH CYCLE   Bacteria reproduce by **binary fission**, a process by which one parent cell divides to form 2 progeny cells. Because one cell gives rise to 2, bacteria are said to undergo exponential growth (logarithmic growth). The concept of exponential growth can be illustrated by the following relationship:

Number of cells	1	2	4	8	16
Exponential	2^0	2^1	2^2	2^3	2^4

Thus, one bacterium will produce 16 bacteria after 4 generations.

The doubling (generation) time of bacteria ranges from as little as 20 minutes for *Escherichia coli* to more than 24 hours for *Mycobacterium tuberculosis*. The exponential growth and the short doubling time of some organisms result in rapid production of very large numbers of bacteria. For example, one *E coli* organism will produce over 1000 progeny in about 3 hours and over 1 million in about 7 hours. A hypothetical growth curve of bacteria grown through 4 generations is shown in Fig 3–1. The doubling time varies not only with the species but also with the amount of nutrients, the temperature, the pH, and other environmental factors.

The growth cycle of bacteria has 4 major phases. If a small number of bacteria are inoculated into a liquid nutrient medium and the bacteria are counted at frequent intervals, the typical phases of a standard growth curve can be demonstrated (Fig 3–2).

(a) The first is the **lag** phase, during which vigorous metabolic activity occurs but cells do not divide. This can last for a few minutes up to many hours.

(b) The **log** (logarithmic) phase is when rapid cell division occurs.

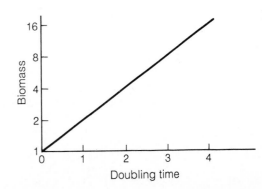

Figure 3–1. Exponential growth of bacteria. (Modified and reproduced, with permission, from Jawetz, E et al: *Review of Medical Microbiology,* 18th ed. Appleton & Lange, 1989.)

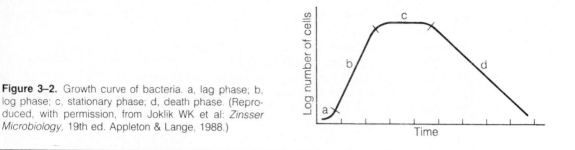

Figure 3–2. Growth curve of bacteria. a, lag phase; b, log phase; c, stationary phase; d, death phase. (Reproduced, with permission, from Joklik WK et al: *Zinsser Microbiology*, 19th ed. Appleton & Lange, 1988.)

(c) The **stationary** phase occurs when nutrient depletion or toxic products cause growth to slow until the number of new cells produced balances the number of cells that die, resulting in a steady state. Cells grown in a special apparatus called a chemostat, into which fresh nutrients are added and from which waste products are removed continuously, can remain in the log phase and do not enter the stationary phase.

(d) The final phase is the **death** phase, which is marked by a decline in the number of viable bacteria.

AEROBIC & ANAEROBIC GROWTH For most organisms, an adequate supply of oxygen enhances metabolism and growth. The oxygen acts as the hydrogen acceptor in the final steps of energy production catalyzed by the flavoproteins and cytochromes. Because the use of oxygen generates 2 toxic molecules, hydrogen peroxide (H_2O_2) and the free radical superoxide ($O_2^{\cdot}$) bacteria require 2 enzymes to utilize oxygen. The first is **superoxide dismutase,** which catalyzes the reaction

$$2O_2^{\cdot} + 2H^+ \rightarrow H_2O_2 + O_2$$

and the second is **catalase,** which catalyzes the reaction

$$2H_2O_2 \rightarrow 2H_2O + O_2$$

The response to oxygen is an important criterion for classifying bacteria and has great practical significance, because specimens from patients must be incubated in the proper atmosphere for the bacteria to grow.

(a) Some bacteria, such as *M tuberculosis*, are **obligate aerobes**, ie, they require oxygen to grow because their ATP-generating system is dependent on oxygen as the hydrogen acceptor.

(b) Other bacteria, such as *E coli*, are **facultative anaerobes (facultatives)**; they utilize oxygen to generate energy by respiration if it is present, but they can use the fermentation pathway to synthesize ATP in the absence of sufficient oxygen.

(c) The third group of bacteria consists of the **obligate anaerobes**, such as *Clostridium tetani*, which cannot grow in the presence of oxygen because they lack either superoxide dismutase or catalase, or both. Obligate anaerobes vary in their response to oxygen exposure; some can survive but are not able to grow, whereas others are killed rapidly.

Review Questions

1. Draw and label a typical bacterial growth curve.
2. Distinguish among aerobic, facultative, and anaerobic growth.
3. Why do certain bacteria die in the presence of oxygen?

Genetics

4

The genetic material of a typical bacterium, *Escherichia coli,* consists of a single circular DNA molecule, with a molecular weight of about 2×10^9 and composed of approximately 5×10^6 base pairs. This amount of genetic information can code for about 2000 proteins with an average molecular weight of 50,000. The DNA of the smallest free-living organism, the wall-less bacterium *Mycoplasma,* has a molecular weight of 5×10^8. Note that bacteria are **haploid,** since they have a single chromosome, in contrast to human cells, which are diploid.

MUTATIONS   A mutation is a change in the base sequence of DNA that usually results in insertion of a different amino acid into a protein and the appearance of an altered phenotype. Mutations result from 3 types of molecular changes:

(1) The first type is the **base substitution.** This occurs when one base is inserted in place of another. It takes place at the time of DNA replication, either because the DNA polymerase makes an error or because a mutagen alters the hydrogen bonding of the base being used as a template in such a manner that the wrong base is inserted. When the base substitution results in a codon that simply causes a different amino acid to be inserted, the mutation is called a **missense mutation**; when the base substitution generates a termination codon that stops protein synthesis prematurely, the mutation is called a **nonsense mutation.** Nonsense mutations almost always destroy protein function.

(2) The second type of mutation is the **frame shift mutation.** This occurs when one or more base pairs are added or deleted, which shifts the reading frame on the ribosome and results in incorporation of the wrong amino acids "downstream" from the mutation and in the production of an inactive protein.

(3) The third type of mutation occurs when **transposons** or **insertion sequences** are integrated into the DNA. These newly inserted pieces of DNA can cause profound changes in the genes into which they insert and in adjacent genes.

Mutations can be caused by chemicals, radiation, or viruses. Chemicals act in several different ways.

(1) Some, such as nitrous acid and alkylating agents, alter the existing base so that it forms a hydrogen bond preferentially with the wrong base; for example, adenine would no longer pair with thymine but with cytosine.

(2) Some chemicals, such as 5-bromouracil, are base analogues, since they resemble normal bases. Because the bromine atom has an atomic radius similar to that of a methyl group, 5-bromouracil can be inserted in place of thymine (5-methyluracil). However, 5-bromouracil has less hydrogen-bonding fidelity than does thymine, and so it binds to guanine with greater frequency. This results in a transition from an A-T base pair to a G-C base pair, thereby producing a mutation. The antiviral drug iododeoxyuridine acts as a base analogue of thymidine.

(3) Some chemicals, such as benzpyrene, which is found in tobacco smoke, bind to the existing DNA bases and cause frame shift mutations. These chemicals, which are frequently carcinogens as well as mutagens, intercalate between the adjacent bases, thereby distorting and offsetting the DNA sequence.

X-rays and ultraviolet light can cause mutations also.

(1) X-rays have high energy and can damage DNA in 3 ways: (a) by breaking the covalent bonds that hold the ribose phosphate chain together, (b) by producing free radicals that can attack the bases, and (c) by altering the electrons in the bases and thus changing their hydrogen bonding.

(2) Ultraviolet radiation, which has lower energy than x-rays, causes the cross-linking of adjacent pyrimidine bases to form dimers. This cross-linking, for example, of adjacent thymines to form a thymine dimer, results in inability of the DNA to replicate properly.

Certain viruses, such as the bacterial virus Mu (mutator bacteriophage), cause a high frequency of mutations when their DNA is inserted into the bacterial chromosome. Since the viral DNA can insert into many different sites, mutations in various genes can occur. These mutations are either frame shift mutations or deletions.

Conditional-lethal mutations are of medical interest, since they may be useful in vaccines, eg, influenza vaccine. The word "conditional" indicates that the mutation is expressed only under certain conditions. The most important conditional-lethal mutations are the temperature-sensitive ones. Temperature-sensitive organisms can replicate at a relatively low, permissive temperature, eg, 32° C, but cannot grow at a higher, restrictive temperature, eg, 37° C. This behavior is due to a mutation that causes an amino acid change in an essential protein, allowing it to function normally at 32° C but not at 37° C owing to an altered conformation at the higher temperature. An example of a conditional-lethal mutant of medical importance is a strain of influenza virus currently used in an experimental vaccine. This vaccine contains a virus that cannot grow at 37° C and hence cannot infect the lungs and cause pneumonia, but it can grow at 32° C in the nose, where it can replicate and induce immunity.

TRANSFER OF DNA BETWEEN CELLS   The transfer of genetic information from one cell to another can occur by 3 methods: conjugation, transduction, and transformation (Table 4–1). From a medical viewpoint, the most important consequence of DNA transfer is that antibiotic resistance genes are spread from one bacterium to another by these processes.

(1) Conjugation is the mating of 2 bacterial cells during which DNA is transferred from the donor to the recipient cell (Fig 4–1). The mating process is controlled by an **F (fertility) plasmid,** which carries the genes for the proteins required for conjugation. One of the most important proteins is pilin, which forms the **sex pilus** (conjugation tube). Mating begins when the pilus of the donor male bacterium carrying the F factor (F^+) attaches to a receptor on the surface of the recipient female bacterium, which does not contain an F plasmid (F^-). The cells are then drawn into direct contact by "reeling in" the pilus. After an enzymatic cleavage of the F factor DNA, one strand is transferred across the conjugal bridge into the recipient cell. The process is completed by synthesis of the complementary strand to form a double-stranded F factor plasmid in both the donor and recipient cells. The recipient is now an F^+ cell that is capable of transmitting the plasmid further. Note that in this instance only the F factor, and not the bacterial chromosome, has been transferred.

Some F^+ cells have their F plasmid integrated into the bacterial DNA and thereby acquire the capability of transferring the chromosome into another cell. These cells are called **Hfr (high-frequency recombination).** During this transfer, the single strand of DNA that enters the recipient F^- cell contains a piece of the F factor at the leading end followed by the bacterial chromosome and then by the remainder of the F factor. The time required for complete transfer of the bacterial DNA is approximately 100 minutes. Most matings result in the transfer of only a portion of the donor chromosome owing to the instability of the mating complex. The donor cell genes that are transferred vary, since the F plasmid can integrate at several different sites in the bacterial DNA. The adjacent bacterial genes downstream from the integration site are the first and therefore the most frequently transferred. The newly acquired DNA can recombine into the recipient's DNA and become a stable component of its genetic material.

Table 4–1. Comparison of conjugation, transduction, and transformation.

Transfer Procedure	Process	Type of Cells Involved	Nature of DNA Transferred
Conjugation	DNA transferred from one bacterium to another	Prokaryotic	Chromosomal or plasmid
Transduction	DNA transferred by a virus from one cell to another	Prokaryotic	Any gene in generalized transduction; only certain genes in specialized transduction
Transformation	Purified DNA taken up by a cell	Prokaryotic or eukaryotic (eg, human)	Any DNA

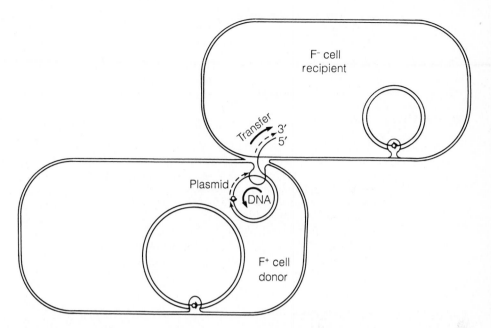

Figure 4–1. Conjugation. An F plasmid is being transferred from an F$^+$ donor bacterium to an F$^-$ recipient. (Modified and reproduced, with permission, from Stanier RY, Doudoroff M, Adelberg EA: *The Microbial World,* 3rd ed. Copyright © 1970. By permission of Prentice-Hall, Inc., Englewood Cliffs, NJ.)

(2) Transduction is the transfer of cell DNA by means of a bacterial virus. During the growth of the virus within the cell, a piece of bacterial DNA is incorporated into the virus particle and is carried into the recipient cell at the time of infection. There are 2 types of transduction.

(a) The **generalized** type occurs when the virus carries a segment from any part of the bacterial chromosome. This occurs because the cell DNA is fragmented after phage infection and pieces of cell DNA the same size as the viral DNA are incorporated into the virus particle at a frequency of about one in every 1000 virus particles.

(b) The **specialized** type occurs when the bacterial virus DNA that has integrated into the cell DNA is excised and carries with it an adjacent part of the cell DNA. Since most lysogenic (temperate) phages integrate at specific sites in the bacterial DNA, the adjacent cellular genes that are transduced are usually specific to that virus.

(3) Transformation is the transfer of DNA itself from one cell to another. This occurs by either of the 2 following methods. In nature, dying bacteria may release their DNA, which may be taken up by recipient cells. There is little evidence that this natural process plays a significant role in disease. In the laboratory, an investigator may extract DNA from one type of bacteria and introduce it into genetically different bacteria.

The experimental use of transformation has revealed important information about DNA. In 1944, it was shown that DNA extracted from encapsulated "smooth" pneumococci could transform nonencapsulated "rough" pneumococci into smooth encapsulated organisms. This demonstration that the "transforming principle" was DNA marked the first evidence that DNA was the genetic material.

RECOMBINATION Once the DNA is transferred from the donor to the recipient cell by one of the 3 processes just described, it can integrate into the host cell chromosome by recombination. There are 2 types of recombination:

(1) homologous recombination, in which 2 pieces of DNA that have extensive homologous regions pair up and exchange pieces by the processes of breakage and reunion, and

(2) nonhomologous recombination, in which little, if any, homology is necessary. Different genetic loci govern these 2 types, and so it is presumed that different enzymes are involved.

Although it is known that a variety of endonucleases and ligases are involved, the precise sequence of events is unknown.

Review Questions

1. Describe the chromosomal DNA of a typical bacterium. Compare it with plasmid DNA.
2. What are the 3 main types of mutations?
3. How do base analogues, eg, iododeoxyuridine, and ultraviolet radiation cause mutations?
4. What is a conditional-lethal mutation?
5. What is conjugation? How does an Hfr cell differ from an F^+ cell? What is the medical importance of conjugation?
6. What is transduction? Why is it important?
7. How does transformation differ from transduction and conjugation?

5   Classification of Medically Important Bacteria

The current classification of bacteria is based primarily on morphologic and biochemical characteristics. A scheme that divides the medically important organisms by genus is shown in Table 5–1. For pedagogical purposes this classification scheme deviates from those derived from strict taxonomic principles in 2 ways:

(1) only organisms that are described in this book in the section on medically important bacteria are included; and

(2) because there are so many gram-negative rods, they are divided into 3 categories: respiratory organisms, zoonotic organisms, and enteric and related organisms.

The initial criterion used in the classification is the nature of the cell wall; ie, is it rigid, flexible, or absent? Bacteria with rigid, thick walls can be subdivided into free-living bacteria, which are capable of growing on laboratory medium in the absence of human or other animal cells, and non-free-living bacteria, which are obligate intracellular parasites and therefore can grow only within human or other animal cells. The free-living organisms are further subdivided according to shape and staining reaction into a variety of gram-positive and gram-negative cocci and rods with different oxygen requirements and spore-forming abilities. Bacteria with flexible, thin walls (the spirochetes) and those without cell walls (the mycoplasmas) form separate units.

Review Question

Describe the criteria used to classify bacteria.

Table 5–1. Classification of medically important bacteria.

Characteristics	Genus	Representative Diseases
I. Rigid, thick-walled cells		
A. Free-living (extracellular)		
1. Gram-positive		
a. Cocci	*Streptococcus*	Pneumonia, pharyngitis, cellulitis
	Staphylococcus	Abscess of skin and other organs
b. Spore-forming rods		
(1) Aerobic	*Bacillus*	Anthrax
(2) Anaerobic	*Clostridium*	Tetanus, gas gangrene, botulism
c. Non-spore-forming rods		
(1) Nonfilamentous	*Corynebacterium*	Diphtheria
	Listeria	Meningitis
(2) Filamentous	*Actinomyces*	Actinomycosis
	Nocardia	Nocardiosis
2. Gram-negative		
a. Cocci	*Neisseria*	Gonorrhea, meningitis
b. Rods		
(1) Facultative		
(a) Straight		
(i) Respiratory organisms	*Haemophilus*	Meningitis
	Bordetella	Whooping cough
	Legionella	Pneumonia
(ii) Zoonotic organisms	*Brucella*	Brucellosis
	Francisella	Tularemia
	Pasteurella	Cellulitis
	Yersinia	Plague
(iii) Enteric and related organisms	*Escherichia*	Urinary tract infection, diarrhea
	Enterobacter	Urinary tract infection
	Serratia	Pneumonia
	Klebsiella	Pneumonia, urinary tract infection
	Salmonella	Enterocolitis, typhoid fever
	Shigella	Enterocolitis
	Proteus	Urinary tract infection
(b) Curved	*Campylobacter*	Enterocolitis
	Vibrio	Cholera
(2) Aerobic	*Pseudomonas*	Pneumonia, urinary tract infection
(3) Anaerobic	*Bacteroides*	Peritonitis
3. Acid-fast	*Mycobacterium*	Tuberculosis, leprosy
B. Non-free-living (obligate intracellular parasites)	*Rickettsia*	Rocky Mountain spotted fever, typhus, Q fever
	Chlamydia	Urethritis, trachoma, psittacosis
II. **Flexible, thin-walled cells** (spirochetes)	*Treponema*	Syphilis
	Borrelia	Lyme disease
	Leptospira	Leptospirosis
III. Wall-less cells	*Mycoplasma*	Pneumonia

Normal Flora

6

The body surfaces support the growth of a variety of bacteria and fungi which collectively are called the **normal flora** (Tables 6–1 and 6–2). The 2 other major groups of microorganisms, the viruses and parasites, are usually not considered members of the normal flora, although they can be present in asymptomatic individuals. The normal flora comprises a permanent population of organisms that vary in both number and kind from one site to another. Although the normal flora extensively populates many areas of the body, the internal organs usually are sterile. Areas such as the central nervous system, blood, lower bronchi and alveoli, liver, spleen, kidneys, and bladder are free of all but the occasional transient organism.

Table 6–1. Summary of the normal flora and the anatomic location.

Members of the Normal Flora[1]	Anatomic Location
Bacteroides species	Colon, throat, vagina
Candida albicans	Mouth, colon, vagina
Clostridium species	Colon
Corynebacterium species (diphtheroids)	Nasopharynx, skin, vagina
Escherichia coli and other coliforms	Colon, vagina, outer urethra
Gardnerella vaginalis	Vagina
Haemophilus species	Nasopharynx, conjunctiva
Lactobacillus species	Mouth, colon, vagina
Neisseria species	Mouth, nasopharynx
Pseudomonas aeruginosa	Colon, skin
Staphylococcus aureus	Nose, skin
Staphylococcus epidermidis	Skin, nose, mouth, vagina, urethra
Streptococcus faecalis (enterococcus)	Colon
Viridans streptococci	Mouth, nasopharynx

[1]In alphabetical order.

There is a distinction between the presence of these organisms and the **carrier state.** In a sense we all are carriers of microorganisms, but that is not the normal use of the term in the medical context. The term ''carrier'' implies that an individual harbors a potential pathogen and therefore can be a source of infection of others. It is most frequently used in reference to asymptomatic infection or to a patient who has recovered from a disease but continues to carry

Table 6–2. Medically important members of the normal flora.

Organ	Important Organisms[1]	Less Important Organisms[2]
Skin	*Staphylococcus epidermidis*	*Staphylococcus aureus*, *Corynebacterium* (diphtheroids), various streptococci, *Pseudomonas aeruginosa*, anaerobes, eg, *Peptococcus*, yeasts, eg, *Candida albicans*
Nose	*Staphylococcus aureus*	*S epidermidis*, *Corynebacterium* (diphtheroids), various streptococci
Mouth	Viridans streptococci	Various streptococci
Dental plaque	*Streptococcus mutans*	
Gingival crevices	Various anaerobes, eg, *Bacteroides*, *Fusobacterium*, streptococci, *Actinomyces*	
Throat	Viridans streptococci	Various streptococci including *Streptococcus pyogenes* and *S pneumoniae*, *Neisseria* species, *Haemophilus influenzae*, *S epidermidis*
Colon	*Bacteroides fragilis*, *Escherichia coli*	*Bifidobacterium*, *Eubacterium*, *Fusobacterium*, *Lactobacillus*, various aerobic gram-negative rods, *Streptococcus faecalis* and other streptococci, *Clostridium*
Vagina	*Lactobacillus*, *E coli*,[3] group B streptococci[3]	Various streptococci, various gram-negative rods, *B fragilis*, *Corynebacterium* (diphtheroids), *C albicans*
Urethra		*S epidermidis*, *Corynebacterium* (diphtheroids), various streptococci, various gram-negative rods

[1]Organisms that are medically significant or present in large numbers.
[2]Organisms that are less medically significant or present in smaller numbers.
[3]These organisms are not part of the normal flora but are important colonizers.

the organism and may shed it for a long period. When an organism establishes more than a temporary relationship, the host is said to be **colonized** by that organism.

The normal flora plays a role both in the maintenance of health and in the causation of disease in 3 significant ways.

(1) These organisms can cause disease, especially in immunocompromised and debilitated individuals. Although organisms of the normal flora are nonpathogens in their usual anatomic location, they can be pathogens in other parts of the body.

(2) They constitute a protective host defense mechanism. The nonpathogenic resident bacteria occupy ecologic niches, and so pathogens have difficulty multiplying efficiently. If the normal flora is suppressed, pathogens may grow and cause disease.

(3) They may serve a nutritional function. The intestinal bacteria produce several B vitamins and vitamin K. Poorly nourished people who are treated with oral antibiotics can suffer vitamin deficiencies as a result of the reduction in the normal flora. However, since germ-free animals are well nourished, the normal flora is not essential for proper nutrition.

NORMAL FLORA OF THE SKIN The predominant organism is *Staphylococcus epidermidis,* which is a nonpathogen on the skin but which can cause disease when it reaches certain sites such as artificial heart valves. It is found on the skin much more frequently than its pathogenic relative, *Staphylococcus aureus* (Table 6–2). There are about 10^3 to 10^4 organisms/cm^2 of skin. Most of them are located superficially in the stratum corneum, but some are found in the hair follicles and act as a reservoir to replenish the superficial flora after hand washing. Anaerobic organisms, such as *Peptococcus* and *Propionibacterium,* are situated in the deeper follicles in the dermis, where oxygen tension is low.

NORMAL FLORA OF THE RESPIRATORY TRACT A wide spectrum of organisms colonize the nose, throat, and mouth, but the lower bronchi and alveoli typically contain few, if any, organisms. The nose is colonized by a variety of streptococcal and staphylococcal species, the most significant of which is the pathogen *S aureus.* Occasional outbreaks of disease due to this organism, particularly in the newborn nursery, can be traced to nasal, skin, or perianal carriage by personnel.

The throat contains a mixture of viridans streptococci, *Neisseria* species, and *S epidermidis* (Table 6–2). These nonpathogens are inhibitory to the growth of the pathogens *Streptococcus pyogenes, Neisseria meningitidis,* and *S aureus,* respectively.

In the mouth, viridans streptococci make up about half of the bacteria. *Streptococcus mutans,* a member of the viridans group, is of special interest since it is found in large numbers (10^{10}/g) in dental plaque, the precursor of caries. The plaque on the enamel surface is composed of gelatinous, high-molecular-weight glucans secreted by the bacteria. The entrapped bacteria produce large amounts of acid which demineralizes the enamel and initiates caries. The viridans streptococci are also the leading cause of subacute bacterial (infective) endocarditis. These organisms can enter the bloodstream at the time of dental surgery and attach to damaged heart valves.

Anaerobic bacteria, such as species of *Bacteroides, Fusobacterium, Clostridium,* and *Peptostreptococcus,* are found in the gingival crevices, where the oxygen concentration is very low. If aspirated, these organisms can cause lung abscesses, especially in debilitated patients with poor dental hygiene. In addition, the gingival crevices are the natural habitat of *Actinomyces israelii,* an anaerobic actinomycete that can cause abscesses of the jaw, lungs, or abdomen.

NORMAL FLORA OF THE INTESTINAL TRACT In normal fasting people, the stomach contains few organisms owing to its low pH and its enzymes. The small intestine usually contains small numbers of streptococci, lactobacilli, and yeasts, particularly *Candida albicans.* Larger numbers of these organisms are found in the terminal ileum.

The colon is the major location of bacteria in the body. Roughly 20% of the feces consists of bacteria, approximately 10^{11} organisms/g. The major bacteria found are shown in Table 6–3.

The normal flora of the intestinal tract plays a significant role in extraintestinal disease. For example, *Escherichia coli* is the leading cause of urinary tract infections, and *Bacteroides*

Table 6–3. Major bacteria found in the colon.

Bacterium[1]	Number/g of Feces	Frequency of Infection
Bacteroides, especially *B fragilis*	10^{10}–10^{11}	Common
Bifidobacterium	10^{10}	Rare
Eubacterium	10^{10}	Rare
Coliforms	10^{7}–10^{8}	Common
Streptococcus, especially *S faecalis*	10^{7}–10^{8}	Common
Lactobacillus	10^{7}	Rare
Clostridium, especially *C perfringens*	10^{6}	Common

[1] *Bacteroides, Bifidobacterium,* and *Eubacterium* (which make up more than 90% of the fecal flora) are anaerobes. Coliforms (*Escherichia coli, Enterobacter* species, and other gram-negative organisms) are the predominant facultative anaerobes.

fragilis is an important cause of peritonitis associated with perforation of the intestinal wall following trauma, appendicitis, or diverticulitis. Other organisms include *Streptococcus faecalis* (an enterococcus), which causes urinary tract infections and endocarditis and *Pseudomonas aeruginosa,* which can cause various infections, particularly in hospitalized patients with decreased host defenses. It is present in 10% of normal stools, as well as in soil and water.

Antibiotic therapy, for example with clindamycin, can suppress the predominant normal flora, thereby allowing a rare organism such as the toxin-producing *Clostridium difficile* to overgrow and cause a severe colitis. Administration of certain antibiotics, such as neomycin orally, prior to gastrointestinal surgery to "sterilize" the gut leads to a marked reduction of the normal flora for several days, followed by a gradual return to normal levels.

NORMAL FLORA OF THE GENITOURINARY TRACT   The flora of the vaginas of adult women consists primarily of Lactobacillus species (Table 6–2). Lactobacilli are responsible for producing the acid which keeps the pH of the adult woman's vagina low. Before puberty and after menopause, when estrogen levels are low, lactobacilli are rare and the vaginal pH is high. Lactobacilli appear to prevent the growth of potential pathogens, since their suppression by antibiotics can lead to overgrowth by *Candida albicans.*

Although the vagina is located close to the anus, it is infrequently significantly colonized by members of the fecal flora. However, women who are prone to recurrent urinary tract infections do harbor organisms such as *E coli* and *Enterobacter* in the introitus. About 15–20% of women of childbearing age carry group B streptococci in the vagina. This organism is an important cause of sepsis and meningitis of the newborn and is acquired during passage through the birth canal.

Urine in the bladder is sterile in the normal person, but during passage through the outermost portions of the urethra it often becomes contaminated with *S epidermidis,* coliforms, diphtheroids, and nonhemolytic streptococci. The area around the urethras of women and uncircumcised men contains secretions which carry *Mycobacterium smegmatis,* an acid-fast organism.

Review Questions

1. What is the difference between the terms "normal flora" and "carrier state"?
2. What are the major organisms of the skin and of the oropharynx? With what diseases are they particularly associated?
3. Describe the important anaerobes and facultative anaerobes in the normal flora of the colon.
4. If the normal flora of the colon is suppressed by certain antibiotics, what disease can result? What is its pathogenesis?
5. What is the importance of the lactobacilli that are part of the vaginal normal flora?

6. The vaginas of some women are colonized by *Escherichia coli*. What is the significance of this observation? If the organisms were group B streptococci, what would be the significance?

7. If a urine culture grew many colonies of *Staphylococcus epidermidis*, what would be your interpretation?

Pathogenesis 7

A microorganism is a **pathogen** if it is capable of causing disease; however, some organisms are frequently pathogens, whereas others cause disease rarely. **Opportunistic** organisms are those that rarely if ever cause disease in immunocompetent people but can cause serious infections in immunocompromised patients. These opportunists are frequently members of the body's normal flora. The origin of the term "opportunistic" refers to the ability of the organism to take the opportunity offered by reduced host defenses to cause disease. **Virulence** is a quantitative measure of pathogenicity and is measured by the number of organisms required to cause disease. The 50% lethal dose (LD_{50}) is the number of organisms needed to kill half the hosts, and the 50% infectious dose (ID_{50}) is the number needed to cause infection in half the hosts.

TYPES OF BACTERIAL INFECTIONS Bacteria cause disease by 2 major mechanisms: (1) toxin production and (2) invasiveness. Toxins fall into 2 general categories: **exotoxins** and **endotoxins.** Exotoxins are polypeptides released by the cell, whereas endotoxins are lipopolysaccharides, which form an integral part of the cell wall. Endotoxins occur only in gram-negative rods and cocci; are not actively released from the cell; and cause fever, shock, and other generalized symptoms. Both exotoxins and endotoxins by themselves can cause symptoms; the presence of the bacteria in the host is not required. Invasive bacteria, on the other hand, grow to large numbers locally and cause symptoms in that area by producing a variety of enzymes that damage adjacent host cells.

Many, but not all, infections are communicable, ie, are spread from host to host. For example, tuberculosis is communicable, as it is spread from person to person by airborne droplets produced by coughing; but botulism is not, as the exotoxin produced by the organism in the contaminated food affects only those eating that food. If a disease is highly communicable, the term "contagious" is applied.

An infection is **epidemic** if it occurs much more frequently than usual; it is **pandemic** if it has a worldwide distribution. An **endemic** infection is constantly present at a low level in a specific population. In addition to infections that result in overt symptoms, many are **inapparent** or **subclinical** and can be detected by the presence of antibodies against the organism or by the presence of the organism itself. Some infections result in a **latent** state, after which reactivation of the growth of the organism and recurrence of symptoms may occur. Certain other infections lead to a **chronic carrier** state, in which the organisms continue to grow with or without producing symptoms in the host. Chronic carriers, eg, Typhoid Mary, are an important source of infection of others and hence are a public health hazard.

The determination of whether an organism recovered from a patient is actually the cause of the disease involves an awareness of 2 phenomena: normal flora and colonization. Members of the normal flora are permanent residents of the body and vary in type according to anatomic site (see Chapter 6). When an organism is obtained from a patient's specimen, the question of whether it is a member of the normal flora is important in interpreting the finding. **Colonization** refers to the presence of new organism that is neither a member of the normal flora nor the cause of symptoms. It can be a difficult clinical dilemma to distinguish between a pathogen and a colonizer, especially in specimens obtained from the respiratory tract, such as throat and sputum cultures.

DETERMINANTS OF BACTERIAL PATHOGENESIS

1. **Transmission**   Although some infections are caused by members of the normal flora, most infections are acquired by transmission from external sources. Pathogens exit the infected patient most frequently from the respiratory and gastrointestinal tracts; hence, transmission to the new host usually occurs through airborne respiratory droplets or fecal contamination of food and water. Organisms can also be transmitted by sexual contact, urine, skin contact, blood transfusions, contaminated needles, or biting insects. There are 4 important portals of entry: respiratory tract, gastrointestinal tract, genital tract, and skin (Table 7–1). The specific mode of transmission of each organism is described in the subsequent section devoted to that organism.

Animals can also be an important source of organisms that infect humans. They can be either the source (**reservoir**) or the mode of transmission (**vector**) of certain organisms. Diseases for which animals are the reservoirs are called **zoonoses**.

Table 7–1. Portals of entry of some common pathogens

Portal of Entry	Pathogen	Type of Organism[1]	Disease
Respiratory tract	*Streptococcus pneumoniae*	B	Pneumonia
	Neisseria meningitidis	B	Meningitis
	Haemophilus influenzae	B	Meningitis
	Mycobacterium tuberculosis	B	Tuberculosis
	Influenza virus	V	Influenza
	Rhinovirus	V	Common cold
	Epstein-Barr virus	V	Infectious mononucleosis
	Coccidioides immitis	F	Coccidiodomycosis
	Histoplasma capsulatum	F	Histoplasmosis
Gastrointestinal tract	*Shigella dysenteriae*	B	Dysentery
	Salmonella typhi	B	Typhoid fever
	Vibrio cholerae	B	Cholera
	Hepatitis A virus	V	Infectious hepatitis
	Poliovirus	V	Poliomyelitis
	Trichinella spiralis	P	Trichinosis
Skin	*Clostridium tetani*	B	Tetanus
	Rickettsia rickettsii	B	Rocky Mountain spotted fever
	Hepatitis B virus	V	Hepatitis B
	Rabies virus	V	Rabies
	Trichophyton rubrum	F	Tinea pedis (athlete's foot)
	Plasmodium vivax	P	Malaria
Genital tract	*Neisseria gonorrhoeae*	B	Gonorrhea
	Treponema pallidum	B	Syphilis
	Chlamydia trachomatis	B	Urethritis
	Candida albicans	F	Vaginitis

[1]B, bacterium; V, virus; F, fungus; P, parasite.

2. **Adherence to Cell Surfaces**   Certain bacteria have specialized structures or contain substances that allow them to adhere to the surface of human cells, thereby enhancing their ability to cause disease. These adherence mechanisms are essential for organisms that attach to mucous membranes; mutants that lack these mechanisms are often nonpathogenic. For example, the pili of *Neisseria gonorrhoeae* and *Escherichia coli* mediate the attachment of the organisms to the urinary tract epithelium.

3. **Invasiveness**   One of the 2 main mechanisms by which bacteria cause disease is their ability to invade surrounding tissue and cause **inflammation**. Several enzymes secreted by invasive bacteria play a role in pathogenesis. Among the most prominent are

(1) **collagenase** and **hyaluronidase,** which degrade their respective intercellular substances, thereby allowing the bacteria to spread through tissue;

(2) coagulase, which is an enzyme produced by *Staphylococcus aureus* the accelerates the formation of a fibrin clot from its precursor, fibrinogen (this clot may protect the bacteria from phagocytosis by walling off the infected area and by coating the organisms with a layer of fibrin);

(3) immunoglobulin A (IgA) protease, which is produced by *N gonorrhoeae* and other organisms and which degrades the secretory immunoglobulin; and

(4) leukocidins, which can destroy both neutrophilic leukocytes and macrophages.

In addition to these enzymes, several factors contribute to invasiveness by limiting the ability of the host defense mechanisms, especially phagocytosis, to operate effectively.
(a) The most important of these factors is the **capsule** external to the cell wall of several important pathogens such as *Streptococcus pneumoniae* and *Neisseria meningitidis*. The polysaccharide capsule prevents the phagocyte from adhering to the bacteria; anticapsular antibodies allow more effective phagocytosis to occur (a process called **opsonization**). The vaccines against *S pneumoniae* and *N meningitidis* contain capsular polysaccharides that induce protective anticapsular antibodies.
(b) A second group of antiphagocytic factors are the cell wall proteins of the gram-positive cocci, such as the M protein of the group A streptococci and protein A of the staphylococci. These virulence factors are summarized in Table 7–2.

Table 7–2. Surface virulence factors important for bacterial pathogenesis.

Organism	Virulence Factor	Used in Vaccine	Comments
Gram-positive cocci			
Streptococcus pneumoniae	Polysaccharide capsule	Yes	Determines serotype
Streptococcus pyogenes	M protein	No	Determines serotype[1]
Staphylococcus aureus	Protein A	No	Binds to Fc region of IgG
Gram-negative cocci			
Neisseria meningitidis	Polysaccharide capsule	Yes	Determines serotype
Gram-positive rods			
Bacillus anthracis	Polypeptide capsule	No	. . .
Gram-negative rods			
Haemophilus influenzae	Polysaccharide capsule	Yes	Determines serotype
Klebsiella pneumoniae	Polysaccharide capsule	No	. . .
Escherichia coli	Protein pili	No	Causes adherence
Salmonella typhi	Polysaccharide capsule	No	Not important for other salmonellae
Yersinia pestis	V and W proteins	No	. . .

[1]Do not confuse the serotype with the grouping of streptococci, which is determined by the polysaccharide in the cell wall.

In addition to **pyogenic** inflammation, **granuloma** formation by certain bacteria, e.g., *M. tuberculosis*, occurs. No enzymes or toxins have been identified in these organisms. Rather, it appears that bacterial antigens stimulate the cell-mediated immune system, resulting in sensitized T-lymphocyte and macrophage activity. Phagocytosis by macrophages kills most of the bacteria, but some survive and grow within the macrophages in the granuloma. It is thought that the organisms reside within phagosomes, which are unable to fuse with lysosomes, resulting in protection from degradative enzymes in the lysosomes. Many fungal diseases also are characterized by granulomatous lesions.

4. Toxin Production   The second major mechanism by which bacteria cause disease is the production of toxins. A comparison of the main features of **exotoxins** and **endotoxins** is shown in Table 7–3.

Exotoxins   Exotoxins are produced by several gram-positive and gram-negative bacteria, in contrast to endotoxins, which are present only in gram-negative bacteria. The essential characteristic of exotoxins is that they are **secreted** by the bacteria, whereas endotoxin is a component of the cell wall. Exotoxins are polypeptides whose genes are frequently located on plasmids or lysogenic bacterial viruses. In general, these polypeptides consist of 2 domains or subunits, one responsible for the binding to the cell membrane and entry into the cell and the other possessing the toxic activity.

Table 7–3. Main features of exotoxins and endotoxins.

Property	Comparison of Properties	
	Exotoxin	**Endotoxin**
Source	Certain species of some gram-positive and gram-negative bacteria	Cell wall of most gram-negative bacteria
Mechanism of release	Secreted by living cells	Released on lysis of cells
Chemistry	Polypeptide	Lipopolysaccharide
Location of genes	Plasmid or bacteriophage	Bacterial chromosome
Toxicity	High (fatal dose on the order of 1 μg)	Low (fatal dose on the order of hundreds of micrograms)
Activity	Different action for each exotoxin (see text)	Fever, shock
Antigenicity	Induces high-titer antibodies called antitoxins	Poorly antigenic
Vaccines	Toxoids used as vaccines	No toxoids formed and no vaccine available
Heat stability	Destroyed rapidly at 60°C (except staphylococcal enterotoxin)	Stable at 100°C for 1 hour
Typical diseases	Tetanus, botulism, diphtheria	Meningococcemia, sepsis by gram-negative rods

Exotoxins are among the **most toxic** substances known. For example, the fatal dose of tetanus toxin for a human is estimated to be less than 1 μg. Because some purified exotoxins can reproduce all aspects of the disease, we can conclude that certain bacteria play no other role in pathogenesis than to synthesize the exotoxin. Exotoxin polypeptides are good antigens and induce the synthesis of protective antibodies called antitoxins, some of which are useful in prevention or treatment of diseases such as botulism and tetanus. When treated with formaldehyde (or acid or heat), the exotoxin polypeptides are converted into **toxoids,** which are used in protective vaccines because they retain their antigenicity but have lost their toxicity.

The mechanisms of action of the important exotoxins produced by toxigenic bacteria differ significantly as described below and summarized in Table 7–4.

(1) Diphtheria toxin, produced by *Corynebacterium diphtheriae,* inhibits protein synthesis by ADP ribosylation of elongation factor 2 (EF-2).*The exotoxin activity depends on 2 functions

Table 7–4. Important bacterial exotoxins.

Organism	Disease	Mode of Action	Toxoid Vaccine
Gram-positive			
Corynebacterium diphtheriae	Diphtheria	Inactivates EF-2 by ADP ribosylation.	Yes
Clostridium tetani	Tetanus	Blocks release of the inhibitory neurotransmitter glycine.	Yes
Clostridium botulinum	Botulism	Blocks release of acetylcholine.	Yes[1]
Clostridium perfringens	Gas gangrene	Alpha toxin is a lecithinase.	No
Bacillus anthracis	Anthrax	One of the toxins is an adenylate cyclase.	No
Streptococcus pyogenes	Scarlet fever	Unknown.	No
Gram-negative			
Escherichia coli	Diarrhea	Labile toxin stimulates adenylate cyclase by ADP ribosylation; stable toxin stimulates guanylate cyclase.	No
Vibrio cholerae	Cholera	Stimulates adenylate cyclase by ADP ribosylation.	No
Bordetella pertussis	Whooping cough	Stimulates adenylate cyclase by ADP ribosylation.	No

[1]For high-risk individuals only.

Pseudomonas aeruginosa exotoxin has the same mode of action.

mediated by different domains of the molecule. The toxin is synthesized as a single polypeptide (MW 62,000) that is nontoxic because the active site of the enzyme is masked (Fig 7–1). A single proteolytic "nick" plus reduction of the sulfhydryl bonds yields 2 active polypeptides. Fragment A, a 22,000-molecular- weight peptide at the amino-terminal end of the exotoxin, is an enzyme that catalyzes the transfer of ADP-ribose from nicotinamide

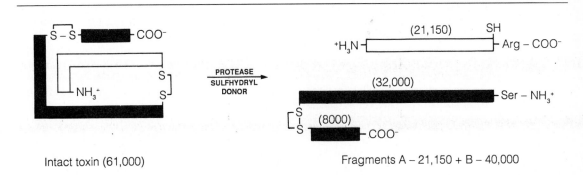

Intact toxin (61,000)   Fragments A – 21,150 + B – 40,000

Figure 7–1. Diphtheria exotoxin. Intact extracellular toxin binds to a eukaryotic cell by its B region (dark fragment). After proteolytic cleavage and reduction of disulfide bond, the A region (light fragment) containing the ribosylating enzyme is activated. (Modified and reproduced, with permission, from Pappenheimer AM Jr: *Microbiology-1979.* American Society for Microbiology, 1979.)

adenine dinucleotide (NAD) to EF-2, thereby inactivating it. The ADP ribosylation of EF-2 freezes the translocation complex, and protein synthesis stops. The reaction is as follows:

$$\text{EF-2 + NAD} \longrightarrow \text{EF-2–ADP-ribose + Nicotinamide + H}^+$$

Fragment B, a 40,000-molecular-weight peptide at the carboxy-terminal end, binds to receptors on the outer membrane of eukaryotic cells and mediates transport of fragment A into the cells.

To summarize, the exotoxin binds to cell membrane receptors via a region near its carboxyl end. The toxin is transported across the membrane, and the proteolytic nick and reduction of the disulfide bonds occur. This releases the active fragment A, which inactivates EF-2. The enzymatic activity is specific for EF-2; no other protein is ADP-ribosylated. The specificity is due to the presence in EF-2 of a unique amino acid, a modified histidine called diphthamide. The reaction occurs in all eukaryotic cells; there is no tissue or organ specificity. Prokaryotic and mitochondrial protein synthesis are not affected, because a different, nonsusceptible elongation factor is involved. The enzyme activity is remarkably potent; a single molecule of fragment A will kill a cell within a few hours. Other organisms whose exotoxins act by ADP ribosylation are *E coli, Vibrio cholerae,* and *Bordetella pertussis.*

The *tox* gene, which codes for the exotoxin, is carried by a temperate bacteriophage. As a result, only *C diphtheriae* strains lysogenized by this phage cause diphtheria. (Nonlysogenized *C diphtheriae* can be found in the throats of some healthy people.) Regulation of exotoxin synthesis is controlled by the interaction of iron in the medium with a repressor of the *tox* gene synthesized by the bacterium. As the concentration of iron increases, the iron-repressor complex inhibits the transcription of the *tox* gene.

(2) Tetanus toxin, produced by *Clostridium tetani,* is a **neurotoxin** that prevents release of the inhibitory neurotransmitter glycine, which causes muscle spasms. Tetanus toxin (tetanospasmin) is composed of 2 polypeptide subunits encoded by plasmid DNA. The heavy chain of the polypeptide binds to gangliosides in the membrane of the neuron; the light chain exerts the toxic activity. The toxin released at the site of the peripheral wound may travel either by retrograde axonal transport or in the bloodstream to the anterior horn and interstitial neurons of the spinal cord. Blockage of release of the inhibitory transmitter leads to convulsive contractions of the voluntary muscles best exemplified by spasm of the jaw and neck muscles ("lockjaw").

(3) Botulinum toxin, produced by *Clostridium botulinum,* is a **neurotoxin** that blocks the release of acetylcholine at the synapse, producing paralysis. The toxin is encoded by the genes of a temperate bacteriophage. Approximately 1 μg is lethal for humans; it is one of the most toxic compounds known. The toxin is composed of 2 polypeptide subunits held together by disulfide bonds. One of the subunits binds to a receptor on the neuron; the mechanism by which the other subunit inhibits acetylcholine release is unknown.

(4) The **heat-labile enterotoxin** produced by *E coli* causes diarrhea by stimulating adenylate cyclase activity in the membrane of cells in the small intestine. The resulting increase in the concentration of cyclic adenosine monophosphate (cAMP) causes excretion of chloride ion, inhibition of sodium ion absorption, and significant fluid and electrolyte loss into the lumen of the gut. The heat-labile toxin, which is inactivated by being heated at 65° C for 30 minutes, is composed of 2 subunits, one of which binds to a ganglioside in the cell membrane while the other enters the cell and mediates the transfer of ADP-ribose from NAD to a stimulatory coupling protein. This results in an increase in guanosine triphosphate (GTP) concentration, which stimulates adenylate cyclase activity. The genes for the heat-labile toxin and for the heat-stable toxin (see below) are carried on a plasmid.

In addition to the labile toxin, there is a **heat-stable toxin**, which is a polypeptide that is not inactivated by boiling for 30 minutes. The heat-stable toxin affects cGMP rather than cAMP. It stimulates guanylate cyclase and thus increases the concentration of cGMP, which inhibits the reabsorption of sodium ions and causes diarrhea. The heat-stable toxin exerts its effect only in intestinal cells, perhaps owing to the presence of receptors only on the membranes of these cells.

The enterotoxins produced by *V cholerae,* the agent of cholera, and *Bacillus cereus,* a cause of diarrhea, act in a manner similar to that of the heat-labile toxin of *E coli. Bordetella pertussis* and *Bacillus anthracis* also produce toxins that increase cAMP concentration, but these toxins act by different mechanisms (see below).

(5) One of the toxins of *B pertussis,* the cause of whooping cough, is an exotoxin that enhances cell membrane adenylate cyclase activity by catalyzing the transfer of ADP-ribose from NAD to an inhibitory coupling component of adenylate cyclase. Inactivation of this inhibitory regulator results in the stimulation of adenylate cyclase activity.

(6) Three exotoxins are produced by *Bacillus anthracis,* the agent of anthrax; edema factor, protective antigen, and lethal factor. Edema factor is an adenylate cyclase that requires protective antigen for its entry into human cells. The bacterial adenylate cyclase raises the cAMP concentration within the cell, resulting in loss of chloride ions and water and consequent edema formation in the tissue. The mode of action of lethal factor is unknown.

(7) Multiple toxins are produced by *Clostridium perfringens* and other species of clostridia that cause gas gangrene. A total of 7 lethal factors and 5 enzymes have been characterized, but no species of *Clostridium* makes all 12 products. The best-characterized is the **alpha toxin**, which is a phospholipase that hydrolyzes lecithin in the cell membrane, resulting in widespread cell death. The other 4 enzymes are collagenase, protease, hyaluronidase, and deoxyribonuclease (DNase). The 7 lethal toxins are a heterogeneous group with hemolytic and necrotizing activity.

(8) Erythrogenic toxin, produced by *Streptococcus pyogenes,* causes the rash characteristic of scarlet fever. The mechanism is unknown. The DNA that codes for the toxin resides on a temperate bacteriophage. Nonlysogenic bacteria do not cause scarlet fever, although they can cause pharyngitis.

Endotoxins Endotoxins are integral parts of the cell walls of both gram-negative rods and cocci, in contrast to exotoxins, which are released from the cell (Table 7–3). In addition, several other features distinguish these substances. Endotoxins are **lipopolysaccharides**, whereas exotoxins are polypeptides; the enzymes that produce the lipopolysaccharide are encoded by genes on the bacterial chromosome, rather than by plasmid or bacteriophage DNA, which usually encodes the exotoxins. The toxicity of endotoxin is low in comparison with that of exotoxins. All endotoxins produce the same generalized effects of **fever and shock**, although the endotoxins of some organisms are more effective than those of others. Endotoxins are weakly antigenic; they induce protective antibodies so poorly that multiple episodes of toxicity can occur. No toxoids have been produced from endotoxins, and endotoxins are not used as antigens in any available vaccine.

The structure of the lipopolysaccharide is shown in Fig 2–6. The toxic portion of the molecule is **lipid A**, which is composed of disaccharides with several fatty acids attached.

β-Hydroxymyristic acid is always one of the fatty acids and is found only in lipid A. The other fatty acids differ according to species. The polysaccharide core in the middle of the molecule protrudes from the surface of the bacteria and has the same chemical composition within members of a genus. The repeat unit of sugars on the terminus differs in each species and frequently differs between strains of a single species. It is an important antigen of some gram-negative rods ("O" or somatic antigen) and is composed of 3, 4, or 5 sugars repeated up to 25 times. Because the number of permutations of this array is very large, many antigenic types exist. For example, more than 1500 antigenic types have been identified for *Salmonella*.

The biologic effects of endotoxin include:

(1) fever due to the release by macrophages of endogenous pyrogen (interleukin-1), which acts on the hypothalamic temperature-regulatory center;

(2) hypotension, shock, and impaired perfusion of essential organs owing to bradykinin-induced vasodilatation and decreased peripheral resistance;

(3) disseminated intravascular coagulation due to activation of the coagulation system through Hageman factor (factor XII);

(4) activation of the alternative pathway of the complement cascade, resulting in tissue damage; and

(5) neutropenia caused by sequestration of neutrophils in the capillaries of the lungs and other organs.

The evidence that endotoxin causes these effects comes from the following 2 findings: (1) purified lipopolysaccharide, free of the organism, reproduces the effects; and (2) antiserum against the core glycolipid of endotoxin can mitigate or block these effects.

Endotoxins do not cause these effects directly. Rather, they elicit the production of host factors such as **cachectin* (tumor necrosis factor)** from macrophages. Cachectin is toxic to vascular endothelium, activates coagulation factors, and has other effects as well. Antiserum against cachectin blocks the effects of the endotoxin. The precise mechanism of action of cachectin is uncertain.

Endotoxins can cause a pyrogenic response in the patient if they are present in intravenous fluids. In the past, intravenous fluids were sterilized by autoclaving, which killed any organisms present but resulted in the release of endotoxins that were not heat-inactivated. For this reason, these fluids are now sterilized by filtration, which physically removes the organism without releasing its endotoxin. The contamination of intravenous fluids by endotoxin is detected by a test based on the observation that nanogram amounts of endotoxin can clot extracts of the horseshoe crab, *Limulus*.

TYPICAL STAGES OF AN INFECTIOUS DISEASE   A typical acute infectious disease has 4 stages:

(1) the **incubation period,** which is the time between the acquisition of the organism (or toxin) and the beginning symptoms (this time can vary from hours to days to weeks depending on the organism);

(2) the **prodrome period,** during which nonspecific symptoms such as fever, malaise, and loss of appetite occur;

(3) the **specific-illness period,** during which the overt characteristic signs and symptoms of the disease occur; and

(4) the **recovery period,** during which the illness abates and the patient returns to the healthy state.

After the recovery period, some individuals become chronic carriers of the organisms and may shed them while remaining clinically well. Others may develop a **latent infection,** which can recur at subsequent times either in the same form as the primary infection or manifesting different signs and symptoms. Although many infections cause symptoms, many others are **subclinical,** ie, the individual remains asymptomatic although infected with the organism.

---

*Cachectin also causes cachexia by inhibiting the synthesis of lipoprotein lipase in adipocytes.

DID THE ISOLATED ORGANISM ACTUALLY CAUSE THE DISEASE? Because people harbor microorganisms as members of the permanent normal flora and as transient passengers, this can be an interesting and sometimes confounding question. The answer depends on the situation. One type of situation relates to the problems of a disease for which no agent has been identified and a candidate organism has been isolated. This is the problem that Robert Koch faced in 1877 when he was among the first to try to determine the cause of an infectious disease, namely anthrax in cattle and tuberculosis in humans. His approach led to the formulation of "**Koch's postulates**," which are criteria that must be satisfied to confirm the causal role of an organism. These criteria are as follows:

(1) the organism must be isolated from every patient with the disease;

(2) the organism must be isolated free from all other organisms and grown in pure culture in vitro;

(3) the pure organism must cause the disease in a healthy, susceptible animal; and

(4) the organism must be recovered from the inoculated animal.

The second type of situation pertains to the practical, everyday problem of a specific diagnosis of a patient's illness. In this instance, the signs and symptoms of the illness usually suggest a constellation of possible causative agents. The recovery of an agent in *sufficient numbers* from the *appropriate specimen* is usually sufficient for an etiologic diagnosis. This approach can be illustrated with 2 examples: (1) in a patient with a sore throat, the presence of a few beta-hemolytic streptococci is insufficient for a microbiologic diagnosis, whereas the presence of many would be sufficient; and (2) in a patient with fever, alpha-hemolytic streptococci in the throat are considered part of the normal flora, whereas the same organisms in the blood could be the cause of bacterial endocarditis.

In some infections, no organism is isolated from the patient, and the diagnosis is made by detecting a rise in antibody titer to an organism. For this purpose, the amount of antibody in the second or late serum sample should be at least 4 times greater than the amount of antibody in the first or early serum sample.

Review Questions

1. What are the main differences between exotoxins and endotoxins?
2. What are the mechanisms of action of the exotoxins of
   (a) *Corynebacterium diphtheriae*
   (b) *Clostridium tetani*
   (c) *Clostridium botulinum*
   (d) *Escherichia coli* (enterotoxin)
   (e) *Vibrio cholerae*
   (f) *Clostridium perfringens* (alpha toxin)
3. What is the chemical nature of endotoxin? What are its main physiologic effects? What host factors mediate its action?
4. What role do the capsular polysaccharide, M protein, A protein, and pili play in pathogenesis?
5. What enzymes and other factors play a role in the invasiveness of certain bacteria?
6. What is the mechanism by which certain bacteria cause granuloma formation?
7. What is the difference between the incubation and prodromal periods of an infectious disease?

Host Defenses

8

Host defenses are composed of 2 complementary, frequently interacting systems: (1) **nonspecific** defenses, which protect against microorganisms in general, and (2) **specific** natural and acquired immunity, which protects against a particular microorganism.

NONSPECIFIC DEFENSES

Skin & Mucous Membranes **Intact skin** is the first line of defense against many organisms. In addition to the physical barrier presented by skin, the fatty acids secreted by sebaceous glands in the skin have antibacterial and antifungal activity. The increased fatty acid production that occurs at puberty is thought to explain the increased resistance to ringworm fungal infections that occurs at that time. The low pH of the skin (between pH 3 and 5), which is due to these fatty acids, also has an antimicrobial effect. Although many organisms live on or in the skin as members of the normal flora, they are harmless as long as they do not enter the body.

A second important defense is the mucous membrane of the respiratory tract, which is lined with cilia and covered with mucus. The coordinated beating of the cilia drives the mucus up to the nose and mouth, where the trapped bacteria can be expelled. This mucociliary apparatus, the "**ciliary elevator**," can be damaged by alcohol, cigarette smoke, and viruses; the damage predisposes the host to bacterial infections. Other protective mechanisms of the respiratory tract involve alveolar macrophages, lysozyme in tears and mucus, hairs in the nose, and the cough reflex, which prevents aspiration into the lung.

The nonspecific protection in the gastrointestinal tract includes hydrolytic enzymes in saliva, acid in the stomach, and various degradative enzymes and macrophages in the small intestine. Vaginas of adult women are protected by the low pH generated by lactobacilli that are part of the normal flora.

The bacteria of the normal flora of the skin, nasopharynx, colon, and vagina occupy these ecologic niches, preventing pathogens from multiplying in these sites. The importance of the normal flora is appreciated in the occasional cases when antimicrobial therapy suppresses these beneficial organisms, thereby allowing organisms such as *Clostridium difficile* and *Candida albicans* to cause diseases such as pseudomembranous colitis and vaginitis, respectively.

Inflammatory Response & Phagocytosis The presence of foreign bodies such as bacteria within the body provokes a protective inflammatory response. This response is characterized by the clinical findings of redness, swelling, warmth, and pain at the site of infection. These signs are due to increased blood flow, increased capillary permeability, and the escape of fluid and cells into the tissue spaces. The increased permeability is due to several chemical mediators, of which histamine is probably the most important. Of the cells that appear at the site, neutrophils and macrophages, both of which perform phagocytic functions, arrive early. Neutrophils predominate in acute pyogenic infections, whereas macrophages are more prevalent in chronic or granulomatous infections. The importance of the inflammatory response in limiting infection is emphasized by the ability of anti-inflammatory agents such as corticosteroids to lower resistance to infection.

As part of the inflammatory response, bacteria are engulfed (phagocytized) by polymorphonuclear neutrophils (PMNs) and macrophages. PMNs make up approximately 60% of the leukocytes in the blood, and their numbers increase significantly during infection (leukocytosis). It should be noted, however, that in certain bacterial infections such as typhoid fever, a decrease in the number of leukocytes (leukopenia) is found.

The process of phagocytosis can be divided into 3 steps: migration, ingestion, and killing. Migration of PMNs to the site of the organisms is due to chemotactic attraction primarily to antigen-antibody complexes, certain components of the complement system such as activated C5a, and kallikrein, which—in addition to being chemotactic—is the enzyme that catalyzes the formation of bradykinin. Increased permeability of capillaries as a result of histamine, kinins, and prostaglandins allows PMNs to migrate through the capillary wall to reach the bacteria. This migration is called **diapedesis** and takes several minutes to occur.

The bacteria are ingested by the invagination of the PMN cell membrane around the bacteria to form a vacuole (**phagosome**). This engulfment is enhanced by the binding of antibodies (**opsonins**) to the surface of the bacteria, a process called **opsonization.** Complement, especially activated C3, enhances opsonization. (The outer cell membranes of both PMNs and macrophages have receptors both for the Fc portion of the antibody molecule and for C3.) Even in the absence of antibody, the activated C3 component of complement, which can be generated by the ''alternative'' pathway, can opsonize. This is particularly important for bacterial and fungal organisms whose polysaccharides activate the alternative pathway.

At the time of engulfment, a new metabolic pathway, known as the **respiratory burst,** is triggered; this results in the production of 2 microbicidal agents, the superoxide radical and hydrogen peroxide. These highly reactive compounds are synthesized by the following reactions:

$$O_2 + 1e^- \rightarrow O_2^-$$
$$2\ O_2^- + 2\ H^+ \rightarrow H_2O_2 + O_2$$

In the first reaction, molecular oxygen is reduced by an electron to form the superoxide radical, which is weakly bactericidal. In the next step, the enzyme superoxide dismutase catalyzes the formation of hydrogen peroxide from 2 superoxide radicals. Hydrogen peroxide is more toxic than superoxide but is not effective against catalase-producing organisms such as staphylococci.

The killing of the organism within the phagosome is a 2-step process that consists of degranulation followed by production of hypochlorite ions (see below), which are probably the most important microbicidal agents. In degranulation, the 2 types of granules in the cytoplasm of the neutrophil fuse with the phagosome, emptying their contents in the process. These granules are lysosomes that contain a variety of enzymes essential to the killing and degradation that occur within the phagolysosome.

(1) The larger lysosomal granules, which constitute about 15% of the total, contain the important enzyme myeloperoxidase, as well as lysozyme and several other degradative enzymes. (Myeloperoxidase, which is green, makes a major contribution to the color of pus.)

(2) The smaller granules, which make up the remaining 85%, contain lactoferrin and additional degradative enzymes such as proteases, nucleases, and lipases. Lysosomal granules can empty into the extracellular space as well as into the phagosome. Outside the cell, the degradative enzymes can attack structures too large to be phagocytized, such as fungal mycelia, as well as extracellular bacteria.

The actual killing of the microorganisms occurs by a variety of mechanisms, which fall into 2 categories: oxygen dependent and oxygen-independent. The most important oxygen-dependent mechanism is the production of the highly reactive **hypochlorite ion** by myeloperoxidase according to the following reaction:

$$Cl^- + H_2O_2 \rightarrow ClO^- + H_2O$$

In this reaction, chloride ion plus H_2O_2, which was produced by the respiratory burst, yields hypochlorite ion in the presence of myeloperoxidase. Hypochlorite by itself damages cell walls but can also react with H_2O_2 to produce singlet oxygen, which damages cells by reacting with double bonds in the fatty acids of membrane lipids.

Rare individuals are genetically deficient in myeloperoxidase, yet their defense systems can kill bacteria, albeit more slowly. In these persons, the respiratory burst that produces H_2O_2 and superoxide ion seems to be sufficient, but with 2 caveats: if an organism produces catalase, H_2O_2 will be ineffective, and if an organism produces superoxide dismutase, superoxide ion will be ineffective.

The oxygen-independent mechanisms are important under anaerobic conditions. These mechanisms involve lactoferrin, which chelates iron from the bacteria; lysozyme, which degrades peptidoglycan in the bacterial cell wall; cationic proteins, which damage bacterial membranes; and low pH.

Macrophages also migrate, engulf, and kill bacteria by using essentially the same processes as PMNs do, but there are several differences.

(1) Macrophages do not possess myeloperoxidase and so cannot make hypochlorite ion; however, they do produce H_2O_2 and superoxide by respiratory burst.

(2) Certain organisms such as the agents of tuberculosis, brucellosis, and toxoplasmosis are preferentially ingested by macrophages rather than PMNs and may remain viable and multiply within these cells; granulomas formed during these infections contain many of these macrophages.

(3) Macrophages secrete plasminogen activator, an enzyme that converts the proenzyme plasminogen to the active enzyme plasmin, which dissolves the fibrin clot.

The importance of phagocytosis as a host defense mechanism is emphasized by the following observations.

(1) Repeated infections occur in children with genetic defects in the phagocytic process. Two examples of these defects are chronic granulomatous disease, in which the phagocyte cannot kill the ingested bacteria owing to a defect in NADPH oxidase and a resultant failure to generate H_2O_2; and Chédiak-Higashi syndrome, in which abnormal lysosomal granules are formed that cannot fuse with the phagosome, so that even though bacteria are ingested, they survive.

(2) Frequent infections occur in patients whose PMN count drops below $500/\mu L$ as a result of immunosuppressive drugs or irradiation. These infections are frequently caused by opportunistic organisms, ie, organisms that rarely cause disease in people with normal immune systems.

Fever Infection causes a rise in the body temperature that is attributed to **endogenous pyrogen** (interleukin-1) released from macrophages. Fever may be a protective response, since a variety of bacteria and viruses grow more slowly at elevated temperatures. The possible beneficial effect of fever has raised questions regarding the use of antipyretics such as aspirin for low-grade fever.

SPECIFIC IMMUNITY There are 2 types of immunity directed against specific organisms: natural immunity, which occurs in the absence of exposure to the organisms, and acquired immunity, which results either from exposure to the organism (active immunity) or from receipt of preformed antibody made in another host (passive immunity).

Natural Immunity Certain species have natural immunity against a particular organism. For example, *Shigella*, the bacterium that causes dysentery, is unable to infect nonprimates; only humans and chimpanzees are affected. In addition, some racial groups are more resistant to certain organisms, eg, light-skinned people are one-tenth as likely to develop the disseminated form of the fungal disease coccidioidomycosis as are dark-skinned people. The age of an individual is also a significant factor. Generally, very young and very old people are most susceptible to infection, but for some viral diseases, such as poliomyelitis, young children get inapparent infections, whereas older children and young adults contract severe disease. The basis for the differences seen with polio is unknown.

Acquired Immunity **Passive acquired immunity** is temporary protection against an organism and is acquired by receiving serum containing preformed antibodies from another person or animal. Passive immunization occurs normally in the form of immunoglobulins passed through the placenta or breast milk from mother to child. This protection is very important during the early days of life, when the child has a reduced capacity to mount an active response.

Passive immunity has the important advantage that its protective abilities are present immediately, whereas active immunity has a delay of a few days to a few weeks depending on whether it is a primary or secondary response. However, passive immunity has the important disadvantage that the antibody concentration decreases fairly rapidly as the proteins are degraded, so that protection usually lasts for only a few weeks. The administration of preformed antibodies can be lifesaving in certain diseases, such as botulism, caused by powerful exotoxins. In addition, they can mitigate but not prevent the symptoms of certain diseases such as hepatitis caused by hepatitis A virus, but they appear to have little effect on bacterial diseases with an invasive form of pathogenesis.

Active acquired immunity is protection based on exposure to the organism in the form of overt disease, subclinical infection without symptoms, or a vaccine. This protection has a slower onset but longer duration than passive immunity. An important advantage of active immunity is that an **anamnestic (secondary)** response occurs; ie, there is a rapid response of large amounts of antibody to an antigen that the immune system has previously encountered. Active immunity is mediated by both immunoglobulins and T cells:

(a) Immunoglobulins protect against organisms by a variety of mechanisms: neutralization of toxins, lysis of bacteria in the presence of complement, opsonization of bacteria to facilitate phagocytosis, and interference with adherence of bacteria and viruses to cell surfaces.

(b) T cells mediate a variety of reactions including cytotoxic destruction of virus-infected cells and bacteria, activation of macrophages, and delayed hypersensitivity. T cells also help B cells to produce antibody against many, but not all, antigens.

Review Questions

1. How do the skin and mucous membranes protect against infection?
2. Describe the 3 steps involved when a neutrophil phagocytizes a bacterium.
3. What is the clinically observed effect of having defective or too few phagocytes?
4. What is the difference between passive and active immunity? What are the advantages and disadvantages of each?

9

Laboratory Diagnosis

In the diagnosis of a disease, several important steps precede the actual laboratory work, namely (1) choosing the appropriate specimen to examine, which requires an understanding of the pathogenesis of the infection; (2) obtaining the specimen properly to avoid contamination from the normal flora; (3) transporting the specimen promptly to the laboratory or storing it correctly; and (4) providing essential information to guide the laboratory personnel.

In general, there are 3 approaches to the laboratory work:

(1) *observing* the organism in the microscope after staining;

(2) *obtaining* a pure culture of the organism by inoculating it onto a bacteriologic medium; and

(3) *identifying* the organism by using biochemical reactions, growth on selective media, or specific antibody reactions. Which of these approaches are used and in what sequence depend on the type of specimen and the organism. After the organism is grown in pure culture, its sensitivity to various antibiotics is determined by procedures described in Chapter 11.

In addition to these bacteriologic procedures, many diagnoses are made by serologic testing, which determines the presence of antibodies specific for the organism. In most cases, a 4-fold rise in antibody titer between the acute- and convalescent-phase serum samples is considered to be significant.

BACTERIOLOGIC METHODS

Blood Cultures Blood cultures are performed most often when sepsis, endocarditis, osteomyelitis, meningitis, or pneumonia is suspected. The organisms most frequently isolated from blood cultures are 2 gram-positive cocci, *Staphylococcus aureus* and *Streptococcus pneumoniae;* and 3 gram-negative rods, *Escherichia coli, Klebsiella pneumoniae,* and *Pseudomonas aeruginosa.*

It is important to obtain at least three 10-mL blood samples in a 24-hour period, because the number of organisms can be small and their presence intermittent. The site for venipuncture must be cleansed with 2% iodine to prevent contamination by members of the flora of the skin, usually *Staphylococcus epidermidis.* The blood obtained is added to 100 mL of a rich growth medium such as brain-heart infusion broth. Whether one or 2 bottles are inoculated varies among hospitals. If 2 bottles are used, one is kept under anaerobic conditions and the other is not. If one bottle is used, the low oxygen tension at the bottom of the bottle permits anaerobes to grow.

Blood cultures are checked for turbidity or for CO_2 production daily for 7 days or longer. If growth occurs, Gram stain, subculture, and antibiotic sensitivity tests are performed. If no growth is observed after 1 or 2 days, blind subculturing onto other media may reveal organisms. Cultures should be held for 14 days when infective endocarditis, fungemia, or infection by slow-growing bacteria, eg, *Brucella,* is suspected.

Throat Cultures Throat cultures are used primarily to detect the presence of group A beta-hemolytic streptococci, an important and treatable cause of pharyngitis. They are also used when diphtheria, gonococcal pharyngitis, or thrush (*Candida*) is suspected.

When the specimen is being obtained, the swab should touch not only the posterior pharynx but both tonsils or tonsillar fossae as well. The material on the swab is inoculated onto a sheep cell blood agar plate and streaked to obtain single colonies. If colonies of beta-hemolytic streptococci are found after 24 hours of incubation at 35 °C, a bacitracin disk is used to determine whether the organism is likely to be a group A streptococcus. If growth is inhibited around the disk, it is a group A streptococcus; if not, it is a non-group A beta-hemolytic streptococcus.

Sputum Cultures Sputum cultures are performed primarily when pneumonia, tuberculosis, or lung abscess is suspected. The most frequent cause of community-acquired pneumonia is *S pneumoniae,* whereas gram-negative rods, such as *K pneumoniae,* are common causes of hospital-acquired pneumonias.

It is important that the specimen for culture really be sputum, not saliva. Examination of a Gram-stained smear of the specimen frequently reveals whether the specimen is satisfactory. A reliable specimen has more than 25 leukocytes and fewer than 10 epithelial cells per 100 × field. An unreliable sample can be misleading and should be rejected by the laboratory. If the patient cannot cough and the need for a microbiologic diagnosis is strong, induction of sputum, transtracheal aspirate, bronchial lavage, or lung biopsy may be necessary. Because these procedures bypass the normal flora of the upper airway, they are more likely to provide an accurate microbiologic diagnosis. A preliminary assessment of the cause of the pneumonia can be made by Gram stain if large numbers of typical organisms are seen.

Culture of the sputum on sheep cell blood agar frequently reveals characteristic colonies, and identification is made by various serologic or biochemical tests. Cultures of *Mycoplasma* are infrequently done; diagnosis is usually confirmed by a rise in antibody titer. If tuberculosis is suspected, an acid-fast stain should be done immediately and the sputum cultured on special media, which are incubated for at least 6 weeks. In diagnosing aspiration pneumonia and lung abscesses, anaerobic cultures are important.

Spinal Fluid Cultures Spinal fluid cultures are performed primarily when meningitis is suspected. Spinal fluid specimens from cases of encephalitis, brain abscess, and subdural empyema usually show negative cultures. The most frequent causes of acute bacterial meningitis are 3 encapsulated organisms: *Neisseria meningitidis, S pneumoniae,* and *Haemophilus influenzae.*

Because acute meningitis is a medical emergency, the specimen should be taken immediately to the laboratory. The Gram-stained smear of the sediment of the centrifuged sample guides the immediate empirical treatment. If organisms resembling *N meningitidis, H influenzae,* or *S pneumoniae* are seen, the quellung test or immunofluorescence with specific antisera can identify the organism rapidly. Cultures are done on blood and on chocolate agar and incubated at 35 °C in a 5% CO_2 atmosphere. Hematin and nicotinamide adenine dinucleotide (NAD) (factors X and V, respectively) are added to enhance the growth of *H influenzae*.

In cases of subacute meningitis. *Mycobacterium tuberculosis* and the fungus *Cryptococcus neoformans* are the most common organisms isolated. Acid-fast stains of the spinal fluid should be done, although *M tuberculosis* may not be seen, because it can be present in small numbers. The fluid should be cultured and the plates held for a minimum of 6 weeks. *C neoformans*, a budding yeast with a prominent capsule, can be seen in spinal fluid when India ink is used.

Immunologic tests to detect the presence of capsular antigen in the spinal fluid can be used to identify *N meningitidis, S pneumoniae, H influenzae,* group B streptococci, *E coli*, and *C neoformans*. The 2 tests most frequently used are latex particle agglutination and counterimmunoelectrophoresis.

Stool Cultures   Stool cultures are performed primarily for cases of gastroenteritis. The most frequent bacterial pathogens causing diarrhea in the USA are *Shigella, Salmonella,* and *Campylobacter*.

A direct microscopic examination of the stool can be informative from 2 points of view: (1) a methylene blue stain that reveals many leukocytes indicates that an invasive organism rather than a toxigenic one is involved; and (2) a Gram stain may reveal large numbers of certain organisms, such as staphylococci, clostridia, or campylobacters.

For culture of *Salmonella* and *Shigella,* a selective, differential medium such as MacConkey or eosin-methylene blue (EMB) agar is used. These media are selective because they allow gram-negative rods to grow but inhibit many gram-positive organisms. Their differential properties are based on the fact that *Salmonella* and *Shigella* do not ferment lactose, whereas many other enteric gram-negative rods do. If non-lactose-fermenting colonies are found, a triple sugar iron (TSI) agar slant is used to distinguish *Salmonella* from *Shigella.* Some species of *Proteus* resemble *Salmonella* on TSI agar but can be distinguished because they produce the enzyme urease, whereas *Salmonella* does not. The organism is further identified as either a *Salmonella* or a *Shigella* species by the use of specific antisera to the organism's cell wall O antigen in an agglutination test. This is usually done in hospital laboratories, but precise identification of the species is performed in public health laboratories.

Campylobacter jejuni is cultured on antibiotic-containing media, eg, Skirrow's agar, at 42 °C in an atmosphere containing 5% O_2 and 10% CO_2. It grows well under these conditions, unlike many other intestinal pathogens. Although the techniques are available, stool cultures are only infrequently performed for organisms such as *Yersinia enterocolitica, Vibrio parahaemolyticus,* and enteropathic or toxigenic *E coli.* Despite the presence of large numbers of anaerobes in feces, they are rarely pathogens in the intestinal tract, and anaerobic cultures of stool specimens are therefore unnecessary.

Urine Cultures   Urine cultures are performed primarily when pyelonephritis or cystitis is suspected. By far the most frequent cause of urinary tract infections is *E coli.* Other common agents are *Enterobacter, Proteus,* and *Streptococcus faecalis* (the enterococcus).

Urine in the bladder of a healthy person is sterile, but it acquires organisms of the normal flora as it passes through the distal portion of the urethra. To avoid these organisms, a midstream specimen, voided after washing the external orifice, is used for urine cultures. In special situations, suprapubic aspiration or catheterization may be required to obtain a specimen. Because urine is a good culture medium, it is essential that the cultures be done within 1 hour after collection or stored in a refrigerator at 4 °C for no more than 18 hours.

It is commonly accepted that a bacterial count of at least 100,000/mL must be found to conclude that significant bacteriuria is present (in asymptomatic persons). There is evidence that as few as 100/mL are significant in symptomatic patients. For this determination to be made, quantitative or semiquantitative cultures must be performed. There are several techniques. (1) A calibrated loop that holds 0.001 mL of urine can be used to streak the culture. (2) Serial 10-fold dilutions can be made and samples from the dilutions streaked. (3) A screening procedure suitable for the physician's office involves an agar-covered "paddle" that is dipped into the urine. After the paddle is incubated, the density of the colonies is compared with standard charts to obtain an estimate of the concentration of bacteria.

Genital Tract Cultures   Genital tract cultures are performed primarily on specimens from individuals with an abnormal discharge or on specimens from asymptomatic contacts of a person with a sexually transmitted disease. One of the most important pathogens in the genital tract is *Neisseria gonorrhoeae*. The laboratory diagnosis of gonorrhea is made by microscopic examination of a Gram-stained smear and by culture of the organism.

Specimens are obtained by swabbing the urethral canal (for men), the cervix (for women), or the anal canal (for men and women). A urethral discharge from the penis is frequently used. Because *N. gonorrhoeae* is very delicate, the specimen should be inoculated directly onto a Thayer-Martin chocolate agar plate or onto a special transport medium (e.g., Trans-grow).

Gram-negative diplococci found *intracellularly* within neutrophils on a smear of a urethral discharge from a man have over 90% probability of being *N gonorrhoeae*. Because smears are less reliable when made from swabs of the endocervix and anal canal, cultures are necessary. The finding of only *extracellular* diplococci suggests that these *Neisseria* may be members of the normal flora and that the patient may have nongonococcal urethritis.

Nongonococcal urethritis and cervicitis are also extremely common infections. The most frequent cause is *Chlamydia trachomatis,* which cannot grow on artificial medium but must be grown in living cells. For this purpose, cultures of human cells or the yolk sacs of embryonated eggs are used. The finding of typical intracytoplasmic inclusions when using Giemsa's stain or fluorescent antibody is diagnostic.

Treponema pallidum, the agent of syphilis, cannot be cultured, and so diagnosis is made by microscopy and serology. The presence of motile spirochetes with typical morphologic features seen by darkfield microscopy of the fluid from a painless genital lesion is sufficient for the diagnosis. The serologic tests fall into 2 groups: the nontreponemal antibody tests such as the Venereal Disease Research Laboratory (VDRL) or rapid plasma reagin (RPR) test, and the treponemal antibody tests such as the fluorescent treponemal antibody-absorption (FTA-ABS) test. These tests are described on p. 38.

Wound & Abscess Cultures   A great variety of organisms are involved in wound and abscess infections. The bacteria most frequently isolated differ according to the anatomic site and predisposing factors. Abscesses of the brain, lungs, and abdomen are frequently associated with anaerobes such as *Bacteroides fragilis* and gram-positive cocci such as *S aureus* and *Streptococcus pyogenes*. Traumatic open wound infections are caused primarily by members of the soil flora such as *Clostridium perfringens;* surgical wound infections are usually due to *S aureus*. Infections of dog or cat bites are commonly due to *Pasteurella multocida,* whereas human bites primarily involve the mouth anaerobes.

Because anaerobes are frequently involved in these types of infection, it is important to place the specimen in anaerobic collection tubes and transport it promptly to the laboratory. Many of these infections are due to multiple organisms, including mixtures of anaerobes and nonanaerobes, and for that reason it is important to culture the specimen on several different media under different atmospheric conditions. The Gram stain will provide valuable information regarding the range of organisms under consideration.

IMMUNOLOGIC METHODS   These methods are described in more detail in Chapter 64. However, it is of interest here to present information on how serologic reactions aid the microbiologic diagnosis. There are essentially 2 basic approaches: (1) using known antibody to identify the microorganism, and (2) using known antigens to detect antibodies in the patient's serum.

Identification of an Organism by Use of Antiserum

A. Capsular Swelling (Quellung) Reaction: Several bacteria can be identified *directly* in clinical specimens by this reaction, which is based on the microscopic observation that the capsule swells in the presence of homologous antiserum. Antisera against the following organisms are available: all serotypes of *S pneumoniae* (Omniserum), *H influenzae* type B, and *N meningitidis* groups A and C.

B. Slide Agglutination Test: Antisera can be used to identify *Salmonella* and *Shigella* by causing agglutination (clumping) of the unknown organism. Antisera directed against the cell wall O antigens of *Salmonella* and *Shigella* are commonly used in hospital laboratories. Antisera against the flagellar H antigens and the capsular Vi antigen of *Salmonella* are used in public health laboratories for epidemiologic purposes.

C. Latex Agglutination Test: Latex beads coated with specific antibody are agglutinated in the presence of the homologous bacteria or antigen. This test is used to determine the presence of the capsular antigen of *H influenzae, N meningitidis,* several species of streptococci, and the yeast *Cryptococcus neoformans.*

D. Counter-immunoelectrophoresis Test: In this test, the unknown bacterial antigen and a known specific antibody move toward each other in an electrical field. If they are homologous, a precipitate forms within the agar matrix. Because antibodies are positively charged at the pH of the test, only negatively charged antigens, usually capsular polysaccharides, can be assayed. The test can be used to detect the presence in the spinal fluid of the capsular antigens of *H influenzae, N meningitidis, S pneumoniae,* and group B streptococci.

E. Enzyme-Linked Immunosorbent Assay: In this test, a specific antibody to which an easily assayed enzyme has been linked is used to detect the presence of the homologous antigen. Because several techniques have been devised to implement this principle, the specific steps used cannot be detailed here (see Chapter 64). This test is useful in detecting a wide variety of bacterial, viral, and fungal infections.

F. Fluorescent-Antibody Tests: A variety of bacteria can be identified by exposure to known antibody labeled with fluorescent dye, which is detected visually in the ultraviolet microscope. Various methods can be used, such as the direct and indirect techniques (see Chapter 64).

Identification of Antibodies in Serum by Use of Known Antigens

A. Slide or Tube Agglutination Test: In this test, serial 2-fold dilutions of a sample of the patient's serum are mixed with standard bacterial suspensions. The highest dilution of serum capable of agglutinating the bacteria is the titer of the antibody. As with most tests of a patient's antibody, at least a 4-fold rise in titer between the early and late samples must be demonsrated for a diagnosis to be made. This test is used primarily to aid in the diagnosis of typhoid fever, brucellosis, tularemia, plague, leptospirosis, and rickettsial diseases.

B. Serologic Tests for Syphilis: The detection of antibody in the patient's serum is frequently used to diagnosis syphilis, because *T pallidum* does not grow on laboratory media. There are 2 kinds of tests.

(1) The nontreponemal tests use a cardiolipin-lecithin-cholesterol mixture as the antigen, not an antigen of the organism. Cardiolipin (diphosphatidylglycerol) is a lipid extracted from normal beef heart. Flocculation (clumping) of the cardiolipin occurs in the presence of antibody to *T pallidum*. The VDRL and RPR tests are nontreponemal tests commonly used as screening procedures. They are not specific for syphilis but are inexpensive and easy to perform.

(2) The treponemal tests use *T pallidum* as the antigen. The most widely used treponemal test is the FTA-ABS test. The patient's serum sample, which has been absorbed with treponemes other than *T pallidum* to remove nonspecific antibodies, is mixed with nonviable *T pallidum* on a slide. Fluorescent-labeled antibody against human immunoglobulin G (IgG) is then used to determine wheter IgG antibody against *T pallidum* is bound to the organism. The most expensive test, which is not performed in hospital laboratories, is the *T pallidum* immobilization (TPI) test. The antigen is live *T pallidum* grown in rabbit testicles. If antibody is present in the patient's serum, the movement of the spirochete is inhibited.

C. Cold Agglutinin Test: Patients with *Mycoplasma pneumoniae* infections develop autoimmune antibodies that agglutinate human red blood in the cold (4 °C) but not at 37 °C. These antibodies are macroglobulins and occur in certain diseases other than *Mycoplasma* infections; thus, false-positive results can occur.

Review Questions

1. Why is the skin treated with 2% iodine before a blood culture specimen is taken?
2. What criteria are used to determine whether a sputum specimen is satisfactory?
3. What immunologic tests can be done on spinal fluid to provide a rapid diagnosis?
4. What is the purpose of EMB agar in stool cultures? What is the basis of its action?
5. In urine cultures, the number of organisms present as well as the species is determined. Why?
6. Describe the microscopic findings in a urethral exudate from a patient with gonorrhea.
7. What test is performed to analyze the fluid from a chancre in a case of primary syphilis? Why?
8. What is the basis for the serologic tests for syphilis?

Antimicrobial Drugs: Mechanisms of Action

10

The most important concept underlying antimicrobial therapy is **selective toxicity**, ie, selective inhibition of the growth of the microorganism without damage to the host. Selective toxicity is achieved by exploiting the differences between the metabolism and structure of the microorganism and the corresponding features of human cells. For example, penicillins and cephalosporins are effective antibacterial agents because they prevent the synthesis of peptidoglycan, thereby inhibiting bacterial, but not human, cell growth.

There are 4 major sites in the bacterial cell that are sufficiently different from the human cell that they serve as the basis for the action of clinically effective drugs: cell wall, ribosomes, nucleic acids, and cell membrane (Table 10–1).

There are far more antibacterial drugs than antiviral drugs. This is a consequence of the difficulty of designing a drug that will selectively inhibit viral replication. Because viruses use many of the normal cellular functions of the host in their growth, it is not easy to develop a drug that specifically inhibits viral functions and does not damage the host cell.

Table 10–1. Modes of action of important antibacterial and antifungal drugs.

Mechanism of Action	Drugs
Inhibition of cell wall synthesis	
Inhibition of cross-linking (transpeptidation) of peptidoglycan	Penicillins, cephalosporins, imipenem, aztreonam
Inhibition of other steps in peptidoglycan synthesis	Vancomycin, cycloserine, bacitracin
Inhibition of protein synthesis	
Action on 50S ribosomal subunit	Chloramphenicol, erythromycin, clindamycin
Action on 30S ribosomal subunit	Tetracyclines and aminoglycosides, eg, streptomycin, tobramycin, gentamicin, amikacin, kanamycin, neomycin, spectinomycin
Inhibition of nucleic acid synthesis	
Blocking of nucleotide synthesis	Sulfonamides, trimethoprim
Blocking of DNA synthesis	Nalidixic acid and quinolones, eg, norfloxacin
Blocking of mRNA synthesis	Rifampin
Alteration of cell membrane function	
Antibacterial Activity	Polymyxin
Antifungal Activity	Amphotericin B, nystatin, ketoconazole
Uncertain site of action	
Unknown mechanism	Isoniazid, metronidazole

Bactericidal & Bacteriostatic Activity

In some clinical situations, it is essential to use a bactericidal drug rather than a bacteriostatic one. A bactericidal drug kills bacteria, whereas a bacteriostatic drug inhibits their growth but does not kill them. The salient features of the behavior of bacteriostatic drugs are that (1) the bacteria can grow again when the drug is withdrawn, and (2) host defense mechanisms, such as phagocytosis, are required to kill the bacteria. Bactericidal drugs are particularly useful in certain infections, eg, those that are immediately life-threatening; those in patients whose polymorphonuclear leukocyte count is below $500/\mu L$; and endocarditis, in which phagocytosis is limited by the fibrinous network of the vegetations and bacteriostatic drugs do not effect a cure.

Mechanisms of Action

INHIBITION OF CELL WALL SYNTHESIS

Penicillins   Penicillins (and cephalosporins) act by inhibiting **transpeptidases,** the enzymes that catalyze the final cross-linking step in the synthesis of peptidoglycan (see Fig 2–5). For example, in *Staphylococcus aureus,* transpeptidation occurs between the amino group on the end of the pentaglycine cross-link and the terminal carboxyl group of the D-alanine on the tetrapeptide side chain. Since the stereochemistry of penicillin is similar to that of a dipeptide, D-alanyl-D-alanine, it can bind to the active site of the transpeptidase and inhibit its activity.

There are 2 additional factors involved in the action of penicillin.

(a) The first is that penicillin binds to a variety of receptors in the bacterial cell membrane and cell wall called **penicillin-binding proteins** (PBPs). Some PBPs are transpeptidases; the function of others is unknown. Changes in PBPs are in part responsible for an organism's becoming resistant to penicillin.

(b) The second factor is that **autolytic enzymes** called murein hydrolases (murein is a synonym for peptidoglycan) are activated in penicillin-treated cells and degrade the peptidoglycan. Some strains of *S aureus* are tolerant to the action of penicillin, since these autolytic enzymes are not activated. A tolerant organism is one that is inhibited but not killed by a usually bactericidal drug, such as penicillin (see Chapter 11).

Penicillin-treated cells die by rupture as a result of the influx of water into the high-osmotic-pressure interior of the bacterial cell. If the osmotic pressure of the medium is raised about 3-fold, by the addition of sufficient KCl for example, rupture will not occur and the organism can survive as a protoplast. Exposure of the bacterial cell to lysozyme, which is present in human tears, results in degradation of the peptidoglycan and osmotic rupture similar to that caused by penicillin.

Penicillin is bactericidal, but it kills cells only when they are growing. When cells are growing, new peptidoglycan is being synthesized and transpeptidation occurs. However, in nongrowing cells, no new cross-linkages are required and penicillin is inactive.

Penicillins (and cephalosporins) are called β-**lactam** drugs because of the importance of the β-lactam ring (Fig 10–1). An intact ring structure is essential for antibacterial activity; cleavage of the ring by penicillinases (β-**lactamases)** inactivates the drug. The most important naturally occurring compound is benzylpenicillin (penicillin G), which is composed of the 6-aminopenicillanic acid nucleus that all penicillins have in common, plus a benzyl side chain (Fig 10–1).

Benzylpenicillin is one of the most widely used and effective antibiotics. However, it has 3 disadvantages, all of which have been successfully overcome by chemical modification of the side chain. These disadvantages are (1) limited effectiveness against many gram-negative rods; (2) hydrolysis by gastric acids, so that it cannot be taken orally; and (3) inactivation by β-lactamases. There is a fourth disadvantage, common to all penicillins, which has *not* been overcome: hypersensitivity, especially anaphylaxis, in some recipients of the drug.

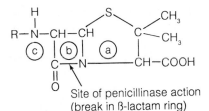
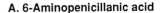
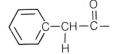

Site of penicillinase action
(break in ß-lactam ring)

A. 6-Aminopenicillanic acid

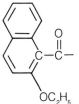

B. Penicillin G (benzylpenicillin)

Figure 10–1. Penicillins. *A:* The 6-aminopenicillanic acid nucleus is composed of a thiazolidine ring (a), a β-lactam ring (b), and an amino group (c). *B:* The benzyl group, which forms benzylpenicillin (penicillin G) when attached at R. *C:* The large aromatic ring substituent that forms nafcillin, a β-lactamase-resistant penicillin, when attached at R.

C. Nafcillin (ethoxynaphthamidopenicillin)

The effectiveness of penicillins against gram-negative rods has been increased by a series of chemical changes in the side chain (Table 10–2). It can be seen that ampicillin and amoxicillin have activity against several gram-negative rods that the earlier penicillins do not have. However, these drugs are not useful against *Pseudomonas aeruginosa* and *Klebsiella pneumoniae.* Hence, other penicillins were introduced. Generally speaking, as the activity against gram-negative bacteria increases, the activity against gram-positive bacteria decreases.

The second important disadvantage—acid hydrolysis in the stomach—also has been addressed by modification of the side chain. The site of acid hydrolysis is the amide bond between the side chain and penicillanic acid nucleus (Fig 10–1). Minor modifications of the side chain in that region, such as addition of an oxygen (to produce penicillin V) or an amino group (to produce ampicillin), prevent hydrolysis and allow the drug to be taken orally.

The inactivation of penicillin G by β-lactamases is another important disadvantage, especially in the treatment of *S aureus* infections. Access of the enzyme to the β-lactam ring is blocked by modification of the side chain with the addition of large aromatic rings containing bulky methyl or ethyl groups (methicillin, oxacillin, nafcillin, etc; Fig 10–1).

Table 10–2. Activity of selected penicillins.

Drug	Major Organisms[1]
Penicillin G	Gram-positive cocci, gram-positive rods, *Neisseria*, spirochetes such as *Treponema pallidum,* and many anaerobes (except *Bacteroides fragilis*) but none of the gram-negative rods listed below
Ampicillin or amoxicillin	Certain gram-negative rods, such as *Haemophilus influenzae, Escherichia coli, Proteus, Salmonella,* and *Shigella* but not *Pseudomonas aeruginosa*
Carbenicillin or ticarcillin	*P aeruginosa,* especially when used in synergistic combination with an aminoglycoside
Piperacillin	Similar to carbenicillin but with greater activity against *P aeruginosa* and *Klebsiella pneumoniae*

[1]The spectrum of activity is intentionally incomplete. It is simplified for the beginning student to illustrate the expanded coverage of gram-negative organisms with successive generations and does not cover all possible clinical uses.

Generally speaking, penicillins are nontoxic at clinically effective levels. The major disadvantage of these compounds is hypersensitivity, which is estimated to occur in 1–10% of patients. The hypersensitivity reactions include anaphylaxis, skin rashes, hemolytic anemia, nephritis, and drug fever. Anaphylaxis, the most serious complication, occurs in 0.5% of patients. Death due to anaphylaxis occurs in 0.002% (1:50,000) patients.

Cephalosporins Cephalosporins are β-lactam drugs that act in the same manner as penicillins; ie, they are bactericidal agents that inhibit the cross-linking of peptidoglycan. The structures, however, are different: The cephalosporins have a 6-membered ring adjacent to the β-lactam ring and are substituted in 2 places on the 7-aminocephalosporanic acid nucleus (Fig 10–2), whereas penicillins have a 5-membered ring and are substituted in only one place.

Similar to the penicillins, new cephalosporins were synthesized with expansion of activity against gram-negative rods as the goal. Cephalosporins are effective against a broad range of organisms, are generally well tolerated, and produce fewer hypersensitivity reactions than do the penicillins. Despite the structural similarity, a patient allergic to penicillin has only about a 10% chance of being hypersensitive to cephalosporins also. Cephalosporins are the products of molds of the genus *Cephalosporium,* except for a few, such as cefoxitin, which is made by the actinomycete *Streptomyces.*

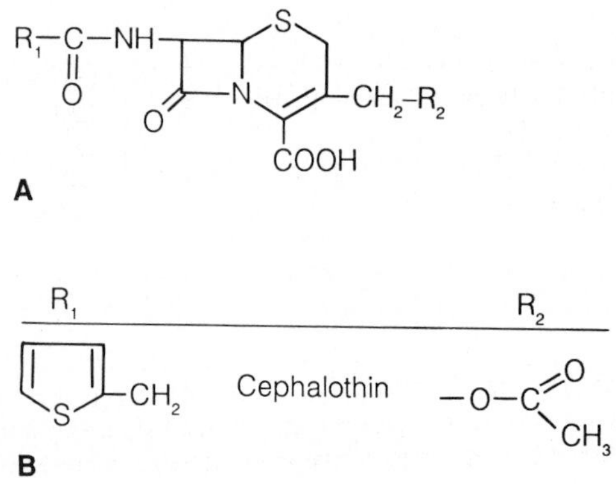

Figure 10–2. Cephalosporins. *A:* The 7-aminocephalosporanic acid nucleus. *B:* The two R groups that form the drug cephalothin.

Carbapenems Carbapenems are β-lactam drugs that are structurally different from penicillins and cephalosporins. For example, imipenem (N-formimidoylthienamycin), the currently used carbapenem, has a methylene group in the ring in place of the sulfur (Fig 10–3). It has excellent bactericidal activity against many gram-positive, gram-negative, and anaerobic bacteria. It is effective against most gram-positive cocci, eg, streptococci and staphylococci; many gram-negative rods, eg, Enterobacteriaceae, *Pseudomonas, Haemophilus,* and *Neisseria;* and various anaerobes, eg, *Bacteroides* and *Clostridium.* It is resistant to most β-lactamases.

Monobactams Monobactams are also β-lactam drugs that are structurally different from penicillins and cephalosporins. Monobactams are characterized by a β-lactam ring without an adjacent fused ring structure, ie, they are monocyclic (Fig 10–3). Aztreonam, currently the most useful monobactam, has excellent activity against many gram-negative rods, such as the Enterobacteriaceae and *Pseudomonas,* but is inactive against gram-positive and anaerobic bacteria. It is resistant to most β-lactamases. It is very useful in patients who are hypersensitive to penicillin, because there is no cross-reactivity.

Vancomycin, Cycloserine, & Bacitracin These 3 drugs inhibit cell wall synthesis by blocking the formation of precursors. Vancomycin binds to the D-alanyl-D-alanine portion of the pentapeptide to prevent the precursor subunit (muramic acid, pentapeptide, and glucosamine) from being incorporated into the growing peptidoglycan. Vancomycin is a bactericidal agent whose most important use is in the treatment of infections by *S aureus* strains that are resistant to the penicillinase-resistant penicillins such as nafcillin. No vancomycin-resistant mutants of *S aureus* have been isolated.

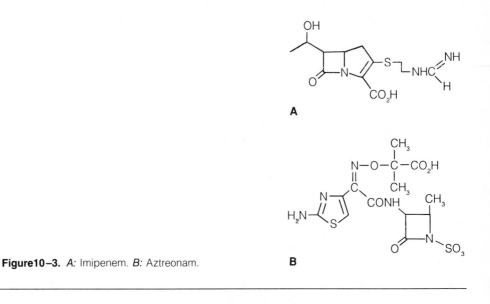

Figure10–3. *A:* Imipenem. *B:* Aztreonam.

Cycloserine is a structural analogue of D-alanine that inhibits the synthesis of the D-alanyl-D-alanine dipeptide. It is used as a second-line drug in the treatment of tuberculosis.

Bacitracin is a cyclic polypeptide antibiotic that prevents the dephosphorylation of the phospholipid that carries the peptidoglycan subunit across the cell membrane. This blocks the regeneration of the lipid carrier and inhibits cell wall synthesis. Bacitracin is a bactericidal drug that is useful in the treatment of superficial skin infections but is too toxic for systemic use.

INHIBITION OF PROTEIN SYNTHESIS Several drugs inhibit protein synthesis in bacteria without significantly interfering with protein synthesis in human cells. This selectivity is due to the differences between bacterial and human ribosomal proteins, RNAs, and associated enzymes. Bacteria have 70S* ribosomes with 50S and 30S subunits, whereas human cells have 80S ribosomes with 60S and 40S subunits. Chloramphenicol, erythromycin, and clindamycin act on the 50S subunit, whereas tetracyclines and aminoglycosides act on the 30S subunit. A summary of the modes of action of these drugs is presented in Table 10–3, and a summary of their clinically useful activity is presented in Table 10–4.

1. Drugs That Act on the 30S Subunit

Aminoglycosides Aminoglycosides are bactericidal drugs that are especially useful against many gram-negative rods. Certain aminoglycosides are used against other organisms; eg,

Table 10–3. Mode of action of antibiotics that inhibit protein synthesis

Antibiotic	Ribosomal Subunit	Mode of Action	Bactericidal or Bacteriostatic
Aminoglycosides	30S	Blocks functioning of initiation complex and causes misreading of mRNA	Bactericidal
Tetracyclines	30S	Blocks tRNA binding to ribosome	Bacteriostatic
Chloramphenicol	50S	Blocks peptidyltransferase	Both[1]
Erythromycin	50S	Blocks translocation	Primarily bacteriostatic
Clindamycin	50S	Blocks peptide bond formation	Primarily bacteriostatic

[1]Chloramphenicol can be either bactericidal or bacteriostatic depending on the organism.

*S stands for Svedberg units, a measure of sedimentation rate in a density gradient. The rate of sedimentation is proportional to the mass of the particle.

streptomycin is used in the multiple-drug therapy of tuberculosis, and gentamicin is used in combination with penicillin G against enterococci. Aminoglycosides are named for the amino sugar component of the molecule, which is connected by a glycosidic linkage to other sugar derivatives (Fig 10–4).

Table 10–4. Spectrum of activity of antibiotics that inhibit protein synthesis.

Antibiotic	Clinically Useful Activity	Comments
Aminoglycosides Streptomycin	Tuberculosis, tularemia, plague, brucellosis	Ototoxic and nephrotoxic.
Gentamicin and tobramycin	Many gram-negative rod infections including *Pseudomonas aeruginosa*	Most widely used aminoglycosides.
Amikacin	Same as gentamicin and tobramycin	Effective against some organisms resistant to gentamicin and tobramycin.
Neomycin	Preoperative bowel preparation	Too toxic to be used systemically; use orally since not absorbed.
Tetracyclines	Rickettsial and chlamydial infections, *Mycoplasma pneumoniae*	Not given during pregnancy or to young children.
Chloramphenicol	*H influenzae* meningitis, typhoid fever, anaerobic infections (especially *Bacteroides fragilis*)	Bone marrow toxicity limits use to severe infections.
Erythromycin	Pneumonia caused by *Mycoplasma* and *Legionella*, infections by gram-positive cocci in penicillin-allergic patients	Toxicity uncommon.
Clindamycin	Anaerobes such as *Clostridium perfringens* and *B fragilis*	Pseudomembranous colitis is a major side effect.

The 2 important modes of action of aminoglycosides have been documented best for streptomycin; other aminoglycosides probably act similarly. Both **inhibition of the "initiation complex"** and **misreading of messenger RNA** (mRNA) occur; the former is probably more important for the bactericidal activity of the drug. An initiation complex composed of a streptomycin-treated 30S subunit, a 50S subunit, and mRNA will not function—ie, no peptide bonds are formed, no polysomes are made, and a frozen "streptomycin monosome" results. Misreading of the triplet codon of mRNA so that the wrong amino acid is inserted into the protein also occurs in streptomycin-treated bacteria. The site of action on the 30S subunit includes both a ribosomal protein and the ribosomal RNA (rRNA). As a result of inhibition of initiation and misreading, membrane damage occurs and the bacterium dies.

One of the major limitations of aminoglycosides is their toxic effect both on the kidney and on the auditory and vestibular portions of the eighth cranial nerve. To avoid toxicity, serum levels of the drug, blood urea nitrogen, and creatinine should be measured. Aminoglycosides are poorly absorbed from the gastrointestinal tract and cannot be given orally. They penetrate the spinal fluid poorly and must be given intrathecally in the treatment of meningitis.

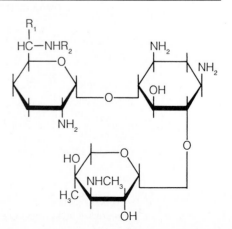

Figure 10–4. Aminoglycosides. Aminoglycosides consist of amino sugars joined by a glycosidic linkage. The structure of gentamicin is shown.

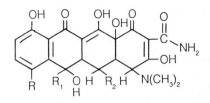

Figure 10-5. Tetracycline structure. The 4-ring structure is depicted with its three R sites. Chlortetracycline, for example, has R = Cl, R_1 = CH_3, and R_2 = H.

Tetracyclines Tetracyclines are a family of antibiotics with bacteriostatic activity against a variety of gram-positive and gram-negative bacteria, mycoplasmas, chlamydiae, and rickettsiae. They inhibit protein synthesis by binding to the 30S ribosomal subunit and blocking the aminoacyl transfer RNA (tRNA) from entering the acceptor site on the ribosome. However, the selective action of tetracycline on bacteria is not at the level of the ribosome, as tetracycline in vitro will inhibit protein synthesis equally well in purified ribosomes from both bacterial and human cells. Its selectivity is based on its greatly increased uptake into susceptible bacterial cells compared with human cells.

Tetracyclines, as the name indicates, have 4 cyclic rings with different substituents at the 4 R groups (Fig 10–5). The various tetracyclines have similar antimicrobial activity but altered pharmacologic properties. In general, tetracyclines have low toxicity but are associated with 2 significant difficulties. One is suppression of the normal flora of the intestinal tract, which can lead to diarrhea and overgrowth by drug-resistant bacteria and fungi. The other is brown staining of the teeth of fetuses and young children owing to deposition of the drug in developing teeth; tetracyclines are avid calcium chelators. For this reason, tetracycline is contraindicated for use in pregnant women and in children under age 8 years.

2. Drugs That Act on the 50S Subunit

Chloramphenicol Chloramphenicol is active against a broad range of organisms, including gram-positive and gram-negative bacteria (including anaerobes). It is bacteriostatic against certain organisms, such as *Salmonella typhi*, but has bactericidal activity against the 3 important encapsulated organisms that cause meningitis: *Haemophilus influenzae, Streptococcus pneumoniae,* and *Neisseria meningitidis.*

Chloramphenicol inhibits protein synthesis by binding to the 50S ribosomal subunit and blocking the action of peptidyltransferase; this prevents the synthesis of new peptide bonds. It inhibits bacterial protein synthesis selectively, because it binds to the catalytic site of the transferase in the 50S bacterial ribosomal subunit but not to the transferase in the 60S human ribosomal subunit. Chloramphenicol inhibits protein synthesis in the mitochondria of human cells to some extent, since mitochondria have a 50S subunit (mitochondria are thought to have evolved from bacteria). This inhibition may be the cause of the dose-dependent toxicity to the bone marrow (discussed below).

Chloramphenicol is a comparatively simple molecule with a nitrobenzene nucleus (Fig 10–6). Nitrobenzene itself is a bone marrow depressant, and so the nitrobenzene portion of the molecule may be involved in the hematologic problems reported with this drug. The most important side effect of chloramphenicol is bone marrow toxicity, of which there are 2 distinct types. One is a dose-dependent suppression, which is more likely to occur in patients on high doses for long periods and which is reversible when administration of the drug is stopped. The other is aplastic anemia, which is caused by an idiosyncratic reaction to the drug. This reaction is not dose-dependent, can occur weeks after administration of the drug has been stopped, and is not reversible. Fortunately, this reaction is rare, occurring in about 1:30,000 patients.

Erythromycin Erythromycin is a bacteriostatic drug with a wide spectrum of activity: it is the treatment of choice for pneumonia caused by *Legionella* (a gram-negative rod) and

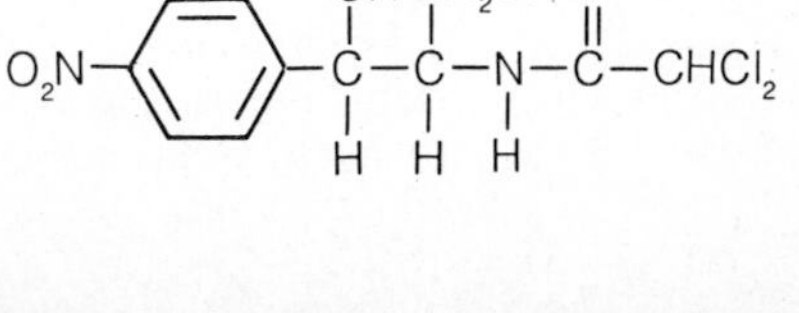

O_2N—⟨benzene ring⟩—$\overset{\overset{OH}{|}}{\underset{\underset{H}{|}}{C}}$—$\overset{\overset{CH_2OH}{|}}{\underset{\underset{H}{|}}{C}}$—$\overset{}{\underset{\underset{H}{|}}{N}}$—$\overset{\overset{O}{||}}{C}$—$CHCl_2$

Figure 10-6. Chloramphenicol.

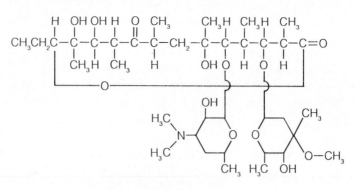

Figure 10–7. Erythromycin.

Mycoplasma (a wall-less bacterium) and is also an effective alternative against a variety of infections caused by gram-positive cocci in penicillin-allergic patients.

Erythromycin binds to the 50S subunit and blocks the translocation step by preventing the release of the uncharged tRNA from the donor site after the peptide bond is formed. It has a macrolide structure composed of a large 13-carbon ring to which 2 sugars are attached by glycosidic linkages (Fig 10–7). Erythromycin is one of the least toxic drugs, with only some gastrointestinal distress associated with oral use.

Clindamycin   The most useful clinical activity of this bacteriostatic drug is against anaerobes, both gram-positive bacteria such as *Clostridium perfringens* and gram-negative bacteria such as *Bacteroides fragilis*.

Clindamycin binds to the 50S subunit and blocks peptide bond formation by an undetermined mechanism. Its specificity for bacteria arises from its inability to bind to the 60S subunit of human ribosomes.

The most important side effect of clindamycin is pseudomembranous colitis, which, in fact, can occur with virtually any antibiotic, whether taken orally or parenterally. The pathogenesis of this potentially severe complication is suppression of the bowel normal flora by the drug and overgrowth of a drug-resistant strain of *Clostridium difficile*. The organism secretes an exotoxin that produces the pseudomembrane in the colon. Oral vancomycin is the treatment of choice for pseudomembranous colitis.

INHIBITION OF NUCLEIC ACID SYNTHESIS

1.   Inhibition of Precursor Synthesis

Sulfonamides   Either alone or in combination with trimethoprim, sulfonamides are useful in a variety of bacterial diseases such as *Escherichia coli* urinary tract infections, otitis media caused by *S pneumoniae* or *H influenzae* in children, shigellosis, nocardiosis, and chancroid. In combination, they are also the drugs of choice for 2 parasitic diseases, toxoplasmosis and *Pneumocystis* pneumonia. The sulfonamides are a large family of bacteriostatic drugs that are produced by chemical synthesis. In 1935, the parent compound, sulfanilamide, became the first clinically effective antimicrobial agent.

The mode of action of sulfonamides is to block the synthesis of tetrahydrofolic acid, which is required as a methyl donor in the synthesis of the nucleic acid precursors adenine, guanine, and thymine. Sulfonamides are **structural analogues of *p*-aminobenzoic acid** (PABA). PABA condenses with a pteridine compound to form dihydropteroic acid, a precursor of tetrahydrofolic acid (Fig 10–8). Sulfonamides compete with PABA for the active site of the enzyme dihydropteroate synthetase. This competitive inhibition can be overcome by an excess of PABA.

The basis of the selective action of sulfonamides on bacteria is that many bacteria synthesize their folic acid from PABA-containing precursors, whereas human cells require preformed folic acid as an exogenous nutrient, since they lack the enzymes to synthesize it. Human cells

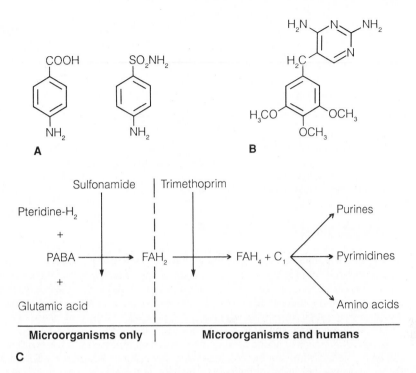

Figure 10–8. Sulfonamide and trimethoprim. **A:** Comparison of PABA (left) and sulfonamide (right). **B:** Trimethoprim. **C:** Inhibition of the folic acid pathway by sulfonamide and trimethoprim (FAH_2 = dihydrofolate; FAH_4 = tetrahydrofolate). (Modified and reproduced, with permission, from Corcoran JW, Hahn FE [editors]: *Mechanism of Action of Antimicrobial and Antitumor Agents.* Vol 3 of: *Antibiotics.* Springer-Verlag, 1975.

therefore bypass the step at which sulfonamides act. Bacteria that can use preformed folic acid are similarly resistant to sulfonamides.

The *p*-amino group on the sulfonamide is essential for its activity. Modifications are therefore made on the sulfonic acid side chain.

Sulfonamides are inexpensive and cause side effects uncommonly. Drug fever, rashes, and bone marrow suppression can occur.

Trimethoprim Trimethoprim also inhibits the production of tetrahydrofolic acid but by a mechanism different from that of the sulfonamides; ie, it inhibits the enzyme dihydrofolate reductase (Fig 10–8). Its specificity for bacteria is based on its much greater affinity for bacterial reductase than for the human enzyme.

Trimethoprim is used most frequently together with sulfamethoxazole. Note that both drugs act on the same pathway—but at different sites—to inhibit the synthesis of tetrafolate. The advantages of the combination are that (1) bacterial mutants resistant to one drug will be inhibited by the other and that (2) the 2 drugs can act **synergistically**—ie, when used together, they cause significantly greater inhibition than the sum of the inhibition caused by each drug separately.

Trimethoprim-sulfamethoxazole is clinically useful in the treatment of urinary tract infections, *Pneumocystis* pneumonia, and shigellosis. It also is used for prophylaxis in granulopenic patients to prevent nosocomial infections.

2. Inhibition of DNA Synthesis

Quinolones Quinolones are bactericidal drugs that block bacterial DNA synthesis by inhibiting **DNA gyrase.** Norfloxacin has low minimum inhibitory concentrations (MICs) against many organisms (Fig 10–9). At present, it is approved only for the treatment of urinary tract infections, but it promises to have wider usage. Side effects are few, and it can be taken

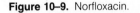

Figure 10–9. Norfloxacin.

orally. Ciprofloxacin is active against a broad range of organisms causing infections of the lower respiratory tract, urinary tract, bones, and joints. Nalidixic acid has a narrower spectrum of activity and higher MICs than norfloxacin. It is effective in the treatment of certain urinary tract infections, but it is not widely used.

3. Inhibition of mRNA Synthesis

Rifampin   Rifampin is used primarily for the treatment of tuberculosis in combination with other drugs and for prophylaxis in close contacts of patients with meningitis caused by either *N meningitidis* or *H influenzae*. It is also used in combination with other drugs in the treatment of prosthetic-valve endocarditis caused by *Staphylococcus epidermidis*. With the exception of the short-term prophylaxis of meningitis, rifampin is given in combination with other drugs, since resistant mutants appear at a high rate when it is used alone.

The selective mode of action of rifampin is based on **blocking mRNA synthesis** by bacterial RNA polymerase without affecting the RNA polymerase of human cells. Rifampin is red, and the urine, saliva, and sweat of patients taking rifampin often turn orange; this is disturbing but harmless. Rifampin is excreted in high concentration in saliva, which accounts for its success in the prophylaxis of bacterial meningitis, as the organisms are carried in the throat.

ALTERATION OF CELL MEMBRANE FUNCTION

1. Bacterial
There are few antimicrobial compounds that act on the cell membrane, because the structural and chemical similarities of bacterial and human cell membranes make it difficult to provide sufficient selective toxicity.

Polymyxins   Polymyxins are a family of polypeptide antibiotics of which the clinically most useful compound is polymyxin E (colistin). It is active against gram-negative rods, especially *P aeruginosa*. Polymyxins are cyclic peptides composed of 10 amino acids, 6 of which are diaminobutyric acid. The positively charged free amino groups act like a cationic detergent to disrupt the phospholipid structure of the cell membrane.

2. Fungal

Amphotericin B & Nystatin   Amphotericin B, the most important antifungal drug, is used in the treatment of a variety of disseminated fungal diseases. It is classified as a polyene compound, because it has a series of 7 unsaturated double bonds in its macrolide ring structure (*poly* means many, and *-ene* is a suffix indicating the presence of double bonds; Fig 10–10). It disrupts the cell membrane of fungi owing to its affinity for **ergosterol** ,a component of fungal membranes but not of bacterial or human cell membranes. Amphotericin B has significant renal toxicity; serum creatinine is used to monitor the dose.

Nystatin is another polyene antifungal agent, which, because of its toxicity, is used topically for infections caused by the yeast *Candida*.

Ketoconazole   Ketoconazole is the most important of a family of imidazole compounds with antifungal activity. They all inhibit ergosterol synthesis. It is useful in the treatment of blastomycosis, chronic mucocutaneous candidiasis, coccidioidomycosis, and skin infections caused by dermatophytes. Miconazole and clotrimazole, 2 other imidazoles, are useful for topical therapy of *Candida* infections and dermatophytoses.

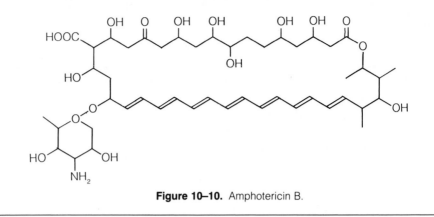

Figure 10–10. Amphotericin B.

UNCERTAIN MECHANISMS OF ACTION

Isoniazid Isoniazid, or isonicotinic acid hydrazide (INH), is a bactericidal drug highly specific for *Mycobacterium tuberculosis* and other mycobacteria. It is used in combination with other drugs to treat tuberculosis and by itself to prevent tuberculosis in exposed persons. Because it penetrates cells well, it is effective against the organisms residing within macrophages.

Despite its widespread use and its availability for over 30 years, its mode of action is unclear. The most likely possibility is that it inhibits mycolic acid synthesis, which explains why it is specific for mycobacteria and relatively nontoxic for humans. Its main side effect is liver toxicity. It is given with pyridoxine to prevent neurologic complications.

Metronidazole Metronidazole exerts its bactericidal activity chiefly against anaerobic organisms, both bacteria and protozoa. This drug has 2 possible mechanisms of action, and it is unclear which is the more important. The first, which explains its specificity for anaerobes, is its ability to act as an electron sink. By accepting electrons, the drug deprives the organism of required reducing power. In addition, when electrons are acquired, the drug ring is cleaved and a toxic intermediate is formed. The precise nature of the intermediate and its action is unknown.

The second mode of action of metronidazole relates to its ability to inhibit DNA synthesis. The drug binds to DNA and causes strand breakage, which prevents its proper functioning as a template for DNA polymerase.

Review Questions

1. What is the basis for the selective ability of the following drugs to affect bacteria but not human cells: (a) penicillins, (b) cephalosporins, (c) aminoglycosides, (d) tetracyclines, (e) erythromycin, (f) chloramphenicol, (g) sulfonamides, (h) rifampin.
2. What is the mode of action of each of the above drugs?
3. What is the difference between a bactericidal and a bacteriostatic drug?
4. What is the essential portion of the penicillin and cephalosporin molecules?
5. Why are sulfonamides and trimethoprim used in combination to treat certain infections?
6. Why is rifampin frequently given in combination with other drugs?
7. Why is amphotericin B selectively active against fungal and not bacterial or human cells?
8. What is the likely reason that isoniazid is selectively active against *Mycobacterium tuberculosis*?

11 Antimicrobial Drugs: Resistance

There are 3 major mechanisms that mediate bacterial resistance to drugs. (1) Bacteria produce enzymes that inactivate the drug; eg, β-lactamases can inactivate penicillins and cephalosporins by cleaving the β-lactam ring of the drug. (2) Bacteria synthesize modified targets against which the drug has no effect; eg, a mutant protein on the 30S ribosomal subunit can result in resistance to streptomycin, and a methylated 23S ribosomal RNA can result in resistance to erythromycin. (3) Bacteria alter their permeability so that an effective intracellular concentration of the drug is not achieved; eg, tetracycline is concentrated less in resistant bacteria than in susceptible ones.

Most drug resistance is due to a genetic change in the organism, either a chromosomal mutation or the acquisition of a plasmid or transposon. Nongenetic changes, which are of lesser importance, are discussed below on page 52.

GENETIC BASIS OF RESISTANCE

Chromosome-Mediated Resistance Chromosomal resistance is due to a mutation in the gene that codes for either the target of the drug or the transport system in the membrane that controls the uptake of the drug. The frequency of spontaneous mutations usually ranges from 10^{-7} to 10^{-9}, which is much lower than the frequency of acquisition of resistance plasmids. Therefore, chromosomal resistance is less of a clinical problem than is plasmid-mediated resistance.

Plasmid-Mediated Resistance Plasmid-mediated resistance is very important from a clinical point of view for 3 reasons:

(1) It occurs in many different species, especially gram-negative rods;

(2) plasmids frequently mediate resistance to multiple drugs; and

(3) plasmids have a high rate of transfer from one cell to another, usually by conjugation.

Resistance plasmids (resistance factors, R factors) are extrachromosomal, circular, double-stranded DNA molecules that carry the genes for a variety of enzymes that can degrade antibiotics and modify membrane transport systems. Table 11–1 describes the most important mechanisms of resistance for several important drugs.

In addition to producing drug resistance, R factors have 2 very important properties: (1) They can replicate independently of the bacterial chromosome, so that a cell can contain many copies; and (2) they can be transferred not only to cells of the same species but also to other species and genera. Note that this conjugal transfer is under the control of the genes of the R plasmid and not of the F (fertility) plasmid, which governs the transfer of the bacterial chromosome.

Table 11–1. R-factor-mediated resistance mechanisms.

Drug	Mechanism of Resistance
Penicillins and cephalosporins	β-Lactamase cleavage of β-lactam ring
Aminoglycosides	Modification by acetylation, adenylylation, or phosphorylation
Chloramphenicol	Modification by acetylation
Erythromycin	Change in receptor by methylation of rRNA
Tetracycline	Reduced uptake into the cell
Sulfonamides	Active export out of the cell and reduced affinity of enzyme

R factors exist in 2 broad size categories: large plasmids with molecular weights of about 60 million and small ones with molecular weights of about 10 million. The large plasmids are conjugative R factors, which contain the extra DNA to code for the conjugation process, whereas small R factors, are not conjugative and contain only the resistance genes.

In addition to conveying antibiotic resistance, R factors impart 2 other traits: (1) resistance to metal ions, such as mercuric ions, by coding for an enzyme that reduces it to elemental mercury; and (2) resistance to certain bacterial viruses by coding for restriction endonucleases that degrade the DNA of the infecting bacteriophages. Resistance to mercuric ions can be important clinically; eg, the active ingredient of the antiseptic Merthiolate is the mercuric ion.

Transposon-Mediated Resistance **Transposons** are genes that are transferred either within or between larger pieces of DNA such as the bacterial chromosome and plasmids. A typical drug resistance transposon is composed of 3 genes flanked on both sides by shorter DNA sequences, usually a series of inverted repeated bases that mediate the interaction of the transposon with the larger DNA (see Fig 2–7). The 3 genes code for (1) transposase, the enzyme that catalyzes excision and reintegration of the transposon; (2) a repressor that regulates synthesis of the transposase; and (3) the drug resistance gene.

SPECIFIC MECHANISMS OF RESISTANCE

Penicillins & Cephalosporins There are several mechanisms of resistance to these drugs. Cleavage by β-**lactamases** (penicillinases and cephalosporinases) is by far the most important (see Fig 10–1). β-Lactamases produced by various organisms have different properties. For example, staphylococcal penicillinase is inducible by penicillin and is secreted into the medium. In contrast, some β-lactamases produced by several gram-negative rods are constitutively produced, are located in the periplasmic space near the peptidoglycan, and are not secreted into the medium. The β-lactamases produced by various gram-negative rods have different specificities; some are more active against cephalosporins, others against penicillins.

Resistance to penicillins can also be due to changes in the **penicillin-binding proteins** in the bacterial cell membrane. These changes probably account for the low-level resistance exhibited by *Streptococcus pneumoniae* to penicillin G and for the resistance of *Staphylococcus aureus* to nafcillin and other β-lactamase-resistant penicillins. The relative resistance of *Streptococcus faecalis* (an enterococcus) to penicillins may be due to altered penicillin-binding proteins. Low-level resistance of *Neisseria gonorrhoeae* to penicillin is attributed to poor permeability to the drug. High-level resistance is due to the presence of a plasmid coding for penicillinase.

Some isolates of *S aureus* demonstrate yet another form of resistance, called **tolerance,** in which growth of the organism is inhibited by penicillin but the organism is not killed. This is attributed to a failure of activation of the autolytic enzymes, murein hydrolases, which degrade the peptidoglycan.

Aminoglycosides Resistance to aminoglycosides occurs by 3 mechanisms: (1) modification of the drugs by plasmid-encoded phosphorylating, adenylylating, and acetylating enzymes (the most important mechanism); (2) chromosomal mutation, eg, a mutation in the gene that codes for the target protein in the 30S subunit of the bacterial ribosome; and (3) decreased permeability of the cell to the drug.

Tetracyclines Resistance to tetracyclines is the result of failure of the drug to reach an inhibitory concentration inside the bacteria. This is due to plasmid-encoded processes that either reduce uptake of the drug or enhance its transport out of the cell.

Chloramphenicol Chloramphenicol resistance is due to a plasmid-encoded acetyltransferase that acetylates the drug, thus inactivating it.

Erythromycin Resistance to erythromycin is due primarily to a plasmid-encoded enzyme that methylates the 23S ribosomal RNA (rRNA), thereby blocking binding of the drug.

Sulfonamides Resistance to sulfonamides is mediated by 2 mechanisms: (1) a plasmid-encoded transport system that actively exports the drug out of the cell; and (2) a chromosomal mutation in the gene coding for the target enzyme, dihydropteroate synthetase, which reduces the binding affinity of the drug.

Rifampin   Resistance to rifampin is due to a chromosomal mutation in the gene for the β subunit of the bacterial RNA polymerase, resulting in ineffective binding of the drug. Resistance occurs at high frequency (10^{-5}), and so rifampin is not usually prescribed alone.

Isoniazid   Resistance of *Mycobacterium tuberculosis* to isoniazid appears to be due to chromosomal mutations that reduce the permeability of the organism to the drug.

NONGENETIC BASIS OF RESISTANCE   There are several nongenetic reasons for the failure of drugs to inhibit the growth of bacteria.

(1) Bacteria can be walled off within an abscess cavity which the drug cannot penetrate effectively. Surgical drainage is therefore a necessary adjunct to chemotherapy.

(2) Bacteria can be in a resting state, ie, not growing; they are therefore insensitive to cell wall inhibitors such as penicillins and cephalosporins. Similarly, *M tuberculosis* can remain dormant in tissues for many years, during which time it is insensitive to drugs. If host defenses are lowered and the bacteria begin to multiply, they are again susceptible to the drugs, indicating that a genetic change did not occur.

(3) Under certain circumstances, organisms that would ordinarily be killed by penicillin can lose their cell walls, survive as **protoplasts,** and be insensitive to cell-wall-active drugs. Later, if such organisms resynthesize their cell walls, they are fully susceptible to these drugs.

(4) There are several artifacts that can make it appear that the organisms are resistant, eg, administration of the wrong drug or the wrong dose, failure of the drug to reach the appropriate site in the body, improper administration of the drug (a good example is the poor penetration into spinal fluid by several early-generation cephalosporins), or failure of the patient to take the drug.

SELECTION OF RESISTANT BACTERIA BY OVERUSE AND MISUSE OF ANTIBIOTICS   Serious outbreaks of diseases caused by gram-negative rods resistant to multiple antibiotics have occurred in many developing countries. In North America, many hospital-acquired infections are caused by multiply resistant organisms. There are 3 main focal points of overuse and misuse of antibiotics that increase the likelihood of these problems by enhancing the selection of resistant mutants:

(1) Some physicians use multiple antibiotics when one would be sufficient, prescribe unnecessarily long courses of antibiotic therapy, use antibiotics in self-limited infections for which they are not needed, and overuse antibiotics for prophylaxis before and after surgery.

(2) In many countries, antibiotics are sold over the counter to the general public; this practice encourages the inappropriate and indiscriminate use of the drugs.

(3) Antibiotics are used in animal feed to prevent infections and promote growth. This selects for resistant organisms in the animals and may contribute to the pool of resistant organisms in humans.

ANTIBIOTIC SENSITIVITY TESTING

Minimal Inhibitory Concentration   For many infections, the results of sensitivity testing are important in the choice of antibiotic. These results are commonly reported as the **minimal inhibitory concentration** (MIC), which is defined as the lowest concentration of drug that inhibits the growth of the organism. The MIC is determined by inoculating the organism isolated from the patient into a series of tubes or cups containing 2-fold dilutions of the drug. After incubation at 35 °C for 18 hours, the lowest concentration of drug that prevents visible growth of the organism is the MIC. This provides the physician with a precise concentration of drug to guide the choice of both the drug and the dose.

A second method of determining antibiotic sensitivity is the disk diffusion method, in which disks impregnated with various antibiotics are placed on the surface of an agar plate that has been inoculated with the organism isolated from the patient (Fig 11–1). After incubation at 35 °C for 18 hours, during which time the antibiotic diffuses outward from the disk, the diameter of the zone of inhibition is determined. The size of the zone of inhibition is used to determine the sensitivity of the organism to the drug, as compared with standards.

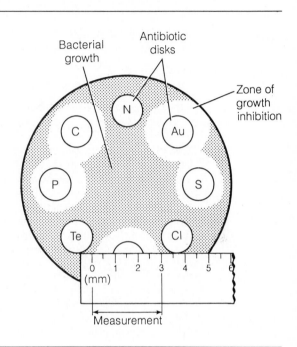

Figure 11–1. Antibiotic sensitivity testing. A zone of inhibition surrounds several antibiotic-containing disks. A zone size of a certain diameter or greater indicates that the organism is sensitive. Some resistant organisms will grow all the way up to the disk. (Modified and reproduced, with permission, from Wistreich GA, Lechtman MD: *Laboratory Exercises in Microbiology,* 5th ed. Macmillan, 1984.)

Minimal Bactericidal Concentration   For certain infections, such as endocarditis, it is important to know the concentration of drug that actually kills the organism rather than the concentration that merely inhibits growth. This concentration, called the **minimal bactericidal concentration** (MBC), is determined by taking a small sample (0.01 or 0.1 mL) from the tubes used for the MIC assay and spreading it over the surface of a drug-free blood agar plate. Any organisms that were inhibited but not killed now have a chance to grow, because the drug has been diluted significantly. After incubation at 35 °C for 48 hours, the lowest concentration that has reduced the number of colonies by 99.9%, compared to the control with no drug, is the MBC. Bactericidal drugs usually have an MBC equal or very similar to the MIC, whereas bacteriostatic drugs usually have an MBC significantly higher than the MIC.

Serum Bactericidal Activity   In the treatment of endocarditis, it can be useful to determine whether the drug is effective by assaying the ability of the drug in the patient's serum to kill the organism. This test, called the **serum bactericidal activity,** is performed in a manner similar to that of the MBC determination, except that it is a serum sample from the patient, rather than a standard drug solution, that is diluted in 2-fold steps. After a standard inoculum of the organism has been added and the mixture incubated at 35 °C for 18 hours, a small sample is subcultured onto blood agar plates, and the serum dilution that kills 99.9% of the organisms is determined. Clinical experience has shown that a peak* serum bactericidal activity of 1:8 or 1:16 is adequate for successful therapy of endocarditis.

β-Lactamase Production   For severe infections caused by certain organisms, such as *S aureus* and *Haemophilus influenzae,* it is important to know as soon as possible whether the organism isolated from the patient is producing β-lactamase. For this purpose, rapid assays for

---

*One of the variables in this test is whether the serum should be drawn shortly after the drug has been administered (at the "peak concentration") or shortly before the next dose is due (at the "trough"). Another is the inoculum size.

the enzyme can be used that yield an answer in a few minutes, as opposed to an MIC test or a disk diffusion test, both of which take 18 hours.

A commonly used procedure is the chromogenic β-lactam method, in which a colored β-lactam drug is added to a suspension of the organisms. If β-lactamase is made, hydrolysis of the β-lactam ring causes the drug to turn a different color in 2–10 minutes. Disks impregnated with a chromogenic β-lactam can also be used.

USE OF ANTIBIOTIC COMBINATIONS   One of the concepts underlying the appropriate use of antimicrobial agents is to select the *single* best drug whenever possible, because this minimizes side effects. However, there are several instances in which 2 or more drugs are commonly given:

(1) to treat serious infections before the identity of the organism is known;

(2) to achieve a synergistic inhibitory effect against certain organisms; and

(3) to prevent the emergence of resistant organisms.

Two drugs can interact in one of several ways (Fig 11–2). They are usually indifferent to each other, ie, additive only. Sometimes there is a **synergistic** interaction, in which the effect of the 2 drugs together is significantly greater than the sum of the effects of the 2 drugs acting separately. Rarely, the effect of the 2 drugs together is **antagonistic**, and the result is significantly lower activity than the sum of the activities of the 2 drugs alone.

A synergistic effect can result from a variety of mechanisms. For example, the combination of a penicillin and an aminoglycoside such as gentamicin has a synergistic action against the enterococcus *S faecalis*, because penicillin damages the cell wall sufficiently to enhance the entry of aminoglycoside. When given alone, neither drug is effective. A second example is the combination of a sulfonamide with trimethoprim. In this instance, the 2 drugs act on the same metabolic pathway, so that if one drug does not inhibit folic acid synthesis sufficiently, the second drug provides effective inhibition by blocking a subsequent step in the pathway.

Although antagonism between 2 antibiotics is unusual, one example is clinically important. This involves the use of penicillin G combined with the bacteriostatic drug tetracycline in the treatment of meningitis caused by *S pneumoniae*. Antagonism occurs because the tetracycline inhibits the growth of the organism, thereby preventing the bactericidal effect of penicillin G, which kills growing organisms only.

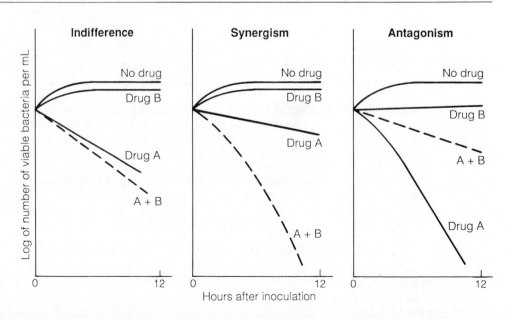

Figure 11–2. Drug interaction. The solid lines represent the response of bacteria to drug A alone, drug B alone, or no drug. The dotted lines represent the response to drug A and drug B together.

Review Questions

1. What are the similarities and differences between chromosome- and plasmid-mediated resistance to antimicrobial drugs?
2. How is plasmid-mediated resistance transmitted from one bacterium to another?
3. How does an R plasmid (R factor) differ from an F plasmid?
4. What are the characteristics of transposons that mediate antibiotic resistance?
5. What are the specific mechanisms of resistance to the following drugs: (a) penicillins, (b) cephalosporins, (c) aminoglycosides, (d) tetracyclines, (e) chloramphenicol, (f) erythromycin, (g) sulfonamides, (h) rifampin?
6. How are (a) the MIC test and (b) the MBC test performed, and what information is obtained?
7. What is the basis for the synergistic effect of penicillin and streptomycin against enterococci?

Bacterial Vaccines

12

Immunity can be acquired by the use of vaccines prepared from bacteria or their products. This chapter will present a summary of the types of vaccines (Table 12–1); detailed information regarding each vaccine is located in the chapters on the specific organisms.

Bacterial vaccines are composed of capsular polysaccharides; inactivated protein exotoxins (toxoids); killed bacteria; or live, attenuated bacteria. The available bacterial vaccines and their indications are as follows.

(1) *Streptococcus pneumoniae* vaccine contains the capsular polysaccharides of the 23 most prevalent types. It is recommended for persons over 60 years of age and patients of any age with chronic diseases such as diabetes and cirrhosis or with compromised spleen function or splenectomy.

(2) *Neisseria meningitidis* vaccine contains capsular polysaccharide of 4 important types (A, C, W-135, and Y). It is given when there is a high risk of meningitis, eg, during an outbreak or when military recruits enter boot camp.

(3) *Haemophilus influenzae* vaccine contains the type b polysaccharide conjugated to diptheria toxoid. It is given to children at the age of 18 months to prevent meningitis.

Table 12–1. Current bacterial vaccines (1990).

Bacterium	Disease	Antigen	Efficacy[1]
Streptococcus pneumonae	Pneumonia	Capsular polysaccharide	3+
Neisseria meningitidis	Meningitis	Capsular polysaccharide	3+
Haemophilus influenzae	Meningitis	Capsular polysaccharide-conjugate	3+
Corynebacterium diphtheriae	Diphtheria	Toxoid	4+
Clostridium tetani	Tetanus	Toxoid	4+
Bordetella pertussis	Whooping cough	Killed organism	4+
Bacillus anthracis	Anthrax	Culture filtrate containing "protective" antigen	3+
Salmonella typhi	Typhoid fever	Killed organism	2+ or 3+
Vibrio cholerae	Cholera	Killed organism	1+
Yersinia pestis	Plague	Killed organism	3+
Mycobacterium bovis (BCG)	Tuberculosis	Live, attenuated organism	1+ or 2+

[1]Efficacy is evaluated as percent protection. Symbols: 1+, 50–65%; 2+, 65–80%; 3+, 80–90%; 4+, more than 90%.

(4) *Corynebacterium diphtheriae* vaccine contains the toxoid (formaldehyde-treated exotoxin). Immunization against diphtheria is indicated for every child and is given in 3 doses at 2, 4, and 6 months of age, with boosters given 1 year later and at intervals thereafter.

(5) *Clostridium tetani* vaccine contains tetanus toxoid and is given to everyone both early in life and later as boosters for protection against tetanus.

(6) *Bordetella pertussis* vaccine contains killed organisms and is indicated for every child as a protection against whooping cough. It is usually given in combination with diphtheria and tetanus toxoids (DPT vaccine).

(7) *Bacillus anthracis* vaccine contains partially purified protein and is given to persons whose occupations place them at risk of anthrax.

(8) *Salmonella typhi* vaccine contains killed organisms and is indicated for persons living in high-risk areas for typhoid fever and for those in close contact with infected patients and carriers.

(9) *Vibrio cholerae* vaccine contains killed organisms and is given to persons traveling to areas where cholera is endemic.

(10) *Yersinia pestis* vaccine contains killed organisms and is indicated for persons at high risk of acquiring plague.

(11) The vaccine against tuberculosis contains a live, attenuated strain of *Mycobacterium bovis* called BCG and is recommended for children at high risk of exposure to active tuberculosis in some countries.

An estimate of the efficacy of the vaccines is presented in Table 12–1.

Review Question

What is the nature of the antigen in the vaccines against each of the following organisms: (a) *Streptococcus pneumoniae*, (b) *Haemophilus influenzae*, (c) *Corynebacterium diphtheriae*, (d) *Clostridium tetani*, (e) *Bordetella pertussis*, (f) *Mycobacterium tuberculosis*?

13

Sterilization & Disinfection

Sterilization is the killing or removal of *all* microorganisms, including bacterial spores, which are highly resistant. Sterilization is usually achieved by autoclaving, which consists of exposure to steam at 121 °C under a pressure of 15 lb/in^2 for 15 minutes. Surgical instruments that can be damaged by moist heat are usually sterilized by exposure to ethylene oxide gas, and most intravenous solutions are sterilized by filtration.

Disinfection is the killing of many, but not all, microorganisms. For adequate disinfection, pathogens must be killed but some organisms and bacterial spores may survive. Disinfectants vary in their tissue-damaging properties from the corrosive phenol-containing compounds, which should be used only on inanimate objects, to less toxic materials such as ethanol and iodine, which can be used on skin surfaces. Chemicals used to kill microorganisms on the surface of skin and mucous membranes are called **antiseptics.**

Rate of Killing of Microorganisms

Death of microorganisms occurs at a certain rate dependent primarily upon 2 variables: the concentration of the killing agent and the length of time it is applied. The rate of killing is defined by the relationship

$$N \propto \frac{1}{CT}$$

which shows that the number of survivors, N, is inversely proportionate to the concentration of the agent, C, and the time of application of the agent, T. Collectively, CT is often referred to as the dose. Stated alternatively, the number of microorganisms killed is directly proportionate to CT. The relationship is usually stated in terms of survivors, as they are easily measured by colony formation. Death is defined as the inability to reproduce. In certain circumstances, the physical remains of dead bacteria can still cause problems (see p. 59).

Chemical Agents

Chemicals vary greatly in their ability to kill microorganisms. A quantitative measure of this variation is expressed as the **phenol coefficient,** which is the ratio of the concentration of phenol to the concentration of the agent required to cause the same amount of killing under the standard conditions of the test.

Chemical agents act primarily by one of 3 mechanisms: disruption of the lipid-containing cell membrane, modification of proteins, or modification of DNA. Each of the following chemical agents has been classified into one of the 3 categories, but some of the chemicals act by more than one mechanism.

DISRUPTION OF CELL MEMBRANES

Alcohols Ethanol is widely used to clean the skin prior to an immunization or venipuncture. It acts mainly by disorganizing the lipid structure in membranes but denatures proteins as well. Ethanol requires the presence of water for maximal activity, ie, it is far less effective at 100% than at 70%.

Detergents Detergents are "surface-active" agents composed of a long-chain, lipid-soluble, hydrophobic portion and a polar hydrophilic group, which can be a cation, an anion, or a nonionic group. These surfactants interact with the lipid in the cell membrane through their hydrophobic chain and with the surrounding water through their polar group and thus disrupt the membrane. Quaternary ammonium compounds, eg, benzalkonium chloride, are cationic detergents widely used for skin antisepsis.

Phenols Phenol was the original disinfectant used in the operating room by Lister in the 1860s, but it is rarely used as a disinfectant today because it is too caustic. Hexachlorophene, which is a biphenol with 6 chlorine atoms, is used in germicidal soaps, but concern over possible neurotoxicity has limited its use. Another phenol derivative is cresol (methylphenol), the active ingredient in Lysol. Phenols not only damage membranes but also denature proteins.

MODIFICATION OF PROTEINS

Chlorine Chlorine is used as a disinfectant to purify the water supply and to treat swimming pools. It is also the active component of hypochlorite (bleach, Clorox), which is used as a disinfectant in the home and in hospitals. Chlorine is a powerful oxidizing agent that kills by cross-linking essential sulfhydryl groups in enzymes to form the inactive disulfide.

Iodine   Iodine is the most effective skin antiseptic used in medical practice. It is supplied in 2 forms.

(1) Tincture of iodine (2% solution of iodine and potassium iodide in ethanol) is used to prepare the skin prior to blood culture. Because tincture of iodine can be irritating to the skin, it should be removed with alcohol.

(2) Iodophors are complexes of iodine with detergents that are frequently used to prepare the skin prior to surgery because they are less irritating than tincture of iodine. Iodine, like chlorine, is an oxidant that inactivates sulfhydryl-containing enzymes. It also binds specifically to tyrosine residues in proteins.

Heavy Metals   Mercury and silver have the greatest antibacterial activity of the heavy metals and are the most widely used in medicine. They act by binding to sulfhydryl groups, thereby blocking enzymatic activity. Thimerosal (Merthiolate) and merbromin (Mercurochrome), which contain mercury, are used as skin antiseptics. Silver nitrate drops are useful in preventing gonococcal ophthalmia neonatorum. Silver sulfadiazine is used to prevent infection of burn wounds.

Hydrogen Peroxide   Hydrogen peroxide is used as an antiseptic to clean wounds and to disinfect contact lenses. Its effectiveness is limited by the organism's ability to produce catalase, an enzyme that degrades H_2O_2. (The bubbles produced when peroxide is used on wounds are formed by oxygen arising from the breakdown of H_2O_2 by tissue catalase.) Hydrogen peroxide is an oxidizing agent that attacks sulfhydryl groups, thereby inhibiting enzymatic activity.

Formaldehyde & Glutaraldehyde   Formaldehyde, which is available as a 37% solution in water (Formalin), denatures proteins and nucleic acids. Both proteins and nucleic acids contain essential -NH_2 and -OH groups, which are the main sites of alkylation by the hydroxymethyl group of formaldehyde. Glutaraldehyde, which has 2 reactive aldehyde groups, is 10 times more effective than formaldehyde and is less toxic. In hospitals, it is used to sterilize respiratory therapy equipment.

Ethylene Oxide   Ethylene oxide gas is used extensively in hospitals for the sterilization of heat-sensitive materials such as surgical instruments and plastics. It kills by alkylating both proteins and nucleic acids, ie, the hydroxyethyl group attacks the reactive hydrogen atoms on essential amino and hydroxyl groups.

Acids & Alkalis   Strong acids and alkalis kill by denaturing proteins. Although most bacteria are susceptible, it is important to note that *Mycobacterium tuberculosis* and other mycobacteria are relatively resistant to 2% NaOH, which is used in the clinical laboratory to liquefy sputum prior to culturing the organism. Weak acids, such as benzoic, propionic, and citric acids, are frequently used as food preservatives because they are bacteriostatic. The action of these acids is partially a function of the organic moiety, eg, benzoate, as well as the low pH.

MODIFICATION OF NUCLEIC ACIDS   A variety of dyes not only stain microorganisms but also inhibit their growth. One of these is crystal violet (gentian violet), which is used as a skin antiseptic. Its action is based on binding of the positively charged dye molecule to the negatively charged phosphate groups of the nucleic acids. Malachite green, a triphenylamine dye like crystal violet, is a component of Löwenstein-Jensen's medium, which is used to grow *M tuberculosis*. The dye inhibits the growth of unwanted organisms in the sputum during the 6-week incubation period.

Physical Agents

The physical agents act either by imparting energy in the form of heat or radiation or by removing organisms through filtration.

HEAT Heat energy can be applied in 3 ways: in the form of moist heat (either boiling or autoclaving) or dry heat or by pasteurization. In general, heat kills by denaturing proteins, but membrane damage and enzymatic cleavage of DNA may also be involved. Moist heat sterilizes at a lower temperature than dry heat, since water aids in the disruption of noncovalent bonds, eg, hydrogen bonds, which hold protein chains together in their secondary and tertiary structures.

Moist-heat sterilization, usually autoclaving, is the most frequently used method of sterilization in medicine. Because most bacterial spores are resistant to boiling (100 °C at sea level), they must be exposed to a higher temperature; this cannot be achieved unless the pressure is increased. For this purpose, an autoclave chamber is used in which steam, at a pressure of 15 lb/in^2, reaches a temperature of 121 °C and is held for 15–20 minutes. This kills even the highly heat-resistant spores of *Clostridium botulinum,* the cause of botulism, with a margin of safety.

Sterilization by dry heat, on the other hand, requires temperatures in the range of 180 °C for 2 hours. This process is used primarily for glassware sterilization and is less frequently used than autoclaving.

Pasteurization, which is used primarily for milk, consists of heating the milk to 62 °C for 30 minutes, followed by rapid cooling. ("Flash" pasteurization at 72 °C for 15 seconds is frequently used.) This is sufficient to kill the vegetative cells of the milk-borne pathogens, eg, *M tuberculosis, Salmonella, Streptococcus,* and *Brucella,* but not to sterilize the milk.

RADIATION The 2 types of radiation used to kill microorganisms are ultraviolet (UV) light and x-rays. The greatest activity of UV light occurs at 250–260 nm, which is the wavelength region of maximum absorption by the purine and pyrimidine bases of DNA. The most significant lesion caused by UV irradiation is the formation of thymine dimers, but addition of hydroxyl groups to the bases also occurs. As a result, DNA replication is inhibited and the organism cannot grow. Cells have repair mechanisms against UV-induced damage that involve either cleavage of dimers in the presence of visible light (photoreactivation) or excision of damaged bases, which is not dependent upon visible light (dark repair). The use of UV irradiation in medicine is limited, as UV radiation can damage the cornea and skin.

X-rays and gamma rays are produced by bombardment of an atom with particles such as electrons and by radioactive decay, respectively; they have a similar amount of energy. They have higher energy and penetrating power than UV radiation and kill mainly by the production of free radicals, eg, production of hydroxyl radicals by the hydrolysis of water. These highly reactive radicals can break covalent bonds in DNA, thereby killing the organism. Sulfhydryl-containing compounds, such as the amino acid cysteine, can protect DNA from free-radical attack. Another mechanism is a direct hit on a covalent bond in DNA, resulting in chain breakage, but this is probably less important than the mechanism involving free radicals.

X-rays kill vegetative cells readily, but spores are remarkably resistant, probably owing to their lower water content. X-rays are used in medicine for sterilization of heat-sensitive items, such as sutures and surgical gloves, and plastic items, such as syringes.

FILTRATION Filtration is the preferred method of sterilizing certain solutions, eg, those with heat-sensitive components. In the past, solutions for intravenous use were autoclaved, but heat-resistant endotoxin in the cell walls of the dead gram-negative bacteria caused fever in recipients of the solutions. Therefore, solutions are now filtered to make them "**pyrogen-free**" prior to autoclaving.

The most commonly used filter is composed of nitrocellulose and has a pore size of 0.22 μm. This size will retain all bacteria and spores. Filters work by physically trapping particles larger than the pore size and by retaining somewhat smaller particles owing to electrostatic attraction of the particles to the filters.

Review Questions

1. What is the difference between sterilization and disinfection?

2. What are the mechanisms of action of the following agents:
   (a) ethanol, (b) detergents, (c) iodine, (d) formaldehyde, (e) UV light?

3. How is pasteurization performed, and what does it accomplish?

14 Overview of the Major Pathogens & Introduction to Anaerobic Bacteria

OVERVIEW OF THE MAJOR PATHOGENS   The major bacterial pathogens are presented in Table 14–1 and described in Chapters 15–26. So that the reader may concentrate on the important pathogens, the bacteria that are less medically important are described in a separate chapter (see Chapter 27).

Table 14–1 is divided into organisms that are readily Gram-stained and those that are not. The readily stained organisms fall into 4 categories: gram-positive cocci, gram-negative cocci, gram-positive rods, and gram-negative rods. Since there are so many kinds of gram-negative rods, they have been divided into 3 groups:

(1) organisms associated with the enteric tract,

(2) organisms associated with the respiratory tract, and

(3) organisms from animal sources (zoonotic bacteria).

For ease of understanding, the organisms associated with the enteric tract are further subdivided into 3 groups: (1) pathogens both inside and outside the enteric tract, (2) pathogens inside the enteric tract, and (3) pathogens outside the enteric tract.

As is true of any classification dealing with biologic entities, this one is not entirely precise. For example, *Campylobacter* causes enteric tract disease but frequently has an animal source. Nevertheless, despite some uncertainties, subdivision of the large number of gram-negative rods into these functional categories should be helpful to the reader.

Table 14–1. Major bacterial pathogens.

Type of Organism	Genus
Readily Gram-stained	
Gram-positive cocci	*Staphylococcus, Streptococcus*
Gram-negative cocci	*Neisseria*
Gram-positive rods	*Corynebacterium, Listeria, Bacillus, Clostridium, Actinomyces, Nocardia*
Gram-negative rods	
Enteric tract organisms	
Pathogenic inside and outside tract	*Escherichia, Salmonella*
Pathogenic primarily inside tract	*Shigella, Vibrio, Campylobacter*
Pathogenic outside tract	*Kiabsiella-Enterobacter-Serratia* group. *Pseudomonas, Proteus-Providencia-Morganella* group, *Bacteroides*
Respiratory tract organisms	*Haemophilus, Legionella, Bordetella*
Organisms from animal sources	*Brucella, Francisella, Pasteurella, Yersinia*
Not readily Gram-stained	
Not obligate intracellular parasites	*Mycobacterium, Mycoplasma, Treponema, Leptospire*
Obligate intracellular parasites	*Chlamydia, Rickettsia*

Table 14–2. Notifiable bacterial diseases in the USA in 1986.[1]

Disease	Number of Cases
Gonorrhea	900,868
Salmonellosis	49,984
Syphilis	27,883
Tuberculosis	22,768
Shigellosis	17,371
Pertussis	4,195
Meningococcal infections	2,594
Legionellosis	948
Rocky Mountain spotted fever	760
Toxic shock syndrome	412

[1]The latest year for which complete data are available.

The organisms that are not readily Gram-stained fall into 6 major categories: *Mycobacterium* species, which are acid-fast rods; *Mycoplasma* species, which have no cell wall and so do not stain with Gram's stain; *Treponema* and *Leptospira* species, which are spirochetes too thin to be seen by Gram's stain; and *Chlamydia* and *Rickettsia* species, which stain well with Giemsa's stain or other special stains but poorly with Gram's stain.

Table 14–2 presents the 10 most common "notifiable" bacterial diseases in the USA for 1986 as compiled by the Centers for Disease Control. Note that only notifiable diseases are included and that certain common conditions such as streptococcal pharyngitis and chlamydial infection are not included. Gonorrhea is by far the most common disease listed, followed by syphilis, salmonellosis, tuberculosis, and shigellosis in the top 5.

INTRODUCTION TO ANAEROBIC BACTERIA

Important Properties   Anaerobes are characterized by their ability to grow only in an atmosphere containing less than 20% oxygen; ie, they grow poorly if at all in room air. They are a heterogeneous group composed of bacteria that can barely grow in 20% oxygen to those that can grow only in less than 0.02% oxygen. Table 14–3 describes the optimal oxygen requirements for several representative groups of organisms. The obligate aerobes, such as *Pseudomonas aeruginosa,* grow best in the 20% oxygen of room air and not at all under anaerobic conditions. Facultative anaerobes such as *Escherichia coli* can grow well under either circumstance. Aerotolerant organisms such as *Clostridium histolyticum* can grow to some extent in air but multiply much more rapidly in a lower oxygen concentration. Microaerophilic organisms such as *Campylobacter jejuni* require a reduced oxygen concentration (approximately 5%) to grow optimally. The obligate anaerobes such as *Bacteroides fragilis* and *Clostridium perfringens* require an almost total absence of oxygen.

The precise reason why the growth of anaerobes is inhibited by oxygen is not understood, but several factors are probably involved (see Chapter 3). One important aspect is the

Table 14–3. Optimal oxygen requirements of representative bacteria.

Bacterial Type	Representative Organism	Growth Under Following Conditions	
		Aerobic	Anaerobic
Obligate aerobes	*Pseudomonas aeruginosa*	3+	0
Facultative anaerobes	*Escherichia coli*	4+	3+
Aerotolerant organisms	*Clostridium histolyticum*	1+	4+
Microaerophiles	*Campylobacter jejuni*	0	1+[1]
Obligate anaerobes	*Bacteroides fragilis*	0	4+

[1]*C jejuni* grows best (3+) in 5% O_2 plus 10% CO_2. It is also called **capnophilic** in view of its need for CO_2 for optimal growth.

production of toxic compounds, such as H_2O_2 and superoxides, and the reduced amount or absence of catalase and superoxide dismutase in anaerobes to detoxify them. A second factor is oxidation of essential sulfhydryl groups in enzymes without sufficient reducing power to regenerate them.

In addition to oxygen concentration, the oxidation-reduction potential (E_h) of a tissue is an important determinant of the growth of anaerobes. Areas with low E_h, such as the periodontal pocket, dental plaque, and colon, support the growth of anaerobes well. Crushing injuries that result in devitalized tissue owing to impaired blood supply produce a low E_h, allowing anaerobes to grow and cause disease.

Anaerobes of Medical Interest   The anaerobes of medical interest are presented in Table 14–4. It can be seen that they include both rods and cocci and both gram-positive and gram-negative organisms. The rods are divided into the spore formers, eg, *Clostridium*, and the nonspore formers, eg, *Bacteroides*. In this book, 3 genera of anaerobes are described as major bacterial pathogens, namely *Clostridium, Actinomyces,* and *Bacteroides. Streptococcus* is a genus of major pathogens composed of both anaerobic and facultative organisms. The remaining anaerobes are less important and are discussed in Chapter 27.

Clinical Infections   Many of the medically important anaerobes are part of the normal human flora. As such, they are nonpathogens in their normal habitat and cause disease only when they leave those sites. The 2 prominent exceptions to this are *Clostridium botulinum* and *Clostridium tetani,* the agents of botulism and tetanus, respectively, which are soil organisms. *C perfringens,* another important human pathogen, is found in the colon and in the soil.

Diseases caused by members of the anaerobic normal flora are characterized by abscesses, which are most frequently located in the brain, lungs, female genital tract, biliary tract, and other intra-abdominal sites. Most abscesses contain more than one organism, either multiple anaerobes or a mixture of anaerobes plus facultative anaerobes. It is thought that the facultative anaerobes consume sufficient oxygen to allow the anaerobes to flourish.

Three important findings on physical examination that arouse suspicion of an anaerobic infection are a foul-smelling discharge, gas in the tissue, and necrotic tissue. In addition, infections in the setting of pulmonary aspiration, bowel surgery, abortion, cancer, or human and animal bites frequently involve anaerobes.

Laboratory Diagnosis   Two aspects of microbiologic diagnosis of an anaerobic infection are important even before the specimen is cultured: (1) obtaining the appropriate specimen, and (2) rapidly transporting the specimen under anaerobic conditions to the laboratory. An appropriate specimen is one that does not contain members of the normal flora to confuse the interpretation. For example, specimens such as blood, pleural fluid, pus, and transtracheal aspirates are appropriate, but sputum and feces are not.

In the laboratory, the cultures are handled and incubated under anaerobic conditions. In addition to the usual diagnostic criteria of Gram's stain, morphology, and biochemical reactions, the special technique of gas chromatography is important. In this procedure, organic acids such as formic, acetic, and propionic acid are measured.

Treatment   In general, surgical drainage of the abscess plus administration of antimicrobial drugs are indicated. Drugs that are commonly used to treat anaerobic infections are penicillin G, cefoxitin, chloramphenicol, clindamycin, and metronidazole. Note, however, that many isolates of the important pathogen *B fragilis* produce β-lactamase and so are resistant to penicillin.

Table 14–4. Anaerobic bacteria of medical interest.

Morphology	Gram Reaction	Genus
Spore-forming rods	+	*Clostridium*
	—	None
Non-spore-forming rods	+	*Actinomyces, Bifidobacterium, Eubacterium, Lactobacillus, Propionibacterium*
	—	*Bacteroides, Fusobacterium*
Non-spore-forming cocci	+	*Peptococcus, Peptostreptococcus, Streptococcus*
	—	None[1]

[1]*Veillonella,* a gram-negative, non-spore-forming coccus, is infrequently involved in human infections.

Review Questions

1. Why is the growth of anaerobes inhibited in the presence of oxygen?
2. *Clostridium* and *Bacteroides* are 2 genera of medically important organisms. What are 2 significant differences between these organisms?
3. What are the characteristics of anaerobic infections?

Gram-Positive Cocci
15

There are 2 medically important genera: *Staphylococcus* and *Streptococcus*. They are nonmotile and do not form spores.

STAPHYLOCOCCUS

Diseases *Staphylococcus aureus* causes abscesses, various pyogenic infections (eg, endocarditis and osteomyelitis), food poisoning, and toxic shock syndrome. *Staphylococcus epidermidis* can cause endocarditis, and *Staphylococcus saprophyticus* is an infrequent cause of urinary tract infections.

Important Properties Staphylococci are spherical cocci often arranged in irregular **grape-like clusters.** All staphylococci produce **catalase,** whereas no streptococci do (catalase degrades H_2O_2 into O_2 and H_2O).

Three species of staphylococci are human pathogens: *S aureus, S epidermidis,* and *S saprophyticus* (Table 15–1). Of the 3, *S aureus* is by far the most important. *S aureus* is distinguished from the others primarily by **coagulase** production (coagulase clots citrated plasma). Furthermore, it usually ferments mannitol and hemolyzes blood, whereas the others do not.

S aureus has several important cell wall components and antigens.

(1) Protein A is the major protein in the cell wall. It may be a virulence factor, since it binds to the Fc portion of IgG, preventing the binding of complement. Protein A is useful in the clinical laboratory because it binds to IgG and can be used to ''coagglutinate'' antigen-antibody complexes.

(2) Teichoic acids are polymers of ribitol phosphate. Antibodies to teichoic acids develop in certain staphylococcal infections, eg, endocarditis.

(3) Surface receptors for specific staphylococcal bacteriophages permit the ''phage typing'' of strains for epidemiologic purposes. Teichoic acids make up part of these receptors.

Table 15–1. Staphylococci of medical importance.

Species	Coagulase Production	Typical Hemolysis	Important Features[1]
S aureus	+	β	Protein A on cell surface; suppurative lesions.
S epidermidis	–	None	Sensitive to novobiocin; common member of skin flora.
S saprophyticus	–	None	Resistant to novobiocin; sometimes causes urinary tract infections.

[1]All staphylococci are catalase-positive.

Transmission Staphylococci are ubiquitous in the human environment and in the normal human flora. *S epidermidis* is regularly present on normal **skin** and mucous membranes. *S aureus* is often found in the **nose** and sometimes on the skin, especially in hospital staff and patients. Additional sources of staphylococcal infection are shedding from human lesions and fomites contaminated by these lesions. Disease production is favored by a heavily contaminated environment (eg, family members with boils) and a compromised immune system.

Pathogenesis Staphylococci cause disease both by producing toxins and by multiplying in tissue and causing inflammation. The typical lesion of *S aureus* infection is an **abscess**. Abscesses undergo central necrosis and usually drain to the outside (eg, furuncles and boils), but organisms may disseminate via the bloodstream as well.

Several important toxins and enzymes are produced by *S aureus*.

(1) Enterotoxin is a protein that causes vomiting and diarrhea. It acts by stimulating centers of gut motility in the brain. It is fairly heat-resistant and so is usually not inactivated by cooking. There are 6 immunologic types of enterotoxin: A–F.

(2) Exfoliatin is a protein produced by staphylococci of phage group II, which causes "scalded-skin" syndrome in young children.

(3) Toxic shock syndrome toxin (TSST-1) is associated with toxic shock in tampon-using menstruating women or in individuals with wound infections. It is indistinguishable from enterotoxin F.

(4) Several toxins can cause death of leukocytes (leukocidins), necrosis of tissues, and other damage in vivo. Other enzymes demonstrable in vitro include hemolysins, proteases, hyaluronidases, lipases, deoxyribonucleases, etc.

Clinical Findings The important clinical manifestations caused by *S aureus* are as follows:

(1) skin infections, including impetigo, furuncles, cellulitis, surgical wound infections, and postpartum breast infections;

(2) bacteremia from any localized lesion, especially wound infection, or as a result of intravenous drug abuse (bacteremia may lead to endocarditis);

(3) endocarditis on normal or prosthetic heart valves, (prosthetic valve endocarditis is often caused by *S epidermidis*);

(4) osteomyelitis, either hematogenous or traumatic;

(5) pneumonia in postoperative patients or following viral (especially influenza) respiratory infection (staphylococcal pneumonia often leads to empyema);

(6) abscesses (metastatic) in any organ, after bacteremia;

(7) food poisoning (characterized mainly by vomiting) due to ingestion of enterotoxin, which is preformed in foods and hence has a short incubation period (1–8 hours); and

(8) toxic shock syndrome, which includes fever, hypotension, a rash that goes on to desquamate, and multisystem involvement.

Coagulase-negative staphylococci, such as *S epidermidis*, are part of the normal human flora on skin and mucous membranes but can cause infections of intravenous catheters and prosthetic implants, eg, heart valves. *S saprophyticus* can cause urinary tract infections.

Laboratory Diagnosis Smears from local lesions or pus reveal gram-positive cocci in grapelike clusters. Cultures yield white or golden-yellow colonies that are usually beta-hemolytic. *S aureus* is coagulase-positive. The 2 coagulase-negative staphylococci are distinguished by their reaction to the antibiotic novobiocin: *S epidermidis* is sensitive, whereas *S saprophyticus* is resistant. There are no generally useful serologic or skin tests.

Treatment In the USA, 80% or more of *S aureus* strains were resistant to penicillin G by 1987. Most of them produce β-**lactamase** under control of transmissible plasmids. Such organisms can be treated with β-lactamase-resistant penicillins, eg, nafcillin or cloxacillin, some cephalosporins, or vancomycin. Some staphylococci are "methicillin-resistant" (or "nafcillin-resistant") by virtue of altered penicillin-binding proteins. Such organisms can produce sizable outbreaks of disease, especially in hospitals. The drug of choice for these staphylococci is vancomycin. Some strains of staphylococci exhibit **tolerance**; ie, they can be inhibited by antibiotics but are not killed (the MBC/MIC ratio is very high). Tolerance may be due to failure of the drugs to inactivate inhibitors of autolytic enzymes that degrade the organism. Tolerant organisms should be treated with drug combinations.

Drainage (spontaneous or surgical) is the cornerstone of abscess treatment. Repeated infections do not give complete immunity to reinfection.

Prevention There is no effective immunization with toxoids or bacterial vaccines. Cleanliness, frequent hand washing, and aseptic management of lesions help to control spread of *S aureus*. Dissemination from the nose or skin of carriers can be reduced by topical application of antimicrobial agents (or by systemic treatment) but is difficult to arrest altogether. Shedders may have to be removed from high-risk areas, eg, operating rooms and newborn nurseries.

STREPTOCOCCUS Streptococci of medical importance are listed in Table 15–2. All but one of these streptococci are discussed here; *Streptococcus pneumoniae* is discussed separately (see p 68).

Diseases Streptococci produce a wide variety of infections, ranging from pharyngitis and cellulitis to sepsis. They also can trigger immunologic disorders such as rheumatic fever and acute glomerulonephritis.

Important Properties Streptococci are spherical cocci usually arranged in chains or pairs. All streptococci are **catalase-negative**, whereas staphylococci are catalase-positive (Table 15–2).

One of the most important criteria for identification is the type of hemolysis.

(a) Alpha-hemolytic streptococci form a green zone around their colonies as a result of incomplete lysis of red blood cells in the agar.

(b) Beta-hemolytic streptococci form a clear zone around their colonies, since complete lysis of the red cells occurs. Beta-hemolysis is due to the production of enzymes called hemolysins (see below).

(c) Some streptococci are nonhemolytic (gamma-hemolysis).

There are 2 important antigens of beta-hemolytic streptococci:

(1) C carbohydrate determines the *group* of beta-hemolytic streptococci. It is located in the cell wall, and its specificity is determined by an amino sugar.

(2) M protein is associated with virulence and determines the *type* of group A beta-hemolytic streptococci. It interferes with ingestion by phagocytes. Antibody to M protein provides type-specific immunity.

Table 15–2. Streptococci of medical importance.

Species	Lancefield Group	Typical Hemolysis	Diagnostic Features[1]
S pyogenes	A	Beta	Bacitracin-sensitive
S agalactiae	B	Beta	Bacitracin-resistant; hippurate hydrolyzed.
S faecalis[2]	D	Alpha or beta or none	Growth in 6.5% NaCl.[3]
S bovis	D	Alpha or none	No growth in 6.5% NaCl.
S pneumoniae	NA[4]	Alpha	Bile-soluble; inhibited by optochin.
Viridans group	NA	Alpha	Not bile-soluble; not inhibited by optochin.

[1]All streptococci are catalase-negative.
[2]Commonly called enterococci; *S bovis* is a nonenterococcal group D organism.
[3]Both *S faecalis* and *S bovis* grow on bile-esculin agar, whereas other streptococci do not. They hydrolyze the esculin, and this results in a characteristic black discoloration of the agar.
[4]NA: not applicable.

The classification of streptococci is as follows.

A. Beta-Hemolytic Streptococci: These are arranged into groups A–U (known as Lancefield groups) on the basis of antigenic differences in C carbohydrate. In the clinical laboratory, the group is determined by precipitin tests with specific antisera or by immuno-fluorescence.

Group A streptococci (*Streptococcus pyogenes*) are among the most important human pathogens. They are the most frequent bacterial cause of pharyngitis. They adhere to pharyngeal epithelium via pili covered with lipoteichoic acid. They are usually **bacitracin-susceptible**, an important diagnostic criterion.

Group B streptococci (*Streptococcus agalactiae*) are normal inhabitants of the female genital tract and can cause neonatal meningitis and sepsis. They are usually bacitracin-resistant.

Group D streptococci include enterococci (eg, *Streptococcus faecalis**) and nonenterococci (eg, *Streptococcus bovis*). Enterococci grow in 6.5% NaCl and are not killed by penicillin G. They occur as part of the normal flora in the gut and are noted for their ability to cause urinary, biliary, and cardiovascular infections. Nonenterococci can produce similar infections but are inhibited by 6.5% NaCl and killed by penicillin G. Note that the hemolytic reaction of group D streptococci is variable: some are beta-hemolytic, whereas others are alpha- or nonhemolytic.

Groups C, E, F, G, H, and K–U streptococci infrequently cause human disease.

Group N "lactic" streptococci produce normal souring of milk.

B. Non-beta-hemolytic Streptococci: Some produce no hemolysis; others produce alpha-hemolysis. The principal alpha-hemolytic organisms are *S pneumoniae* and the viridans group of streptococci. The viridans streptococci (eg, *Streptococcus mitis* and *Streptococcus mutans*) are *not* bile-soluble and *not* inhibited by optochin—in contrast to *S pneumoniae*. Viridans streptococci are part of the normal flora of the human pharynx and intermittently reach the bloodstream to cause infective endocarditis. *S mutans* synthesizes polysaccharides (dextrans) that are found in dental plaque and lead to dental caries.

C. Peptostreptococci: These grow under anaerobic or microaerophilic conditions and produce variable hemolysis. Peptostreptococci are members of the normal flora of the gut and the female genital tract and participate in mixed anaerobic infections.

Transmission Most streptococci are part of the normal flora of the human throat, skin, and intestines but produce disease when they gain access to tissues or blood. Viridans streptococci and *S pneumoniae* are found chiefly in the **oropharynx**; *S pyogenes* is found on the **skin** and in the oropharynx in small numbers; *S agalactiae* occurs in the **female genital tract**; and both the enterococci and anaerobic streptococci are located in the **lower intestinal tract**.

Pathogenesis & Immunity Streptococci produce the following 6 important toxins and enzymes:

(1) Streptokinase (fibrinolysin) activates plasmin in blood, which can dissolve clots, thrombi, and emboli.

(2) Streptodornase (streptococcal DNase) depolymerizes DNA in exudates or necrotic tissue. Antibody to DNase develops during pyoderma; this can be used for diagnostic purposes. Streptokinase-streptodornase mixtures applied as a skin test give a positive reaction in most adults, indicating normal cell-mediated reactivity.

(3) Hyaluronidase hydrolyzes the ground substance of connective tissue, which aids the spread of streptococci.

(4) Erythrogenic toxin is produced only by certain group A streptococci lysogenized by a bacteriophage carrying the gene for the toxin. It acts as a capillary poison and causes the rash of scarlet fever. The injection of a skin test dose of erythrogenic toxin (Dick test) gives a positive result in persons lacking antitoxin (ie, susceptible persons).

(5) Streptolysin O is a hemolysin that is inactivated by oxidation (oxygen-labile). It causes beta-hemolysis only when colonies grow under the surface of a blood agar plate. It is antigenic, and antibody to it (ASO) develops after group A streptococcal infections. The titer of ASO antibody can be important in the diagnosis of rheumatic fever.

(6) Streptolysin S (oxygen-stable) is *not* antigenic but is responsible for beta-hemolysis when colonies grow on the surface of a blood agar plate.

S faecalis was recently renamed *Enterococcus faecalis*.

Resistance or immunity to group A streptococci is due to type-specific antibody to **M protein**. Resistance to group B infection of neonates is due to transplacentally passed antibody developed by the mother.

Clinical Findings   *S pyogenes* (group A beta-hemolytic streptococcus) is the most common bacterial cause of sore throat. Pharyngitis is characterized by edema, exudate, fever, leukocytosis, and tender cervical lymph nodes. If untreated, spontaneous recovery occurs in 10 days. However, it may extend to otitis, sinusitis, mastoiditis, and meningitis. If the infecting streptococci produce erythrogenic toxin and the host lacks antitoxin, scarlet fever may result. Rheumatic fever may occur, especially following pharyngitis (see below).

Group A streptococci can enter skin defects to produce cellulitis, erysipelas, lymphangitis, or bacteremia. They can enter the uterus after delivery to produce endometritis and sepsis (puerperal fever). Streptococcal pyoderma (impetigo) is a superficial infection of abraded skin that forms pus or crusts. It is communicable among children, especially in hot, humid climates. Glomerulonephritis may occur, especially following skin infections (see below).

Infective endocarditis is commonly caused by viridans streptococci that intermittently enter the bloodstream from the oropharynx (as a result of poor dentition or after dental surgery). Signs of endocarditis are fever, anemia, heart murmur, and embolic events. It is 100% fatal unless effectively treated with antimicrobial agents. About 10% of endocarditis cases are caused by enterococci, but any organism causing bacteremia may settle on deformed valves. At least 3 blood cultures are necessary to ensure recovery of the organism in over 90% of cases.

Streptococci also cause other infections. Enterococci cause urinary tract infections, endocarditis, and abdominal sepsis; peptostreptococci participate in mixed anaerobic infections of the abdomen, pelvis, lungs, or brain; and group B streptococci cause neonatal sepsis and meningitis.

Poststreptococcal (Nonsuppurative) Diseases   These are disorders in which a local infection with group A streptococci is followed weeks later by inflammation in an organ that was *not* infected by the streptococci.

A. Acute Glomerulonephritis (AGN):   Acute glomerulonephritis typically occurs 2–3 weeks after skin infection by certain group A streptococcal types in children (eg, M protein type 49 causes AGN most frequently). AGN is more frequent after skin infections than after pharyngitis. The most striking clinical features are hypertension, edema of the face and ankles, and "smoky" urine (owing to red cells in the urine). Most patients recover completely. Reinfection with streptococci rarely leads to recurrence of acute glomerulonephritis.

The disease is initiated by antigen-antibody complexes on the glomerular basement membrane, and soluble antigens from streptococcal membranes may be the inciting antigen. It can be prevented by early eradication of nephritogenic streptococci from skin colonization sites but *not* by administration of penicillin after onset of the process.

B. Rheumatic Fever: At 1–4 weeks after any type of group A streptococcal infection— usually pharyngitis—fever, migratory polyarthritis, and carditis may develop, leading to myocardial and valve damage. ASO titers and the erythrocyte sedimentation rate are elevated.

Rheumatic fever is due to an immunologic reaction resulting from cross-reactions between streptococcal antigens and antigens of joint and heart tissue. This causes an autoimmune disease, greatly exacerbated by recurrence of streptococcal infections. If streptococcal infections are treated within 8 days after onset, rheumatic fever is usually prevented. After a heart-damaging attack of rheumatic fever, reinfection must be prevented by long-term prophylaxis. In the USA, less than 0.5% of group A streptococcal infections lead to rheumatic fever but in developing tropical countries, the rate is over 5%.

Laboratory Diagnosis

A. Microbiologic: Smears are useless in pharyngitis because viridans streptococci are members of the normal flora and cannot be visually distinguished from the pathogenic *S pyogenes*. However, stained smears from skin lesions or wounds that reveal streptococci are diagnostic. Cultures of swabs from the pharynx or lesion on blood agar plates show small, translucent beta-hemolytic colonies in 18–48 hours. If inhibited by bacitracin disk, they are likely to be group A streptococci. Group B streptococci are characterized by their ability to hydrolyze hippurate and by the production of a protein that causes enhanced hemolysis on sheep blood agar when combined with beta-hemolysin of *S aureus* (CAMP test). Group D streptococci hydrolyze esculin in the presence of bile, eg, they produce a black pigment on bile-esculin agar. The group D organisms are further subdivided: the enterococci grow in hypertonic (6.5%) NaCl, whereas the nonenterococci do not.

B. Serologic: ASO titers are high soon after group A streptococcal infections. Titers of antihyaluronidase and anti-DNase are high in group A streptococcal skin infections.

Treatment & Prevention All group A streptococci are susceptible to penicillin G, but neither rheumatic fever nor acute glomerulonephritis patients benefit from penicillin treatment *after* onset. Endocarditis caused by most viridans streptococci is curable by prolonged penicillin treatment. However, enterococcal endocarditis can be eradicated only by a penicillin combined with an aminoglycoside. Many group B streptococci are tolerant to penicillin and may require combined-drug treatment for their eradication in neonatal infections.

Prevention of rheumatic fever involves prompt treatment of group A streptococcal pharyngitis with penicillin. Prevention of streptococcal infections (usually with benzathine penicillin once each month for several years) in persons who have had rheumatic fever is important to prevent recurrence of the disease. There is no evidence that patients who have had acute glomerulonephritis require similar penicillin prophylaxis.

There are no vaccines available against streptococcal infections.

STREPTOCOCCUS PNEUMONIAE

Diseases Pneumococci cause pneumonia, bacteremia, meningitis, and infections of the upper respiratory tract such as otitis and sinusitis.

Important Properties Pneumococci are lancet-shaped or spherical cocci arranged in pairs (**diplococci**) or short chains. On blood agar they produce alpha-hemolysis. In contrast to viridans streptococci, they are lysed by bile or deoxycholate and their growth is inhibited by optochin.

Pneumococci possess **polysaccharide capsules** of more than 85 antigenically distinct types. With type-specific antiserum, capsules swell (**quellung reaction**), and this can be used to identify the type. Capsules are virulence factors; ie, they interfere with phagocytosis and favor invasiveness. Specific antibody to the capsule opsonizes the organism, facilitates phagocytosis, and promotes resistance. Such antibody develops in humans as a result either of infection (asymptomatic or clinical) or of administration of polysaccharide vaccine. Capsular polysaccharide elicits primarily a B cell (ie, T-independent) response.

Transmission Pneumococcal infections are not considered to be communicable, since a proportion (5–50%) of the healthy population harbor virulent organisms in their **upper respiratory tract**. Resistance is high in healthy young people, and disease results most often when predisposing factors (see below) are present.

Pathogenesis Pneumococci produce no toxins known to play a role in pathogenesis. They do produce IgA protease that may enhance the organism's ability to colonize the mucosa of the upper respiratory tract. Pneumococci multiply in tissues and cause inflammation. When they reach alveoli, there is outpouring of fluid and red and white cells, resulting in consolidation of the lung. During recovery, pneumococci are phagocytized, mononuclear cells ingest debris, and the consolidation resolves.

Factors that lower resistance and predispose persons to pneumococcal infection include (1) alcohol or drug intoxication or other cerebral impairment that can depress the cough reflex and increase aspiration of secretions; (2) abnormality of the respiratory tract (eg, viral infections), pooling of mucus, bronchial obstruction, and respiratory tract injury due to irritants (which disturb the integrity and movement of the mucociliary blanket); (3) abnormal circulatory dynamics (eg, pulmonary congestion and heart failure); and (4) chronic diseases (eg, sickle cell anemia, hyposplenism, debility, malnutrition, and nephrosis).

Clinical Findings Pneumonia often begins with a sudden chill, fever, cough, and pleuritic pain. Sputum is a red or brown "rusty" color. Bacteremia occurs in 15–25% of cases. Spontaneous recovery may begin in 5–10 days with development of anticapsular antibodies. Pneumococci are a prominent cause of otitis media, sinusitis, purulent bronchitis, and bacterial meningitis.

Laboratory Diagnosis In sputum, pneumococci can be seen as predominant organisms in Gram-stained smears or in the quellung reaction with multitype antiserum. On blood agar, pneumococci form small **alpha-hemolytic** colonies. The colonies are **bile-soluble**, and growth is **inhibited by optochin**. Blood cultures are positive in 15–25% of pneumococcal infections. Culture of cerebrospinal fluid is usually positive in meningitis.

Treatment Most pneumococci are susceptible to penicillins and erythromycin. Some isolates exhibit low-level resistance to penicillin, primarily as a result of changes in penicillin-binding proteins. Rare isolates show high-level resistance, the mechanism of which is unknown. They do not produce β-lactamase.

Prevention In spite of the efficacy of antimicrobial drug treatment, the mortality rate is high in elderly or debilitated persons. They should be immunized with the polyvalent (23-type) **polysaccharide vaccine**. The vaccine is safe and fairly effective and provides long-lasting protection (at least 5 years).

Review Questions

1. What are the differences in appearance on Gram-stained smears between staphylococci, streptococci, and pneumococci?
2. What is the typical pathologic lesion caused by staphylococci?
3. What laboratory test distinguishes *Staphylococcus aureus* from *Staphylococcal epidermidis?*
4. Which staphylococcal species is usually associated with (a) endocarditis in drug addicts, (b) endocarditis in patients with prosthetic heart valves, (c) osteomyelitis, (d) lower urinary tract infections, and (e) carbuncle?
5. What is the pathogenesis of staphylococcal food poisoning?
6. What are the virulence factors produced by *S aureus*, and what is their postulated mode of action?
7. Many *S aureus* infections are unsuccessfully treated with benzylpenicillin (penicillin G). Why? What 2 drugs can be used instead? Why?
8. Distinguish between the grouping and typing of streptococci.
9. Which streptococcal species is usually associated with (a) pharyngitis, (b) neonatal sepsis, (c) infective (subacute) endocarditis, (d) pyoderma, (e) urinary tract infection, (f) glomerulonephritis, and (g) rheumatic fever?
10. What is the role of hemolysis in the classification of streptococci?
11. What are the natural habitat and special growth characteristics of enterococci?
12. What is the role of various streptococcal enzymes and toxins in pathogenesis?
13. Describe the pathogenesis of (a) rheumatic fever and (b) acute glomerulonephritis.
14. How would you distinguish *Streptococcus pyogenes* (group A) from *Streptococcus agalactiae* (group B) in the clinical laboratory?
15. How would you distinguish between pneumocci (*Streptococcus pneumoniae*) and viridans streptococci in the clinical laboratory?
16. Pneumococci have many serologic types. What is the nature of the antigen, and what role does it play in pathogenesis?
17. What is the pathogenesis of pneumococcal pneumonia?
18. How can pneumococcal pneumonia and bacteremia be prevented?

Gram-Negative Cocci

NEISSERIA

Diseases   The genus *Neisseria* contains 2 important human pathogens: *Neisseria meningitidis* and *Neisseria gonorrhoeae*. *N meningitidis* mainly causes meningitis and meningococcemia. *N gonorrhoeae* causes gonorrhea, the most common notifiable bacterial disease in the USA (Table 16–1).

Important Properties   Neisseriae are gram-negative cocci that resemble paired kidney beans.

(a) *N meningitidis* (meningococcus) has a prominent polysaccharide capsule that enhances virulence by its antiphagocytic action and induces protective antibodies. Meningococci are divided into at least 13 serologic groups based on the antigenicity of their capsular polysaccharides. (Table 16-2)

(b) *N gonorrhoeae* (gonococcus) has no polysaccharide capsule but has multiple serotypes based on the antigenicity of its pilus protein. There is marked antigenic variation in the gonococcal pili as a result of chromosomal rearrangement; more than 100 serotypes are known. Gonococci have 3 outer membrane proteins (proteins I, II, and III). Protein II plays a role in attachment of the organism to cells and varies antigenically as well. Because neisseriae are gram-negative organisms, they contain endotoxin in their cell walls similar to that found in the wall of gram-negative rods.

The growth of both organisms is inhibited by toxic trace metals and fatty acids found in certain culture media, eg, blood agar plates. They are therefore cultured on "chocolate" agar containing blood heated to 80 °C, which inactivates the inhibitors. Growth is stimulated by an atmosphere containing 5% CO_2 in a candle jar. (Room air has 0.03% CO_2.) Neisseriae are **oxidase-positive,** ie, they possess the enzyme cytochrome C. This is an important laboratory diagnostic test in which colonies exposed to phenylenediamine turn black as a result of oxidation of the reagent by the enzyme.

The genus *Neisseria* is one of several in the family Neisseriaceae. A separate genus contains the organism *Branhamella catarrhalis,* which is part of the normal throat flora and an occasional opportunistic pathogen. Members of other genera, such as *Moraxella, Kingella,* and *Acinetobacter,* are described in Chapter 27.

1. Neisseria meningitidis

Pathogenesis & Epidemiology   Humans are the only natural hosts for meningococci. The organisms are transmitted by **airborne droplets**; they colonize the membranes of the nasopharynx and become part of the transient flora of the upper respiratory tract. Carriers are usually asymptomatic. From the nasopharynx, the organism can enter the bloodstream and spread to specific sites, such as the meninges or joints, or be disseminated throughout the body (meningococcemia). About 5% of people become chronic carriers and serve as a source of infection for others. The carriage rate can be as high as 35% in people who live in close quarters, eg, military recruits; this explains the high frequency of outbreaks of meningitis in the armed forces. The carriage rate is also high in close (family) contacts of patients.

Table 16–1. Gram-negative cocci (*Neisseria*) of medical importance.[1]

Species	Portal of Entry	Polysaccharide Capsule	Maltose Fermentation	β-Lactamase Production	Available Vaccine
N meningitidis (meningococcus)	Respiratory tract	+	+	None	+
N gonorrhoeae (gonococcus)	Genital tract	–	–	Some	–

[1]All neisseriae are oxidase-positive.

Table16–2. Properties of the polysaccharide capsule of the meningococcus.[1]

Property
(1) Enhances virulence by its antiphagocytic action
(2) Is the antigen that defines the serologic groups
(3) Is the antigen detected in the spinal fluid of patients with meningitis
(4) Is the antigen in the vaccine

[1]The same 4 features apply to the capsule of the pneumococcus and *Haemophilus influenzae*.

Three organisms cause more than 80% of cases of bacterial meningitis in persons over 2 months of age: *Haemophilus influenzae, Streptococcus pneumoniae*, and *N meningitidis*. Of these organisms, meningococci, especially those in group A, are most likely to cause epidemics of meningitis. As a cause of sporadic cases, meningococci rank second to *H influenzae* in causing meningitis in children aged 6 months to 6 years and are similar in frequency to *S pneumoniae* infections in adults.

Meningococci have 3 important virulence factors:

(1) a **polysaccharide capsule** that enables the organism to resist phagocytosis by polymorphonuclear leukocytes (PMNs);

(2) endotoxin, which causes fever, shock, and other pathophysiologic changes (in purified form, endotoxin can reproduce many of the clinical manifestations of meningococcemia); and

(3) an immunoglobulin A **(IgA) protease**, which, by cleaving secretory IgA, helps the bacteria to attach to the membranes of the upper respiratory tract.

Resistance to disease correlates with the presence of antibody to the capsular polysaccharide. Most carriers develop protective antibody titers within 2 weeks of colonization. Immunity is group-specific, and so it is possible to have protective antibodies to one group of organisms yet be susceptible to infection by organisms of the other groups. Complement is an important feature of the host defenses, because people with complement deficiencies, particularly in the **late-acting complement components** (C5–C8), have an increased incidence of meningococcal bacteremia.

Clinical Findings The 2 most important manifestations of disease are **meningococcemia** and **meningitis.** The most severe form of meningococcemia is the life-threatening **Waterhouse-Friderichsen syndrome**, which is characterized by high fever, shock, widespread purpura, disseminated intravascular coagulation, and adrenal insufficiency. Bacteremia can result in the seeding of many organs, especially the meninges. The symptoms of meningococcal meningitis are those of a typical bacterial meningitis—namely fever, headache, stiff neck, and an increased level of PMNs in spinal fluid.

Laboratory Diagnosis The principal laboratory procedures are smear and culture of blood and spinal fluid samples. A presumptive diagnosis of meningococcal meningitis can be made if gram-negative cocci are seen in a smear of spinal fluid. The organism grows best on chocolate agar incubated at 37 °C in a 5% CO_2 atmosphere. A presumptive diagnosis of *Neisseria* can be made if oxidase-positive colonies of gram-negative diplococci are found. The differentiation between *N meningitidis* and *N gonorrhoeae* is made on the basis of sugar fermentation: meningococci ferment maltose, whereas gonococci do not (both organisms ferment glucose). Immunofluorescence can also be used to identify these species. Tests for serum antibodies are not useful for clinical diagnosis. However, a procedure that can assist in the rapid diagnosis of meningococcal meningitis is the latex agglutination test, which detects capsular polysaccharide in the spinal fluid.

Treatment Penicillin G is the treatment of choice for meningococcal infections. Strains resistant to penicillin have not emerged, but sulfonamide resistance is common.

Prevention Chemoprophylaxis and immunization are both used to prevent meningococcal disease. Rifampin is used for prophylaxis in household and other close contacts. It is preferred because it is efficiently secreted into the saliva, in contrast to penicillin G. The meningococcal vaccine, which contains the capsular polysaccharides of group A, C, Y, and W-135 strains, is effective in preventing epidemics of meningitis and in reducing the carrier rate, especially in military personnel. The vaccine does not contain the group B polysaccharide, which is poorly immunogenic in humans.

2. Neisseria gonorrhoeae

Pathogenesis & Epidemiology Gonococci, like meningococci, cause disease only in humans. The organism is usually transmitted **sexually**; newborns can be infected during birth. Because the gonococcus is quite sensitive to dehydration and cool conditions, sexual transmission favors its survival. Gonorrhea is usually symptomatic in men but often asymptomatic in women. Infections of the anorectal area and pharynx, as well as those of the genital tract, can act as the source of the organisms.

Pili constitute one of the most important virulence factors, because they mediate attachment to mucosal cell surfaces and are antiphagocytic. Piliated gonococci are usually virulent, whereas nonpiliated strains are avirulent. Two virulence factors in the cell wall are endotoxin and the outer membrane proteins. The organism's **IgA protease** can hydrolyze secretory IgA, which could otherwise block attachment to the mucosa. Gonococci have no capsules.

Certain strains of gonococci cause disseminated infections more frequently than others. These strains are characterized by 3 features: (1) resistance to the bactericidal action of serum; (2) marked sensitivity to penicillin; and (3) auxotrophy for arginine, uracil, and hypoxanthine; ie, for growth, they require that these substances be present in the medium.

The occurrence of a disseminated infection is a function not only of the strain of gonococcus but also of the effectiveness of the host defenses. Persons with a deficiency of the late-acting complement components (C5–C8) are at risk for disseminated infections, as are women during menses and pregnancy. Disseminated infections usually arise from asymptomatic infections, indicating that local inflammation may deter dissemination.

Clinical Findings Gonococci cause both localized infections, usually in the genital tract, and disseminated infections with seeding of various organs. Gonorrhea in men is characterized primarily by urethritis accompanied by dysuria and a purulent discharge. In women, infection is located primarily in the endocervix, causing a purulent vaginal discharge and intermenstrual bleeding. The most frequent complication in women is an ascending infection of the uterine tubes (salpingitis, pelvic inflammatory disease), which can result in sterility due to scarring of the tubes. Disseminated infections commonly manifest as arthritis or dermatitis.

Other infected sites include the anorectal area and the throat. Anorectal infections occur chiefly in women and homosexual men. They are frequently asymptomatic, but a bloody or purulent discharge (proctitis) can occur. In the throat, pharyngitis occurs but many patients are asymptomatic. In newborn infants, a purulent conjunctivitis (ophthalmia neonatorum) is the result of gonococcal infection acquired from the mother during passage through the birth canal. The incidence of gonococcal ophthalmia has declined markedly in recent years owing to the widespread use of prophylactic erythromycin eye ointment (or silver nitrate) given shortly after birth.

Other sexually transmitted infections, eg, syphilis and nongonococcal urethritis caused by *Chlamydia trachomatis,* can coexist with gonorrhea; therefore, appropriate diagnostic and therapeutic measures must be taken.

Laboratory Diagnosis The diagnosis of localized infections depends on Gram staining and culture of the discharge. The finding of gram-negative diplococci **within PMNs** in a sample of urethral discharge from a man is sufficient for diagnosis. Because the Gram stain is often falsely negative in women, culture must be done. Cultures must also be used in diagnosing suspected pharyngitis or anorectal infections.

Specimens are cultured on Thayer-Martin medium, which is a chocolate agar containing antibiotics (vancomycin, colistin, trimethoprim, and nystatin) to suppress the normal flora, and are incubated at 37 °C in a 5% CO_2 atmosphere. The finding of an oxidase-positive colony composed of gram-negative diplococci is sufficient to diagnose *Neisseria*. Specific identification of the gonococcus can be made either by its fermentation of glucose (but not maltose) or by fluorescent-antibody staining. Serologic tests are not useful for diagnosis of gonorrhea.

Treatment Oral amoxicillin or I.M. ceftriaxone is the treatment of choice in uncomplicated gonococcal infections. Oral probenecid is given to retard the renal excretion of penicillin. Spectinomycin should be used if the patient is allergic to penicillin. In addition, tetracycline is recommended for treating *C trachomatis,* as mixed infections are common. A follow-up culture should be done 1 week after completion of treatment to determine whether gonococci are still present.

Prior to the mid 1950s, all gonococci were highly sensitive to penicillin. Subsequently, isolates emerged with low-level resistance to penicillin and to other antibiotics such as tetracycline and chloramphenicol. This type of resistance is encoded by the bacterial chromosome and is due to reduced uptake of the drug or to altered binding sites rather than to enzymatic degradation of the drug. Then, in 1976, β-**lactamase**-producing strains that exhibited high-level resistance were isolated. This enzyme, which is encoded by a plasmid, is active against both penicillins and cephalosporins. Fortunately, these strains remain rare in the USA; however, they are prevalent in the Philippines and western Africa.

Prevention The prevention of gonorrhea involves the use of condoms and the prompt treatment of symptomatic patients and their contacts. Cases of gonorrhea must be reported to the public health department to ensure proper follow-up. A major problem is the detection of asymptomatic carriers. Gonococcal conjunctivitis in newborns is prevented most often by the use of erythromycin ointment. Silver nitrate drops are used less frequently. No vaccine is available.

Review Questions

1. What role does the polysaccharide capsule of *Neisseria meningitidis* play in pathogenesis?
2. *Neisseria gonorrhoeae* does not have a capsule, but it does have pili. What role do the pili play in pathogenesis?
3. Why is chocolate agar used to culture neisseriae?
4. What is the meaning of the phrase, "Neisseriae are oxidase-positive"?
5. Meningococci colonize the oropharynx. How do they reach the meninges to cause meningitis?
6. What role does endotoxin play in meningococcal disease?
7. What 3 organisms cause most of the cases of meningitis in persons over the age of 2 months?
8. What immunologic deficiency predisposes individuals to bacteremia caused by meningococci and gonococci?
9. How can meningococci and gonococci be distinguished in the clinical laboratory?
10. What means are available to prevent meningococcal meningitis?
11. What role does IgA protease play in gonococcal disease?
12. What is the risk to the newborn of gonorrhea in the mother?
13. What is the significance of finding gram-negative diplococci within neutrophils in a urethral exudate?
14. Why is Thayer-Martin medium used to culture gonococci?
15. Why does penicillin fail to cure gonorrhea in some patients?

17

Gram-Positive Rods

There are 4 medically important genera of gram-positive rods: *Bacillus, Clostridium, Corynebacterium,* and *Listeria. Bacillus* and *Clostridium* form spores, whereas *Corynebacterium* and *Listeria* do not. Members of the genus *Bacillus* are aerobic, whereas those of the genus *Clostridium* are anaerobic (Table 17–1).

Spore-Forming Gram-Positive Rods

BACILLUS There are 2 medically important *Bacillus* species: *Bacillus anthracis* and *Bacillus cereus.*

1. Bacillus anthracis

Disease *B anthracis* causes anthrax, which is common in animals but rare in humans.

Important Properties *B anthracis* is a large gram-positive rod with square ends, frequently found in chains. Its antiphagocytic capsule is composed of **D-glutamate.** (This is unique—capsules of other bacteria are polysaccharides.) It is nonmotile, whereas other members of the genus are motile.

Transmission Spores of the organism persist in soil for years. Humans are infected by **spores on animal products** such as hides, bristles, and wool or by contact with sick animals. The portals of entry are the skin, mucous membranes, and respiratory tract.

Pathogenesis *B anthracis* invades the host and produces **anthrax toxin,** which consists of 3 components: protective antigen, lethal factor, and edema factor. Edema factor, an exotoxin, is an **adenylate cyclase** dependent on protective antigen for its binding and entry into the cell. Lethal factor in the presence of protective antigen is rapidly fatal for mice. The mode of action of lethal factor is unknown.

Clinical Findings The typical lesion is a painless ulcer with a black, necrotic eschar. Local edema is striking. Untreated cases progress to bacteremia and death. ''Woolsorter's disease'' (pulmonary anthrax) is a life-threatening pneumonia caused by inhalation of spores.

Laboratory Diagnosis Smears show large, gram-positive rods in chains. Colonies form on blood agar aerobically. No serologic tests are useful.

Treatment Penicillin is the most effective treatment. No resistant strains have been isolated clinically.

Prevention Soil contamination is prevented by sterilizing dead animals and animal products from endemic areas. Protective clothing should be worn by persons at risk of exposure.

Table 17–1. Gram-positive rods of medical importance.

Genus	Anaerobic Growth	Spore Formation	Exotoxins Important in Pathogenesis
Bacillus	–	+	+
Clostridium	+	+	+
Corynebacterium	–	–	+
Listeria	–	–	–

Persons at high risk can be immunized with cell-free vaccine containing purified protective antigen as immunogen.

2. Bacillus cereus

Disease   *B cereus* causes food poisoning.

Transmission   Spores on grains such as rice survive steaming and rapid frying. The spores germinate when rice is kept warm (**reheated fried rice**). The portal of entry is the gastrointestinal tract.

Pathogenesis   *B cereus* produces 2 enterotoxins. Their mode of action is unclear.

Clinical Findings   There are 2 syndromes: (1) one involves a short incubation period (4 hours) with nausea and vomiting and is similar to staphylococcal food poisoning; (2) the other involves a long incubation period (18 hours) with diarrhea and resembles clostridial gastroenteritis.

Laboratory Diagnosis   This is not usually done.

Treatment   Only symptomatic treatment is given.

Prevention   Rice should not be reheated.

CLOSTRIDIUM   There are 4 medically important *Clostridium* species: *C tetani, C botulinum, C perfringens* (which causes either gas gangrene or food poisoning), and *C difficile*. All clostridia are anaerobic, spore-forming, gram-positive rods.

1. Clostridium tetani

Disease   *C tetani* causes tetanus (lockjaw).

Transmission   Spores are widespread in soil. The portal of entry is a **wound** site. Germination of spores is favored by necrotic tissue and poor blood supply in the wound.

Pathogenesis   **Tetanus toxin** (tetanospasmin) is an exotoxin produced by vegetative cells at the wound site. This polypeptide toxin is carried intra-axonally (retrograde) to the central nervous system, where it binds to ganglioside receptors and blocks release of inhibitory mediators (eg, glycine) at spinal synapses. Tetanospasmin, along with botulinus toxin, is among the most toxic substances known.

Clinical Findings   Violent muscle spasms; **lockjaw** (trismus) due to rigid contraction of the jaw muscles, which prevents the mouth from opening; a characteristic grimace known as "**risus sardonicus**"; and exaggerated reflexes occur. Respiratory failure ensues. A high mortality rate is associated with this disease.

Laboratory Diagnosis   There is no microbiologic or serologic diagnosis. Organisms are rarely isolated from the wound site.

Treatment   Treatment involves penicillin, respiratory support, and muscle relaxants.

Prevention   Tetanus is prevented by immunization with tetanus **toxoid** (formaldehyde-treated toxin) in childhood and every 10 years thereafter. When trauma occurs, the wound should be cleaned and debrided and tetanus toxoid booster should be given. If the wound is grossly contaminated, tetanus immune globulin, as well as the toxoid booster, should be given and penicillin administered.

2. Clostridium botulinum

Disease *C botulinum* causes botulism.

Transmission Spores, widespread in soil, contaminate vegetables and meats. When these foods are canned or vacuum-packed without adequate sterilization, spores survive and germinate in the anaerobic environment. Toxin is produced within the canned food and **ingested preformed**. The highest-risk foods are (1) alkaline vegetables such as green beans, peppers, and mushrooms and (2) smoked fish. Toxin is relatively heat-labile; it is inactivated by cooking, eg, boiling for 10 minutes.

Pathogenesis **Botulinus toxin** is absorbed from the gut and carried via the blood to peripheral nerve synapses, where it blocks release of acetylcholine. The toxin is a polypeptide encoded by a lysogenic phage. Along with tetanus toxin, it is among the most toxic substances known. There are 8 immunologic types of toxin; types A, B, and E are the most common in humans.

Clinical Findings Descending weakness and paralysis including diplopia, dysphagia, and respiratory muscle failure are seen. No fever is present. Two special clinical forms occur: (1) wound botulism, in which spores contaminate a wound, germinate, and produce toxin at the site; and (2) infant botulism, in which the organisms grow in the gut and produce toxins. Ingestion of honey containing the organism is implicated in transmission of infant botulism. Affected infants develop weakness or paralysis and may need respiratory support but usually recover spontaneously.

Laboratory Diagnosis The organism is usually not cultured. Botulinus toxin is demonstrable in uneaten food and the patient's serum by mouse protection tests. Mice are inoculated with a sample of the clinical specimen and will die unless protected by antitoxin.

Treatment Trivalent antitoxin (types A, B, and E) is given, along with respiratory support.

Prevention Proper sterilization of all canned and vacuum-packed foods is essential. Food must be adequately cooked to inactivate the toxin. Swollen cans must be discarded (clostridial proteolytic enzymes cause gas formation that swells cans).

3. Clostridium perfringens   *C perfringens* causes 2 distinct diseases: gas gangrene and food poisoning.

A. Gas Gangrene (Myonecrosis):*

Transmission Spores are located in the **soil**; vegetative cells are members of the **normal flora of the colon and vagina**. Gas gangrene is associated with war wounds, automobile accidents, and septic abortions.

Pathogenesis Organisms grow in traumatized tissue (especially muscle) and produce a variety of toxins. The most important is **alpha toxin** (lecithinase), which damages cell membranes, including those of erythrocytes, resulting in hemolysis. Degradative enzymes produce gas in tissues.

Clinical findings Pain and edema occur in the wound area. Crepitation indicates the presence of gas in tissues. Hemolysis and jaundice are common, as are blood-tinged exudates. Shock and death can ensue. Mortality rates are high.

Laboratory diagnosis Smears of tissue and exudate samples show large gram-positive rods. Spores are not usually seen because they are formed primarily under nutritionally deficient conditions. The organisms are cultured anaerobically and then identified by sugar fermentation reactions and organic acid production. Serologic tests are not useful.

---

*Gas gangrene is also caused by other histotoxic clostridia such as *C histolyticum, C septicum,* and *C novyi.*

Treatment   Penicillin is the antibiotic of choice. Wounds should be debrided.

Prevention   Wounds should be cleansed and debrided.

B. Food Poisoning:

Transmission   Spores are located in **soil** and on **food**. They survive cooking, and the organisms grow to large numbers in reheated foods, especially meat dishes.

Pathogenesis   During sporulation (spore formation) in the gastrointestinal tract, an **enterotoxin** is produced. The enterotoxin is identical to a protein in the spore coat. The mode of action of the enterotoxin is unknown.

Clinical findings   The disease has an 8- to 16-hour incubation period and is characterized by watery diarrhea with cramps and little vomiting. It resolves in 24 hours.

Laboratory diagnosis   This is not usually done. There is no assay for the toxin. Large numbers of the organisms can be isolated from uneaten food.

Treatment   Symptomatic treatment is given; no antimicrobial drugs are administered.

Prevention   There are no specific preventive measures. Food should be adequately cooked to kill the organism.

4. Clostridium difficile

Disease   *C difficile* causes antibiotic-associated pseudomembranous colitis.

Transmission   The organism is part of the **normal flora of the gastrointestinal tract** in approximately 3% of the general population.

Pathogenesis   Antibiotics suppress drug-sensitive normal flora, allowing *C difficile* to multiply and produce toxin. Clindamycin and ampicillin are 2 of many antibiotics that cause this disease. The mechanism of action of the toxin is uncertain.

Clinical Findings   *C difficile* causes diarrhea, associated with **pseudomembranes** (yellow-white plaques) on the colonic mucosa. The pseudomembranes are visualized by sigmoidoscopy.

Laboratory Diagnosis   The toxin is detected in stool samples by its cytotoxic effect on cultured cells. It is identified by inhibition of cytotoxicity by specific antibody. Anaerobic culture is usually not done.

Treatment   The causative antibiotic should be withdrawn. Oral vancomycin should be given and fluids replaced.

Prevention   There are no specific preventive measures.

Non-Spore-Forming Gram-Positive Rods

There are 2 important pathogens in this group: *Corynebacterium diphtheriae* and *Listeria monocytogenes*.

CORYNEBACTERIUM DIPHTHERIAE

Disease   *C diphtheriae* causes diphtheria. Other *Corynebacterium* species (diphtheroids) are implicated in opportunistic infections.

Important Properties   Corynebacteria are gram-positive rods that appear **club-shaped** (tapered at one end) and are arranged in palisades or in V- or L-shaped formations, resembling Chinese characters. The rods have a beaded appearance. The beads consist of granules of highly polymerized polyphosphate, a storage mechanism for high-energy phosphate bonds. The granules stain **metachromatically**, ie, a dye that stains the rest of the cell blue will stain the granules red.

Transmission   Humans are the only natural host of *C diphtheriae*. Both toxigenic and nontoxigenic organisms reside in the upper respiratory tract and are transmitted by **airborne droplets**. The organism can also infect the skin at the site of a preexisting skin lesion. This occurs primarily in the tropics but can occur worldwide in indigent persons with poor skin hygiene.

Pathogenesis & Epidemiology   Although exotoxin production is essential for pathogenesis, invasiveness is also necessary because the organism must first establish and maintain itself in the throat. Diphtheria toxin inhibits protein synthesis by **ADP ribosylation of elongation factor 2** (EF-2). The toxin affects all eukaryotic cells regardless of tissue type but has no effect on the analogous factor in prokaryotic cells.

The toxin is a single polypeptide with 2 functional domains. One domain mediates binding of the toxin to glycoprotein receptors on the cell membrane. The other domain possesses enzymatic activity that cleaves nicotinamide from nicotinamide adenine dinucleotide (NAD) and transfers the remaining ADP-ribose to EF-2, thereby inactivating it. Other organisms whose exotoxins act by ADP ribosylation are listed on page 27.

The DNA that codes for diphtheria toxin is part of the genetic material of a temperate bacteriophage. During the lysogenic phase of viral growth, the DNA of this virus integrates into the bacterial chromosome and the toxin is synthesized. *C diphtheriae* cells that are not lysogenized by this phage do not produce exotoxin and are nonpathogenic.

The host response to *C diphtheriae* consists of

(1)   local inflammation in the throat, with a fibrinous exudate that forms the tough, adherent, gray "pseudomembrane" characteristic of the disease; and

(2)   antibody that can neutralize exotoxin activity by blocking the interaction of fragment B with the receptors, thereby preventing entry into the cell. The immune status of a person can be assessed by Schick's test. The test is performed by intradermal injection of 0.1 mL of purified standardized toxin. If the patient has no antitoxin, the toxin will cause inflammation at the site 4–7 days later. If no inflammation occurs, antitoxin is present and the patient is immune. The test is rarely performed in the USA except under special epidemiologic circumstances.

Clinical Findings   Although diphtheria is rare in the USA, physicians should be aware of its most prominent sign, the thick, gray, adherent membrane over the tonsils and throat. The other aspects are nonspecific: fever, sore throat, and cervical adenopathy. There are 3 prominent complications:

(1)   extension of the membrane into the larynx and trachea, causing airway obstruction;

(2)   myocarditis accompanied by arrhythmias and circulatory collapse; and

(3)   recurrent laryngeal nerve palsy.

Cutaneous diphtheria causes ulcerating skin lesions and does not cause systemic symptoms.

Laboratory Diagnosis   Laboratory diagnosis involves both isolating the organism and demonstrating toxin production. It should be emphasized that the decision to treat with antitoxin is a clinical one and cannot wait for the laboratory results. A throat swab should be cultured on Löffler's medium, a **tellurite plate**, and a blood agar plate. The tellurite plate contains a tellurium salt that is reduced to elemental tellurium within the organism. The typical gray-black color of tellurium in the colony is a telltale diagnostic criterion. If *C diphtheriae* is recovered from the cultures, either animal inoculation or a gel diffusion precipitin test is performed to document toxin production.

Smears of the throat swab should be stained with both Gram's stain and methylene blue. Although the diagnosis of diphtheria cannot be made by examination of the smear, the finding of many tapered, pleomorphic gram-positive rods can be suggestive. The methylene blue stain is excellent for revealing the typical metachromatic granules.

Treatment   The treatment of choice is **antitoxin**, which should be given immediately on the basis of clinical impression because there is a delay in laboratory diagnostic procedures. The toxin binds rapidly and irreversibly to cells and, once bound, cannot be neutralized by antitoxin. The function of antitoxin is therefore to neutralize unbound toxin in the blood. Because the antiserum is made in horses, the patient must be tested for hypersensitivity and medications for the treatment of anaphylaxis must be available.

Treatment with penicillin or erythromycin is recommended also, but neither is a substitute for antitoxin. Antibiotics inhibit growth of the organism, reduce toxin production, and decrease the incidence of chronic carriers.

Prevention   The small number of cases of diphtheria in the USA is due to immunization of children with **diphtheria toxoid** (usually given as a combination of diphtheria toxoid, tetanus toxoid, and killed pertussis organisms). Diphtheria toxoid is prepared by treating the exotoxin with formaldehyde. This treatment inactivates the toxic effect but leaves the antigenicity intact. Immunization consists of 3 doses given at 2, 4, and 6 months of age, with a booster at 1 and 6 years of age. Because immunity wanes, a booster every 10 years is recommended. Immunization does not prevent nasopharyngeal carriage of the organism.

LISTERIA MONOCYTOGENES

Diseases   *L monocytogenes* causes meningitis and sepsis in newborns and immunosuppressed adults.

Important Properties   *L monocytogenes* is a small gram-positive rod arranged in a clumped, ''Chinese character'' configuration similar to corynebacteria. The organism exhibits an unusual **tumbling** movement that distinguishes it from the corynebacteria, which are nonmotile. Colonies on a blood agar plate produce a narrow zone of beta-hemolysis that resembles the hemolysis of some streptococci.

Pathogenesis & Epidemiology   *Listeria* infections occur primarily in 2 clinical settings: (1) in the fetus or newborn as a result of transmission **across the placenta or during delivery**; and (2) in immunosuppressed adults, especially renal transplant patients. The organism is distributed worldwide in animals, plants, and soil. From these reservoirs, it is transmitted to humans by contact with animals or their feces, by unpasteurized milk, and by contaminated vegetables. The **gastrointestinal tract** is the most likely source of infections that arise endogenously. The pathogenesis of *Listeria* is dependent upon the organism's ability to parasitize mononuclear phagocytic cells and to induce granuloma formation.

Clinical Findings   Infection during pregnancy can cause abortion, premature delivery, or sepsis during the peripartum period. Newborns infected at the time of delivery can have acute meningitis 1–4 weeks later. The infected mother is either asymptomatic or has an influenzalike illness. *L monocytogenes* infections in immunocompromised adults can be either sepsis or meningitis.

Laboratory Diagnosis   Laboratory diagnosis is made primarily by Gram stain and culture. The appearance of gram-positive rods resembling **diphtheroids** and the formation of small, gray colonies with a narrow zone of beta-hemolysis on a blood agar plate suggest the presence of *Listeria*. The isolation of *Listeria* is confirmed by the presence of motile organism, which differentiate them from the nonmotile corynebacteria. Identification of the organism as *L monocytogenes* is made by sugar fermentation tests.

Treatment   Penicillin is the drug of choice, and resistant strains are rare.

Prevention   Prevention is difficult because there is no immunization. Limiting the exposure of immunosuppressed patients to potential sources such as infected animals and their products and contaminated vegetables is recommended.

Review Questions

1. How is the capsule of *Bacillus anthracis* different from that of most other bacteria?
2. What is the natural habitat of *B anthracis,* and how does it persist there for long periods?
3. How does *B anthracis* cause disease?
4. *Bacillus cereus* causes food poisoning. How is it transmitted? What is the pathogenesis?
5. How is tetanus acquired? What is its pathogenesis?
6. What are the 3 important components of tetanus prevention?
7. How is botulism acquired? What is its pathogenesis? How is it prevented?
8. *Clostridium perfringens* can cause gas gangrene. Under what circumstances does this occur, and what is the role of alpha toxin in the disease? How can the disease be prevented?
9. In an exudate from a patient with gas gangrene, what would you see on Gram stain? How would you culture the organism?
10. What is the pathogenesis of food poisoning caused by *C perfringens?*
11. What is the pathogenesis of diarrhea caused by *Clostridium difficile?*
12. What is the appearance of *Corynebacterium diphtheriae* on Gram's stain?
13. What is the mechanism of action of diphtheria toxin?
14. Only lysogenized strains of *C diphtheriae* are pathogenic. Why?
15. Why is diphtheria rare in the USA?
16. What is the role of antitoxin in the treatment of diphtheria?
17. In what 2 population groups do *Listeria* infections primarily occur?
18. How is *Listeria monocytogenes* transmitted, and what is its mode of pathogenesis?

18

Gram-Negative Rods Related to the Enteric Tract

Overview

Gram-negative rods are a large group of diverse organisms. In this book, these bacteria are subdivided into 3 clinically relevant categories, each in a separate chapter, according to whether the organism is related primarily to the enteric or the respiratory tract or to animal sources (Table 18–1). Although this approach leads to some overlaps, it should be helpful because it allows general concepts to be emphasized.

Gram-negative rods related to the enteric tract include a large number of genera. These genera have therefore been divided into 3 groups depending on the major anatomic location of

Table 18–1. Categories of gram-negative rods.

Chapter	Source of Site of Infection	Genus
18	Enteric tract 1. Both within and outside	*Escherichia, Salmonella*
	2. Primarily within	*Shigella, Vibrio, Campylobacter*
	3. Outside only	*Klebsiella-Enterobacter-Serratia* group, *Proteus-Providencia-Morganella* group, *Pseudomonas, Bacteroides*
19	Respiratory tract	*Haemophilus, Legionella, Bordetella*
20	Animal sources	*Brucella, Francisella, Pasteurella, Yersinia*

Table 18–2. Frequency of diseases caused in the USA by gram-negative rods related to the enteric tract.

Site of Infection	Frequent Pathogens	Less-Frequent Pathogens
Enteric tract	*Salmonella, Shigella, Campylobacter*	*Escherichia, Vibrio, Yersinia*
Urinary tract	*Escherichia*	*Enterobacter, Klebsiella, Proteus, Pseudomonas*

disease, namely (1) pathogens both within and outside the enteric tract, (2) pathogens primarily within the enteric tract, and (3) pathogens outside the enteric tract (Table 18–1).

The frequency with which the organisms related to the enteric tract cause disease in the USA is shown in Table 18–2. *Salmonella, Shigella,* and *Campylobacter* are frequent pathogens in the gastrointestinal tract, whereas *Escherichia, Vibrio, and Yersinia* are less so. Enterotoxigenic strains of *Escherichia coli* are a common cause of diarrhea in developing countries but are less common in the USA. Urinary tract infections are caused primarily by *E coli:* the other organisms occur less commonly.

Before describing the specific organisms, it is appropriate to describe the family Enterobacteriaceae, to which many of these gram-negative rods belong.

ENTEROBACTERIACEAE & RELATED ORGANISMS

The Enterobacteriaceae are a large family of gram-negative rods found primarily in the colons of humans and other animals, many as part of the normal flora. They are the major facultative anaerobes in the large intestine but are present in relatively small numbers compared with anaerobes such as *Bacteroides*. Although the Enterobacteriaceae are classified together taxonomically, they cause a variety of diseases with different pathogenetic mechanisms. The organisms and some of the diseases they cause are listed in Table 18–3.

Members of this heterogeneous family are united both by their anatomic location and by the following 4 metabolic processes: (1) they are all facultative anaerobes; (2) they all ferment glucose (fermentation of other sugars varies); (3) none have cytochrome oxidase, ie, they are oxidase-negative; and (4) they reduce nitrates to nitrites as part of their energy-generating processes.

These 4 reactions can be used to distinguish the Enterobacteriaceae from another medically significant group of organisms, the nonfermenting gram-negative rods, the most important of which is *Pseudomonas aeruginosa.** P aeruginosa,* a significant cause of urinary tract infections and sepsis in hospitalized patients, does not ferment glucose or reduce nitrates and is oxidase-positive. In contrast to the Enterobacteriaceae, it is a strict aerobe and derives its energy from oxidation, not fermentation.

Pathogenesis All Enterobacteriaceae, being gram-negative, contain endotoxin in their cell walls. In addition, several exotoxins are produced; eg, *E coli* and *Vibrio cholerae* secrete exotoxins, called enterotoxins, that activate adenylate cyclase within the cells of the small intestine, causing diarrhea.

Table 18–3. Diseases caused by Enterobacteriaceae.

Major Pathogens	Representative Diseases	Minor Related Genera
Escherichia	Urinary tract infection, traveler's diarrhea, neonatal meningitis	
Shigella	Dysentery	
Salmonella	Typhoid fever, enterocolitis	*Arizona, Citrobacter, Edwardsiella*
Klebsiella	Pneumonia, urinary tract infection	
Enterobacter	Pneumonia, urinary tract infection	*Hafnia*
Serratia	Pneumonia, urinary tract infection	
Proteus	Urinary tract infection	*Providencia, Morganella*
Yersinia	Plague, enterocolitis, mesenteric adenitis	

---

*The other less frequently isolated organisms in this group are members of the following genera: *Achromobacter, Acinetobacter, Alcaligenes, Eikenella, Flavobacterium, Kingella,* and *Moraxella;* see p. 120.

Antigens   The antigens of several Enterbacteriaceae, especially *Salmonella* and *Shigella,* are important; they are used for identification purposes both in the clinical laboratory and in epidemiologic investigations. The 3 surface antigens are as follows.

(1) The cell wall antigen (also known as the somatic or O antigen) is the outer polysaccharide portion of the lipopolysaccharide (see Fig 2–6). The O antigen, which is composed of repeating oligosaccharides consisting of 3 or 4 sugars repeated 15 or 20 times, is the basis for the serologic typing of many enteric rods. The number of different O antigens is very large; eg, there are approximately 1500 types of *Salmonella* and 150 types of *E coli.*

(2) The H antigen is on the flagellar protein. Only flagellated organisms, such as *Escherichia* and *Salmonella,* have H antigens, whereas the nonmotile ones, such as *Klebsiella* and *Shigella,* do not. The H antigens of certain *Salmonella* species are unusual, because the organisms can reversibly alternate between 2 types of H antigens called phase 1 and phase 2. The organisms may use this change in antigenicity to evade the immune response.

(3) The capsular or K polysaccharide antigen is particularly prominent in heavily encapsulated organisms such as *Klebsiella.* The K antigen is identified by the quellung (capsular swelling) reaction in the presence of specific antisera and is used to serotype *E coli* and *Salmonella typhi* for epidemiologic purposes. In *S typhi,* the cause of typhoid fever, it is called the Vi (or virulence) antigen.

Laboratory Diagnosis   Specimens suspected of containing Enterobacteriaceae and related organisms are usually inoculated onto 2 media, a blood agar plate and a selective differential medium such as MacConkey's agar or eosin-methylene blue (EMB) agar. The *differential* ability of these latter media is based on **lactose fermentation,** which is the most important metabolic criterion used in the identification of these organisms (Table 18–4). On these media, the nonlactose fermenters, eg, *Salmonella* and *Shigella,* form colorless colonies, whereas the lactose fermenters form colored colonies. The *selective* effect of the media in suppressing unwanted gram-positive organisms is exerted by bile salts or bacteriostatic dyes in the agar.

An additional set of screening tests, consisting of triple sugar iron (TSI) agar and urea medium, is done prior to the definitive identification procedures. The rationale for the use of these media and the reactions of several important organisms are presented in the box and in Table 18–5. The results of the screening process are frequently sufficient to identify the genus of an organism; however, an array of 20 or more biochemical tests is required to identify the species.

Triple Sugar Iron Agar

The important components of this medium are ferrous sulfate and the 3 sugars—glucose, lactose, and sucrose. The glucose is present in one-tenth the concentration of the other 2 sugars. The medium in the tube is produced so that there is a solid, poorly oxygenated area on the bottom, called the butt, and an angled, well-oxygenated area on top, called the slant. The organism is inoculated into the butt and across the surface of the slant.

The interpretation of the test is as follows: (1) If lactose (or sucrose) is fermented, a large amount of acid is produced, which turns the phenol red indicator yellow both in the butt and on the slant. Some organisms generate gases, which produce bubbles in the butt. (2) If lactose is not fermented but the small amount of glucose is, the oxygen-deficient butt will be yellow, but on the slant the acid will be oxidized to CO_2 and H_2O by the organism and the slant will be red (neutral or alkaline). (3) If neither lactose nor glucose is fermented, both the butt and the slant will be red. The slant can become a deeper red-purple (more alkaline) owing to the production of ammonia from the oxidative deamination of amino acids. (4) If H_2S is produced, the black color of ferrous sulfide is seen.

The reactions of some of the important organisms are presented in Table 18-5. Because several organisms can give the same reaction, TSI agar is only a screening device.

Urea Agar

The important components of this medium are urea and the pH indicator phenol red. If the organism produces urease, the urea is hydrolyzed to NH_3 and CO_2. Ammonia turns the medium alkaline, and the color of the phenol red changes from light orange to reddish purple. The important organisms that are urease-positive are *Proteus* species and *K pneumoniae.*

Table 18–4. Lactose fermentation by Enterobacteriaceae and related organisms.

Fermentation	Genera
Occurs	*Escherichia, Klebsiella, Enterobacter*
Does not occur	*Shigella, Salmonella, Proteus, Pseudomonas*
Occurs slowly	*Serratia, Vibrio*

Another valuable piece of information used to identify some of these organisms is their motility, which is dependent on the presence of flagella. *Proteus* species are very motile and characteristically **"swarm"** over the blood agar plate, obscuring the colonies of other organisms. Motility is also an important diagnostic criterion in the differentiation of *Enterobacter cloacae,* which is motile from *Klebsiella pneumoniae,* which is nonmotile.

If the results of the screening tests suggest the presence of a *Salmonella* or *Shigella* strain, an agglutination test can be used to identify the genus of the organism and to determine whether it is a member of group A, B, C, or D.

Table 18–5. Agar reactions.

Reactions[1]				Representative Genera
Slant	Butt	Gas	H$_2$S	
Acid	Acid	+	−	*Escherichia, Enterobacter, Klebsiella*
Alkaline	Acid	−	−	*Shigella, Serratia*
Alkaline	Acid	+	+	*Salmonella, Proteus*
Alkaline	Alkaline	−	−	*Pseudomonas*[2]

[1]Acid production causes the phenol red indicator to turn a yellow color; the indicator is red under alkaline conditions. The presence of black FeS in the butt indicates H$_2$S production. Not every species within the various genera will give the above appearance on TSI agar. For example, some *Serratia* strains can ferment lactose slowly and give an acid reaction on the slant.
[2]*Pseudomonas,* although not a member of the Enterobacteriaceae, is included in this table because its reaction on TSI agar is a useful diagnostic criterion.

Coliforms & Public Health   Contamination of the public water supply system by sewage is detected by the presence of coliforms in the water. In a general sense, the term "coliform" includes not only *E coli* but also other inhabitants of the colon such as *Enterobacter* and *Klebsiella.* However, because only *E coli* is exclusively a large-intestine organism, whereas the others are found in the environment also, it is used as the indicator of fecal contamination. In water-quality testing, *E coli* is identified by its ability to ferment lactose with the production of acid and gas, its ability to grow at 44.5°C, and its characteristic colony type on EMB agar. An *E coli* colony count above 4/dL in municipal drinking water is indicative of unacceptable fecal contamination. Because *E coli* and the enteric pathogens are killed by chlorination of the drinking water, there is rarely a problem with meeting this standard. Disinfection of the public water supply is one of the most important advances of public health in this century.

Antibiotic Therapy   The appropriate treatment for infections caused by the Enterobacteriaceae and related organisms must be individually tailored to the antibiotic sensitivity of the organism. Generally speaking, a wide range of antimicrobial agents are potentially effective, eg, some penicillins and cephalosporins, aminoglycosides, chloramphenicol, tetracyclines, and sulfonamides. The specific choice usually depends upon the results of antibiotic sensitivity tests.

Pathogens Both Within and Outside the Enteric Tract

ESCHERICHIA

Diseases   *E coli* is the most common cause of urinary tract infections and gram-negative rod sepsis. It is one of the 2 important causes of neonatal meningitis and the agent most frequently associated with "traveler's diarrhea" (Tables 18–6 and 18–7).

Table 18–6. Gram-negative rods causing diarrhea.

Species	Fever	Leukocytes in Stool	Infective Dose	Typical Bacteriologic or Epidemiologic Findings
Enterotoxin-mediated				
1. *Escherichia coli*	–	–	?	Ferments lactose.
2. *Vibrio cholerae*	–	–	10^7	Comma-shaped organisms.
Invasive-inflammatory				
1. *Salmonella,* eg, *S typhimurium*	+	+	10^5	Does not ferment lactose.
2. *Shigella,* eg, *S dysenteriae*	+	+	10^4	Does not ferment lactose.
3. *Campylobacter jejuni*	+	+	10^4	Comma or gull-shaped organisms; growth at 42°C.
Mechanism uncertain				
1. *Vibrio parahaemolyticus*[1]	+	+	?	Transmitted by seafood.
2. *Yersinia enterocolitica*[1]	+	+	10^8	Usually transmitted from pets, eg, puppies.

[1]Some strains produce enterotoxin, but its pathogenetic role is not clear.

Important Properties   *E coli* is the most abundant facultative anaerobe in the colon and feces. It is, however, greatly outnumbered by the obligate anaerobes such as *Bacteroides.*

E coli **ferments lactose,** a property that distinguishes it from the 2 major intestinal pathogens, *Shigella* and *Salmonella.* It has 3 antigens that are used to identify the organism in epidemiologic investigations: the O or cell wall antigen, the H or flagellar antigen, and the K or capsular antigen. Because there are more than 150 O, 50 H, and 90 K antigens, the various combinations result in more than 1000 antigenic types of *E coli.* Specific serotypes are associated with certain diseases, eg, O55 and O111 cause outbreaks of neonatal diarrhea.

Pathogenesis   *E coli* has several clearly identified components that contribute to its ability to cause disease: pili, a capsule, endotoxin, and 2 exotoxins (enterotoxins).

A. Intestinal Tract Infection: The first step is the adherence of the organism to the cells of the jejunum and ileum by means of **pili** that protrude from the bacterial surface. Once attached, the bacteria synthesize **enterotoxins** (exotoxins genetically determined by plasmids), which act on the cells of the jejunum and ileum to cause diarrhea. The toxins are strikingly cell-specific; the cells of the colon are not susceptible, probably because they lack receptors for the toxin. Enterotoxigenic strains of E coli can produce either or both of 2 enterotoxins.

(a) The high-molecular-weight, heat-labile toxin (LT) acts by stimulating **adenylate cyclase**. Both LT and cholera toxin act by catalyzing the addition of ADP-ribose to the coupling protein that stimulates the cyclase. The resultant increase in intracellular cyclic AMP (cAMP) concentration causes an outpouring of fluid, potassium, and chloride from the enterocytes.

(b) The other enterotoxin is a low-molecular-weight, heat-stable toxin (ST), which stimulates guanylate cyclase.

Table 18–7. Gram-negative rods causing urinary tract infection[1] or sepsis.[2]

Species	Lactose Fermented	Features of the Organism
Escherichia coli	+	Colonies show metallic sheen on EMB agar.
Enterobacter sp	+	Often nosocomial and drug-resistant.
Klebsiella pneumoniae	+	Has large mucoid capsule and hence viscous colonies.
Serratia marcescens	–	Some strains produce red pigment; often nosocomial and drug-resistant.
Proteus mirabilis	–	Motility causes "swarming" on agar; produces urease.
Pseudomonas aeruginosa	–	Blue-green pigment and fruity odor produced; usually nosocomial and drug-resistant.

[1]Diagnosed by quantitative culture of urine.
[2]Diagnosed by culture of blood or pus.

The enterotoxin-producing strains do not invade the intestinal mucosa. However, certain strains of *E coli* are enteropathogenic and cause disease not by enterotoxin formation but by invasion of the epithelium of the large intestine, causing bloody diarrhea (dysentery).

B. Systemic Infection: The other 2 structural components, the **capsule** and the **endotoxin**, play a more prominent role in the pathogenesis of systemic, rather than intestinal tract, disease. The capsular polysaccharide interferes with phagocytosis, thereby enhancing the organism's ability to cause infections in various organs. For example, *E coli* strains that cause neonatal meningitis usually have a specific capsular type called the K1 antigen. The endotoxin of *E coli* is the cell wall lipopolysaccharide that causes several features of gram-negative sepsis such as fever, hypotension, and disseminated intravascular coagulation.

Clinical Findings *E coli* causes a variety of diseases both within and outside the intestinal tract. It is the leading cause of community-acquired urinary tract infections. These occur primarily in women; this finding is attributed to 3 features that facilitate ascending infection into the bladder, namely a short urethra, the proximity of the urethra to the anus, and colonization of the vagina by members of the fecal flora. It is also the most frequent cause of nosocomial (hospital-acquired) urinary tract infections, which occur equally frequently in both men and women and are associated with the use of indwelling urinary catheters. Urinary tract infections can be limited to the bladder or extend up the collecting system to the kidneys. If only the bladder is involved, the disease is called cystitis, whereas infection of the kidney is called pyelonephritis. The most prominent symptoms of cystitis are pain (dysuria) and frequency of urination; pyelonephritis is characterized by fever, chills, and flank pain.

E coli is also a major cause, along with the group B streptococci, of neonatal meningitis. Exposure of the newborn to *E coli* and group B streptococci occurs during birth as a result of colonization of the vagina by these organisms in approximately 25% of pregnant women. *E coli* is the organism isolated most frequently from patients with hospital-acquired sepsis, which arises primarily from urinary, biliary, or peritoneal infections.

Diarrhea caused by enterotoxigenic *E coli* is usually self-limited and of short duration (1–3 days). It is frequently associated with travel (traveler's diarrhea, or ''turista''). Infection with enteropathogenic *E coli,* on the other hand, results in a dysenterylike syndrome characterized by bloody diarrhea, abdominal cramping, and fever similar to that caused by *Shigella.*

Laboratory Diagnosis Specimens suspected of containing enteric gram-negative rods such as *E coli* are grown initially on a blood agar plate and on a differential medium, such as EMB agar or MacConkey's agar. *E coli,* which ferments lactose, forms pink colonies, whereas lactose-negative organisms are colorless. On EMB agar, *E coli* colonies have a characteristic green sheen. Some of the important features that help to distinguish *E coli* from other lactose-fermenting gram-negative rods are as follows: (1) It produces indole from tryptophan, (2) it decarboxylates lysine, (3) it utilizes acetate as its only source of carbon, and (4) it is motile. The isolation of enterotoxigenic or enteropathogenic *E coli* from patients with diarrhea is not a routine diagnostic procedure.

Treatment Treatment of *E coli* infections depends on the site of disease and the resistance pattern of the specific isolate. For example, an uncomplicated lower urinary tract infection can be treated for just 1–3 days with an oral sulfonamide (either alone or in combination with trimethoprim) or an oral penicillin, eg, ampicillin. However, *E coli* sepsis requires treatment with parenteral antibiotics (eg, the aminoglycoside gentamicin) or a cephalosporin. For the treatment of neonatal meningitis, a combination of ampicillin and gentamicin is usually given. Antibiotic therapy is usually *not* indicated in *E coli* diarrheal diseases. However, administration of trimethoprim-sulfamethoxazole may shorten the duration of symptoms. Rehydration is typically all that is necessary in this self-limited disease.

Prevention There is no specific prevention for *E coli* infections, such as active or passive immunization. However, various general measures can be taken to prevent certain infections caused by *E coli* and other organisms. For example, the incidence of urinary tract infections can be lowered by the judicious use and prompt withdrawal of catheters and, in recurrent infections, by prolonged prophylaxis with urinary antiseptic drugs, eg, nitrofurantoin. Some cases of sepsis can be prevented by prompt removal of or switching the site of intravenous lines. Traveler's diarrhea can sometimes be prevented by the prophylactic use of doxycycline (a tetracycline), trimethoprim-sulfamethoxazole, or Pepto-Bismol. Caution regarding uncooked foods and unpurified water while traveling in certain countries is also advisable.

SALMONELLA

Diseases *Salmonella* species cause enterocolitis, enteric fevers such as typhoid fever, and septicemia with metastatic abscesses. They are one of the most common causes of bacterial enterocolitis in the USA.

Important Properties Salmonellae are gram-negative rods that **do not ferment lactose** but do produce H_2S—features that are used in their laboratory identification. Their antigens—cell wall O, flagellar H, and capsular Vi (virulence)—are important for taxonomic and epidemiologic purposes. The O antigens, which are the outer polysaccharides of the cell wall, are used to subdivide the salmonellae into groups A–I. There are 2 forms of the H antigens, phases 1 and 2. Only one of the 2 H proteins is synthesized at any one time, depending on which gene sequence is in the correct alignment for transcription into mRNA. The Vi antigens are used primarily for the typing of *S typhi*, the agent of typhoid fever.

There are 2 methods for naming the salmonellae. Ewing divides the genus into 3 species: *S typhi*, *Salmonella choleraesuis*, and *Salmonella enteritidis*. In this scheme there is one serotype in each of the first 2 species and 1500 serotypes in the third. Kaufman and White assign different species names to each serotype; there are roughly 1500 different species, usually named for the city in which they were isolated. *Salmonella dublin* according to Kaufman and White would be *S enteritidis* serotype *dublin* according to Ewing. Both forms are used in the literature; the Centers for Disease Control use the Ewing system.

Pathogenesis & Epidemiology The 3 types of *Salmonella* infections (enterocolitis, enteric fevers, and septicemia) have different pathogenetic features.

(a) Enterocolitis is characterized by an invasion of the epithelial and subepithelial tissue of the small and large intestines. Strains that do not invade do not cause disease. The organisms penetrate both through and between the mucosal cells into the lamina propria, with resulting inflammation and diarrhea. A polymorphonuclear leukocyte response limits the infection to the gut and the adjacent mesenteric lymph nodes; bacteremia is infrequent in enterocolitis. In contrast to *Shigella* enterocolitis, in which the infectious dose is very small (on the order of 10 organisms), the dose of *Salmonella* required is much higher, at least 100,000 organisms. Gastric acid is an important host defense; gastrectomy or use of antacids lowers the infectious dose significantly.

(b) In **typhoid** and other enteric fevers, infection begins in the small intestine but few gastrointestinal symptoms occur. The organisms enter, multiply in the mononuclear phagocytes of Peyer's patches, and then spread to the phagocytes of the liver, gallbladder, and spleen. This leads to bacteremia, which is associated with the onset of fever and other symptoms, probably due to endotoxin. Survival and growth of the organism in phagocytic cells are a striking feature of this disease, as is the predilection for invasion of the gallbladder, which can result in establishment of the carrier state and excretion of the bacteria in the feces for long periods.

(c) Septicemia accounts for only about 5–10% of *Salmonella* infections and occurs in one of 2 settings: a patient with an underlying chronic disease such as sickle cell anemia or cancer or a child with enterocolitis. The septic course is more indolent than that with many other gram-negative rods. Bacteremia results in the seeding of many organs, with osteomyelitis, pneumonia, and meningitis as the most common sequelae. Previously damaged tissues, such as infarcts and aneurysms, are the most frequent sites of metastatic abscesses.

The epidemiology of *Salmonella* infections is related to the ingestion of food and water contaminated by human and animal wastes. *S typhi*, the cause of typhoid fever, is **transmitted only by humans**, but all other species have a significant animal as well as human reservoir. Human sources are either persons who temporarily excrete the organism during or shortly after an attack of enterocolitis or chronic carriers who excrete the organism for years. The most frequent **animal source is poultry and dried eggs**, but meat products that are inadequately cooked have been implicated as well. Dogs and other pets, including turtles, are additional sources.

Clinical Findings After an incubation period of 6–48 hours, symptoms begin with nausea and vomiting and then progress to abdominal pain and diarrhea, which can vary from mild to severe, with or without blood. Usually the disease lasts a few days, is self-limited, causes nonbloody diarrhea, and does not require medical care except in the very young and very old. The most common cause of enterocolitis is *Salmonella typhimurium*, but virtually every species has been implicated.

In typhoid fever, caused by *S typhi*, and in enteric fever, caused by organisms such as *Salmonella paratyphi* A, B, and C (*S paratyphi* B and C are also known as *Salmonella schottmuelleri* and *Salmonella hirschfeldii*, respectively), the onset of illness is slow, with fever and constipation rather than vomiting and diarrhea predominating. After the first week, as the bacteremia becomes sustained, high fever, delirium, tender abdomen, and enlarged spleen occur. "**Rose spots**," ie, rose-colored papules on the abdomen, are associated with typhoid fever but occur only rarely. The disease begins to resolve by the third week, but severe complications such as intestinal hemorrhage or perforation can occur. About 3% of typhoid fever patients become chronic carriers. The carrier rate is higher among women, especially those with previous gall bladder disease.

Septicemia is most often caused by *S choleraesuis*. The symptoms begin with fever but little or no enterocolitis and then proceed to focal symptoms associated with the affected organ, frequently bone, lung, or meninges.

Laboratory Diagnosis   In enterocolitis, the organism is most easily isolated from a stool sample. However, in the enteric fevers, a blood culture is the procedure most likely to reveal the organism during the first 2 weeks of illness.

Salmonellae form non-lactose-fermenting (colorless) colonies on MacConkey's or EMB agar. On TSI agar, an alkaline slant and an acid butt, frequently with both gas and H_2S (black color in the butt), are produced. *S typhi* is the major exception; it does not form gas and produces only a small amount of H_2S. If the organism is urease-negative (*Proteus* organisms, which can produce a similar reaction on TSI agar, are urease-positive), the *Salmonella* can be identified and grouped by the slide agglutination test. Definitive serotyping of the O, H, and Vi antigens is done by special public health laboratories for epidemiologic purposes. Salmonellosis is a notifiable disease, and an investigation to determine its source should be undertaken. In certain cases of enteric fever and sepsis, when the organism may be difficult to recover, the diagnosis can be made serologically by detecting a rise in antibody titer in the patient's serum (Widal test).

Treatment   Enterocolitis is usually a self-limited disease that resolves without treatment. Fluid and electrolyte replacement may be required. Antibiotic treatment does not shorten the illness or reduce the symptoms; in fact, it may prolong excretion of the organisms, increase the frequency of the carrier state, and select mutants resistant to the antibiotic. Antimicrobial agents are indicated only for neonates or persons with chronic diseases who are at risk of septicemia and disseminated abscesses. Drugs that retard intestinal motility (ie, that reduce diarrhea) appear to prolong the duration of symptoms and the fecal excretion of the organisms.

The treatment of choice for enteric fevers and septicemia is either ampicillin or chloramphenicol. Ampicillin should be used in patients who are chronic carriers of *S typhi*. Cholecystectomy may be necessary to abolish the chronic carrier state. Focal abscesses should be drained surgically whenever feasible.

Prevention   *Salmonella* infections are prevented mainly by public health and personal hygiene measures. Proper sewage treatment, a chlorinated water supply that is monitored for contamination by coliform bacteria, cultures of stool samples from food handlers to detect carriers, hand washing prior to food handling, pasteurization of milk, and proper cooking of poultry and meat are all important.

A vaccine is available that confers some protection against *S typhi* but not against *S paratyphi* A and B serotypes. The preferred vaccine consists of acetone-killed *S typhi* organisms only. A booster dose is indicated every 3 years in endemic areas. The protection is relative and can be overcome by a large dose of organisms.

Pathogens Primarily Within the Enteric Tract

SHIGELLA

Disease   *Shigella* species cause enterocolitis (dysentery).

Important Properties   Shigellae are **non-lactose-fermenting**, gram-negative rods that can be distinguished from salmonellae by 3 criteria: they produce no gas from the fermentation of glucose, they **do not produce H₂S**, and they are **nonmotile**. All shigellae have O antigens (polysaccharide) in their cell walls, and these antigens are used to divide the genus into 4 groups: A, B, C, and D.

Pathogenesis & Epidemiology   Shigellae are the most effective pathogens among the enteric bacteria. Ingestion of as few as 10 organisms causes disease in 10% of healthy volunteers, whereas at least 10^5 *Vibrio cholerae* or *Salmonella* organisms are required to produce symptoms.

Shigellosis is only **a human disease**.* The organism is transmitted from person to person, usually by asymptomatic carriers. The 4 F's—fingers, flies, food, and feces—are the principal factors in transmission. Food-borne outbreaks outnumber water-borne outbreaks by 2 to 1. Outbreaks occur in day-care nurseries and in mental hospitals, where **fecal-oral** transmission is likely to occur. Children under 10 years of age account for approximately half of *Shigella*-positive stool cultures.

Shigellae, which cause disease almost exclusively in the gastrointestinal tract, produce bloody diarrhea (dysentery) by invading the mucosa of the distal ileum and colon. Local inflammation accompanied by ulceration occurs, but the organisms rarely penetrate the wall or enter the bloodstream, unlike salmonellae. Although the organisms produce an enterotoxin, it is thought that invasion is the critical factor in pathogenesis. The evidence for this is that mutants that fail to produce enterotoxin but are invasive can still cause disease, whereas noninvasive mutants are nonpathogenic.

Clinical Findings   After an incubation period of 1–4 days, symptoms begin with fever and abdominal cramps, followed by diarrhea, which may be watery at first but later contains blood and mucus. The disease varies from mild to severe depending on 2 major factors: the species of *Shigella* and the age of the patient, with young children and elderly people being the most severely affected. *Shigella dysenteriae,* which causes the most severe disease, is usually seen in the USA only in travelers returning from abroad. *Shigella sonnei,* which causes mild disease, is isolated from approximately 75% of all individuals with shigellosis in the USA. The diarrhea frequently resolves in 2 or 3 days; in severe cases, antibiotics can shorten the course. Serum agglutinins appear after recovery but are not protective, because the organism does not enter the blood. The role of intestinal IgA in protection is uncertain.

Laboratory Diagnosis   Shigellae form non-lactose-fermenting (colorless) colonies on MacConkey's or EMB agar. On TSI agar, they cause an alkaline slant and an acid butt, with no gas and no H₂S. Confirmation of the organism as *Shigella* and determination of its group are done by slide agglutination.

One important adjunct to laboratory diagnosis is methylene blue stain of a fecal sample to determine whether PMNs are present. If they are found, an invasive organism such as *Shigella, Salmonella,* or *Campylobacter* is involved rather than a toxin-producing organism such as *V cholerae, E coli,* or *Clostridium perfringens.* (Certain viruses and the parasite *Entamoeba histolytica* can also cause diarrhea without PMNs in the stool.)

Treatment   The main treatment for shigellosis is fluid and electrolyte replacement. In mild cases, no antibiotics are indicated; in severe cases, either trimethoprim-sulfamethoxazole or ampicillin is the drug of choice, but the occurrence of plasmids conveying multiple drug resistance is high enough that antibiotic sensitivity tests must be performed. Antiperistaltic drugs are contraindicated in shigellosis, because they prolong the fever, diarrhea, and excretion of the organism.

Prevention   Prevention of shigellosis is dependent on interruption of fecal-oral transmission by proper sewage disposal, chlorination of water, and personal hygiene (hand washing by food handlers). There is no vaccine, and prophylactic antibiotics are not recommended.

---

*However, some primates, such as monkeys, contract shigellosis but have little impact on the epidemiology of the disease in humans.

VIBRIO

Diseases   *Vibrio cholerae,* the major pathogen in this genus, is the cause of cholera. *Vibrio parahaemolyticus* causes diarrhea associated with eating raw or improperly cooked seafood.

Important Properties   Vibrios are curved, "**comma-shaped**" gram-negative rods. *V cholerae* is divided into 2 groups according to the nature of its O cell wall antigen. Members of the O1 group cause epidemic disease, whereas non-O1 organisms either cause sporadic disease or are nonpathogens. The O1 organisms have 2 biotypes, called El Tor and cholerae; and 3 serotypes, called Ogawa, Inaba, and Hikojima. (Biotypes are based on differences in biochemical reactions, whereas serotypes are based on antigenic differences.) These features are used to characterize isolates in epidemiologic investigations.

V parahaemolyticus is primarily a **marine** organism adapted to life in the high-salt concentration of the ocean. For growth in the laboratory, it requires at least 2% NaCl in the medium (human serum contains 0.9% NaCl). There are 11 O antigen serotypes; no serotype is the predominant pathogen.

1. Vibrio cholerae

Pathogenesis & Epidemiology   *V cholerae* infects **only humans** and is transmitted by **fecal contamination** of water and food. Human carriers are frequently asymptomatic and include individuals who are either in the incubation period or convalescing.

The most recent epidemic of cholera, which spanned the 1960s and 1970s, began in Southeast Asia and spread over 3 continents to areas of Africa, Europe, and the rest of Asia. The organism isolated most frequently was the El Tor biotype of O1 *V cholerae,* usually of the Ogawa serotype. The factors that predispose to epidemics are poor sanitation, malnutrition, overcrowding, and inadequate medical services. Quarantine measures failed to prevent the spread of the disease, because there were many asymptomatic carriers.

The pathogenesis of cholera is dependent on colonization of the small intestine by the organism and secretion of enterotoxin. For colonization to occur, large numbers of bacteria, approximately 1 billion, must be ingested, because the organism is particularly sensitive to stomach acid. Persons with little or no stomach acid, such as those taking antacids or those who have had a gastrectomy, are much more susceptible. Adherence to the cells of the brush border of the gut, which is a requirement for colonization, is related to secretion of the bacterial enzyme mucinase, which dissolves the protective glycoprotein coating over the intestinal cells.

After adhering, the organism multiples and secretes an **enterotoxin** called choleragen. This exotoxin can reproduce the symptoms of cholera even in the absence of the *Vibrio* organisms. Choleragen first binds to a sialic acid-containing ganglioside receptor on the surface of the enterocyte and then catalyzes the addition of ADP-ribose to the coupling protein, resulting in the activation of **adenylate cyclase**. The increase in cAMP stimulates a secretion of chloride ion and water, leading to a massive watery diarrhea without inflammatory cells. Morbidity and death are due to dehydration and electrolyte imbalance. However, if treatment is instituted promptly, the disease runs a self-limited course in up to 7 days.

Non-O1 *V cholerae* is an occasional cause of diarrhea associated with eating shellfish obtained from the coastal waters of the USA.

Clinical Findings   Watery diarrhea in large volumes is the hallmark of cholera. The "**rice-water**" stool is the classic description applied to the nonbloody effluent, because it resembles water in which rice has been cooked. There is no abdominal pain, and subsequent symptoms are referable to the marked dehydration. The loss of fluid and electrolytes leads to cardiac and renal failure. Acidosis and hypokalemia also occur as a result of loss of bicarbonate and potassium in the stool. The mortality rate without treatment is 40%.

Laboratory Diagnosis   The approach to laboratory diagnosis depends on the situation. During an epidemic, a clinical judgment is made and there is little need for the laboratory. In an endemic area or for the detection of carriers, a variety of selective media* that are not in

---

*Media such as thiosulfate-citrate-bile salts agar or tellurite-taurocholate-gelatin are used.

common use in the USA are used in the laboratory. For diagnosis of sporadic cases in this country, a culture of the diarrhea stool containing *V cholerae* will show colorless colonies on MacConkey's agar because lactose is fermented slowly. The organism is oxidase-positive, which distinguishes it from the Enterobacteriaceae. On TSI agar, an acid slant and an acid butt without gas or H_2S are seen because the organism ferments sucrose. A presumptive diagnosis of *V cholerae* can be confirmed by agglutination of the organism by polyvalent O1 or non-O1 antiserum. A retrospective diagnosis can be made serologically by detecting a rise in antibody titer in acute- and convalescent-phase sera.

Treatment D The treatment for cholera consists of prompt, adequate replacement of water and electrolytes, either orally or intravenously. Antibiotics such as tetracycline are not necessary, but they do shorten the duration of symptoms and reduce the time of excretion of the organisms.

Prevention Prevention is achieved mainly by public health measures that ensure a clean water and food supply. The vaccine, composed of killed organisms, has limited usefulness; it is only 50% effective in preventing disease for 3–6 months and does not interrupt transmission. The use of tetracycline for prevention is effective in close contacts but cannot prevent the spread of a major epidemic. Prompt detection of carriers is important in limiting outbreaks.

2. **Vibrio parahaemolyticus** *V parahaemolyticus* is a marine organism transmitted by **contaminated seafood**. It is a major cause of diarrhea in Japan, where raw fish is eaten in large quantities, but is an infrequent pathogen in the USA, although several outbreaks have occurred aboard cruise ships in the Caribbean. Little is known about its pathogenesis, except that an enterotoxin similar to choleragen is secreted and limited invasion sometimes occurs.

The clinical picture caused by *V parahaemolyticus* varies from mild to quite severe watery diarrhea, nausea and vomiting, abdominal cramps, and fever. The illness is self-limited, lasting about 3 days. *V parahaemolyticus* can be distinguished from *V cholerae* mainly on the basis of growth in NaCl: *V parahaemolyticus* grows in 8% NaCl solution (as befits a marine organism), whereas *V cholerae* does not. No specific treatment is indicated, because the disease is relatively mild and self-limited. Disease can be prevented by proper refrigeration and cooking of seafood.

CAMPYLOBACTER

Diseases *Campylobacter* is a frequent cause of enterocolitis, especially in children, and a rare cause of systemic infection, particularly bacteremia.

Important Properties Campylobacters are curved, gram-negative rods that appear either **comma- or S-shaped.** They are **microaerophilic,** growing best in 5% oxygen rather than the 20% present in the atmosphere. *Campylobacter jejuni* grows well at 42 °C, whereas *Campylobacter intestinalis** does not—an observation that is useful in microbiologic diagnosis.

Pathogenesis & Epidemiology **Domestic animals** such as cattle, chickens, and dogs serve as a source of the organisms for humans. Person-to-person transmission is usually **fecal-oral**, particularly among small children. *C jejuni* is a major cause of diarrhea in the USA; it was recovered in 4.6% of patients with diarrhea, compared with 2.3 and 1% for *Salmonella* and *Shigella,* respectively.

The pathogenesis of both the enterocolitis and the systemic diseases is unclear. The presence of watery diarrhea suggests an enterotoxin-mediated syndrome, but no enterotoxin has been demonstrated. Invasion often occurs, accompanied by blood in stools, Systemic infections, eg, bacteremia, occur most often in neonates or debilitated adults.

Clinical Findings Enterocolitis, caused primarily by *C jejuni,* begins as watery, foul-smelling diarrhea followed by bloody stools accompanied by fever and severe abdominal pain. The pain is periumbilical and can resemble that of appendicitis.

---

*Also known as *Campylobacter fetus* subsp *fetus.*

Systemic infections, most commonly bacteremia, are caused by *C intestinalis*. The symptoms of bacteremia, eg, fever and malaise, are associated with no diagnostic physical findings. Stillbirths and neonatal sepsis occur in offspring whose mothers were infected during pregnancy.

Laboratory Diagnosis   If the patient has diarrhea, a stool specimen is cultured on a blood agar plate containing antibiotics* that inhibit most other fecal flora. The plate is incubated at 42 °C in a microaerophilic atmosphere containing 5% oxygen and 10% carbon dioxide, which favors the growth of *C jejuni*. It is identified by failure to grow at 25 °C, oxidase positivity, and sensitivity to nalidixic acid. If bacteremia is suspected, a blood culture incubated under standard temperature and atmospheric conditions will reveal the growth of the characteristically S-shaped, motile, gram-negative rods. Identification of the organism as *C intestinalis* is confirmed by its failure to grow at 42°C, its ability to grow at 25 °C, and its resistance to nalidixic acid.

Treatment   Erythromycin is used successfully in *C jejuni* enterocolitis. The treatment of choice for *C intestinalis* bacteremia is an aminoglycoside.

Prevention   There is no vaccine or other specific preventive measure. Proper sewage disposal and personal hygiene (hand washing) are important.

Pathogens Outside the Enteric Tract

KLEBSIELLA-ENTEROBACTER-SERRATIA GROUP

Diseases   These organisms are usually opportunistic pathogens that cause nosocomial infections, especially pneumonia and urinary tract infections. *Klebsiella pneumoniae* is an important respiratory tract pathogen outside hospitals as well.

Important Properties   *K pneumoniae*, *E cloacae*, and *Serratia marcescens* are the species most often involved in human infections. They are frequently found in the **large intestine** but are also present in soil and water. These organisms have very similar properties and are usually distinguished on the basis of several biochemical reactions and motility. *K pneumoniae* has a **very large capsule**, which gives its colonies a striking mucoid appearance.

Pathogenesis & Epidemiology   Of the 3 organisms, *K pneumoniae* is most likely to be a primary, nonopportunistic pathogen; this property is related to its antiphagocytic capsule. Although this organism is a primary pathogen, patients with *K pneumoniae* infections frequently have predisposing conditions such as advanced age, chronic respiratory disease, diabetes, or alcoholism. The organism is carried in the respiratory tracts of about 10% of normal people, who are prone to pneumonia if host defenses are lowered.

Enterobacter and *Serratia* infections are clearly related to hospitalization, especially to invasive procedures such as intravenous catheterization, respiratory intubation, and urinary tract manipulations. In addition, outbreaks of *Serratia* pneumonia have been associated with contamination of the water in respiratory therapy devices. Prior to the extensive use of these procedures, *S marcescens* was a harmless organism most frequently isolated from environmental sources such as water. Because certain strains produce easily recognized red-pigmented colonies, the organism was intentionally introduced into the air and water many years ago as a marker in epidemiologic and engineering studies.

As with many other gram-negative rods, the pathogenesis of septic shock caused by these organisms is related to the endotoxins in their cell walls.

Clinical Findings   Urinary tract infections and pneumonia are the usual clinical entities associated with these 3 bacteria, but bacteremia and secondary spread to other areas such as

---

*For example, Skirrow's medium contains vancomycin, trimethoprim, cephalothin, polymyxin, and amphotericin B.

the meninges occur. It is difficult to distinguish infections caused by these organisms on clinical grounds, with the exception of pneumonia caused by *Klebsiella,* which produces a thick, bloody sputum and can progress to necrosis and abscess formation.

There are 2 other species of *Klebsiella* that cause unusual human infections rarely seen in the USA. *Klebsiella ozaenae* is associated with atrophic rhinitis, and *Klebsiella rhinoscleromatis* causes a destructive granuloma of the nose and pharynx.

Laboratory Diagnosis   Organisms of this group produce lactose-fermenting (colored) colonies on differential agar such as MacConkey's or EMB, although *Serratia,* which is a late lactose fermenter, can give a negative reaction. These organisms are separated by the use of biochemical tests.

Treatment   Because the antibiotic resistance of these organisms can vary greatly, the choice of drug depends on the results of sensitivity testing. Isolates from hospital-acquired infections are frequently resistant to multiple antibiotics. An aminoglycoside such as gentamicin, tobramycin, or amikacin, together with a cephalosporin, is used empirically until the results of testing are known.

Prevention   Some hospital-acquired infections caused by gram-negative rods can be prevented by such general measures as changing the site of intravenous catheters, removing urinary catheters when they are no longer needed, and taking proper care of respiratory therapy devices. There is no vaccine.

PROTEUS-PROVIDENCIA-MORGANELLA GROUP

Diseases   These organisms primarily cause urinary tract infections, both community- and hospital-acquired.

Important Properties   These gram-negative rods are distinguished from other Enterobacteriaceae by their ability to produce the enzyme phenylalanine deaminase. In addition, they produce the enzyme **urease**, which cleaves urea to form NH_3 and CO_2. Certain species are very motile and produce a striking "**swarming**" effect on blood agar, characterized by expanding rings (waves) of organisms over the surface of the agar.

The cell wall O antigens of certain strains of *Proteus,* such as OX-2, OX-19, and OX-K, cross-react with antigens of several species of rickettsiae. These *Proteus* antigens can be used in laboratory tests to detect the presence of antibodies against certain rickettsiae in patients' serum. This test, called the Weil-Felix reaction after its originators, is being used less frequently as more specific procedures are found.

In the past, there were 4 medically important species of *Proteus.* However, molecular studies of DNA relatedness showed that 2 of the 4 were significantly different. These species have been renamed: *Proteus morganii* is now *Morganella morganii,* and *Proteus rettgeri* is now *Providencia rettgeri.* In the clinical laboratory, these organisms are distinguished from *Proteus vulgaris and Proteus mirabilis* on the basis of several biochemical tests.

Pathogenesis & Epidemiology   The organisms are present in the **human colon** as well as in soil and water. Their tendency to cause urinary tract infections is probably due to their presence in the colon and to colonization of the urethra, especially in women. The vigorous motility of *Proteus* organisms may contribute to their ability to invade the urinary tract.

Production of the enzyme urease is an important feature of the pathogenesis of urinary tract infections by this group. Urease hydrolyzes the urea in urine to form ammonia, which raises the pH and encourages the formation of stones (calculi) composed of calcium and magnesium hydroxides. Because alkaline urine also favors growth of the organisms and more extensive renal damage, treatment involves keeping the urine at a low pH.

Clinical Findings   The signs and symptoms of urinary tract infections caused by these organisms cannot be distinguished from those caused by *E coli* or other Enterobacteriaceae. *Proteus* species can also cause pneumonia, wound infections, and septicemia. *P mirabilis* is the species of *Proteus* that causes most community- and hospital-acquired infections, but *P rettgeri* is emerging as an important agent of nosocomial infections.

Laboratory Diagnosis   These organisms usually are highly motile and produce a "swarming" overgrowth on blood agar, which can frustrate efforts to recover pure cultures of other organisms. Growth on blood agar containing phenylethyl alcohol inhibits swarming, thus allowing isolated colonies of *Proteus* and other organisms to be obtained. They produce non-lactose-fermenting (colorless) colonies on MacConkey's or EMB agar. *P vulgaris* and *P mirabilis* produce H_2S, which blackens the butt of TSI agar, whereas neither *M morganii* nor *P rettgeri* does. These 4 medically important species are urease-positive. Identification of these organisms in the clinical laboratory is based on a variety of biochemical reactions.

Treatment   Most strains are sensitive to aminoglycosides and trimethoprim-sulfamethoxazole, but because individual isolates can vary, antibiotic sensitivity tests should be performed. *P mirabilis* is the species most frequently sensitive to ampicillin. *P rettgeri* is frequently resistant to multiple antibiotics.

Prevention   There are no specific preventive measures, but many hospital-acquired urinary tract infections can be prevented by prompt removal of urinary catheters.

PSEUDOMONAS

Diseases   *Pseudomonas aeruginosa* causes infections (eg, sepsis, pneumonia, and urinary tract infections) primarily in patients with lowered host defenses. *Pseudomonas cepacia* and *Pseudomonas maltophilia* also cause these infections but much less frequently. *Pseudomonas pseudomallei*, the cause of melioidosis, is described in Chapter 27.

Important Properties   Pseudomonads are gram-negative rods that resemble the Enterobacteriaceae but differ in that they are strict aerobes; ie, they derive their energy only by oxidation of sugars rather than by fermentation. Because they do not ferment glucose, they are called "**nonfermenters**," in contrast to the Enterobacteriaceae, which do ferment glucose. Oxidation involves electron transport by cytochrome C, ie, they are **oxidase-positive**.

Pseudomonads are able to grow in **water** containing only traces of nutrients, eg, tap water, and this favors their persistence in the hospital environment. *P aeruginosa* and *P cepacia* have a remarkable ability to withstand disinfectants, accounting in part for their role in hospital-acquired infections. They have been found growing in hexachlorophene-containing soap solutions, in antiseptics, and in detergents.

P aeruginosa produces 2 pigments useful in clinical and laboratory diagnosis: (1) **pyocyanin**, which can color the pus in a wound blue; and (2) pyoverdin (fluorescein), a yellow-green pigment that fluoresces under ultraviolet light, a property that can be used in the early detection of skin infection in burn patients. In the laboratory, these pigments diffuse into the agar, imparting a blue-green color that is useful in identification. *P aeruginosa* is the only species of *Pseudomonas* that synthesizes pyocyanin.

Pathogenesis & Epidemiology   *P aeruginosa* is found chiefly in soil and water, although approximately 10% of people carry it in the normal flora of the colon. It is found on the skin in moist areas and can colonize the upper respiratory tract of hospitalized patients. Its ability to grow in simple aqueous solutions has resulted in contamination of respiratory therapy and anesthesia equipment, intravenous fluids, and even distilled water.

P aeruginosa is primarily an opportunistic pathogen that causes infections in hospitalized patients, eg, those with extensive burns, in which the skin host defenses are destroyed; those with chronic respiratory disease (eg, cystic fibrosis), in which the normal clearance mechanisms are impaired; those who are immunosuppressed; those with neutrophil counts of less than 500/µL; and those with indwelling catheters. It causes 10–20% of hospital-acquired infections.

Both endotoxin and an exotoxin play important roles in pathogenesis. *P aeruginosa* produces exotoxin A, which inhibits eukaryotic protein synthesis by the same mechanism as diphtheria exotoxin, namely ADP ribosylation of elongation factor 2. The 2 pigments, pyocyanin and fluorescein, are nontoxic.

Clinical Findings   *P aeruginosa* can cause infections virtually anywhere in the body, but urinary tract infections, pneumonia, and wound infections (especially burns) predominate.

From these sites, the organism can enter the blood, causing sepsis. Patients with *P aeruginosa* sepsis have a mortality rate of over 50%. A severe external otitis and other skin lesions occur in users of swimming pools and hot tubs in which the chlorination is inadequate.

Laboratory Diagnosis   *P aeruginosa* grows as non-lactose-fermenting (colorless) colonies on MacConkey's or EMB agar. It is **oxidase-positive**. A typical metallic sheen of the growth on TSI agar, coupled with the blue-green pigment on ordinary nutrient agar and a fruity aroma, is sufficient to make a presumptive diagnosis. The diagnosis is confirmed by biochemical reactions. Identification for epidemiologic purposes is done by bacteriophage or pyocin* typing.

Treatment   Because *P aeruginosa* is resistant to many antibiotics, treatment must be tailored to the sensitivity of each isolate and monitored frequently; resistant strains can emerge during therapy. Several new antibiotics have enhanced activity against *P aeruginosa;* these include azlocillin (a penicillin) and ceftazidime (a cephalosporin). They are usually administered with an aminoglycoside.

Prevention   Prevention of *P aeruginosa* infections involves keeping neutrophil counts above 500/μL, removing indwelling catheters promptly, taking special care of burned skin, and taking other similar measures to limit infection in patients with reduced host defenses.

BACTEROIDES

Diseases   *Bacteroides* is the most common cause of serious anaerobic infections, eg, sepsis, peritonitis, and abscesses. *Bacteroides fragilis* is the most frequent pathogen.

Important Properties   *Bacteroides* organisms are anaerobic, non-spore-forming, gram-negative rods. Of the 22 species of *Bacteroides,* 3 are human pathogens: *B fragilis,*[†] *Bacteroides melaninogenicus,* and *Bacteroides corrodens.*

Members of the *B fragilis* group are the predominant organisms in the human colon, numbering approximately 10^{11}/g of feces, and are found in the vaginas of approximately 60% of women. *B melaninogenicus* and *B corrodens* occur primarily in the oral cavity.

Pathogenesis & Epidemiology   Because *Bacteroides* species are part of the normal flora, **infections are endogenous**, usually arising from a break in a mucosal surface, and are not communicable. These organisms cause a variety of infections, such as local abscesses at the site of a mucosal break, metastatic abscesses by hematogenous spread to distant organs, or lung abscesses by aspiration of oral flora.

Predisposing factors such as surgery, trauma, and chronic disease play an important role in pathogenesis. Local tissue necrosis, impaired blood supply, and growth of facultative anaerobes at the site contribute to anaerobic infections. The facultative anaerobes, such as *E coli,* utilize the oxygen, thereby reducing it to a level that allows the anaerobic *Bacteroides* strains to grow. As a result, many anaerobic infections contain mixed facultative and anaerobic flora. This has important implications for therapy; both the facultative anaerobes and the anaerobes should be treated.

The polysaccharide capsule of *B fragilis* is an important virulence factor. Many of the symptoms of *Bacteroides* sepsis resemble those of sepsis caused by bacteria with endotoxin, but the lipopolysaccharide of *Bacteroides* is chemically different from the typical endotoxin. No exotoxins have been found.

Clinical Findings   The *B fragilis* group of organisms is most frequently associated with intra-abdominal infections, either peritonitis or localized abscesses. Pelvic abscesses and bacteremia occur as well. Oral, pharyngeal, and pulmonary abscesses are more commonly

---

*A pyocin is a type of bacteriocin produced by *P aeruginosa*. Different strains produce various pyocins, which can serve to distinguish the organisms.

†*B fragilis* is divided into 5 subspecies, the most important of which is *B fragilis* subsp *fragilis*. The other 4 subspecies are *B fragilis* subspp *distasonis, ovatus, thetaiotaomicron,* and *vulgatus.* It is proper, therefore, to speak of the *B fragilis* group rather than simply *B fragilis*.

caused by *B melaninogenicus,* a member of the normal oral flora, but *B fragilis* is found in about 25% of lung abscesses.

Laboratory Diagnosis *Bacteroides* species can be isolated anaerobically on blood agar plates containing kanamycin and vancomycin to inhibit unwanted organisms. They are identified by biochemical reactions (eg, sugar fermentations) and by production of certain organic acids (eg, formic, acetic, and propionic acids), which are detected by gas chromatography.

Treatment Members of the *B fragilis* group are resistant to penicillins, first-generation cephalosporins, and aminoglycosides, making them among the most antibiotic-resistant of the anaerobic bacteria. Clindamycin is the drug of choice, with cefoxitin, metronidazole, and chloramphenicol as alternatives. Aminoglycosides are frequently combined to treat the facultative gram-negative rods in mixed infections. *B melaninogenicus,* by contrast, is highly susceptible to penicillin G, which is the drug of choice. Surgical drainage of abscesses usually accompanies antibiotic therapy, but lung abscesses often heal without drainage.

Prevention Prevention of *Bacteroides* infections centers on perioperative administration of a cephalosporin, frequently cefoxitin, for abdominal or pelvic surgery. There is no vaccine.

Review Questions

1. What are the important characteristics of the Enterobacteriaceae?
2. What are the differences between the O and H antigens of the Enterobacteriaceae?
3. What is the importance of lactose fermentation in distinguishing between certain members of the Enterobacteriaceae?
4. Why is the incidence of urinary tract infections caused by *Escherichia coli* higher in women than in men?
5. *E coli* is one of the 2 main causes of neonatal meningitis. What predisposes to this disease?
6. What is the pathogenesis of *E coli*-induced diarrhea?
7. *E coli* sepsis is frequently accompanied by shock. What is the pathogenesis of the shock?
8. Salmonellae can change their flagellar antigens by DNA rearrangement. What is the pathogenetic significance of this?
9. Is *Salmonella* enterocolitis caused by toxins or by invasion of the gut epithelium?
10. Is the infectious dose of *Salmonella* higher or lower than that of *Shigella?*
11. What is the pathogenesis of typhoid fever?
12. Where are salmonellae found in nature, and how are they transmitted?
13. In enteric fevers caused by salmonellae, what are the 2 most important cultures to perform?
14. What measures are appropriate to prevent *Salmonella* infections?
15. What is the natural habitat and mode of transmission for shigellae?
16. Is *Shigella* enterocolitis caused by toxins or by invasion of the gut epithelium? Are fecal leukocytes usually found in shigellosis?
17. What is the appearance of *Vibrio cholerae* on Gram's stain?
18. What is the mode of action of cholera toxin?
19. Does cholera occur in the USA? in developing countries?
20. What is the relative importance of fluid and electrolyte replacement and of antibiotics in the treatment of cholera?
21. What is the appearance of *Campylobacter* on Gram's stain?
22. What is the natural reservoir for *Campylobacter?* What is its mode of transmission?
23. How can *Campylobacter* infections be prevented?
24. Why are *Klebsiella, Enterobacter,* and *Serratia* grouped together? In general, which of these 3 generally cause(s) opportunistic infections?
25. *Klebsiella pneumoniae* has a very prominent capsule. What are 2 important functions of this capsule?
26. The O antigens of certain *Proteus* strains cross-react with which organisms in the Weil-Felix test?
27. *Proteus* species resemble *Salmonella* species on TSI agar but can be distinguished by the production of which enzyme?

28. *Proteus* species are motile and produce urease. How might these features contribute to pathogenesis?
29. *Pseudomonas* is not a member of the Enterobacteriaceae. What is the major metabolic feature that accounts for this?
30. Pus from wound infections caused by *Pseudomonas aeruginosa* can be blue. Why?
31. In the hospital, *P aeruginosa* is usually found in what environment?
32. Does a neutrophil count of less than 500µL predispose to *P aeruginosa* infection? Is the organism an opportunist?
33. What is the natural habitat of *Bacteroides fragilis?*
34. Why do an impaired blood supply and the presence of E *coli* contribute to infection by *B fragilis?*
35. *B fragilis* infections frequently do not respond to penicillin G. Why?

19 Gram-Negative Rods Related to the Respiratory Tract

There are 3 medically important gram-negative rods typically associated with the respiratory tract, namely *Haemophilus influenzae, Legionella pneumophila,* and *Bordetella pertussis* (Table 19–1).

HAEMOPHILUS

Diseases *H influenzae* is the leading cause of meningitis in young children. It is also an important cause of upper respiratory tract infections (otitis media, sinusitis, and epiglottitis) and sepsis in children. It causes pneumonia in adults, particularly those with chronic obstructive lung disease. *Haemophilus ducreyi,* the agent of chancroid, is discussed in Chapter 27.

Important Properties *H influenzae* is a small gram-negative rod (coccobacillus) with a polysaccharide capsule. It is one of the 3 important **encapsulated pyogens**, along with the pneumococcus and the meningococcus. Serologic typing is based on the antigenicity of the capsular polysaccharide. Of the 6 serotypes, **type b** causes most of the severe, invasive diseases, such as meningitis and sepsis. The type b capsule is composed of polyribitol phosphate. Unencapsulated and therefore untypeable strains can also cause disease but are usually noninvasive. Growth of the organism on laboratory media requires the addition of 2 components, **heme (factor X)** and **NAD (factor V)**, for adequate energy production.

Pathogenesis & Epidemiology *H influenzae* enters the body through the **upper respiratory tract**, resulting in either asymptomatic colonization or infections such as otitis media, sinusitis, or pneumonia. The organism produces an IgA protease that degrades secretory IgA, thus facilitating attachment to the respiratory mucosa. After becoming established in the upper

Table 19–1. Gram-negative rods associated with the respiratory tract.

Species	Major Disease	Diagnosis	Factors X and V Required for Growth	Vaccine Available	Rifampin Prophylaxis for Contacts
H influenzae	Meningitis	Culture.	+	+	+
L pneumophila	Pneumonia	Serology; culture not usually done.	–	–	–
B pertussis	Whooping cough	Clinical plus culture.	–	+	–

respiratory tract, the organism can enter the bloodstream and spread to the meninges. Meningitis is caused primarily by the encapsulated strains (95% of which possess the type b capsule), but nonencapsulated strains are frequently involved in otitis media, sinusitis, and pneumonia. Pathogenesis involves the antiphagocytic capsule and endotoxin; no exotoxin is produced.

Most infections occur in children between the ages of 6 months and 6 years, with a peak in the age group from 6 months to 1 year. This age distribution is attributed to a decline in maternal IgG in the child coupled with the inability of the child to generate sufficient antibody until the age of approximately 2 years.

Clinical Findings Meningitis caused by *H influenzae* cannot be distinguished on clinical grounds from that caused by other bacterial pathogens, eg, pneumococci or meningococci. The rapid onset of fever, headache, and stiff neck along with drowsiness is typical. Sinusitis and otitis media cause pain in the affected area, opacification of the infected sinus, and redness with bulging of the tympanic membrane. *H influenzae* is second only to the pneumococcus as a cause of these 2 infections. Rarely, epiglottitis, which can obstruct the airway, occurs. This life-threatening disease of young children is caused almost exclusively by *H influenzae*. Pneumonia in elderly adults, especially those with chronic respiratory disease, can be caused by untypeable strains of *H influenzae*.

Laboratory Diagnosis Laboratory diagnosis depends on isolation of the organism on heated-blood (''chocolate'') agar enriched with 2 growth factors required for bacterial respiration, namely factor X (a heme compound) and factor V (NAD). The blood used in chocolate agar is heated to inactivate nonspecific inhibitors of *H influenzae* growth.

An organism that grows only in the presence of both growth factors is presumptively identified as *H influenzae;* other species of *Haemophilus*, such as *H parainfluenzae*, do not require both factors. Definitive identification can be made with either biochemical tests or the capsular swelling (quellung) reaction. Additional means of identifying encapsulated strains include fluorescent-antibody staining of the organism and counterimmunoelectrophoresis or latex agglutination tests, which detect the capsular polysaccharide.

Treatment The early (empirical) treatment of *H influenzae* meningitis involves both ampicillin and chloramphenicol. Because approximately 15% of isolates are resistant to ampicillin owing to a plasmid-encoded β-**lactamase**, chloramphenicol is added until the antibiotic sensitivity is determined. If the isolate is sensitive to ampicillin, chloramphenicol should be discontinued because of its potential toxicity. Alternatively, a single drug, cefuroxime, can be used. It is important to institute antibiotic treatment promptly, because the incidence of neurologic sequelae, eg, subdural empyema, is high. Persons with untreated *H influenzae* meningitis have a fatality rate of approximately 90%. *H influenzae* upper respiratory tract infections, such as otitis media and sinusitis, are treated with either ampicillin or a cephalosporin, eg, cefaclor.

Prevention Meningitis in close contacts of the patient can be prevented with rifampin. Rifampin is used because it is secreted in the saliva to a greater extent than ampicillin. Rifampin decreases respiratory carriage of the organism, thereby reducing transmission. The vaccine contains the capsular polysaccharide of *H influenzae* type b conjugated to diptheria toxoid. It is given at 18 months of age. However, its scope is limited; it induces protective antibody primarily in children over the age of 18 months, whereas most disease occurs in children younger than that.

LEGIONELLA

Disease *Legionella pneumophila* (and other legionellae) cause pneumonia, both in the community and in hospitalized immunocompromised patients. The genus is named after the famous outbreak of pneumonia among people attending the American Legion convention in Philadelphia in 1976 (Legionnaire's disease).

Important Properties Legionellae are gram-negative rods that **stain faintly with the standard Gram stain**. They do, however, have a gram-negative type of cell wall, and increasing the time of the safranin counterstain enhances visibility. In lung biopsy sections, they do not stain with the standard hematoxylin-and-eosin (H&E) procedure, and so special methods, such as the Dieterle silver impregnation stain, are used.

Initial attempts to grow the organisms on ordinary culture media from specimens obtained from the legionnaires failed. This is due to the organism's requirement for a high concentration of iron and cysteine; culture media supplemented with these nutrients will support growth.

In addition to *L pneumophila,* which is the most important species, 23 other *Legionella* species have been identified, most of which cause **atypical pneumonia,** eg, these species include *Legionella micdadei* (Pittsburgh pneumonia agent) and *Legionella bozemanii.*

Pathogenesis & Epidemiology Legionellae are associated chiefly with **environmental water sources** such as air conditioners and water-cooling towers. Outbreaks of pneumonia in hospitals have been attributed to the presence of the organism in water taps, sinks, and showers. The portal of entry is the respiratory tract, and pathologic changes occur primarily in the lung.

The typical candidate for Legionnaires' disease is an older man who smokes and consumes substantial amounts of alcohol. Cancer and immunosuppression (renal transplants) are major risk factors. Despite airborne transmission of the organism, person-to-person spread does not occur, as shown by the failure of secondary cases to occur in close contacts of patients.

Clinical Findings The clinical picture can vary from a mild flulike illness to a severe pneumonia accompanied by mental confusion, nonbloody diarrhea, proteinuria, and microscopic hematuria. Although cough is a prominent symptom, sputum is frequently scanty and nonpurulent. Most cases resolve spontaneously in 7–10 days, but in older or immunocompromised patients the infection can be fatal.

Legionellosis is an atypical pneumonia* and must be distinguished from other similar pneumonias such as *Mycoplasma* pneumonia, viral pneumonia, psittacosis, and Q fever. Pontiac fever is a mild, flulike form of *Legionella* infection that does not result in pneumonia. The name "Pontiac" is derived from the city in Michigan that was the site of an outbreak in 1968.

Laboratory Diagnosis The organism **fails to grow on ordinary media** in a culture of sputum or blood. Diagnosis usually depends on a significant increase in antibody titer in convalescent-phase serum by the indirect immunofluorescence assay. Since there are 6 serotypes of *L pneumophila,* a pool of antigens is used. The diagnosis can also be made by growing this fastidious organism on medium supplemented with iron and cysteine. However, this is rarely successful with sputum cultures, because other organisms present in sputum usually overgrow the agar. If tissue is available, it is possible to demonstrate *Legionella* antigens in infected lung tissue by using fluorescent-antibody staining. The cold-agglutinin titer does not rise in *Legionella* pneumonia, in contrast to pneumonia caused by *Mycoplasma.*

Treatment Erythromycin is the treatment of choice; it is effective not only against *L pneumophila* but also against *Mycoplasma pneumoniae* and *Streptococcus pneumoniae.* The organism frequently produces β-lactamase, and so penicillins and cephalosporins are less effective.

Prevention Prevention involves reducing cigarette and alcohol consumption, eliminating aerosols from water sources, and reducing *Legionella* in hospital water supplies by using high temperatures and hyperchlorination.

BORDETELLA

Disease *Bordetella pertussis* causes whooping cough (pertussis).

Important Properties *B pertussis* is a small, encapsulated gram-negative rod. Its polysaccharide capsule is essential for virulence; strains that have lost this capsule do not cause disease.

---

*A pneumonia is atypical when its causative agent cannot be isolated on ordinary laboratory media or when its clinical picture does not resemble that of typical pneumococcal pneumonia.

Pathogenesis & Epidemiology   *B pertussis*, a pathogen **only for humans**, is transmitted by **airborne droplets**. The organisms attach to the ciliated epithelium of the upper respiratory tract but do not invade the underlying tissue. Decreased cilia activity and epithelial cell death occur. The mechanism of pathogenesis is uncertain, but several factors play a role.

(1) **Pertussis toxin*** stimulates adenylate cyclase by catalyzing the addition of ADP-ribose to the inhibitory coupling protein of the cyclase. The toxin also has a domain that mediates its binding to target cell receptors. Antibodies against the toxin prevent the disease in experimental animals.

(2) The organisms also synthesize and export adenylate cyclase. This enzyme, when taken up by phagocytic cells, eg, neutrophils, can inhibit their bactericidal activity. Bacterial mutants that lack cyclase activity are avirulent.

(3) Attachment of the organism to the cilia of the epithelial cells is mediated by a protein on the pili. Antibody against pilus protein also protects against disease.

(4) Endotoxin is implicated in the pathogenesis.

The disease occurs primarily in infants and young children and has a worldwide distribution. It occurs infrequently in the USA because use of the vaccine is widespread.

Clinical Findings   Whooping cough is an acute tracheobronchitis that begins with mild upper respiratory tract symptoms followed by the typical paroxysmal cough, which lasts from 1 to 4 weeks. The paroxysmal pattern is characterized by a series of hacking coughs, accompanied by production of copious amounts of mucus, that end with an inspiratory "whoop" as air rushes past the narrowed glottis. Despite the severity of the symptoms, the organism is restricted to the respiratory tract and blood cultures are negative. A pronounced leukocytosis with up to 70% lymphocytes is seen. Central nervous system anoxia and exhaustion can occur, although death is due mainly to pneumonia.

Laboratory Diagnosis   The organism can be isolated from throat swabs taken during the paroxysmal stage. Bordet-Gengou[†] medium used for this purpose contains a high percentage of blood (20–30%) to inactivate inhibitors in the agar. Specific identification is made either by agglutination with specific antiserum or by fluorescent-antibody staining.

Treatment   Erythromycin reduces the number of organisms in the throat and decreases the risk of secondary complications but has little influence on the course of the disease. This drug is also useful in the prevention of disease in exposed, unimmunized individuals. Supportive care during the paroxysmal stage, especially in infants, is important.

Prevention   Whooping cough can be prevented by active immunization with **killed B pertussis** organisms. It is usually given combined with diphtheria and tetanus toxoids in 3 doses beginning at 2 months of age. A booster at 1 year of age and another at the time of entering school are recommended. Neither the vaccine nor the actual disease provides lifelong immunity, and there is little protection from maternal IgG. There is controversy about whether to continue using the vaccine, because it produces postvaccine encephalopathy at a rate of about one case per million doses administered. Most public health officials agree that in view of the high morbidity of the disease, including central nervous system complications, the immunization program should continue.

---

*Also known as lymphocytosis-promoting factor.
[†]The French scientists who first isolated the organism in 1906.

Review Questions

1. Type b *Haemophilus influenzae* is responsible for most of the invasive disease caused by this species. What determine the serotype?
2. What are the 3 most common bacteria that cause meningitis? What important pathogenetic feature do they share?

3. Factors X (heme) and V (NAD) are required for *H influenzae* growth. Why?
4. What are 2 methods of preventing *H influenzae* meningitis?
5. What 2 features of *Legionella pneumophila* account for the difficulty in isolating the organism during the 1976 outbreak at the American Legion Convention?
6. What is the natural habitat of *L pneumophila?* What is its usual mode of transmission?
7. What is the most common method of making the diagnosis of *L pneumophila* pneumonia in the clinical laboratory? Why?
8. What is the pathogenesis of whooping cough?
9. What is the nature of *Bordetella pertussis* vaccine? What are the problems associated with the vaccine?

20

Gram-Negative Rods Related to Animal Sources (Zoonotic Organisms)

There are 4 medically important gram-negative rods that have significant animal reservoirs: *Brucella* species, *Francisella tularensis, Yersinia pestis,* and *Pasteurella multocida* (Table 20–1).

BRUCELLA

Disease *Brucella* species cause brucellosis (undulant fever).

Important Properties Brucellae are small gram-negative rods without a capsule. The 3 major human pathogens and their animal reservoirs are *Brucella melitensis* (goats and sheep), *Brucella abortus* (cattle), and *Brucella suis* (pigs).

Pathogenesis & Epidemiology The organisms enter the body either by ingestion of **contaminated milk products or through the skin** by direct contact in an occupational setting such as an abattoir. They localize in the **reticuloendothelial system,** namely the lymph nodes, liver, spleen, and bone marrow. Many organisms are killed by macrophages, but some survive within these cells, where they are protected from antibody. The host response is granulomatous, with lymphocytes and epithelioid giant cells, which can progress to form focal abscesses and caseation. The mechanism of pathogenesis of these organisms is not well defined, except that endotoxin is involved; ie, when the O antigen polysaccharides are lost from the external portion of the endotoxin, the organism loses its virulence. No exotoxins are produced.

Table 20–1. Gram-negative rods associated with animal sources.

Species	Disease	Source of Human Infection	Mode of Transmission From Animal to Human	Diagnosis
Brucella species	Brucellosis	Pigs, cattle, goats	Dairy products; contact with animal tissues	Serology
F tularensis	Tularemia	Rabbits, deer, ticks	Contact with animal tissues; ticks.	Serology
Y pestis	Plague	Rodents	Flea bite.	Immunofluorescence
P multocida	Cellulitis	Cats, dogs	Cat or dog bite.	Wound culture

Imported cheese made from unpasteurized goats' milk produced in either Mexico or the Mediterranean region has been a source of *B melitensis* infection in the USA. The disease occurs worldwide but is rare in the USA, because pasteurization of milk kills the organism.

Clinical Findings   After an incubation period of 1–3 weeks, nonspecific symptoms resembling influenza occur. The undulating (rising and falling) fever pattern that gives the disease its name occurs in a minority of patients. Weakness and fatigue are marked. Enlarged lymph nodes, liver, and spleen are frequently found. *B melitensis* infections tend to be more severe and prolonged, whereas those caused by *B abortus* are more self-limited. Osteomyelitis is the most frequent complication. Secondary spread from person to person rarely occurs.

Laboratory Diagnosis   Recovery of the organism requires the use of enriched culture media and incubation in 10% CO_2. The organisms can be presumptively identified by using a slide agglutination test with *Brucella* antiserum, and the species can be identified by biochemical tests. If organisms are not isolated, analysis of a serum sample from the patient for a rise in antibody titer to *Brucella* can be used to make a diagnosis. In the absence of an acute-phase serum specimen, a titer of at least 1:160 in the convalescent-phase serum sample is diagnostic.

Treatment   The treatment of choice is tetracycline.

Prevention   Prevention of brucellosis involves pasteurization of milk, immunization of animals, and slaughtering of infected animals. There is no human vaccine.

FRANCISELLA

Disease   *Francisella tularensis* causes tularemia.

Important Properties   *F tularensis* is a small, pleomorphic gram-negative rod. It has a single serologic type.

Pathogenesis & Epidemiology   *F tularensis* is remarkable in the wide variety of animals that it infects and in the breadth of its distribution in the USA. It is enzootic (endemic in animals) in every state, but most human cases occur in the rural areas of Arkansas and Missouri. It has been isolated from more than 100 different species of **wild animals**, the most important of which are rabbits, deer, and a variety of rodents. The bacteria are transmitted among these animals by vectors such as **ticks**, mites, and lice, especially the *Dermacentor* ticks that feed on the blood of wild rabbits. The tick maintains the chain of transmission by passing the bacteria to its offspring by the transovarian route. In this process, the bacteria are passed through ovum, larva, and nymph stages to adult ticks capable of transmitting the infection.

Humans are accidental "dead-end" hosts who acquire the infection most often by being bitten by the animal vector or by having skin contact with the animal during removal of the hide. Rarely, the organism is ingested in infected meat, causing gastrointestinal tularemia, or is inhaled, causing pneumonia. There is no person-to-person spread. The main type of tularemia in the USA is tick-borne tularemia from a rabbit reservoir.

The organism enters through the skin, forming an ulcer at the site in most cases. It then localizes to the cells of the reticuloendothelial system, and granulomas are formed. Caseation necrosis and abscesses can also occur.

Clinical Findings   Presentation can vary from sudden onset of an influenzalike syndrome to prolonged onset of a low-grade fever and adenopathy. Approximately 75% of cases are of the "ulceroglandular" type, in which the site of entry ulcerates and the regional lymph nodes are swollen and painful. Other, less frequent forms of tularemia include glandular, oculoglandular, typhoidal, gastrointestinal, and pulmonary. Disease usually confers lifelong immunity.

Laboratory Diagnosis   Attempts to culture the organism in the laboratory are rarely undertaken, because there is a high risk to laboratory workers of infection by inhalation and the special cysteine-containing medium required for growth is not usually available. The most frequently used diagnostic method is the agglutination test with acute- and convalescent-phase serum samples. Fluorescent-antibody staining of infected tissue can be used if available.

Treatment   Streptomycin is the drug of choice.

Prevention   Prevention involves avoiding both being bitten by ticks and handling wild animal skins. There is a live, attenuated bacterial vaccine that is given only to persons, such as fur trappers, whose occupation brings them into close contact with wild animals. This and the BCG vaccine for tuberculosis are the only 2 live bacterial vaccines for human use.

YERSINIA*

Disease   *Yersinia pestis* is the cause of plague, also known as the black death, the scourge of the Middle Ages. It is also a 20th century disease, occurring in the western USA and in many other countries around the world.

Important Properties   *Y pestis* is a small gram-negative rod that exhibits bipolar staining; ie, it resembles a safety pin, with a central clear area. Freshly isolated organisms possess a capsule, which can be lost with passage in the laboratory; loss of the capsule is accompanied by a loss of virulence.

Pathogenesis & Epidemiology   The plague bacillus has been endemic in the wild rodents of Europe and Asia for thousands of years but entered North America in the early 1900s, probably carried by a rat that jumped ship at a California port. It is now endemic in the wild rodents in the western USA, although 99% of cases of plague occur in Southeast Asia.

The enzootic (sylvatic) cycle consists of transmission among **wild rodents by fleas**. In the USA, prairie dogs are the main reservoir. Rodents are relatively resistant to disease; most are asymptomatic. Humans are accidental hosts, and cases of plague in this country occur as a result of being bitten by a flea that is part of the sylvatic cycle.

The urban cycle, which does not occur in the USA, consists of transmission of the bacteria among urban rats, with the **rat flea** as vector. This cycle predominates during times of poor sanitation, eg, wartime, when rats proliferate and come in contact with the wild fleas in the sylvatic cycle.

The events within the flea are fascinating as well as essential. The flea ingests the bacteria while taking a blood meal from a bacteremic rodent. The blood clots in the flea's stomach owing to the action of the enzyme coagulase, which is made by the bacteria. The bacteria are trapped in the fibrin and proliferate to large numbers. The mass of organisms and fibrin block the proventriculus of the flea's intestinal tract, and during its next blood meal the flea regurgitates the organisms into the next animal. Because the proventriculus is blocked, the flea gets no nutrition, becomes hungrier, loses its natural host selectivity for rodents, and more readily bites a human.

The organisms inoculated at the time of the bite spread to the regional lymph nodes, which become swollen and tender. These swollen lymph nodes are the **buboes** that have led to the name **bubonic plague.** The organisms can reach high concentrations in the blood and disseminate to form abscesses in many organs. The endotoxin-related symptoms, including disseminated intravascular coagulation and cutaneous hemorrhages, probably were the genesis of the term "black death."

In addition to the sylvatic and urban cycles of transmission, respiratory droplet transmission of the organism from patients with pneumonic plague can occur.

The organism has 5 factors that contribute to its virulence: (1) the envelope antigen, called F-1, which protects against phagocytosis; (2) endotoxin; (3) an exotoxin; and 2 proteins known as (4) V antigen and (5) W antigen. The action of these last 3 proteins is unknown. Two additional correlates of virulence are the formation of pigmented colonies on certain media and the ability to synthesize purines.

Clinical Findings   Bubonic plague, which is the most frequent form, begins with pain and swelling of the lymph nodes draining the site of the flea bite and systemic symptoms such as high fever, myalgias, and prostration. The affected nodes enlarge and become exquisitely tender. These buboes are an early characteristic finding. Septic shock and pneumonia are the main life-threatening subsequent events. Pneumonic plague can arise either from inhalation of

---

* *Yersinia enterocolitica* and *Yersinia pseudotuberculosis,* which cause enterocolitis and mesenteric adenitis, are described in Chapter 27.

an aerosol or from septic emboli that reach the lung. Untreated bubonic plague is fatal in approximately half of cases, and untreated pneumonic plague is invariably fatal.

Laboratory Diagnosis   Smear and culture of blood or pus from the bubo is the best diagnostic procedure. Great care must be taken by the physician during aspiration of the pus and by laboratory workers doing the culture not to create an aerosol that might transmit the infection. Giemsa's or Wayson's stain reveals the typical safety-pin appearance of the organism better than does Gram's stain. Fluorescent-antibody staining can be used to identify the organism in tissues. A rise in antibody titer to the envelope antigen can be useful retrospectively.

Treatment   The treatment of choice is a combination of streptomycin and tetracycline, although streptomycin alone can be used. In view of the rapid progression of the disease, treatment should not wait for the results of the bacteriologic culture. Incision and drainage of the buboes are not usually necessary.

Prevention   Prevention of plague involves controlling the spread of rats in urban areas, preventing rats from entering the country by ship or airplane, and avoiding both flea bites and contact with dead wild rodents. A patient with plague must be placed in strict isolation (quarantine) for 72 hours after antibiotic therapy is started. Only close contacts need receive prophylactic tetracycline, but all contacts should be observed for fever. Reporting a case of plague to the public health authorities is mandatory.

A vaccine consisting of formalin-killed organisms provides partial protection against bubonic but not pneumonic plague. It was used in the armed forces during the Vietnam war but is not recommended for tourists traveling to Southeast Asia.

PASTEURELLA

Disease   *Pasteurella multocida* causes wound infections associated with cat and dog bites.

Important Properties   *P multocida* is a short, encapsulated gram-negative rod that exhibits bipolar staining.

Pathogenesis & Epidemiology   The organism is part of the normal flora in the mouths of many animals, particularly **domestic cats and dogs**, and is transmitted by **biting**. About 25% of animal bites become infected with the organism, with sutures acting as a predisposing factor to infection. Most bite infections are polymicrobial, with a variety of facultative anaerobes and anaerobic organisms present in addition to *P multocida*. Pathogenesis is not well understood, except that the capsule is a virulence factor and endotoxin is present in the cell wall. No exotoxins are made.

Clinical Findings   The rapid onset of cellulitis at the site of an animal bite is indicative of *P multocida* infection. Osteomyelitis can complicate cat bites in particular, because cats' sharp, pointed teeth can implant the organism under the periosteum.

Laboratory Diagnosis   The diagnosis is made by finding the organism in a culture of a sample from the wound site.

Treatment   Penicillin G is the treatment of choice.

Prevention   The use of ampicillin as prophylaxis, especially for cat bites, appears to be warranted.

Review Questions

1. How is brucellosis acquired?
2. In brucellosis, the organism is located primarily in which organ system and cells?

3. How can brucellosis be prevented?
4. How is tularemia acquired? How can it be prevented?
5. Infections caused by cat bites are associated with what organism?
6. What is the epidemiology of plague; ie, what is the reservoir, how is it transmitted, and where in the USA does it occur?
7. What is the pathogenesis of plague?

21

Mycobacteria

Mycobacteria are aerobic, **acid-fast** bacilli (rods). They are neither gram-positive nor gram-negative; ie, they are stained poorly by the dyes used in Gram's stain. They are virtually the only organisms that are acid-fast. (One exception is *Nocardia asteroides,* the major cause of nocardiosis, which is also acid-fast.) The term ''acid-fast'' refers to an organism's ability to retain the carbolfuchsin stain despite subsequent treatment with an ethanol-hydrochloric acid mixture. The high lipid content (approximately 60%) of their cell wall makes mycobacteria acid-fast.

The major pathogens are *Mycobacterium tuberculosis,* the cause of tuberculosis, and *Mycobacterium leprae,* the cause of leprosy. Atypical mycobacteria, such as *Mycobacterium avium-intracellulare* complex and *Mycobacterium kansasii,* can cause tuberculosislike disease but are less frequent pathogens. Rapidly-growing mycobacteria, such as *Mycobacterium chelonei,* are saprophytes that occasionally cause human disease in immunocompromised hosts. (Table 21–1).

MYCOBACTERIUM TUBERCULOSIS

Disease This organism causes tuberculosis.

Important Properties *M tuberculosis* **grows slowly** (ie, it has a doubling time of 18 hours, in contrast to most bacteria, which can double in number in 1 hour or less). Because growth is so slow, cultures of clinical specimens must be held for 6–8 weeks before being recorded as negative. *M tuberculosis* can be cultured on bacteriologic media, whereas *M leprae* cannot. Media used for its growth (eg, Löwenstein-Jensen medium) contain complex nutrients (eg, egg yolk) and dyes (eg, malachite green). The dyes inhibit the unwanted normal flora present in sputum samples.

M tuberculosis is an **obligate aerobe**; this explains its predilection for causing disease in highly oxygenated tissue such as the upper lobe of the lung and the kidney. Its cell wall

Table 21–1. Mycobacteria.

Species	Growth on Bacteriologic Media	Preferred Temperature in Vivo (°C)	Source or Mode of Transmission
M tuberculosis	Slow (weeks)	37	Respiratory droplets
M bovis	Slow (weeks)	37	Milk from infected animals
M leprae	None	32	Prolonged close contact
Atypical mycobacteria[1] M kansasii	Slow (weeks)	37	Environment
M marinum	Slow (weeks)	37	Water
M avium-intracellulare complex	Slow (weeks)	37	Environment
M fortuitum	Rapid (days)	37	Soil and water

[1]Only representative examples are given.

contains several complex lipids: (1) long-chain (C_{78}–C_{90}) fatty acids called **mycolic acids**, which contribute to the organism's acid-fastness; (2) wax D, one of the active components in Freund's adjuvant, which is used to enhance the immune response to many antigens in experimental animals; and (3) phosphatides, which play a role in caseation necrosis.

Cord factor (trehalose dimycolate) is correlated with virulence of the organism. Virulent strains grow in a characteristic "serpentine" cordlike pattern, whereas avirulent strains do not. The organism also contains several proteins, which, when combined with waxes, elicit delayed hypersensitivity. These proteins are the antigens in the PPD (purified protein derivative) skin test.

M tuberculosis is relatively resistant to acids and alkalis. NaOH is used to concentrate clinical specimens; it destroys unwanted bacteria, human cells, and mucus but not the organism. It is resistant to dehydration and so survives in dried, expectorated sputum; this property may be important in its transmission.

Transmission & Epidemiology *M tuberculosis* is transmitted from person to person by **respiratory aerosol**, and its initial site of infection is the lung. In the body, it resides chiefly within cells of the reticuloendothelial system.

In the USA, tuberculosis is almost exclusively a human disease. In developing countries, cows infected with *M bovis* constitute a reservoir for the human disease. Unless pasteurized, cows' milk can spread *M bovis,* causing gastrointestinal tuberculosis in humans. The disease tuberculosis occurs in only a small proportion of infected individuals. In the USA, most tuberculosis is due to reactivation in elderly, malnourished men. The risk of infection and disease is highest among socioeconomically disadvantaged people, who have poor housing and poor nutrition. These factors, rather than genetic ones, probably account for the high rate of infection among Native Americans, blacks, and Eskimos.

Pathogenesis *M tuberculosis* produces no exotoxins and does not contain endotoxin in its cell wall. In fact, no mycobacteria produce toxins. Lesions are dependent on the presence of the organism and the host response. There are 2 types of lesions:

(1) exudative lesions, which consist of an acute inflammatory response and occur chiefly in the lungs at the initial site of infection; and

(2) granulomatous lesions, which consist of a central area of giant cells containing tubercle bacilli surrounded by a zone of epithelioid cells. A **tubercle** is a granuloma surrounded by fibrous tissue that has undergone central caseation necrosis. Tubercles heal by fibrosis and calcification.

The primary lesion of tuberculosis usually occurs in the lungs. The parenchymal exudative lesion and the draining lymph nodes together are called a **Ghon complex.** Primary lesions usually occur in the lower lobes, whereas reactivation lesions usually occur in the apices. Reactivation lesions also occur in other well-oxygenated sites such as the kidneys, brain, and bone. Reactivation is seen primarily in immunocompromised or debilitated patients.

Spread of the organism within the body occurs by 2 methods:

(1) A tubercle can erode into a brochus, empty its caseous contents, and thereby spread the organism to other parts of the lungs, to the gastrointestinal tract if swallowed, and to other persons if expectorated.

(2) It can disseminate via the bloodstream to many internal organs.

Immunity & Hypersensitivity After recovery from the primary infection, resistance to the organism is acquired; this is mediated by cellular immunity. Circulating antibodies also form, but they play no role in resistance and are not used for diagnostic purposes.

Prior infection can be detected by a positive **tuberculin skin test**, which is due to a delayed hypersensitivity reaction. **PPD** is used as the antigen in the tuberculin skin test. The intermediate-strength preparation of PPD, which contains 5 tuberculin units, is usually used. The test is positive if 10 mm of induration occurs 48–72 hours after intradermal injection of the PPD. **Induration** (thickening), not simply erythema (reddening), must be observed.

A positive skin test indicates previous infection by the organism but not necessarily active disease. The tuberculin test becomes positive 4–6 weeks after infection. Immunization with BCG vaccine also causes a positive test. The skin test itself does not induce a positive response. Tuberculin reactivity is mediated by the cellular arm of the immune system; it can be transferred by lymphoid cells but not by serum.

Clinical Findings   Clinical findings are protean; many organs can be involved. Fever, fatigue, night sweats, and weight loss are common. Pulmonary tuberculosis causes cough and hemoptysis. Miliary tuberculosis is characterized by multiple disseminated lesions that resemble millet seeds.

Laboratory Diagnosis   Acid-fast staining of sputum or other specimens is the usual initial test. For rapid screening purposes, auramine stain, which can be visualized by fluorescence microscopy, can be used.

After digestion and concentration by treatment with NaOH, the material is cultured on special media, such as Löwenstein-Jensen medium, for up to 8 weeks. It will not grow on a blood agar plate. If growth in the culture occurs, the organism can be identified by biochemical tests. For example, *M tuberculosis* produces **niacin**, whereas almost no other mycobacteria do. Because drug resistance, especially to isoniazid (see below), is a problem, susceptibility tests should be performed.

Treatment   **Multiple-drug** therapy is used to prevent the emergence of drug-resistant mutants. **Isoniazid** (isonicotinic acid hydrazide, INH), a bactericidal drug, is the mainstay of treatment. Rifampin or ethambutol (or both) is frequently combined with isoniazid. Therapy usually is given for 9 months, but the patient's sputum becomes noninfectious within 2–3 weeks. The necessity for protracted therapy is attributed to (1) the intracellular location of the organism; (2) caseous material, which blocks penetration by the drug; and (3) metabolically inactive "persisters" within the lesion.

Resistance to isoniazid and other antituberculosis drugs is being seen with increasing frequency in the USA, especially in immigrants from Southeast Asia.

Prevention   The incidence of tuberculosis began to decrease markedly even before the advent of drug therapy in the 1940s. This is attributed to better housing and nutrition and other socioeconomic factors.

The most important current mode of prevention is chemoprophylaxis with isoniazid. It is prescribed for (1) asymptomatic patients whose PPD skin test has recently converted to positive, (2) children exposed to patients with symptomatic pulmonary tuberculosis, and (3) patients with a positive PPD skin test who undergo immunosuppression. Patients receiving isoniazid prophylaxis should be evaluated for drug-induced hepatitis, especially those over age 35 years, in view of their increased risk of hepatotoxicity.

A vaccine containing a strain of live, attenuated *M bovis* (bacillus Calmette-Guérin or **BCG**) can be used to induce partial resistance to tuberculosis. Although in use in Europe and other areas of the world, it is not given in the USA because vaccinees become skin test-positive; hence, an important diagnostic tool is lost. Pasteurization of milk and destruction of infected cattle are important in preventing intestinal tuberculosis.

ATYPICAL MYCOBACTERIA   Several species of mycobacteria are characterized as atypical, because they differ in certain respects from typical *M tuberculosis*. For example, atypical mycobacteria are widespread in the **environment** and are not pathogenic for guinea pigs, whereas *M tuberculosis* is found only in humans and is highly pathogenic for guinea pigs.

The atypical mycobacteria are classified into 4 groups according to their rate of growth and whether they produce pigment under certain conditions (Table 21–2). Group I organisms produce a yellow-orange pigmented colony only when exposed to light (**photochromogens**), whereas group II organisms produce the pigment chiefly in the dark (**scotochromogens**). Group III mycobacteria produce little or no yellow-orange pigment, irrespective of the

Table 21–2. Runyon's classification of atypical mycobacteria.

Group	Growth Rate	Pigment Formation in Light	Dark	Typical Species
I	Slow	+	−	*M kansasii, M marinum*
II	Slow	+	+	*M scrofulaceum*
III	Slow	−	−	*M avium-intracellulare complex*
IV	Rapid	−	−	*M fortuitum-chelonei complex*

presence or absence of light (nonchromogens). In contrast to the organisms in the previous 3 groups, which grow slowly, group IV organisms grow rapidly, producing colonies in less than 7 days.

Group I (Photochromogens)   *M kansasii* causes lung disease clinically resembling tuberculosis. It is antigenically similar to *M tuberculosis,* and so patients are frequently tuberculin skin test-positive. Its habitat in the environment is unknown, but infections by this organism are localized to the midwestern states and Texas. It is susceptible to the standard antituberculosis drugs.

Myobacterium marinum causes "swimming pool granuloma." These granulomatous, ulcerating lesions occur in the skin at the site of abrasions incurred at swimming pools. The natural habitat of the organism is both fresh and salt water. Treatment with tetracycline is effective.

Group II (Scotochromogens)   *Mycobacterium scrofulaceum* causes scrofula, a granulomatous cervical adenitis, usually in children. The organism enters through the oropharynx and affects the draining lymph nodes. Its natural habitat is environmental water sources, but it has also been isolated as a saprophyte from the human respiratory tract. Scrofula can often be cured by surgical excision of the affected lymph nodes.

Group III (Nonchromogens)   *M avium-intracellulare* complex is composed of 2 species, *M avium* and *M intracellulare,* that are very difficult to distinguish by standard laboratory tests. They cause pulmonary disease clinically indistinguishable from tuberculosis, especially in immuno-compromised patients such as those with AIDS. The organisms are widespread in the environment, including water and soil, particularly in the southeastern USA. They are highly resistant to antituberculosis drugs, and 6 drugs in combination are frequently required for adequate treatment.

Group IV (Rapidly Growing Mycobacteria)   *Mycobacterium fortuitum-chelonei* complex is composed of 2 similar species, *M fortuitum* and *M chelonei.* They are saprophytes, found chiefly in soil and water, which rarely cause human disease. Infections occur chiefly in 2 populations: (1) immunocompromised patients and (2) individuals with prosthetic heart valves and hip joints. They are frequently resistant to antituberculosis therapy, and therapy with 6 drugs in combination plus surgical excision may be required for effective treatment.

Mycobacterium smegmatis is a rapidly growing mycobacterium that is not associated with human disease. It is part of the normal flora of smegma, the material that collects under the foreskin of the penis.

MYCOBACTERIUM LEPRAE

Disease   This organism causes leprosy.

Important Properties   *M leprae* has **not been grown** in the laboratory, either on artificial media or in cell culture. It can be grown in the mouse footpad or in the armadillo. Humans are the natural hosts. The optimal temperature for growth is **lower** than body temperature; it therefore grows preferentially in the skin and superficial nerves.

Transmission   Infection is acquired by **prolonged contact with patients** with lepromatous leprosy, who excrete *M leprae* in large numbers in secretions.

Pathogenesis   The organism replicates intracellularly, typically within skin histiocytes, endothelial cells, and the Schwann cells of nerves. There are 2 distinct forms of leprosy—**tuberculoid and lepromatous**—with several intermediate forms between the 2 extremes.

(a) In tuberculoid leprosy, the cell-mediated immune response to the organism limits its growth, very few acid-fast bacilli are seen, granulomas containing giant cells form, and the lepromin skin test is positive.

(b) In lepromatous leprosy, the cell-mediated response to the organism is poor, the skin and mucous membrane lesions contain large number of organisms, foamy histiocytes rather than granulomas are found, and the lepromin skin test is negative.

Whether an individual gets tuberculoid or lepromatous leprosy may be, in part, genetically determined; individuals with HLA gene DR2 are predisposed to tuberculoid leprosy. Note that the cell-mediated response to other immunogens is unaffected and the serologic response to *M leprae* is intact. However, these antibodies are not protective.

Clinical Findings   The incubation period averages several years, and the onset of the disease is gradual. In tuberculoid leprosy, hypopigmented macular skin lesions, thickened superficial nerves, and significant anesthesia of the skin lesions occur. In lepromatous leprosy, multiple nodular skin lesions occur, resulting in the typical **leonine** (lionlike) **facies**.

The disfiguring appearance of the disease is due to several factors: (1) the skin anesthesia results in burns and other traumas, which often become infected; (2) resorption of bone leads to loss of features such as the nose and fingertips; and (3) infiltration of the skin and nerves leads to thickening and folding of the skin. In the majority of patients with a single skin lesion, the disease resolves spontaneously. Patients with forms of the disease intermediate between tuberculoid and lepromatous can progress to either extreme.

Laboratory Diagnosis   In lepromatous leprosy, the bacilli are easily demonstrated by performing an acid-fast stain of skin lesions or nasal scrapings. In the tuberculoid form, very few organisms are seen and the appearance of typical granulomas is sufficient for diagnosis. No serologic tests are useful. False-positive serologic tests for syphilis occur frequently.

Treatment   The mainstay of therapy is **dapsone** (diaminodiphenylsulfone), but sufficient resistance to the drug has emerged that combination therapy is now recommended, eg, dapsone, rifampin, and clofazimine for lepromatous leprosy and dapsone and rifampin for the tuberculoid form. Treatment is given for at least 2 years or until the lesions are free of organisms.

Prevention   Isolation of all lepromatous patients, coupled with chemoprophylaxis with dapsone for exposed children, is required. At present, the use of BCG vaccine is not recommended.

Review Questions

1. What feature of mycobacteria makes them acid-fast?
2. *Mycobacterium tuberculosis* grows very slowly and has complex nutritional requirements. What are the practical implications of these facts on diagnosis by the clinical laboratory?
3. What components of the organism play a role in pathogenesis?
4. How is tuberculosis acquired, and what are the main features of its pathogenesis?
5. Regarding the tuberculin skin test, what is the antigen and what is the interpretation of the results?
6. How is the diagnosis of *M tuberculosis* infection made in the clinical laboratory?
7. Why is multiple-drug therapy used for tuberculosis?
8. How can tuberculosis be prevented?
9. Why are certain mycobacteria called "atypical"? What is the basis for their classification?
10. What are the predisposing factors to disease caused by (1) *Mycobacterium avium-intracellulare* complex and (2) *Mycobacterium fortuitum-cheloni* complex?
11. What is unusual about the drug susceptibility of *M avium-intracellulare* complex?
12. How is the pathogenesis of lepromatous leprosy different from that of tuberculoid leprosy?
13. *Mycobacterium leprae* cannot be grown in culture. How is the diagnosis made in the laboratory?

Actinomycetes

22

Actinomycetes are true bacteria (related to corynebacteria and mycobacteria), but they form **long, branching filaments** that resemble the hyphae of fungi. They are gram-positive, but some are also acid-fast (Table 22–1).

ACTINOMYCES ISRAELII

Disease *Actinomyces israelii* causes actinomycosis.

Important Properties & Pathogenesis *A israelii* is an **anaerobe** that forms part of the **normal flora of the oral cavity.** After local trauma, it may invade tissues, forming filaments surrounded by areas of inflammation. Hard, yellow granules (**"sulfur granules"**) composed of a mass of filaments are formed in pus.

Clinical Findings Actinomycosis appears as a hard, nontender swelling that develops slowly and eventually drains pus through sinus tracts. In about 50% of cases, the initial lesion involves the face and neck; in the rest, the chest or abdomen is the site. *A israelii* and *Arachnia* species are the most common causes of actinomycosis in humans. The disease is not communicable.

Laboratory Diagnosis Diagnosis in the laboratory is made by (1) seeing gram-positive branching rods, especially in the presence of sulfur granules; and (2) seeing growth when pus or tissue specimens are cultured under anaerobic conditions. Organisms can be identified by immunofluorescence. There are no serologic tests.

Treatment & Prevention Treatment consists of prolonged administration of penicillin G, coupled with surgical drainage. No vaccine or prophylactic drug is available.

NOCARDIA ASTEROIDES

Disease *Nocardia asteroides* causes nocardiosis.

Important Properties & Pathogenesis *Nocardia* species are **aerobes** and are found in the **environment,** particularly in the **soil.** In immunocompromised individuals, they can produce lung infection and may disseminate. In tissues, *Nocardia* species are thin, branching filaments that may fragment into bacillary forms. Many isolates are **acid-fast,** especially *N asteroides*. Sulfur granules are not formed.

Clinical Findings *N asteroides* and *Nocardia brasiliensis* are the most common causes of human nocardiosis. The disease begins as a pulmonary infection and may progress to form abscesses and sinus tracts. In immunocompromised persons, the organism may spread to the brain or kidneys. The disease is not communicable.

Table 22–1. Actinomycetes.

Species	Disease	Habitat	Growth in Media	Diagnosis	Treatment
A israelii	Actinomycosis (abscess with draining sinuses)	Oral cavity	Strictly anaerobic	Gram-positive branching filaments; "sulfur granules" in pus; culture (anaerobic).	Penicillin G
N asteroides	Nocardiosis (abscesses in brain and kidneys in immunodeficient patients, pneumonia)	Environment	Aerobic	Gram-positive filaments that fragment into rods; often acid-fast; culture (aerobic).	Sulfonamides

Laboratory Diagnosis   Diagnosis in the laboratory involves (1) seeing branching rods or filaments that are gram-positive or acid-fast and (2) seeing aerobic growth on bacteriologic media in a few days.

Treatment & Prevention   Treatment is with sulfonamides. Surgical drainage may also be needed. Occasional drug resistance occurs. No vaccine or prophylactic drug is available.

Review Questions

1. What is the distinctive morphologic feature of the actinomycetes?
2. What is the natural habitat of (a) *Actinomyces israelii* and (b) *Nocardia asteroides?*
3. What is the pathogenesis of infections caused by (a) *A israelii* and (b) *N asteroides?*
4. Which of these organisms is usually acid-fast?
5. What are sulfur granules?

23

Mycoplasmas

Mycoplasmas are a group of small, **wall-less** organisms of which *Mycoplasma pneumoniae* is the major pathogen.

MYCOPLASMA PNEUMONIAE

Disease   *M pneumoniae* causes "atypical" pneumonia.

Important Properties   Mycoplasmas are the **smallest free-living organisms;** many are as small as 0.3 μm in diameter. Their most striking feature is the absence of a cell wall.* Consequently, mycoplasmas stain poorly with Gram's stain, and antibiotics that inhibit cell wall synthesis, eg, penicillins and cephalosporins, are ineffective. Their outer surface is a flexible 3-layer cell membrane; hence, these organisms can assume a variety of shapes. Theirs is the only bacterial membrane that contains **cholesterol,** a sterol usually found in eukaryotic cell membranes.

Mycoplasmas can be grown in the laboratory on artificial media, but they have complex nutritional requirements, including several lipids. They grow slowly and require at least 1 week to form a visible colony. The colony frequently has a characteristic "fried-egg" shape, with a raised center and a thinner outer edge.

Pathogenesis & Epidemiology   *M pneumoniae,* a pathogen **only for humans,** is transmitted by **respiratory droplets.** In the lungs, the organism is rod-shaped, with a tapered tip that contains specific proteins which serve as the point of attachment to the respiratory epithelium. The respiratory mucosa is not invaded, but ciliary motion is inhibited and necrosis of the epithelium occurs. The mechanism by which *M pneumoniae* causes inflammation is uncertain.

---

*Other types of bacteria, in the presence of penicillin, can exist in a wall-less state called an "L form" but can resynthesize their cell walls when penicillin is removed.

Infections by *M pneumoniae* resolve spontaneously in 10–14 days owing to the action of IgM and IgG antibodies and alveolar macrophages. Humoral antibody provides protection against disease for about 5 years, after which reinfection can occur. *M pneumoniae* has only one serotype and is antigenically distinct from other species of *Mycoplasma*. During *M pneumoniae* infection, autoantibodies are produced against red cells (**cold agglutinins**) and brain, lung, and liver cells. These antibodies may be the source of the extrapulmonary manifestations of infection.

M pneumoniae infections occur worldwide, with an increased incidence in the winter. This organism is the most frequent cause of pneumonia in young adults and is responsible for outbreaks in groups with close contacts such as families, military personnel, and college students. It is estimated that only 10% of infected individuals actually get pneumonia. *Mycoplasma* pneumonia accounts for about 5–10% of all community-acquired pneumonia.

Clinical Findings *Mycoplasma* pneumonia is the most common type of atypical pneumonia. It was formerly called primary **atypical pneumonia.** (Other atypical pneumonias are legionnaires' disease, Q fever, psittacosis, and viral pneumonias such as influenza. The term "atypical" means that a causative bacterium cannot be isolated on routine media in the diagnostic laboratory or that the disease does not resemble pneumococcal pneumonia.) After an incubation period of 2–3 weeks, the onset of *Mycoplasma* pneumonia is gradual, usually beginning with a nonproductive cough, sore throat, or earache. Small amounts of whitish, nonbloody sputum are produced. Constitutional symptoms of fever, headache, malaise, and myalgias are pronounced. The paucity of findings on chest examination is in marked contrast to the prominence of the chest x-ray infiltrates. The disease resolves spontaneously in 10–14 days.

Laboratory Diagnosis Diagnosis is usually not made by culturing sputum samples; it takes at least 1 week for colonies to appear on special media. Culture on regular media reveals only normal flora.

Serologic testing is the mainstay of diagnosis. A cold-agglutinin titer of 1:128 or higher is indicative of recent infection. Cold agglutinins are IgM autoantibodies against type O red blood cells that agglutinate these cells at 4 °C but not at 37 °C. However, only half of patients with *Mycoplasma* pneumonia will be positive for cold agglutinins. The test is nonspecific. The diagnosis of *M pneumoniae* infection can be confirmed by a 4-fold or greater rise in specific antibody titer in the complement fixation test.

Treatment The treatment of choice is erythromycin, which can shorten the duration of symptoms, although, as mentioned above, the disease resolves spontaneously. Penicillins and cephalosporins are inactive because the organism has no cell wall.

Prevention There are no specific preventive measures.

OTHER MYCOPLASMAS *Mycoplasma hominis* has been implicated as an infrequent cause of pelvic inflammatory disease. *Ureaplasma urealyticum* is one of several causes of nongonococcal urethritis. Ureaplasmas can be distinguished from mycoplasmas by their ability to produce the enzyme urease, which degrades urea to ammonia and carbon dioxide.

Review Questions

1. What are the unusual structural features of mycoplasmas?
2. How is *Mycoplasma pneumoniae* transmitted, and how does it cause disease?
3. What are cold agglutinins?
4. Why can penicillin not be used to treat *M pneumoniae* infections?

24

Spirochetes

Three genera of spirochetes cause human infection: (1) *Treponema*, which causes syphilis and the nonvenereal treponematoses; (2) *Borrelia*, which causes relapsing fever and Lyme disease; and (3) *Leptospira*, which causes leptospirosis (Table 24–1). Spirochetes are thin-walled, **flexible, spiral rods.** They are motile through the undulation of an axial filament that lies under the outer sheath. Treponemes and leptospirae are so thin that they are seen only by darkfield microscopy, silver impregnation, or immunofluorescence. Borreliae are larger, accept Giemsa's and other blood stains, and can be seen in the standard light microscope.

TREPONEMA

1. Treponema pallidum

Disease   *Treponema pallidum* causes syphilis.

Important Properties   *T pallidum* has **not been grown** on bacteriologic media or in cell culture. Nonpathogenic treponemes, which are part of the normal flora of human mucous membranes, can be cultured.

The antigens of *T pallidum* induce specific antibodies, which can be detected by immunofluorescence tests in the clinical laboratory. They also induce nonspecific antibodies (**reagin**)*, which can be detected by the flocculation of lipids (cardiolipin) extracted from normal mammalian tissues, eg, beef heart. Both specific antitreponemal antibody and nonspecific reagin are used in the serologic diagnosis of syphilis.

Transmission & Epidemiology   *T pallidum* is transmitted from spirochete-containing lesions of skin or mucous membranes (eg, genitalia, mouth, and rectum) of an infected person to other persons by **intimate contact.** It can also be transmitted from pregnant women to their fetuses. Rarely, blood for transfusions collected during early syphilis is also infectious.

Syphilis occurs worldwide, and its incidence is increasing. It is one of the leading notifiable diseases in the USA. Many cases are believed to go unreported, which limits public health

*Syphilitic reagin (IgM and IgG) should not be confused with the reagin (IgE) antibody involved in allergy.

Table 24–1. Spirochetes.

Species	Disease	Mode of Transmission	Diagnosis	Morphology	Growth in Bacteriologic Media	Treatment
T pallidum	Syphilis	Intimate (sexual) contact	Microscopy; serologic tests.	Thin, tight, spirals, seen by darkfield illumination, silver impregnation or immunofluorescent stain.	–	Penicillin G
B recurrentis	Relapsing fever	Louse bite	Clinical observations; microscopy.	Large, loosely coiled; stain with Giemsa's stain.	+	Tetracycline
B burgdorferi	Lyme disease	Tick bite	Clinical observations; microscopy.	Large, loosely coiled; stain with Giemsa's stain.	+	Tetracycline
L interrogans	Leptospirosis	Food or drink contaminated by urine of infected animals (rats, pigs, cows)	Serologic tests.	Thin, tight spirals, seen by darkfield illumination.	+	Tetracycline

efforts. There has been a marked increase in incidence of the disease in homosexual men in recent years.

Pathogenesis & Clinical Findings   *T pallidum* produces no important toxins or enzymes. At the site of inoculation, the spirochetes multiply and a local, nontender ulcer (**chancre**) usually forms in 2–10 weeks. This is known as "**primary**" syphilis. The ulcer heals spontaneously, but spirochetes spread widely in tissues; 1–3 months later, "**secondary**" lesions may appear as a maculopapular rash or as moist papules on skin and mucous membranes, or there may be organ involvement (meningitis, nephritis, hepatitis, etc). These lesions are rich in spirochetes and are highly infectious, but they also heal spontaneously. These stages may be asymptomatic, and yet progression of the disease may occur.

About one-third of these early syphilis cases progress to cure without treatment. Another third remain "**latent**"; ie, no lesions appear, but positive serologic tests indicate infection. In the remainder the disease progresses to the late, "**tertiary**" stage. Tertiary syphilis may show granulomas (gummas), especially of skin and bones, central nervous system involvement (eg, tabes, paresis), or cardiovascular lesions (eg, aortitis, aneurysm). In tertiary lesions, treponemes are very rare.

An infected woman can transmit *T pallidum* to her fetus after the third month of pregnancy. This is known as "**congenital syphilis.**" Unless treated promptly, stillbirth or multiple fetal abnormalities, primarily in skin, bone, and liver, result.

Immunity to syphilis is incomplete. Antibodies to the organism are produced but do not stop the progression of the disease. Patients with early syphilis who have been treated can contract syphilis again. Patients with late syphilis are relatively resistant to reinfection.

Laboratory Diagnosis   There are 3 important approaches.

A. Microscopy: Spirochetes are demonstrated in early lesions by **darkfield** or immunofluorescence microscopy. They are not seen on a Gram-stained smear.

B. Nonspecific Serologic Tests: These tests involve the use of **nontreponemal** antigens. Extracts of normal mammalian tissues (eg, **cardiolipin** from beef heart) react with antibodies in serum samples from patients with syphilis. These antibodies, which are a mixture of IgG and IgM, are called "reagin" antibodies (see above). Flocculation tests, eg, VDRL (Venereal Disease Research Laboratory) and RPR (rapid plasma reagin) tests, detect the presence of these antibodies. The antibodies are detectable in the majority of patients at the time the primary lesion appears and are virtually always present in secondary syphilis. False-positive reactions occur in infections such as hepatitis and infectious mononucleosis and in various autoimmune diseases. Therefore, positive results have to be confirmed by specific tests (see below). Results of nonspecific tests usually become negative after treatment. These tests can also be falsely negative as a result of the "**prozone**" phenomenon. In the prozone, the titer of antibody is too high (antibody excess) and no flocculation will occur. On dilution of the serum, however, the test becomes positive.

C. Specific Serologic Tests: These tests involve the use of **treponemal** antigens. *T pallidum* extracted from experimentally infected rabbits reacts in immunofluorescence (FTA-ABS)* or hemagglutination (TPHA)† tests with specific antitreponemal antibodies, which arise within 2–3 weeks of syphilitic infection.

Treponemal antibody tests are specific for treponematoses, are fairly expensive, and remain positive after adequate treatment.

Treatment   *T pallidum* and other treponemes are susceptible to penicillin G. A single injection of benzathine penicillin G (2.4 million units) can eradicate *T pallidum* and cure early syphilis. As alternative treatment, tetracycline or erythromycin can be used but must be given for prolonged periods to effect a cure.

---

*FTA-ABS is the fluorescent treponemal antibody-absorbed test. The patient's serum is absorbed with nonpathogenic treponemes to remove cross-reacting antibodies prior to reacting with *T pallidum*.

†TPHA is the *Treponema pallidum* hemagglutination assay.

Prevention Prevention depends on early diagnosis and adequate treatment, sex hygiene, administration of antibiotic after suspected exposure, and serologic follow-up of infected individuals and their contacts. The presence of any sexually transmitted diseases makes testing for syphilis mandatory, because several different infections are often transmitted simultaneously. There is no vaccine against syphilis.

2. Nonvenereal Treponematoses

These are infections caused by spirochetes that are virtually indistinguishable from *T pallidum*. They are endemic in populations and are transmitted by direct contact. All of these infections result in positive (nontreponemal and treponemal) serologic tests for syphilis. None of the spirochetes have been grown on bacteriologic media. The diseases include bejel in Africa, yaws (caused by *T pallidum* subspecies *pertenue*) in many humid tropical countries, and pinta (caused by *T carateum*) in Central and South America. All can be cured by penicillin.

BORRELIA

Borrelia species are irregular, loosely coiled spirochetes which stain readily with Giemsa's and other stains. They can be cultured in bacteriologic media containing serum or tissue extracts. They are transmitted by **arthropods.** They cause 2 major diseases, relapsing fever and Lyme disease.

Borrelia recurrentis & Borrelia hermsii *Borrelia recurrentis, Borrelia hermsii* and several other borreliae cause relapsing fever. During infection, the **antigens** of these organisms **undergo variation.** As antibodies develop against one antigen, variants emerge and produce relapses of the illness. This can be repeated 3–10 times.

B recurrentis is transmitted from person to person by the **human body louse.** Humans are the only hosts. *B hermsii* and many other *Borrelia* species are transmitted to humans by soft **ticks** (Ornithodorus). Rodents and other small animals are the main reservoirs. These species of *Borrelia* are passed transovarially in the ticks, a phenomenon that plays an important role in maintaining the organism in nature.

During infection, the arthropod bite introduces spirochetes, which then multiply in many tissues, producing fever, chills, headaches, and multiple organ dysfunction. Each attack is terminated as antibodies arise.

Diagnosis is usually made by seeing the large spirochetes in stained smears of peripheral blood. They can be cultured in special media. Serologic tests are rarely useful. Tetracycline may be beneficial early in the illness and may prevent relapses. Avoidance of arthropod vectors is the best means of prevention.

Borrelia burgdorferi *Borrelia burgdorferi* causes Lyme disease (named after a town in Connecticut), which occurs mainly in summer and is transmitted by **tick bite.** *Ixodes dammini* is the vector on the East Coast and in the Midwest; *Ixodes pacificus* is involved on the West Coast. Mice and deer are the important reservoirs.

Early in the disease, fever, severe headache, myalgia, stiff neck, and a typical skin lesion (**erythema chronicum migrans**) occur. If untreated, neurologic and cardiac abnormalities ensue weeks later and arthritis follows months to years later. Immune complexes are found in the affected joints.

Diagnosis is usually made by detecting IgM antibodies by immunofluorescence tests or ELISA. Cultures are not typically done. The treatment of choice is either penicillin or tetracycline. Penicillin in high doses is most effective in Lyme arthritis. Prevention centers on avoiding tick bites, eg, by wearing protective clothing.

LEPTOSPIRA

Leptospiras are tightly coiled, fine spirochetes that are not stained by dyes but are seen in darkfield microscopy. They grow in bacteriologic media containing serum.

Leptospira interrogans is the cause of leptospirosis. It is divided into serogroups that occur in different animals and geographic locations. Each serogroup is subdivided into serovars by the response to agglutination tests.

Leptospirae infect various animals including **rats** and other rodents, domestic livestock, and household pets. Animals excrete leptospirae in **urine,** which contaminates water and the environment. Swimming in contaminated water or consuming contaminated food or drink can result in human infection. Miners, farmers, and people who work in sewers are at high risk. Person-to-person transmission is rare.

Human infection results when leptospirae are ingested or pass through mucous membranes or skin. They circulate in the blood and multiply in various organs, producing fever and dysfunction of the liver (jaundice, hemorrhage), kidneys (uremia), and central nervous system (aseptic meningitis). Subclinical infection is common. Serovar-specific immunity develops with infection.

Diagnosis is based on history of possible exposure, suggestive clinical signs, and marked rise in agglutinating antibodies. Occasionally, leptospirae are isolated from blood and urine cultures.

Infected persons may benefit from being given tetracycline during the first days of illness. Prevention primarily involves avoiding contact with the contaminated environment. Doxycycline is effective in preventing the disease in exposed persons.

OTHER SPIROCHETES Anaerobic saprophytic spirochetes are prominent in the normal flora of the human mouth. Such spirochetes participate in mixed anaerobic infections, infected human bites, stasis ulcers, etc.

Spirillum minor causes one type of rat bite fever in humans.

Review Questions

1. *Treponema pallidum* cannot be seen on Gram's stain. Why?
2. How is syphilis transmitted to an adult? To a newborn?
3. What are the number and distribution of the organisms in (a) primary, (b) secondary, and (c) late syphilis?
4. What are the differences between the treponemal and nontreponemal antibody tests?
5. How can syphilis be prevented?
6. What is the mode of transmission of (a) relapsing fever, (b) Lyme disease, and (c) leptospirosis?

Chlamydiae

CHLAMYDIA PSITTACI & CHLAMYDIA TRACHOMATIS

Diseases *Chlamydia psittaci* causes psittacosis; *Chlamydia trachomatis* causes ocular, respiratory, and genital tract infections (Table 25–1).

Table 25–1. *Chlamydiae.*

Medically Important Species	Disease	Natural Hosts	Mode of Transmission to Humans	Number of Immunologic Types	Diagnosis	Treatment
C psittaci	Psittacosis (pneumonia)	Birds	Inhalation of dried bird feces.	1	Serologic test (cell culture rarely done)	Tetracyclines
C trachomatis	Urethritis, pneumonia, conjunctivitis	Humans	Sexual contact; perinatal transmission.	More than 15	Inclusions in epithelial cells seen with Giemsa's stain or by immunofluorescence; also cell culture.	Erythromycin, tetracyclines

Important Properties   Chlamydiae are **obligate intracellular bacteria** with a distinct cycle of replication. They lack some mechanism for the production of energy and can therefore grow only inside host cells. Their cell walls resemble those of gram-negative bacteria but lack muramic acid.

The distinctive replicative cycle begins when the extracellular, inert, small **elementary body** enters the cell and reorganizes into a larger, metabolically active **reticulate body.** The latter undergoes repeated binary fission to form daughter elementary bodies, which are released from the cell. Within cells, *C trachomatis* induces the formation of glycogen-containing inclusions, whereas *C psittaci* does not. This observation is useful in the diagnosis of these organisms in the clinical laboratory.

All chlamydiae share a group-specific lipopolysaccharide antigen, which is detected by complement fixation tests. They also possess species-specific and immunotype-specific antigens (proteins), which are detected by immunofluorescence. *C psittaci* has one immunotype, whereas *C trachomatis* has at least 15.

Transmission & Epidemiology   *C psittaci* infects **birds** and many mammals. Humans are infected primarily by **inhaling** organisms in dry bird feces. Recently, a new strain of *C psittaci,* designated TWAR, was described. It is transmitted from person to person without a bird intermediate and causes upper and lower respiratory tract infections in young adults. *C trachomatis* infects **only humans** and is usually transmitted by close personal contact, eg, **sexually** or by **passage through the birth canal.**

Disease caused by both organisms occurs worldwide, but trachoma is most frequently found in developing countries in tropical regions. Nongonococcal urethritis caused by *C trachomatis* is said to occur more frequently in higher socioeconomic groups, in contrast to gonorrhea, which is found predominantly in lower socioeconomic groups. However, the 2 diseases commonly occur simultaneously in the same individual.

Pathogenesis & Clinical Findings   *C psittaci* infects the lungs primarily. The infection may be asymptomatic (detected only by a rising antibody titer) or may produce high fever and pneumonia. Human psittacosis is not generally communicable.

C trachomatis exists in more than 15 immunotypes (A–L). Types A, B, and C cause **trachoma,** a chronic conjunctivitis endemic in Africa and Asia. Trachoma may recur over many years and may lead to blindness but causes no systemic illness. Types D–K cause **genital tract infections,** which are occasionally transmitted to the eyes or the respiratory tract. These types are the cause of what is probably the most common sexually transmitted disease. In men, it is a common cause of nongonococcal urethritis, which may progress to epididymitis, prostatitis, or proctitis. In women, cervicitis develops and may progress to salpingitis and pelvic inflammatory disease. Infants born to infected mothers often develop mucopurulent eye infections (neonatal inclusion conjunctivitis) 7–12 days after delivery, and some may develop chlamydial pneumonitis 2–12 weeks after birth.

C trachomatis L1–L3 immunotypes cause **lymphogranuloma venereum,** a sexually transmitted disease with lesions on genitalia and in lymph nodes.

Infection by *C trachomatis* leads to formation of antibodies and cell-mediated reactions but not to resistance to reinfection or elimination of organisms.

Laboratory Diagnosis   Chlamydiae form **cytoplasmic inclusions,** which can be seen with special stains (eg, Giemsa's stain) or by immunofluorescence. Particles in exudates can also be seen by immunofluorescence microscopy. Chlamydiae can be grown in cell cultures treated with cycloheximide. In culture, *C trachomatis*-infected cells contain glycogen-filled inclusions, whereas *C psittaci*-infected cells do not. These inclusions are visualized by staining with iodine. Exudates from eyes, respiratory tract, or genital tract give positive cultures in about half of cases.

Antibodies to chlamydiae develop in most infected persons, and a rise in titer of immunotype-specific antibodies may be diagnostic. However, the presence of antibodies in a single specimen is rarely helpful because of the frequency of infection.

Treatment   All chlamydiae are susceptible to tetracyclines and erythromycin. Treatment suppresses signs and symptoms but does not regularly eradicate the organisms. Chronic infections, with persistence of organisms and recurrence of clinical activity, are common.

Prevention   Psittacosis in humans is controlled by restriction on import of psittacine birds, destruction of sick birds, and addition of tetracycline to feed. Domestic flocks of turkeys and ducks are surveyed for the presence of *C psittaci*.

C trachomatis infection in humans should be diagnosed and treated early both in clinically manifest cases and in asymptomatic sexual contacts. Several types of sexually transmitted diseases are often present simultaneously. Thus, diagnosis of one requires a search for other etiologic agents. Erythromycin given to newborn infants of infected mothers can prevent inclusion conjunctivitis and pneumonitis.

Review Questions

    1. Why are chlamydiae obligate intracellular parasites?
    2. Describe the life cycle of chlamydiae.
    3. Contrast the natural reservoirs of *Chlamydia psittaci* and *Chlamydia trachomatis*.
    4. What is the relationship of serotype to disease with (a) *C psittaci* and (b) *C trachomatis?*
    5. How are chlamydial infections diagnosed in the clinical laboratory?

Rickettsiae 26

Rickettsiae are small bacteria, all but one of which are obligate intracellular parasites. They are the agents of typhus, spotted fevers, and Q fever.

Diseases   In the USA, there are 2 rickettsial diseases of significance: Rocky Mountain spotted fever, caused by *Rickettsia rickettsii*, and Q fever, caused by *Coxiella burnetii*. Several other rickettsial diseases such as epidemic, endemic, and scrub typhus are important in developing countries. Rickettsialpox, caused by *Rickettsia akari*, is a rare disease found in certain densely populated cities in the USA. Trench fever is a rare disease caused by *Rochalimaea quintana*.

Important Properties   Rickettsiae are very short rods that are barely visible in the light microscope. Structurally, their cell wall resembles that of gram-negative rods, but they stain poorly with the standard Gram stain.

With one exception, rickettsiae are **obligate intracellular parasites;** they are unable to synthsize sufficient energy to replicate extracellularly. The exception is *R quintana*, which is able to grow on blood agar supplemented with specific nutrients. Other rickettsiae must be grown in cell culture, embryonated eggs, or experimental animals. Rickettsiae divide by binary fission within the host cell, in contrast to chlamydiae, which are also obligate intracellular parasites but replicate by a distinctive intracellular cycle.

Several rickettsiae, such as *Rickettsia prowazekii, Rickettsia tsutsugamushi*, and *R rickettsii*, possess antigens that cross-react with antigens of the OX strains of *Proteus vulgaris*. The **Weil-Felix** test, which detects antirickettsial antibodies in a patient's serum by agglutination of the *Proteus* organisms, is based on this cross-reaction.

Transmission   The most striking aspect of the life cycle of the rickettsiae is that they are maintained in nature in certain arthropods such as ticks, lice, fleas, and mites and, with one exception, are transmitted to humans by the **bite of the anthropod.** The exception to arthropod transmission is *C burnetii*, the cause of Q fever, which is transmitted by aerosol and inhaled into the lungs. Virtually all rickettsial diseases are zoonoses (ie, they have an animal

reservoir), with the prominent exception of **epidemic typhus, which occurs only in humans.**
A summary of the vectors and reservoirs for selected rickettsial diseases is presented in Table
26–1.

The incidence of the disease depends upon the geographic distribution of the arthropod
vector and on the risk of exposure, which is enhanced by such things as poor hygienic
conditions and camping in wooded areas. These factors are discussed below with the
individual diseases.

Pathogenesis   The typical lesion caused by the rickettsiae is a **vasculitis,** particularly in the
endothelial lining of the vessel wall where the organism can be found. Damage to the vessels
of the skin results in the characteristic rash and in edema and hemorrhage due to increased
capillary permeability. The basis for pathogenesis by these organisms is unclear. There is some
evidence that endotoxin is involved, which is in accord with the nature of some of the lesions
such as fever and petechiae, but its role has not been confirmed. No exotoxins or cytolytic
enzymes have been found.

Clinical Findings & Epidemiology   This section is limited to the 2 rickettsial diseases that
are most common in the USA, ie, Rocky Mountain spotted fever and Q fever, and to the other
major rickettsial disease, typhus.

A. Rocky Mountain Spotted Fever: This disease is characterized by the acute onset of
nonspecific symptoms, eg, fever, severe headache, myalgias, and prostration. The typical
rash, which appears 2–6 days later, begins with macules that frequently progress to petechiae.
The rash usually appears first on the hands and feet, then moves inward to the trunk. In
addition to headache, other profound central nervous system changes such as delirium and
coma can occur. Disseminated intravascular coagulation, edema, and circulatory collapse may
ensue in severe cases. The diagnosis must be made on clinical grounds and therapy started
promptly, because the laboratory diagnosis is delayed until a rise in antibody titer can be
observed.

The name of the disease is misleading, because it occurs primarily along the **East Coast** of
the USA where the dog tick, *Dermacentor variabilis,* is located. The name ''Rocky Mountain
spotted fever'' is derived from the region in which the disease was first found.* The **tick** is the
reservoir of *R rickettsii* as well as the vector; the organism is passed by the transovarian route
from tick to tick, and a lifetime infection results. Humans are accidental hosts and are not
required for the perpetuation of the organism in nature; there is no person-to-person
transmission. Most cases occur in children during spring and early summer, when the ticks are
active. Rocky Mountain spotted fever accounts for 95% of the rickettsial disease in the USA;
there are about 1000 cases per year. It can be fatal if untreated, but if it is diagnosed and
treated, a prompt cure results.

---

*In the western USA, it is transmitted by the wood tick, *Dermacentor andersoni.*

Table 26–1. Summary of selected rickettsial diseases.

Disease	Organism	Arthropod Vector	Arthropod Reservoir	Mammalian Reservoir	Important in the USA
Spotted fevers Rocky Mountain spotted fever	*R rickettsii*	Ticks	Yes	Dogs, rodents	Yes (especially on the East Coast)
Rickettsialpox	*R akari*	Mites	Yes	Mice	No
Typhus group Epidemic	*R prowazekii*	Lice	No	Humans	No
Endemic	*R typhi*	Fleas	No	Rodents	No
Scrub	*R tsutsugamushi*	Mites	Yes	Rodents	No
Others Q fever	*C burnetii*	None	No	Cattle, sheep, goats	Yes
Trench fever	*R quintana*	Lice	No	Humans	No

B. Q Fever[†]: Unlike the other rickettsial diseases, the main focus of disease in Q fever is in the lungs. It begins suddenly with fever, severe headache, and influenzalike symptoms. In many patients, this is all that occurs, but in about half, pneumonia ensues. Hepatitis is frequent enough that the combination of pneumonia and hepatitis should suggest Q fever. A rash is rare, unlike in the other rickettsial diseases. In general, Q fever is an acute disease and recovery is expected even in the absence of antibiotic therapy. Rarely, chronic Q fever characterized by a life-threatening endocarditis occurs.

Q fever is the one rickettsial disease that is **not** transmitted to humans by the bite of an arthropod. The important reservoirs for human infection are cattle, sheep, and goats. The agent *C burnetii*, which causes an inapparent infection in these reservoir hosts, is found in high concentrations in the urine, feces, placental tissue, and amniotic fluid of the animals. It is transmitted to humans by the **inhalation of aerosols** of these materials. The disease occurs worldwide, chiefly in individuals whose occupations expose them to livestock, such as shepherds, abattoir employees, and farm workers. Cows' milk is usually responsible for subclinical infections rather than disease in humans. Pasteurization of milk kills the organism.

C. Typhus: There are several different forms of typhus, namely louse-borne epidemic typhus caused by *R prowazekii*, flea-borne endemic typhus caused by *Rickettsia typhi*, chigger-borne scrub typhus caused by *R tsutsugamushi,* and several other quite rare forms. The following description is limited to epidemic typhus, the most important of the typhus group of diseases.

Typhus begins with the sudden onset of chills, fever, headache, and other influenzalike symptoms approximately 1–3 weeks after the louse bite occurs. Between the fifth and ninth days after the onset of symptoms, the rash begins on the trunk and spreads peripherally. It is macular or maculopapular in appearance. Signs of severe meningoencephalitis, including delirium and coma, begin with the rash and continue into the second and third weeks. In untreated cases, death occurs from peripheral vascular collapse or from the most frequent complication, bacterial pneumonia.

Epidemic typhus is transmitted from person to person by the **human body louse,** *Pediculus.* When a bacteremic patient is bitten, the organism is ingested by the louse and multiplies in the gut epithelium. It is excreted in the feces of the louse during the act of biting the next person and autoinoculated by the person while scratching the bite. The infected louse dies after a few weeks, and there is no louse-to-louse transmission, so that human infection is an obligatory stage in the cycle. Epidemic typhus is associated with wars and poverty; at present it is found in developing countries in Africa and South America but not in the USA. The last case of louse-borne typhus in the USA was in 1922, although the organism was isolated recently from flying squirrels in the eastern USA, and so human infection may occur.

A recurrent form of epidemic typhus is called Brill-Zinsser disease. The signs and symptoms are similar to those of epidemic typhus but are less severe, of shorter duration, and rarely fatal. Recurrences can appear as long as 50 years later and can be precipitated by another intercurrent infectious disease. In the USA, the disease is seen in older people who had epidemic typhus during World War II in Europe. Brill-Zinsser disease is epidemiologically interesting; persistently infected patients can serve as a source of the organism should a louse bite occur.

Laboratory Diagnosis Laboratory diagnosis of rickettsial diseases is based on serologic analysis rather than isolation of the organism. Although rickettsiae can be grown in cell culture or embryonated eggs, it is a hazardous procedure that is not available in the standard clinical laboratory.

Of the 2 serologic tests, complement fixation is more frequently used and provides more specific data than the Weil-Felix reaction. (A microagglutination test is used by public health laboratories but is not widely available.) As usual, a 4-fold rise in antibody titer found in a convalescent-phase serum sample is significant. However, in the presence of the clinical picture of Rocky Mountain spotted fever, a single acute-phase serum titer of 1:16 or greater is diagnostic.

The Weil-Felix test is based on the cross-reaction of an antigen present in many rickettsiae with the O antigen polysaccharide found in *P vulgaris* strains OX-2, OX-19, and OX-K. The

---

[†]Q stands for ''Query''; the cause of this disease was a question mark, ie, was unknown, when the disease was first described in Australia in 1937.

test measures the presence of antibodies against the rickettsiae in the patient's serum by its ability to agglutinate *Proteus* bacteria. The specific rickettsial organism can be identified by the agglutination observed with one or another of these 3 different strains of *P vulgaris*. However, since there can be false-positive reactions following *Proteus* urinary tract infections and false-negative reactions due to variable antibody responses, and since no Weil-Felix agglutinins are made in Q fever, the test is of limited value.

Treatment   The treatment of choice for all rickettsial diseases is tetracycline, with chloramphenicol as the second choice.

Prevention   Prevention of many of these diseases is based on reducing exposure to the arthropod vector by wearing protective clothing and insect repellent. Frequent examination of the skin for ticks is important in preventing Rocky Mountain spotted fever; the tick must be attached for several hours to transmit the disease. Prevention of typhus is based on personal hygiene and "delousing" with DDT. A typhus vaccine containing formalin-killed *R prowazekii* organisms is effective and useful in the military during wartime but is not available in the USA. Persons at high risk of contracting Q fever, such as veterinarians, shepherds, abattoir workers, and laboratory personnel exposed to *C burnetii,* should receive the vaccine that consists of the killed organism.

Review Questions

1. Why are most rickettsiae obligate intracellular parasites?
2. What is the common mode of transmission for all rickettsiae except *Coxiella burnetii?* How is *C burnetii* transmitted?
3. What is the pathogenesis of most rickettsial diseases (except Q fever)? Why do they cause a rash?
4. Contrast Rocky Mountain spotted fever and Q fever.
5. Why is epidemic typhus not a zoonotic disease?
6. What is the Weil-Felix test, and what is its role in diagnosis?

Minor Bacterial Pathogens

The bacterial pathogens of lesser medical importance are briefly described in this chapter. Experts may differ on their choice of which organisms to put in this category. Nevertheless, separating the minor from the major pathogens should allow the reader to focus on the more important pathogens while providing at least some information about the less important ones.

These organisms are presented in alphabetical order. Table 27–1 lists the organisms according to their appearance on Gram's stain.

Achromobacter   *Achromobacter* species are gram-negative coccobacillary rods found chiefly in water supplies. They are opportunistic pathogens and are involved in sepsis, pneumonia, and urinary tract infections.

Acinetobacter   *Acinetobacter* species are gram-negative coccobacillary rods found commonly in soil and water, but they can be part of the normal flora. They are opportunistic pathogens that readily colonize patients with compromised host defenses. *Acinetobacter calcoaceticus,* the species usually involved in human infection, causes disease chiefly in a

Table 27–1. Minor bacterial pathogens.

Gram Reaction and Shape	Genus or Species
Gram-positive cocci	*Micrococcus, Peptococcus, Peptostreptococcus, Sarcina*
Gram-positive rods	*Arachnia, Bifidobacterium, Erysipelothrix, Eubacterium, Gardnerella, Lactobacillus, Propionibacterium*
Gram-negative cocci	*Branhamella, Veillonella*
Gram-negative rods	*Achromobacter, Acinetobacter, Actinobacillus, Aeromonas, Alcaligenes, Arizona, Bartonella, Calymmatobacterium, Capnocytophaga, Cardiobacterium, Cat-scratch fever bacillus, Chromobacterium, Citrobacter, Edwardsiella, Eikenella, Erwinia, Flavobacterium, Fusobacterium, Haemophilus ducreyi, Hafnia, Kingella, Moraxella, Pseudomonas pseudomallei, Spirillum, Streptobacillus, Yersinia enterocolitica, Yersinia pseudotuberculosis*

hospital setting usually associated with respiratory therapy equipment and indwelling catheters. Sepsis, pneumonia, and urinary tract infections are the most frequent manifestations. Previous names for this organism include *Herellea* and *Mima*.

Actinobacillus *Actinobacillus* species are gram-negative coccobacillary rods. *Actinobacillus actinomycetemcomitans* is found as part of the normal flora in the upper respiratory tract. It is a rare opportunistic pathogen, causing endocarditis on damaged heart valves and sepsis.

Aeromonas *Aeromonas* species are gram-negative rods found in water, soil, food, and animal and human feces. *Aeromonas hydrophila* causes wound infections and sepsis, especially in immunocompromised patients.

Alcaligenes *Alcaligenes* species are gram-negative coccobacillary rods that are found in soil and water and are associated with water-containing materials such as respirators in hospitals. *Alcaligenes faecalis* is an opportunistic pathogen, causing sepsis and pneumonia.

Arachnia *Arachnia* species are anaerobic gram-positive rods that form long, branching filaments similar to those of *Actinomyces*. They are found primarily in the mouth (associated with dental plaque) and in the tonsillar crypts. Arachnia propionica, the major species, causes abscesses similar to those of *Actinomyces israelii*, including the presence of ''sulfur granules'' in the lesions.

Arizona *Arizona* species are gram-negative rods in the family Enterobacteriaceae; they ferment lactose slowly. Arizona hinshawii is found in the feces of chickens and other domestic animals and causes diseases similar to those caused by *Salmonella*, such as enterocolitis and enteric fevers. The organism is usually transmitted by contaminated food, eg, dried eggs.

Bartonella *Bartonella bacilliformis* is a pleomorphic gram-negative rod. It causes 2 rare diseases which occur only in humans: Oroya fever and verruga peruana, both of which are stages of Carrión's disease. The disease occurs only in certain areas of the Andes Mountains, and an animal reservoir is suspected.

Bifidobacterium *Bifidobacterium eriksonii* is a gram-positive, filamentous, anaerobic rod found as part of the normal flora in the mouth and gastrointestinal tract. It occurs in mixed anaerobic infections.

Branhamella *Branhamella catarrhalis* is a gram-negative diplococcus morphologically indistinguishable from the neisseriae. Although considered to be a member of the normal flora in the human nasopharynx, it can cause sinusitis, otitis, bronchitis, and pneumonia, particularly in immunocompromised patients. Most clinical isolates produce β-lactamase.

Calymmatobacterium *Calymmatobacterium granulomatis* is a gram-negative rod that causes granuloma inguinale, a sexually transmitted disease characterized by genital ulceration and soft-tissue and bone destruction. The diagnosis is made by visualizing the stained organisms (Donovan bodies) within large macrophages from the lesion. Tetracycline is the treatment of choice for this disease, which is rare in the USA but endemic in many developing countries.

Capnocytophaga   *Capnocytophaga gingivalis* is a gram-negative fusiform rod that is associated with periodontal disease, but it can also be an opportunistic pathogen, causing sepsis.

Cardiobacterium   *Cardiobacterium hominis* is a gram-negative pleomorphic rod. It is a member of the normal flora of the human colon, but it can be an opportunistic pathogen, causing mainly endocarditis.

Cat-Scratch Fever Bacillus   Cat-scratch fever is characterized by localized lymphade-nopathy in a person who reports being in contact with or being scratched by a cat. This diagnosis is supported by characteristic histopathology on a biopsied lymph node and a positive skin test with sterile pus. The disease is mild and self-limited, and no antibiotic therapy is recommended. It is caused by a gram-negative (or gram-variable) small rod that has not been classified.

Chromobacterium   *Chromobacterium violaceum* is a gram-negative rod that produces a violet pigment. It is found in soil and water and can cause wound infections, especially in subtropical parts of the world.

Citrobacter   *Citrobacter* species are gram-negative rods (members of the Enterobacteriaceae) related to *Salmonella* and *Arizona*. They occur in the environment and in the human colon and can cause sepsis in immunocompromised patients.

Edwardsiella   *Edwardsiella* species are gram-negative rods (members of the Entero-bacteriaceae) resembling *Salmonella*. They can cause enterocolitis, sepsis, and wound infections.

Eikenella   *Eikenella corrodens* is a gram-negative rod that is a member of the normal flora in the human mouth, but it can cause sepsis and soft-tissue infections of the head and neck, especially in immunocompromised patients.

Erwinia   *Erwinia* species are gram-negative rods (members of the Enterobacteriaceae) found in soil and water and are rarely involved in human disease.

Erysipelothrix   *Erysipelothrix rhusiopathiae* is a gram-positive rod that causes erysipeloid, a skin infection that resembles erysipelas (caused by streptococci). Erysipeloid usually occurs on the hands of meat and fish handlers.

Eubacterium   *Eubacterium* species are gram-positive, anaerobic, non-spore-forming rods that are present in large numbers as part of the normal flora of the human colon. They rarely cause human disease.

Flavobacterium   *Flavobacterium* species are gram-negative rods found in soil and water. They can be opportunistic pathogens, causing meningitis and sepsis especially in premature infants.

Fusobacterium   *Fusobacterium* species are anaerobic gram-negative rods with pointed ends. They are part of the human normal flora of the mouth, colon, and female genital tract and are sometimes isolated from pulmonary, intra-abdominal, and pelvic abscesses. They are frequently found in mixed infections with other anaerobes and facultative anaerobes. *Fusobacterium nucleatum* occurs in cases of Vincent's angina (trench mouth), along with various spirochetes.

Gardnerella   *Gardnerella vaginalis* is a gram-variable rod associated with nonspecific vaginitis, characterized by a malodorous vaginal discharge and "clue cells," which are vaginal epithelial cells covered with bacteria.

Haemophilus ducreyi   This small gram-negative rod causes the sexually transmitted disease chancroid (soft chancre), which is common in tropical countries but rare in the USA. The disease begins with penile lesions, which are painful, nonindurated (soft) ulcers, and local lymphadenitis (bubo). The diagnosis is made by isolating *Haemophilus ducreyi* from the ulcer or from pus aspirated from a lymph node. The organism requires heated (chocolate) blood agar supplemented with X factor (heme) but, unlike *Haemophilus influenzae,* does not require V factor (NAD). Chancroid can be treated with tetracycline, erythromycin, or a sulfonamide.

Hafnia   *Hafnia* species are gram-negative rods (members of the Enterobacteriaceae) found in soil and water and are rare opportunistic pathogens.

Kingella   *Kingella kingae* is a gram-negative rod in the normal flora of the human oropharynx. It is a rare cause of opportunistic infection.

Lactobacillus   Lactobacilli are gram-positive non-spore-forming rods found as members of the normal flora in the mouth, colon, and female genital tract. In the mouth, they may play a role in the production of dental caries. In the vagina, they are the main source of lactic acid, which keeps the pH low. Lactobacilli are rare causes of opportunistic infection.

Micrococcus   Micrococci are gram-positive cocci that are part of the normal flora of the skin. They are rare human pathogens.

Moraxella   *Moraxella* species are gram-negative coccobacillary rods resembling neisseriae. They are members of the normal flora of the upper respiratory tract. *Moraxella nonliquefaciens* is one of the 2 common causes of blepharitis (infection of the eyelid); *Staphylococcus aureus* is the other. The usual treatment is local application of antibiotic ointment, such as erythromycin.

Peptococcus   Peptococci are anaerobic gram-positive cocci, resembling staphylococci, found as members of the normal flora of the mouth and colon. They are also isolated from abscesses of various organs, usually from mixed anaerobic infections.

Peptostreptococcus   Peptostreptococci are anaerobic gram-positive cocci found as members of the normal flora of the mouth and colon. They are also isolated from abscesses of various organs, usually from mixed anaerobic infections.

Propionibacterium   Propionibacteria are anaerobic gram-positive rods sometimes called ''diphtheroids,'' because they are similar to *Corynebacterium diphtheriae. Propionibacterium acnes* is part of the normal flora of the skin and can cause opportunistic infections. Its lipase contributes to the genesis of acne.

Pseudomonas pseudomallei   *Pseudomonas pseudomallei* is a gram-negative rod that causes melioidosis, a rare disease found primarily in Southeast Asia, where the organism is a soil inhabitant. This disease has been seen in the USA since infections acquired by members of the armed forces during the Vietnam War have reactivated many years later. The acute disease is characterized by high fever and bloody, purulent sputum. Untreated cases can proceed to sepsis and death. In the chronic form, the disease can appear as pneumonia or lung abscess or may resemble tuberculosis. Diagnosis is made by culturing the organism from blood or sputum. The treatment of choice is usually either tetracycline or chloramphenicol, which is administered for several months.

Sarcina   *Sarcina* species are anaerobic gram-positive cocci grouped in packets of 8. They are minor members of the normal flora of the colon and are rarely pathogens.

Spirillum   *Spirillum minor* is a gram-negative, spiral-shaped rod that causes rat-bite fever (''sodoku''). The disease is characterized by a reddish brown rash spreading from the bite, accompanied by fever and local lymphadenopathy. The diagnosis is made by a combination of microscopy and animal inoculation.

Streptobacillus   *Streptobacillus moniliformis* is a gram-negative rod that causes another type of rat-bite fever (see *Spirillum,* above).

Veillonella   *Veillonella parvula* is an anaerobic gram-negative diplococcus that is part of the normal flora of the mouth, colon, and vagina. It is a rare opportunistic pathogen that causes abscesses of the sinuses, tonsils, and brain, usually in mixed anaerobic infections.

Yersinia enterocolitica & Yersinia pseudotuberculosis *Yersinia enterocolitica* and *Yersinia pseudotuberculosis* are gram-negative oval rods that are larger than *Yersinia pestis*. The virulence factors produced by *Y pestis* are not made by these species. These organisms are transmitted to humans by contamination of food with the excreta of domestic animals such as dogs, cats, and cattle. *Yersinia* infections are relatively infrequent in the USA, but the number of documented cases has increased during the past few years, perhaps as a result of improved laboratory procedures.

Y enterocolitica causes enterocolitis that is clinically indistinguishable from enterocolitis caused by *Salmonella* or *Shigella*. Both *Y enterocolitica* and *Y pseudotuberculosis* can cause mesenteric adenitis that clinically resembles acute appendicitis. Rarely, these organisms are involved in bacteremia or abscesses of the liver or spleen, mainly in persons with underlying diseases.

Y enterocolitica is usually isolated from stool specimens and forms a lactose-negative colony on MacConkey's agar. It grows better at 25 °C than at 37 °C; most biochemical tests are positive at 25 °C and negative at 37 °C. Incubation of a stool sample at 4 °C for 1 week, a technique called "cold enrichment," increases the frequency of recovery of the organism. *Y enterocolitica* can be distinguished from *Y pseudotuberculosis* by biochemical reactions.

The laboratory is usually not involved in the diagnosis of *Y pseudotuberculosis;* cultures are rarely performed in cases of mesenteric adenitis, and the organism is rarely recovered from stool specimens. Serologic tests are not available in most hospital clinical laboratories.

Enterocolitis and mesenteric adenitis caused by these organisms do not require treatment. In cases of bacteremia or abscess, aminoglycosides are usually effective. There are no preventive measures except to guard against contamination of food by the excreta of domestic animals.

(1) Viruses are particles composed of an internal core which contains *either* DNA or RNA (but not both), covered by a protective protein coat. Some viruses have an outer lipoprotein membrane, called an envelope, external to the coat.

(2) Viruses must grow within cells, because they cannot generate energy or synthesize proteins.

(3) Viruses replicate in a manner different from that of cells; ie, viruses do not undergo binary fission.

Table 1 compares some of the attributes of viruses and cells.

Table 1. Comparison of viruses and cells.

Property	Viruses	Cells
Type of nucleic acid	DNA or RNA but not both	DNA and RNA
Proteins	Few	Many
Lipoprotein membrane	Envelope present in some viruses	Cell membrane present in all cells
Ribosomes	Absent[1]	Present
Mitochondria	Absent	Present in eukaryotic cells
Enzymes	None or Few	Many
Multiplication by binary fission	No	Yes (most cells)

[1]Arenaviruses have a few nonfunctional ribosomes.

28   Structure

SIZE & SHAPE   Viruses range from 20 to 300 nm in diameter; this corresponds roughly to a spectrum of sizes from that of the largest protein to that of the smallest cell (see Fig. 2–2). Their shapes are frequently referred to in colloquial terms, eg, spheres, rods, bullets, or bricks, but in reality they are complex structures made up of repeating subunits of precise geometric symmetry. The shapes and sizes of some important viruses are depicted in Fig. 28–1.

VIRAL NUCLEIC ACIDS   The anatomy of 2 representative types of virus particles is shown in Fig 28–2. The viral nucleic acid is located internally and can be either single- or double-stranded DNA or single- or double-stranded RNA.* The existence of genetic material as single-stranded DNA and as double-stranded RNA is unique to viruses. The nucleic acid can be either linear or circular. The DNA is always a single molecule; the RNA can exist either as a single molecule or in several pieces. With the exception of the retroviruses, which are diploid, viruses are haploid; ie, they contain only one copy of their genes.

CAPSID & SYMMETRY   The nucleic acid is surrounded by a protein coat called a **capsid,** made up of subunits called capsomers. Each capsomer, consisting of one or several proteins, can be seen

---

*The nature of the nucleic acid of each virus is listed in Tables 31–1 and 31–2.

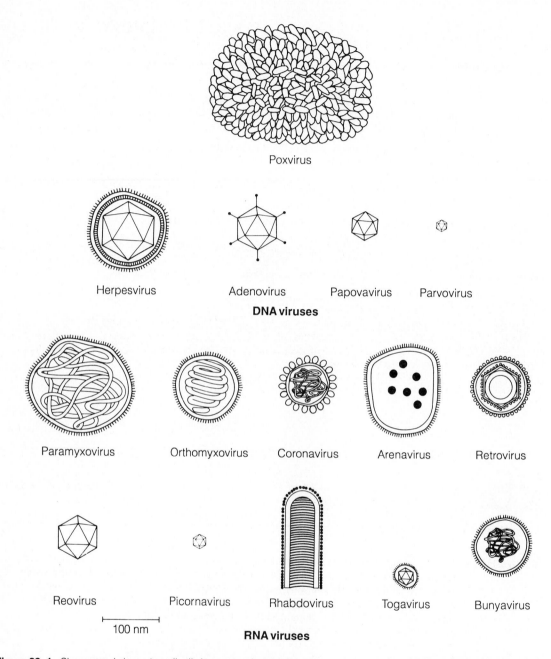

Poxvirus

Herpesvirus   Adenovirus   Papovavirus   Parvovirus

DNA viruses

Paramyxovirus   Orthomyxovirus   Coronavirus   Arenavirus   Retrovirus

Reovirus   Picornavirus   Rhabdovirus   Togavirus   Bunyavirus

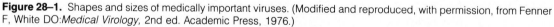

100 nm

RNA viruses

Figure 28–1. Shapes and sizes of medically important viruses. (Modified and reproduced, with permission, from Fenner F, White DO:*Medical Virology,* 2nd ed. Academic Press, 1976.)

in the electron microscope as a spherical particle, sometimes with a central hole. The arrangement of capsomers gives the virus structure its geometric symmetry. There are 2 forms of symmetry in virus capsids: (1) **icosahedral,** in which the capsomers are arranged in 20 triangles that form a symmetric figure (an icosahedron) with the approximate outline of a sphere; and (2) **helical,** in which the capsomers are arranged in a hollow coil that appears rod-shaped. The helix can be either rigid or flexible. Both the icosahedral and the helical forms can exist either ''naked'' or with an outer envelope layer.

The advantage of building the virus particle from identical protein subunits is 2-fold: (1) it reduces the need for genetic information, and (2) it promotes self-assembly; ie, no enzyme or energy is required. In fact, functional virus particles have been assembled in the test tube by combining the purified nucleic acid with the purified proteins in the absence of cells, energy source, and enzymes.

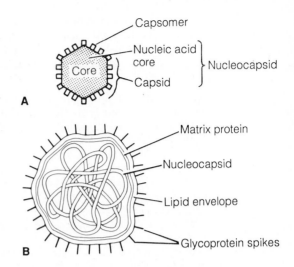

Figure 28–2. Cross section of 2 types of virus particles. *A:* Nonenveloped virus with icosahedral symmetry. *B:* Enveloped virus with helical symmetry. (Modified and reproduced, with permission, from Jawetz E et al: *Review of Medical Microbiology,* 18th ed. Appleton & Lange, 1989.)

VIRAL PROTEINS   Viral proteins serve several important functions. The outer capsid proteins **protect** the genetic material and **mediate the attachment** of the virus to specific receptors on the host cell surface. This interaction of the viral proteins with the cell receptor is the major determinant of species and organ **specificity.** Some of the internal proteins are associated with the nucleic acid, eg, nucleic acid polymerases, which are essential for replication, and histonelike proteins, which may have a regulatory function or may neutralize the negative charge on the nucleic acid during assembly of the virus particle.

ENVELOPE   In addition to the capsid and internal proteins, there are 2 other types of proteins, both of which are associated with the envelope. The **envelope** is a **lipoprotein** membrane composed of lipid derived from the host cell membrane and protein that is virus-specific. Furthermore, there are frequently glycoproteins in the form of spikelike projections on the surface, which attach to host cell receptors during the entry of the virus into the cell. Another protein, the **matrix** protein, mediates the interaction between the capsid proteins and the envelope.

In general, the presence of an envelope confers **instability** on the virus. Enveloped viruses are more sensitive to heat, detergents, and lipid solvents such as alcohol and ether than are nonenveloped (nucleocapsid) viruses, which are composed only of nucleic acid and capsid proteins.

The surface proteins of the virus, whether they are the capsid proteins or the envelope glycoproteins, are the principal **antigens** against which the host mounts its immune response to viruses. They are also the determinants of type specificity. For example, poliovirus types 1, 2, and 3 are distinguished by the antigenicity of their capsid proteins. It is important to know the number of serotypes of a virus, since vaccines should contain the prevalent serotypes. There is often little cross protection between different serotypes.

ATYPICAL VIRUSES   There are 4 exceptions to the typical virus as described above:

(1) Defective viruses are composed of viral nucleic acid and proteins but cannot replicate without a "helper" virus, which provides the missing function. Defective viruses usually have a mutation or a deletion of part of their genetic material. During the growth of most human viruses, many more defective than infectious virus particles are produced. The ratio of defective to infectious particles can be as high as 100:1. Because these defective particles can interfere with the growth of the infectious particles, it has been hypothesized that the defective viruses may aid in recovery from an infection by limiting the ability of the infectious particles to grow.

(2) Pseudovirions contain host cell DNA instead of viral DNA within the capsid. They are formed during infection with certain viruses when the host cell DNA is fragmented and pieces of it are incorporated within the capsid protein. Pseudovirions can infect cells, but they do not replicate.

(3) Viroids consist solely of a single molecule of circular RNA without a protein coat or envelope. There is extensive homology between bases in the viroid RNA, leading to large double-stranded regions. The RNA is quite small (MW 1 $\times$ 10^5) and apparently does not code for any protein. Nevertheless, viroids replicate but the mechanism is unclear. They cause several plant diseases but are not implicated in any human disease.

(4) Prions are infectious protein particles that are composed solely of protein ie, they contain no detectable nucleic acid. They are implicated as the cause of certain "slow" diseases such as Creutzfeldt-Jakob disease in humans and scrapie in sheep (see Chapter 44). Since neither DNA nor RNA has been detected in prions, they are clearly different from viruses. Furthermore, electron microscopy reveals filaments rather than virus particles. Prions are much more resistant to inactivation by ultraviolet light, heat, and acid than are viruses. They are remarkably resistant to formaldehyde and nucleases. However, they are inactivated by hypochlorite and autoclaving. Hypochlorite is now used to sterilize surgical instruments and other medical supplies that cannot be autoclaved.

Prions are composed of a single glycoprotein with a molecular weight of 27,000–30,000. With scrapie prions as the model, it was found that this protein is encoded by a single cellular gene. This gene is found in equal numbers in the cells of both infected and uninfected animals. Furthermore, the amount of prion protein mRNA is the same in uninfected as in infected cells. In view of these findings, posttranslational modifications of the prion protein are hypothesized to be the important distinction between the protein found in infected and uninfected cells. Because prion proteins are found associated with cell membranes, their pathogenicity may be related to alterations of membrane function.

The observation that the prion protein is the product of a normal cellular gene may explain why no immune response is formed against this protein, ie, tolerance occurs. Similarly, there is no inflammatory response in infected brain tissue. A vacuolated (spongiform) appearance is found, without inflammatory cells. Prion proteins in infected brain tissue form rod-shaped particles that are morphologically and histochemically indistinguishable from amyloid, a substance found in the brain tissue of individuals with various central nervous system diseases (as well as diseases of other organs).

The role of prions in the pathogenesis of "slow" diseases such as Creutzfeldt-Jakob disease remains unclear. The central question is: are prions the cause of these diseases or a pathologic byproduct? At present, prions are the most plausible causative agents and no alternative explanation has gathered much support.

Review Questions

1. What are the 2 types of symmetry of viral capsids?
2. What are the functions of viral proteins?
3. What is the composition of the viral envelope, and how is it formed?
4. Which proteins of the virus induce protective antibody?
5. Distinguish between defective viruses, pseudovirions, viroids, and prions.

Replication

The viral replication cycle is described below in 2 different ways. The first approach is a growth curve, which shows the amount of virus produced at different times after infection. The second is a stepwise description of the specific events within the cell during virus growth.

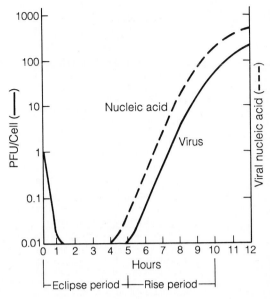

Figure 29–1. Viral growth curve. (Modified and reproduced, with permission, from Joklik WK et al: *Zinsser Microbiology,* 19th ed. Appleton & Lange, 1988.)

VIRAL GROWTH CURVE   A typical growth curve is depicted in Fig 29–1. The amount of virus produced is plotted on a logarithmic scale as a function of time after infection. Note that the time required for the growth cycle varies; it is minutes for some bacterial viruses and hours for some human viruses. In this example, the amount of infecting virus is arbitrarily set at one.

The first event is quite unusual: the virus disappears, as represented by the solid line dropping to the *X* axis. Although the virus particle, as such, is no longer present, the viral nucleic acid continues to function and begins to accumulate within the cell, as indicated by the dotted line. The time during which no virus is found inside the cell is known as the **eclipse period.** The eclipse period ends with the appearance of virus (solid line). The **latent period,** in contrast, is defined as the time from the onset of infection to the appearance of virus extracellularly. Note that infection begins with one virus particle and ends with several hundred virus particles having been produced; this type of reproduction is unique to viruses. Alterations of cell morphology accompanied by marked derangement of cell function begin toward the end of the latent period. This **cytopathic effect** (CPE) culminates in the lysis and death of cells. Not all viruses cause CPE; some can replicate while causing little morphologic or functional change in the cell.

SPECIFIC EVENTS DURING THE GROWTH CYCLE   An overview of the events is described in Table 29–1 and presented in diagrammatic fashion in Fig 29–2. The infecting parental virus particle attaches to the cell membrane and then penetrates the host cell. The capsid proteins are "uncoated," and the viral genetic material is free to function. Early mRNA and proteins are synthesized; the proteins are enzymes used to replicate the viral genome. Late mRNA and proteins are then synthesized. These late proteins are the structural, capsid proteins. The progeny virions are assembled from the replicated genetic material, and the newly made capsid proteins are then released from the cell.

Another, more general way to describe this sequence is as follows: (1) early events, ie, **attachment, penetration, and uncoating;** (2) middle events, ie, **gene expression** and **genome replication;** and (3) late events, ie, **assembly and release**. With this cycle in mind, each stage will be described in more detail.

Attachment, Penetration, & Uncoating   The proteins on the surface of the virion attach to specific receptor proteins on the cell surface through weak, noncovalent bonding. The **specificity** of attachment determines the **host range** of the virus. Some viruses have a narrow range, whereas others have quite a broad range. For example, poliovirus can enter only the cells of humans and other primates, whereas rabies virus can grow in all mammalian cells. The organ specificity of the virus is thought to be governed by receptor interaction as well.

Table 29–1. Stages of the viral growth cycle.

Attachment and penetration by parental virion
↓
Uncoating of the viral genome
↓
Early[1] viral mRNA synthesis[2]
↓
Early viral protein synthesis
↓
Viral genome replication
↓
Late viral mRNA synthesis
↓
Late viral protein synthesis
↓
Progeny virion assembly
↓
Virion release from cell

[1]"Early" is defined as the period before genome replication. Not all viruses exhibit a distinction between early and late functions. In general, early proteins are enzymes, whereas late proteins are structural components of the virus.
[2]In some cases, the viral genome is functionally equivalent to mRNA; thus, early mRNA need not be synthesized.

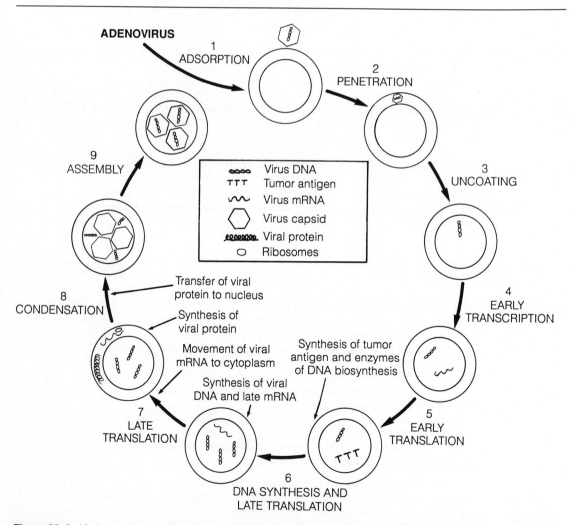

Figure 29–2. Viral growth cycle. The growth cycle of adenovirus, a nonenveloped DNA virus, is shown. (Reproduced, with permission, from Jawetz E, Melnick JL, Adelberg EA: *Review of Medical Microbiology,* 16th ed. Appleton & Lange, 1989.)

The virus particle penetrates by being engulfed in a pinocytotic vesicle, within which the process of uncoating begins. Rupture of the vesicle or fusion of the outer layer of virus with the vesicle membrane deposits the inner core of the virus into the cytoplasm.

Certain bacterial viruses (bacteriophages) have a special mechanism for entering bacteria that has no counterpart in either human viruses or those of animals or plants. Some of the T group of bacteriophages infect *Escherichia coli* by attaching several tail fibers to the cell surface and then using lysozyme from the tail to degrade a portion of the cell wall. At this point, the tail sheath contracts, driving the tip of the core through the cell wall. The viral DNA then enters the cell through the tail core, while the capsid proteins remain outside.

It is appropriate at this point to describe the phenomenon of **infectious nucleic acid,** since it provides a transition between the concepts of host specificity described above and early genome functioning, which is discussed below. Infectious nucleic acid is purified viral DNA or RNA (without any protein) that can carry out the entire viral growth cycle and result in the production of complete virus particles. This is interesting from 3 points of view:

(1) The observation that purified nucleic acid is infectious is the definitive proof that nucleic acid, not protein, is the genetic material.

(2) Infectious nucleic acid can bypass the host range specificity provided by the viral protein-cell receptor interaction. For example, although intact poliovirus can grow only in primate cells, purified poliovirus RNA can enter nonprimate cells, go through its usual growth cycle, and produce normal poliovirus. The poliovirus produced in the nonprimate cells can infect only primate cells, since it now has its capsid proteins. These observations indicate that the internal functions of the nonprimate cells are capable of supporting viral growth once entry has occurred.

(3) Only certain viruses yield infectious nucleic acid. The reason for this is discussed below.

Gene Expression & Genome Replication   The first step in viral gene expression is **mRNA synthesis.** It is at this point that viruses follow different pathways depending on the nature of their nucleic acid and the part of the cell in which they replicate.

DNA viruses, with one exception, replicate in the nucleus and use the host cell DNA-dependent RNA polymerase to synthesize their mRNA. The poxviruses are the exception because they replicate in the cytoplasm, where they do not have access to the host cell RNA polymerase. They therefore carry their own polymerase within the virus particle.

RNA viruses fall into 4 groups with quite different strategies (Table 29–2).

(1) The simplest strategy is illustrated by poliovirus, which has **single-stranded** RNA of **positive polarity*** as its genetic material. These viruses use their RNA genome directly as mRNA.

(2) The second group has **single-stranded** RNA of **negative polarity** as its genetic material. An mRNA must be transcribed by using the negative strand as a template. Because the cell does not have an RNA polymerase capable of using RNA as a template, the virus carries its own **RNA-dependent RNA polymerase.** There are 2 subcategories of negative-polarity RNA

---

*Positive polarity is defined as an RNA with the same base sequence as the mRNA, RNA with negative polarity has a base sequence that is complementary to the mRNA. For example, if the mRNA sequence is A-C-U-G, an RNA with negative polarity would be U-G-A-C and an RNA with positive polarity would be A-C-U-G.

Table 29–2. Synthesis of viral mRNA.

Genome	Polarity	Virion Polymerase	Source of mRNA	Infectivity of Genome	Prototype Human Virus
Single strand, nonsegmented	+	No	Genome	+	Poliovirus
Single strand Nonsegmented	–	Yes	Transcription	–	Measles virus, rabies virus
Segmented	–	Yes	Transcription	–	Influenza virus
Double strand, segmented	±	Yes	Transcription	–	Reovirus
Single strand, diploid	+	Yes[1]	Transcription[2]	–[3]	T-cell leukemia virus

[1]Retroviruses contain an RNA-dependent, DNA polymerase.
[2]mRNA transcribed from DNA intermediate.
[3]Although the retroviral genome RNA is not infectious, the DNA intermediate is.

viruses: those that have a single piece of RNA, eg, measles virus (a paramyxovirus) or rabies virus (a rhabdovirus), and those that have multiple pieces of RNA, eg, influenza virus (a myxovirus).

(3) The third group has **double-stranded RNA** as its genetic material. Because the cell has no enzyme capable of transcribing this RNA into mRNA, the virus carries its own polymerase. Reovirus, the best-studied member of this group, has 10 segments of double-stranded RNA.

(4) The fourth group, exemplified by the RNA tumor viruses (retroviruses), has single-stranded RNA of positive polarity that is transcribed into double-stranded DNA by the RNA-dependent DNA polymerase **(reverse transcriptase)** carried by the virus. This DNA copy is then transcribed into viral mRNA by the regular host cell RNA polymerase (polymerase II).

These differences explain why some viruses yield infectious nucleic acid and others do not. Viruses that do not require a polymerase in the virion can produce infectious DNA or RNA. By contrast, viruses such as the poxviruses, the negative-stranded RNA viruses, the double-stranded RNA viruses, and the retroviruses, which require a virion polymerase, cannot yield infectious nucleic acid. Several additional features of viral mRNA are described in the box.

Viral mRNA

There are 4 interesting aspects of viral mRNA and its expression in eukaryotic cells. (1) Viral mRNAs have 3 attributes in common with cellular mRNAs: on the 5′ end there is a methylated GTP "cap," which is linked by an "inverted" (3′– to 5′–) bond instead of the usual 5′– to 3′– bond; on the 3′ end there is a tail of 100 – 200 adenosine residues (poly[A]); and the mRNA is generated by splicing from a larger transcript of the genome. In fact, these 3 modifications were first observed in studies on viral mRNAs and then extended to cellular mRNAs. (2) Some viruses use their genetic material to the fullest extent by making more than one type of mRNA from the same piece of DNA by "shifting the reading frame." This is done by starting transcription 1 or 2 bases downstream from the original initiation site. (3) With some DNA viruses, there is temporal control over the region of the genome that is transcribed into mRNA. During the beginning stages of the growth cycle, before DNA replication begins, only the early region of the genome is transcribed and, therefore, only certain early proteins are made. One of the early proteins is a repressor of the late genes; this prevents transcription until the appropriate time. (4) Three different processes are used to generate the monocistronic mRNAs that will code for a single protein from the polycistronic viral genome:

(a) Individual mRNAs are transcribed by starting at many specific initiation points along the genome, which is the same mechanism used by eukaryotic cells and by herpesviruses, adenoviruses, and the DNA and RNA tumor viruses;

(b) in the reoviruses and influenza viruses, the genome is segmented into multiple pieces, each of which codes for a single mRNA; and

(c) in polioviruses, their entire RNA genome is translated into one long polypeptide, which is then cleaved into specific proteins by a protease.

Once the viral mRNA of either DNA or RNA viruses is synthesized, it is translated by host cell ribosomes into viral proteins, some of which are the early proteins required for replication of the viral genome. The most important of the early proteins for many RNA viruses is the polymerase that will synthesize many copies of viral genetic material for the progeny virus particles.

Replication of the viral genome is governed by the principle of **complementarity**, which requires that a strand with a complementary base sequence be synthesized; this strand then serves as the template for the synthesis of the actual viral genome. The following examples from Table 29–3 should make this clear: (1) poliovirus makes a negative-strand intermediate, which is the template for the positive-strand genome; (2) influenza, measles, and rabies viruses make a positive-strand intermediate, which is the template for the negative-strand genome; (3) reovirus makes a positive strand that acts both as mRNA and as the template for the negative

Table 29–3. Complementarity in viral genome replication.

Prototype Virus	Parental Genome[1]	Intermediate Form	Progeny Genome
Poliovirus	+ ssRNA	− ssRNA	+ ssRNA
Influenza virus, measles virus, rabies virus	− ssRNA	+ ssRNA	− ssRNA
Reovirus	± dsRNA	+ ssRNA	± dsRNA
Retrovirus	+ ssRNA	± dsDNA	+ ssRNA
Hepatitis B virus	± dsDNA	+ ssRNA	± dsDNA
Papovirus, adenovirus, herpesvirus, poxvirus	± dsDNA		± dsDNA

[1]Code: ss, single-stranded; ds, double-stranded.

strand in the double-stranded genome RNA; (4) retroviruses use the negative strand of the DNA intermediate to make positive-strand progeny RNA; (5) hepatitis B virus uses its mRNA as a template to make progeny double-stranded DNA; and (6) the other double-stranded DNA viruses replicate their DNA by the same semiconservative process by which cell DNA is synthesized.

As the replication of the viral genome proceeds, the structural capsid proteins to be used in the progeny virus particles are synthesized. In some cases, the newly replicated viral genomes can serve as templates for the late mRNA to make these capsid proteins.

Assembly & Release   The progeny particles are assembled by packaging the viral nucleic acid within the capsid proteins. Little is known about the precise steps in the assembly process. Surprisingly, certain viruses can be assembled in the test tube by using only purified RNA and purified protein. This indicates that the specificity of the interaction resides within the RNA and protein and that the action of enzymes and expenditure of energy are not required.

The release of virus from the cell occurs by one of 2 processes. The first is rupture of the cell membrane and release of the mature particles. This usually occurs with unenveloped viruses. Enveloped viruses, on the other hand, are released by **"budding"** through the outer cell membrane (Fig. 29–3). (An exception is the herpesvirus family, whose members acquire their envelopes from the nuclear membrane rather than from the outer cell membrane.) The budding process begins when virus-specific proteins enter the cell membrane at specific sites. The viral nucleocapsid then interacts with the specific membrane site mediated by the matrix protein. The cell membrane evaginates at that site, and an enveloped particle buds off from the membrane. Budding frequently does not damage the cell, and in certain instances the cell survives while producing large numbers of budding virus particles.

LYSOGENY   The typical replicative cycle described above occurs most of the time, but not always, when viruses infect cells. Some viruses can use an alternative pathway, called the **lysogenic cycle,** in which the viral DNA becomes integrated into the host cell chromosome and no progeny virus particles are produced at that time. The viral nucleic acid continues to function in the

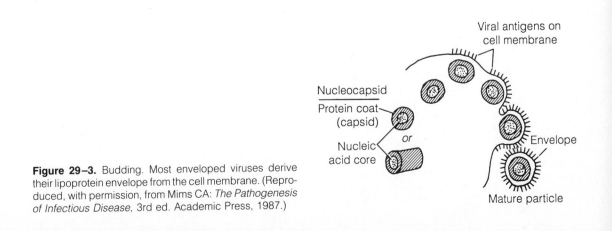

Figure 29–3. Budding. Most enveloped viruses derive their lipoprotein envelope from the cell membrane. (Reproduced, with permission, from Mims CA: *The Pathogenesis of Infectious Disease,* 3rd ed. Academic Press, 1987.)

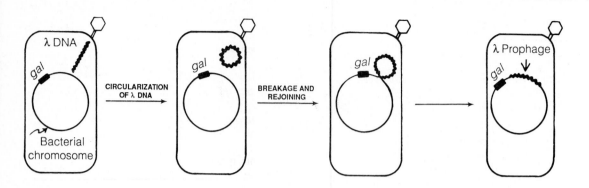

Figure 29–4. Lysogeny. The linear lambda phage genome circularizes within the infected bacterium and integrates into host cell DNA. (Reproduced, with permission, from Jawetz E et al: *Review of Medical Microbiology,* 17th ed. Appleton & Lange, 1989.)

integrated state in a variety of ways. One of the most important functions from a medical point of view is the synthesis of several exotoxins, such as diphtheria and botulinum toxins, coded for by the genes of the integrated bacteriophage (prophage). **Lysogenic conversion** is the term applied to the new properties that a bacterium acquires as a result of expression of the integrated prophage genes.

The lysogenic or "temperate" cycle is described for lambda bacteriophage, because it is the best-understood model system (Fig 29–4). Several aspects of infections by tumor viruses and herpesviruses are similar to the events in the lysogenic cycle of lambda phage.

Infection by lambda phage in *E coli* begins with injection of the linear, double-stranded DNA genome through the phage tail into the cell. The linear DNA becomes a circle as the single-stranded regions on the 5′ end and the 3′ end pair their complementary bases. A ligating enzyme makes a covalent bond in each strand to close the circle. Circularization is important, because it is the circular form that integrates into host cell DNA.

The choice between the pathway leading to lysogeny and that leading to full replication is made as early protein synthesis begins. Simply put, the choice depends on the balance between 2 proteins, the **repressor** produced by the *cI* gene and the **antagonizer of the repressor** produced by the *cro* gene (Fig 29–5). If the repressor predominates, transcription of other early genes is shut off and lysogeny ensues. Transcription is inhibited by binding of the repressor to the 2 operator sites that control early protein synthesis. If the *cro* gene product prevents the synthesis of sufficient repressor, replication and lysis of the cell result. One correlate of the lysogenic state is that the repressor can also prevent the replication of additional lambda phages that infect subsequently. This is called "immunity" and is specifically directed against lambda phage, because the repressor binds only to the operator sites in lambda DNA; other phages are not affected.

The next important step in the lysogenic cycle is the **integration** of the viral DNA into the cell DNA. This occurs by the matching of a specific attachment site on the lambda DNA to a homologous site on the *E coli* DNA and the integration (breakage and rejoining) of the 2 DNAs

Integration genes	cIII	N	P_L	O_L	cI	P_{RM}	O_R	P_R	CRO	cII	DNA replication and capsid protein genes

Figure 29–5. Control of lysogeny. Shortly after infection, transcription of the *N* and *cro* genes begins. The *N* protein is an antiterminator that allows transcription of *cII* and *cIII* and the genes to the right of *cII* and to the left of *cIII*. The *cII* protein enhances the production of the *cI* repressor protein. *cI* has 2 important functions: (1) It inhibits transcription at P_RO_R and P_LO_L, thereby preventing phage replication; and (2) it is a positive regulator of its own synthesis by binding to P_{RM}. The crucial decision point in lysogeny is the binding of either *cI* repressor or the *cro* protein to the O_R site. If *cI* repressor occupies O_R, lysogeny ensues; if *cro* protein occupies O_R, viral replication occurs. *N*, antiterminator gene; *cI*, repressor gene; *cII* and *cIII*, genes that influence the production of *cI*; P_LO_L, left promoter and operator; P_RO_R, right promoter and operator; P_{RM}, promoter for repressor maintenance; *cro*, gene that antagonizes the *cI* repressor.

mediated by a phage-encoded recombination enzyme. The integrated viral DNA is called a **prophage**. Most lysogenic phages integrate at one or a few specific sites, but some, such as the Mu (or mutator) phage, can integrate their DNA at many sites, and other phages, such as the P1 phage, never actually integrate but remain in a ''temperate'' state extrachromosomally, similar to a plasmid.

Because the integrated viral DNA is replicated along with the cell DNA, each daughter cell inherits a copy. However, the prophage is not permanently integrated. It can be induced to resume its replicative cycle by the action of UV light and certain chemicals. UV light induces the synthesis of a protease, which cleaves the repressor. Early genes then function, including the genes coding for the enzymes that excise the prophage from the cell DNA. The virus then completes its replicative cycle, leading to the production of progeny virus and lysis of the cell.

Review Questions

1. What are the differences between the way viruses and bacteria multiply?
2. What is the eclipse period of viral replication?
3. Describe the sequence of events in the viral growth cycle.
4. What is the major determinant of the host range of viruses?
5. What is infectious nucleic acid? If a virus has a virion polymerase, why is it unlikely to yield infectious nucleic acid?
6. Some viruses have an RNA polymerase in the virion. What is the function of this enzyme?
7. In general, what are the differences between ''early'' and ''late'' proteins? What separates early from late?
8. What is the underlying principle by which viruses replicate their genomes?
9. What is the role of budding in the growth cycle of some viruses?
10. What determines whether a virus enters the lysogenic cycle?
11. In lysogeny, where is the viral DNA located?
12. In general, what occurs during the induction of lysogenic prophage?

Genetics

The study of viral genetics falls into 2 general areas: (1) mutations and their effect on replication and pathogenesis, and (2) the interaction of 2 genetically distinct viruses that infect the same cell.

MUTATIONS Mutations in viral DNA and RNA occur by the same processes of base substitution, deletion, and frame shift as those described for bacteria in Chapter 4. Probably the most important practical use of mutations is in the production of vaccines containing live, attenuated virus. These attenuated mutants have lost their pathogenicity but have retained their antigenicity, so that they induce immunity without causing disease.

Conditional-lethal mutations are extremely valuable in determining the function of viral genes. These mutations function normally under permissive conditions but fail to replicate or to express the mutant gene under restrictive conditions. For example, temperature-sensitive conditional-lethal mutants express their phenotype normally at a low (permissive) temperature, but at a higher (restrictive) temperature the mutant gene product is inactive. To give a specific example, temperature-sensitive mutants of Rous sarcoma virus can transform cells to malignancy at the permissive temperature of 37 °C. When the transformed cells are grown at the restrictive temperature of 41 °C, their phenotype reverts to normal appearance and behavior. The malignant phenotype is regained when the permissive temperature is restored. Temperature-sensitive mutants of influenza virus can be used to make a vaccine, because this virus will grow in the cooler, upper airways where it causes few symptoms and induces antibodies but will not grow in the warmer, lower airways where it can cause pneumonia.

Some deletion mutants have the unusual property of being **defective interfering particles.** They are defective because they cannot replicate unless the deleted function is supplied by a "helper" virus. They also interfere with the growth of normal virus if they infect first and preempt the required cellular functions. Defective interfering particles may play a role in recovery from viral infection; they interfere with the production of progeny virus, thereby limiting the spread of the virus to other cells.

There are 2 other kinds of mutants of interest. The first are antigenic variants such as those that occur frequently with influenza viruses, which have an altered surface protein and are therefore no longer inhibited by a person's preexisting antibody. The variant can thus cause disease, whereas the original strain cannot. The second are drug-resistant mutants, which are insensitive to an antiviral drug because the target of the drug, usually a viral enzyme, has been modified.

INTERACTIONS   When 2 genetically distinct viruses infect a cell, 3 different phenomena can ensue.

(1) Recombination is the exchange of genes between 2 chromosomes that is based on crossing over within regions of significant base sequence homology. Recombination can be readily demonstrated for viruses with double-stranded DNA as the genetic material and has been used to determine their genetic map. However, recombination by RNA viruses occurs at a very low frequency, if at all. **Reassortment** is the term used when viruses with segmented genomes, such as influenza virus, exchange segments. This usually results in a much higher frequency of gene exchange than does recombination. Reassortment of influenza RNA segments is involved in the major antigenic changes in the virus that are the basis for recurrent influenza epidemics.

(2) Complementation can occur when one of the 2 viruses that infects the cell has a mutation that results in a nonfunctional protein (Fig 30–1). The nonmutated virus "complements" the mutated one by making a functional protein that serves for both viruses. Complementation is an important method by which a helper virus permits replication of a defective virus. This phenomenon is the basis for the complementation test, which can be used to determine how many genes exist in a viral genome. It is performed by determining whether mutant virus A can complement mutant virus B. If it can, the 2 mutations are in separate genes because they make different, complementary proteins. If it cannot, the 2 mutations are in the same gene and both proteins are nonfunctional. By performing many of these paired tests with different mutants, it is possible to determine functional domains of complementation groups that correspond to genes. Appropriate controls are needed to obviate the effects of recombination.

(3) In phenotypic mixing, the genome of virus type A can be coated with the surface proteins of virus type B (Fig 30–2). This phenotypically mixed virus can infect cells as determined by

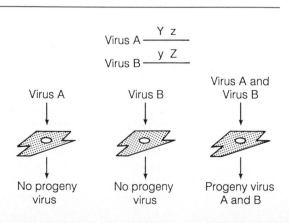

Figure 30–1. Complementation. If either virus A or virus B infects a cell, no virus is produced because each has a mutated gene. If virus A and virus B infect a cell, the protein product of gene Y of virus A will complement virus B and progeny virus will be produced. Note that no recombination has occurred and that the virus B progeny will contain the mutant y gene. Y, Z = functional genes; y, z = mutated, nonfunctional genes.

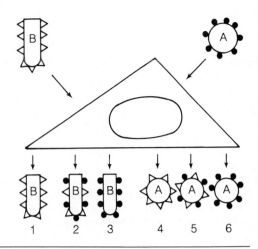

Figure 30-2. Phenotypic mixing. A retrovirus (**A**) and a rhabdovirus (**B**) infect the same cell. The progeny viruses include phenotypically mixed particles (2, 3, 4, and 5) and normal progeny virions (1 and 6). (Modified and reproduced, with permission, from .Boettiger D: Animal virus pseudotypes. *Prog Med Virol* 1979;**25**:37.)

its type B protein coat. However, the progeny virus from this infection has a type A coat; it is encoded solely by its type A genetic material. An interesting example of phenotypic mixing is that of **pseudotypes,** which consist of the nucleocapsid of one virus and the envelope of another. Pseudotypes composed of the nucleocapsid of vesicular stomatitis virus (a rhabdovirus) and the envelope of human immunodeficiency virus (HIV, a retrovirus) are currently being used to study the immune response to HIV.

Review Questions

1. What are temperature-sensitive conditional-lethal mutants?
2. What are defective interfering particles?
3. Distinguish between complementation and phenotypic mixing.

Classification of Medically Important Viruses

31

The classification of viruses is based on chemical and morphologic criteria. The 2 major components of the virus used in classification are (1) the nucleic acid (its molecular weight and structure); and (2) the capsid (its size and symmetry and whether it is enveloped). A classification scheme based on these factors is presented in Tables 31–1 and 31–2 for DNA and RNA viruses, respectively. This scheme was simplified from the complete classification to emphasize organisms of medical importance. Only the virus families are listed; subfamilies are described in the chapter on the specific virus.

DNA VIRUSES The 6 families of DNA viruses are described in Table 31–1. The 3 **naked** (ie, nonenveloped) icosahedral virus families—the parvoviruses, papovaviruses, and adenoviruses—are presented

Table 31–1. Classification of DNA viruses.

Virus Family	Envelope Present	Capsid Symmetry	Particle Size (nm)	DNA MW ($\times 10^6$)	DNA Structure[1]	Medically Important Viruses
Parvovirus	No	Icosahedral	22	2	SS, linear	B19 virus
Papovavirus	No	Icosahedral	55	3–5	DS, circular, supercoiled	Papilloma virus
Adenovirus	No	Icosahedral	75	23	DS, linear	Adenovirus
Hepadnavirus	Yes	Icosahedral	42	1.5	DS, incomplete circular	Hepatitis B virus
Herpesvirus	Yes	Icosahedral	100[2]	100–150	DS, linear	Herpes simplex virus, varicella-zoster virus, cytomegalovirus, Epstein-Barr virus
Poxvirus	Yes	Complex	250 × 400	125–185	DS, linear	Smallpox virus, vaccinia virus

[1]SS, single-stranded; DS, double-stranded.
[2]The herpesvirus nucleocapsid is 100 nm, but the envelope varies in size. The entire virus can be as large as 200 nm in diameter.

Table 31–2. Classification of RNA viruses.

Virus Family	Envelope Present	Capsid Symmetry	Particle Size (nm)	RNA MW ($\times 10^6$)	RNA Structure[1]	Medically Important Viruses
Picornavirus	No	Icosahedral	28	2–3	SS linear, nonsegmented, positive polarity	Poliovirus, rhinovirus, hepatitis virus
Reovirus	No	Icosahedral	75	15	DS linear, 10 segments	Reovirus, rotavirus
Togavirus	Yes	Icosahedral	40–70	4	SS linear, nonsegmented, positive polarity	Rubella virus, yellow fever virus
Retrovirus	Yes	Icosahedral	100	7[2]	SS linear, 2 segments, positive polarity	Leukemia virus, sarcoma virus
Orthomyxovirus	Yes	Helical	80–120	4	SS linear, 8 segments, negative polarity	Influenza virus
Paramyxovirus	Yes	Helical	150	6	SS linear, nonsegmented, negative polarity	Measles virus, mumps virus
Rhabdovirus	Yes	Helical	75 × 180	3–4	SS linear, nonsegmented, negative polarity	Rabies virus
Coronavirus	Yes	Helical	100	5	SS linear, nonsegmented, positive polarity	Coronavirus
Arenavirus	Yes	Helical	80–130	5	SS circular, 2 segments with cohesive ends, negative polarity	Lymphocytic choriomeningitis virus
Bunyavirus	Yes	Helical	100	5	SS circular, 3 segments with cohesive ends, negative polarity	Bunyamwera virus

[1]SS, single-stranded; DS, double-stranded.
[2]Retrovirus RNA contains 2 identical molecules of MW 3.5 $\times 10^6$.

in increasing order of particle size, as are the 3 **enveloped** families. The hepadnavirus family, which includes hepatitis B virus, and the larger herpesviruses are enveloped icosahedral viruses. The largest viruses, the poxviruses, have a complex internal symmetry.

Parvoviruses These are very small (22 nm in diameter) naked icosahedral viruses with single-stranded linear DNA. There are 2 types of parvoviruses: defective and nondefective. The defective parvoviruses, eg, adenoassociated virus, require a helper virus for replication. The DNA of defective parvoviruses is unusual, because plus-strand DNA and minus-strand DNA are carried in separate particles. The nondefective parvoviruses are best illustrated by B19 virus, which is associated with aplastic crises in sickle cell anemia patients and with erythema infectiosum, an innocuous childhood disease characterized by a ''slapped-cheeks'' rash.

Hepadnaviruses These are double-shelled viruses (42 nm in diameter) with an icosahedral capsid covered by an envelope. The DNA is a double-stranded circle that is unusual because the complete strand is not a covalently closed circle and the other strand is missing approximately 25% of its length. Hepatitis B virus is the human pathogen in this family.

Papovaviruses   These are naked icosahedral viruses (55 nm in diameter) with double-stranded circular supercoiled DNA. The name "papova" is an acronym of *pa*pilloma, *po*lyoma, and simian *va*cuolating viruses. Three human papovaviruses are JC virus, isolated from patients with progressive multifocal leukoencephalopathy; BK virus, isolated from the urine of immunosuppressed kidney transplant patients; and the human papillomavirus. Polyomavirus and simian virus 40 are papovaviruses of mice and monkeys, respectively, that induce malignant tumors in a variety of species.

Adenoviruses   There are naked icosahedral viruses (75 nm in diameter) with double-stranded linear DNA. They cause pharyngitis, upper and lower respiratory tract disease, and a variety of other less common infections. There are 31 antigenic types, some of which cause sarcomas in animals but no tumors in humans.

Herpesviruses   These are enveloped viruses (100 nm in diameter) with an internal icosahedral nucleocapsid and double-stranded linear DNA. They are the most important agents of latent infections. The 5 important human pathogens are herpes simplex virus types 1 and 2, varicella-zoster virus, cytomegalovirus, and Epstein-Barr virus (the cause of infectious mononucleosis).

Poxviruses   These are the largest viruses, with a bricklike shape, an envelope with an unusual appearance, and a complex capsid symmetry. They are named for the skin lesions, or "pocks," that they cause. Smallpox virus and vaccinia virus are the 2 important members. The latter virus is used in the smallpox vaccine.

RNA VIRUSES   The 10 families of RNA viruses are described in Table 31–2. The 2 **naked icosahedral** virus families, the picornaviruses and the reoviruses, are listed first and are followed by the 2 **enveloped icosahedral** viruses. The remaining 6 families are **enveloped helical** viruses; the first 4 have single-stranded linear RNA as their genome, whereas the last 2 have single-stranded circular RNA.

Picornaviruses   These are the smallest (28 nm in diameter) RNA viruses. They have single-stranded, linear, nonsegmented, positive-polarity RNA within a naked icosahedral capsid. The name "picorna" is derived from *pico* (small), *RNA*-containing. There are 2 subgroups of human pathogens: (1) enteroviruses such as poliovirus, coxsackievirus, echovirus, and hepatitis A virus; and (2) rhinoviruses.

Reoviruses   These are naked viruses (75 nm in diameter) with 2 icosahedral capsid coats. They have 10 segments of double-stranded linear RNA. The name is an acronym of *r*espiratory *e*nteric *o*rphan, because they were originally found in the respiratory and enteric tracts and were not associated with any human disease. The main human pathogen is rotavirus, which causes diarrhea, mainly in infants.

Togaviruses   These are enveloped viruses with an icosahedral capsid and single-stranded, linear, nonsegmented, positive-polarity RNA. There are 3 major groups of human pathogens: the alphaviruses and rubiviruses (50–70 nm in diameter) and the flaviviruses (40–50 nm in diameter). The alphavirus group comprises the mosquito-borne encephalitis viruses; the rubivirus group consists only of rubella virus. The flaviviruses include the mosquito-borne yellow fever, dengue, and encephalitis viruses and the tick-borne encephalitis viruses. The alphaviruses and flaviviruses are the former arbovirus groups A and B, respectively.

Retroviruses   These are enveloped viruses with an icosahedral capsid and 2 identical strands of single-stranded, linear, positive-polarity RNA. The term "retro" pertains to the reverse transcription of the RNA genome into DNA. The leukemia and sarcoma viruses of many animals are retroviruses, as are several "slow" viruses such as visna virus. Human T-cell leukemia viruses and human immunodeficiency viruses are also retroviruses.

Orthomyxoviruses These viruses (myxoviruses) are enveloped, with a helical nucleocapsid and 8 segments of linear, single-stranded, negative-polarity RNA. The term ''myxo'' refers to the affinity of these viruses for mucins, and ''ortho'' is added to distinguish them from the paramyxoviruses. Influenza virus is the main human pathogen.

Paramyxoviruses These are enveloped viruses with a helical nucleocapsid and single-stranded, linear, nonsegmented, negative-polarity RNA. The important human pathogens are measles, mumps, parainfluenza, and respiratory syncytial viruses.

Rhabdoviruses These are bullet-shaped enveloped viruses with a helical nucleocapsid and a single-stranded, linear, nonsegmented, negative-polarity RNA. The term ''rhabdo'' refers to the bullet shape. Rabies virus is the only important human pathogen.

Coronaviruses These are enveloped viruses with a helical nucleocapsid and a single-stranded, linear, nonsegmented, positive-polarity RNA. The term ''corona'' refers to the prominent halo of spikes protruding from the envelope. Coronaviruses cause respiratory tract infections (eg, the common cold) in humans.

Arenaviruses These are enveloped viruses with a helical nucleocapsid and a single-stranded, circular, negative-polarity RNA in 2 segments. The term ''arena'' means ''sand'' and refers to granules on the virion surface that are nonfunctional ribosomes. Two human pathogens are lymphocytic choriomeningitis and Lassa fever viruses.

Bunyaviruses These are enveloped viruses with a helical nucleocapsid and a single-stranded, circular, negative-polarity RNA in 3 segments. The term ''bunya'' refers to the prototype, Bunyamwera virus, which is named for the place in Africa where it was isolated. These viruses cause encephalitis and various fevers such as Korean hemorrhagic fever.

Review Question

Describe the criteria used to classify viruses.

32

Pathogenesis

The ability of viruses to cause disease can be viewed on 2 distinct levels: (1) the changes that occur within individual cells and (2) the process that takes place in the infected patient.

THE INFECTED CELL There are 4 main effects of virus infection on the cell: (1) death, (2) fusion of cells to form multinucleated cells, (3) malignant transformation, and (4) no apparent morphologic or functional change.

Death of the cell is probably due to inhibition of macromolecular synthesis. Inhibition of host cell protein synthesis frequently occurs first and is probably the most important. Inhibition of DNA and RNA synthesis may be a secondary effect. It is important to note that synthesis of **cellular** proteins is inhibited, but **viral** protein synthesis still occurs. The molecular basis for this selectivity is not clearly understood.

Infected cells frequently contain **inclusion bodies**, which are discrete areas containing viral proteins or viral particles. They have a characteristic intranuclear or intracytoplasmic location and appearance depending on the virus. One of the best examples of inclusion bodies that can assist in clinical diagnosis is that of Negri bodies, which are eosinophilic cytoplasmic inclusions found in rabies virus-infected brain neurons. Electron micrographs of inclusion bodies can also aid in the diagnosis when virus particles of typical morphology are visualized.

Fusion of virus-infected cells produces **multinucleated giant cells**, which characteristically form after infection with herpesviruses and paramyxoviruses. Fusion occurs as a result of cell membrane changes, which are probably due to the insertion of viral proteins into the membrane. The clinical diagnosis of herpesvirus skin infections is aided by the finding of multinucleated giant cells with eosinophilic intranuclear inclusions in skin scrapings.

A hallmark of viral infection of the cell is the **cytopathic effect (CPE)**. This change in the appearance of the infected cell usually begins with a rounding and darkening of the cell and culminates in either lysis (disintegration) or giant cell formation. Detection of virus in a clinical specimen frequently is based on the appearance of CPE in cell culture. In addition, CPE is the basis for the plaque assay, an important method for quantifying the amount of virus in a sample.

Infection with certain viruses causes malignant transformation, which is characterized by unrestrained growth, prolonged survival, and morphologic changes such as focal areas of rounded, piled-up cells. These changes are described in more detail in the chapter on tumor viruses.

Infection of the cell accompanied by virus production can occur without morphologic or gross functional changes. This observation highlights the wide variations in the nature of the interaction between the virus and the cell, ranging from rapid destruction of the cell to a symbiotic relationship in which the cell survives and multiplies despite the replication of the virus.

THE INFECTED PATIENT   Pathogenesis in the infected patient involves (1) transmission of the virus and its entry into the host; (2) replication of the virus and damage to cells; (3) spread of the virus to other cells and organs; (4) the immune response, both as a host defense and as a contributing cause of certain diseases; and (5) persistence of the virus in some instances.

Transmission   Viruses are transmitted to the individual by many different routes. For example, person-to-person spread occurs by transfer of respiratory secretions, saliva, blood, or semen and by fecal contamination of water or food. Transmission can occur also between mother and offspring either in utero across the placenta, at the time of delivery, or during breast feeding. Animal-to-human transmission can take place either directly from a bite of a reservoir host as in rabies or indirectly through the bite of an insect vector, such as a mosquito, which transfers the virus from an animal reservoir to the person. In addition, activation of a latent, nonreplicating virus to form an active, replicating virus can occur within the individual, with no transmission from an external source.

Portal of Entry & Dissemination   Viral infections are either **localized** to the portal of entry (see Table 7–1) or spread **systemically** through the body. The best example of the localized infection is the common cold, which involves only the upper respiratory tract. Influenza infects both the upper and lower respiratory tract primarily. One of the best-understood systemic viral infections is poliomyelitis (Fig 32–1). After poliovirus is ingested, it infects the cells of the small intestine and then spreads to the mesenteric lymph nodes, where it multiplies again. It then enters the bloodstream and is transmitted to the central nervous system, where damage to the anterior horn cells occurs, resulting in the characteristic muscle paralysis. It is during this obligatory viremia that circulating IgG antibodies induced by the polio vaccine can prevent the virus from infecting the central nervous system. Viral replication in the gastrointestinal tract results in the presence of poliovirus in the feces, thus perpetuating its transmission to others.

Some of the molecular determinants of pathogenesis have been determined by using reovirus infection in mice as a model system. This virus has 3 different outer capsid proteins, each of which has a distinct function in determining the course of the infection. One of the proteins binds to specific receptors on the cell surface and thereby determines tissue tropism. A second protein conveys resistance to proteolytic enzymes in the gastrointestinal tract and acts as the antigen that stimulates the cellular immune response. The third protein inhibits cellular RNA

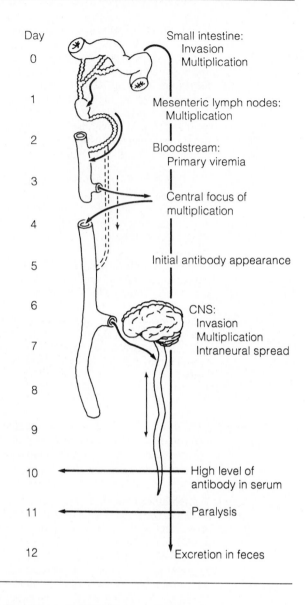

Figure 32–1. Systemic viral infection (poliomyelitis). (Modified from Fenner.)

and protein synthesis, leading to death of the cell. This third protein also plays an important role in initiation of persistent viral infection.

Immunopathogenesis   The signs and symptoms of most viral diseases undoubtedly are the result of cell killing by virus-induced inhibition of macromolecular synthesis. However, there are certain diseases in which cell killing by **immunologic attack** plays an important role in pathogenesis.

(a) The best-studied system is lymphocytic choriomeningitis (LCM) in mice; LCM occurs in humans also. When LCM virus is inoculated into the brain of an adult mouse, virus replication occurs and death follows. However, when LCM virus is inoculated into the brain of an immunosuppressed adult mouse or a newborn mouse, the animal remains well despite extensive virus replication. When immune lymphocytes are inoculated into these infected, healthy mice, death ensues. It appears that death of the cells is caused by immune attack by cytotoxic T cells on the new viral antigens in the cell membrane rather than by virus-induced inhibition of cell functions.

(b) A second example of immune-mediated pathogenesis occurs when virus-antibody-complement complexes form and are deposited in various tissues. This occurs in hepatitis B virus infection, in which immune complexes play a role in producing the chronic hepatitis and arthritis characteristic of this disease.

Persistent Viral Infections In most viral infections, the virus does not remain in the body for a significant period after clinical recovery. However, in certain instances, the virus persists for long periods either intact or in the form of a subviral component, eg, the genome. The mechanisms that may play a role in the persistence of viruses include (1) integration of a DNA provirus into host cell DNA, as occurs with retroviruses; (2) immune tolerance, because neutralizing antibodies are not formed; (3) formation of virus-antibody complexes, which remain infectious; (4) location within an immunologically sheltered "sanctuary," eg, the brain; (5) rapid antigenic variation; (6) intracellular spread so that virus is not exposed to antibody; and (7) immunosuppression, as in AIDS.

There are 3 types of persistent viral infections of clinical importance. They are distinguished primarily by whether virus is usually produced by the infected cells and by the timing of the appearance both of the virus and of the symptoms of disease.

A. Chronic-Carrier Infections: Some patients who have been infected with certain viruses continue to produce significant amounts of the virus for long periods. This **carrier state** can follow an asymptomatic infection as well as the actual disease and can itself either be asymptomatic or result in chronic illness. Important clinical examples are chronic hepatitis, which occurs in hepatitis B virus carriers, and neonatal rubella virus and cytomegalovirus infections, in which carriers can produce virus for as long as 2 years.

B. Latent Infections: In these infections, best illustrated by the herpesvirus group, the patient recovers from the initial infection and virus production stops. Subsequently, a **recurrence** of symptoms may occur that is accompanied by the production of virus. In herpes simplex virus infections, the virus enters the latent state in the cells of the sensory ganglia. The molecular nature of the latent state is unknown. Herpes simplex virus type 1, which causes infections primarily of the eyes and face, is latent in the trigeminal ganglion, whereas herpes simplex virus type 2, which causes infections primarily of the genitals, is latent in the lumbar and sacral ganglia. Varicella-zoster virus, another member of the herpesvirus family, causes varicella (chickenpox) as its initial manifestation and then remains latent, primarily in the trigeminal or thoracic ganglion cells. It can recur later in the form of the painful vesicles of zoster (shingles), usually on the face or trunk.

C. Slow Virus Infections: The term "slow virus" refers to the **prolonged period** between the initial infection and the onset of disease, which is usually measured in years. In instances in which the cause has been identified, the virus has been shown to have a normal, not prolonged, growth cycle. It is not, therefore, that virus growth is slow; rather, the incubation period and the progression of the disease are prolonged. Two of these diseases are caused by conventional viruses, namely subacute sclerosing panencephalitis, which follows several years after measles virus infections, and progressive multifocal leukoencephalopathy (PML), which is associated with infection by JC virus, a papovavirus. PML occurs primarily in patients who have lymphomas or are immunosuppressed. Other slow virus infections in humans, eg, Creutzfeldt-Jakob disease and kuru, may be caused by unconventional agents called **prions** (see p 128). Slow virus infections are described in Chapter 44.

Review Questions

1. What are inclusion bodies? Why are they important in viral diagnosis?
2. How are giant cells formed in viral infection? What is their importance in viral diagnosis?
3. What is the cytopathic effect? How is it used in viral diagnosis?
4. Describe immunopathogenesis.
5. Distinguish between chronic carrier infections and latent infections.
6. What are slow virus infections?

Host defenses against viruses fall into 2 major categories: (1) **nonspecific,** of which the most important are interferons; and (2) **specific,** including both humoral and cell-mediated immunity.

NONSPECIFIC DEFENSES

1. Interferons Interferons are a heterogeneous group of glycoproteins[*] produced by human and other animal cells after viral infection (or after exposure to other inducers). They inhibit the growth of viruses by **blocking the translation of viral proteins.** Interferons are divided into 3 groups based on the cell of origin, namely leukocyte, fibroblast, or lymphocyte. They are also known as alpha, beta, and gamma interferons, respectively. Alpha and beta interferons are induced by viruses, whereas gamma (T cell) interferon is induced by antigens and is one of the effectors of cell-mediated immunity (see Chapter 58). The following discussion of alpha and beta interferons focuses on 2 aspects: induction and action (Fig. 33–1).

Induction of Alpha & Beta Interferons The strong inducers of these interferons are **viruses** and **double-stranded RNAs.** Induction is not specific for a particular virus; many DNA and RNA viruses of humans, other animals, plants, and bacteria are competent, although they differ in effectiveness. The finding that double-stranded RNA, but not single-stranded RNA or DNA, is a good inducer has led to the hypothesis that a double-stranded RNA is synthesized as part of the replicative cycle of all inducing viruses. The double-stranded RNA, poly(rI-rC), is one of the strongest inducers and was under consideration as an antiviral agent, but toxic side effects prevented its clinical use. The weak inducers of microbiologic interest include a variety of intracellular bacteria and protozoa, as well as certain bacterial substances such as endotoxin.

This extensive list of inducers makes it clear that **induction** of these interferons is **not specific.** Similarly, their inhibitory **action** is **not specific** for any particular virus. However, they are **specific** in regard to the **host species** in which they act; ie, interferons produced by human cells are active in human cells but act poorly, if at all, in cells of other species. It is clear, therefore, that other animals cannot be used as a source of interferons for human therapy. Rather, the genes for human interferons have been cloned and material for medical trials is now produced by genetic engineering techniques.

---

[*]Molecular weights between 20,000 and 40,000.

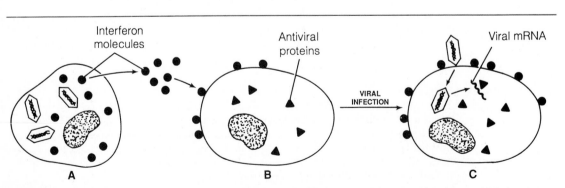

Figure 33–1. Induction and action of interferon. **A:** Virus infection induces the synthesis of interferon, which then leaves the cell. **B:** Interferon binds to the surface of an uninfected cell and induces the synthesis of 3 new enzymes (antiviral proteins). **C:** Antiviral proteins block the translation of viral mRNA. (Modified and reproduced, with permission, from Tortora G, Funk B, Case C: *Microbiology: An Introduction,* 2nd ed. Benjamin/Cummings, 1986.)

Action of Alpha & Beta Interferons   Interferons inhibit the intracellular replication of a wide variety of viruses. They act by inducing 3 proteins that prevent the translation of viral mRNA without affecting the translation of cellular mRNA: (1) a protein kinase that phosphorylates an initiation factor for cell protein synthesis, thereby inactivating it; (2) a 2,5-oligonucleotide synthetase that synthesizes an adenine trinucleotide; and (3) an endonuclease that is activated by the adenine trinucleotide and that degrades viral but not cellular mRNAs. Interferons have no direct effect on extracellular virus particles.

Because interferons are produced within a few hours of the initiation of viral replication, they may act in the early phase of viral diseases to limit the spread of virus. In contrast, antibody begins to appear in the blood several days after infection.

2. Phagocytosis   Macrophages, particularly fixed macrophages of the reticuloendothelial system and alveolar macrophages, are the important cell types in limiting virus infection. In contrast, polymorphonuclear leukocytes are the predominant cellular defense in bacterial infections.

3. Fever   Elevated body temperature may play a role in host defenses, but its importance is uncertain. Fever may act in 2 ways. (1) The higher body temperature may directly inactivate the virus particles, particularly enveloped viruses, which are more heat-sensitive than nonenveloped viruses. (2) Replication of some viruses is reduced at higher temperatures, and so fever may inhibit replication.

4. Mucociliary Clearance   The mucociliary clearance mechanism of the respiratory tract may protect the host. Its damage, eg, from smoking, results in an increased frequency of viral respiratory tract infections, especially influenza.

5. Factors that Modify Host Defenses   Several factors influence host defenses in a nonspecific or multifactorial way.

(1) Age is a significant variable in the outcome of viral infections. In general, infections are more severe in infants and in older people than in children. For example, paralytic polio occurs less often in young children than in teenagers, and encephalitis following chickenpox is much less frequent in children than in adults.

(2) Increased corticosteroid levels predispose to more severe infections with some viruses, such as varicella-zoster virus; the use of topical cortisone in herpetic keratitis can exacerbate eye damage. It is not clear how these effects are mediated, because corticosteroids can cause a variety of pertinent effects, namely lysis of lymphocytes, decreased recruitment of monocytes, inhibition of interferon production, and stabilization of lysosomes.

(3) Malnutrition leads to more severe viral infections; eg, there is a much higher death rate from measles in developing countries than in developed ones. Poor nutrition causes decreased immunoglobulin production and phagocyte activity as well as reduced skin and mucous membrane integrity.

SPECIFIC DEFENSES   There is evidence for natural resistance to some viruses in certain species, which is probably based on the absence of receptors on the cells of the resistant species. However, by far the most important type of defense is **acquired immunity**, both actively acquired by exposure to the virus and passively acquired by the transfer of immune serum. Active immunity can be elicited by contracting the actual disease, by having an inapparent infection with no symptoms, or by being vaccinated.

1. Active Immunity   Active immunity is important in the **prevention** of disease, but its ability to enhance the patient's **recovery** from a viral disease is limited. Disease prevention is chiefly due to the presence of immunoglobulins e.g. passive transfer of serum containing specific antibodies is typically protective.

The duration of protection varies; disseminated viral infections such as measles and mumps confer lifelong immunity against recurrences, but localized infections such as the common cold usually impart only a brief immunity of several months. IgA confers protection against viruses that enter through the respiratory and gastrointestinal mucosa, and IgM and IgG protect against viruses that enter or are spread through the blood. The lifelong protection against systemic viral infections such as the childhood diseases measles, mumps, rubella, and chickenpox (varicella) is a function of the anamnestic (secondary) response of IgG. For certain respiratory viruses such as parainfluenza and respiratory syncytial viruses, the IgA titer in respiratory secretions correlates with protection, whereas the IgG titer does not. Unfortunately, protection by IgA against most respiratory tract viruses usually lasts less than 5 years.

The role of active immunity in recovery from a viral infection is uncertain. Because recovery usually precedes the appearance of detectable humoral antibody, immunoglobulins may not be important. Also, children with agammaglobulinemia recover from measles infections normally and can be immunized against measles successfully, indicating that cell-mediated immunity plays an important role. This is supported by the observation that children with congenital T cell deficiency are vulnerable to severe infections with measles virus and herpesviruses. T cells are important in recovery from many but not all viral illnesses.

The protection offered by active immunity can be affected by the phenomenon of **"original antigenic sin."** This term refers to the observation that when a person is exposed to a virus that cross-reacts with another virus to which that individual was previously exposed, more antibody may be produced against the original virus than against the current one. It appears that the immunologic memory cells can respond to the original antigenic exposure to a greater extent than to the subsequent one. This was observed in people with antibodies to the A_1 type of influenza virus, who, when exposed to the A_2 type, produced large amounts of antibody to A_1 but very little antibody to the A_2 virus. It is also the underlying cause of severe hemorrhagic dengue fever (see **Chapter 42**). This phenomenon has 2 practical consequences as well: (1) Attempts to vaccinate people against the different influenza virus strains may be less effective than expected, and (2) epidemiologic studies based on measurement of antibody titers may yield misleading results.

How does antibody inhibit viruses? There are 2 main mechanisms. The first is **neutralization** of the infectivity of the virus by antibody binding to the proteins on the outer surface of the virus. This binding has 2 effects: (1) It can prevent the interaction of the virus with cell receptors, and (2) it can cross-link the viral proteins and stabilize the virus so that uncoating does not occur. The virus, therefore, cannot replicate. Furthermore, antibody-coated virus is more rapidly phagocytized than normal virus, a process similar to the opsonizing effect of antibody on bacteria. Antibody does not degrade the virus particle; fully infectious virus can be recovered by dissociating the virus-antibody complex. Incomplete or "blocking" antibody can interfere with neutralization and form immune complexes, which are important in the pathogenesis of certain diseases. Some viruses, such as herpesviruses, can spread from cell to cell across intercellular bridges, eluding the neutralizing effect of antibody.

The second mechanism is the **lysis of virus-infected cells** in the presence of antibody and complement. Antibody binds to new virus-specific antigens on the cell surface and then binds complement, which enzymatically degrades the cell membrane. Because the cell is killed before the full yield of virus is produced, the spread of virus is significantly reduced. Cytotoxic T cells can also cause lysis of virus-infected cells. Recognition by cytotoxic T cells is dependent not only on the viral antigen but also on cellular HLA class I proteins.

Not all virus infections induce antibodies. **Tolerance** to viral antigens can occur when the virus infection develops in a fetus or newborn infant. The model system in which tolerance has been demonstrated is lymphocytic choriomeningitis (LCM) infection in mice. If LCM virus is inoculated into a newborn mouse, the virus replicates widely but no antibodies are formed during the lifetime of the animal. The virus is recognized as "self," because it was present at the time of maturation of the immune system. If LCM virus is given to an adult mouse, antibodies are formed normally. There is no example of total tolerance to a virus in humans; even in congenital rubella syndrome, in which the virus infects the fetus, some antibody against rubella virus is made. However, virus production and shedding can go on for months or years.

Suppression of the cell-mediated response can occur during infection by certain viruses. The best-known example is the loss of tuberculin skin test reactivity during measles infection. Infection by cytomegalovirus or human immunodeficiency virus can also cause suppression.

2. Passive Immunity Transfer of human serum containing the appropriate antibodies provides prompt short-term immunity for individuals exposed to certain viruses. The term "passive" refers to the administration of **preformed antibodies.** Two types of immune globulin preparations are used for this purpose. One has a high titer of antibody against a specific virus, and the other is a pooled sample from plasma donors that contains a heterogeneous mixture of antibodies with lower titers. The immune globulins are prepared by alcohol fractionation, which removes any viruses in the serum. The 3 most frequently used high-titer preparations are used after exposure to hepatitis B, rabies, and varicella-zoster viruses. Low-titer immune globulin is used mainly after exposure to hepatitis A virus.

Review Questions

1. Describe interferons from the following points of view: (a) the distinction between alpha, beta, and gamma interferons; (b) the induction, specificity, and mechanism of action of the antiviral effect.
2. Explain the distinction between active and passive immunity. What are their advantages and disadvantages?
3. Does antibody inhibit viruses directly or by destroying virus-infected cells, or both?
4. Does tolerance to viral antigens occur?

Laboratory Diagnosis

34

There are 3 approaches to the diagnosis of viral diseases by the use of clinical specimens: (1) identification of the virus in cell culture, (2) microscopic identification directly in the specimen, and (3) serologic procedures to detect a rise in antibody titer or the presence of IgM antibody.

IDENTIFICATION IN CELL CULTURE The growth of viruses requires cell cultures, because they grow only in living cells, not on cell-free media the way most bacteria can. Because many viruses are inactivated at room temperature, it is important to inoculate the specimen into the cell culture as soon as possible; brief transport or storage at 4 °C is acceptable. Virus growth in cell culture frequently produces a characteristic **cytopathic effect** (**CPE**) that can provide a preliminary diagnosis. The time taken for the CPE to appear and the type of cell in which the virus produces the CPE are important clues in the preliminary identification.

If the virus does not produce a CPE, its presence can be detected by several other techniques:

(1) Hemadsorption, ie, attachment of erythrocytes to the surface of virus-infected cells. This technique is limited to viruses with a hemagglutinin protein on their envelope, such as mumps, parainfluenza, and influenza viruses.

(2) Interference with the formation of a CPE by a second virus. For example, rubella virus, which does not cause a CPE, can be detected by interference with the formation of a CPE by certain enteroviruses such as echovirus or coxsackievirus.

(3) A decrease in acid production by infected, dying cells. This can be detected visually by the color change in the phenol red (a pH indicator) in the culture medium. The indicator remains red (alkaline) in the presence of virus-infected cells but turns yellow in the presence of metabolizing normal cells as a result of the acid produced. This can be used to detect certain enteroviruses.

A definitive identification of the virus grown in cell culture is made by using known antibody in one of several tests. Complement fixation, hemagglutination inhibition, and neutralization of the CPE are the most frequently used tests. Other procedures such as fluorescent antibody, radioimmunoassay, enzyme-linked immunosorbent assay, and immuno-electron microscopy are also used in special instances. A brief outline of these tests follows. They are described in more detail in the section on immunology.

Complement Fixation   If the antigen (the unknown virus in the culture fluid) and the known antibody are homologous, complement will be fixed (bound) to the antigen-antibody complex. This makes it unavailable to lyse the "indicator" system, which is composed of sensitized red blood cells.

Hemagglutination Inhibition   If the virus and antibody are homologous, the virus is blocked from attaching to the erythrocytes and no hemagglutination occurs. Only viruses that agglutinate red blood cells can be identified by this method.

Neutralization   If the virus and antibody are homologous, the antibody bound to the surface of the virus blocks its entry into the cell. This neutralizes viral infectivity, because it prevents viral replication and subsequent CPE formation or animal infection.

Fluorescent Antibody   If the virus-infected cells and the fluorescein-tagged antibody are homologous, then the typical apple-green color of fluorescein is seen in the cells by UV microscopy.

Radioimmunoassay   If the virus and the antibody are homologous, there is less antibody remaining to bind to the known radiolabeled virus.

Enzyme-Linked Immunosorbent Assay   First, the antibody is bound to a surface. If the virus is homologous, it will be bound also. A sample of the antibody linked to an enzyme is added, and the amount of enzyme is assayed.

Immunoelectron Microscopy   If the antibody is homologous to the virus, aggregates of virus-antibody complexes are seen in the electron microscope.

MICROSCOPIC IDENTIFICATION   The second approach to detecting and identifying viruses is direct microscopic examination of clinical specimens such as biopsy material or skin lesions. Three different procedures can be used: (1) Light microscopy can reveal characteristic inclusion bodies or multinucleated giant cells. The Tzanck smear, which shows herpes simplex virus-induced multinucleated giant cells in vesicular skin lesions, is a good example. (2) UV microscopy is used for fluorescent-antibody staining of the virus in infected cells. (3) Electron microscopy detects virus particles, which can be preliminarily characterized by their size and morphology.

SEROLOGIC PROCEDURES   In the third approach, a rise in the titer of antibody to the virus is used to indicate current infection. A serum sample is obtained as soon as a viral etiology is suspected, and a second sample is obtained 10–14 days later. It is important to realize that an antibody titer on a single sample does not distinguish between a previous infection and a current one. The antibody titer can be determined by many of the immunologic tests mentioned above. These serologic diagnoses are usually made retrospectively, because the disease has frequently run its course by the time the results are obtained.

In certain viral diseases, the presence of IgM antibody is used to diagnose current infection. For example, the presence of IgM antibody to core antigen indicates infection by hepatitis B virus.

Other nonspecific serologic tests are available. For example, the heterophil antibody test (Monospot) can be used to diagnose infectious mononucleosis (see Chapter 37).

Review Questions

1. Distinguish between cytopathic effect and hemadsorption in the laboratory diagnosis of viruses.
2. What is the viral neutralization test?
3. Distinguish between the complement fixation and hemagglutination inhibition tests.
4. In the serologic diagnosis of viral diseases, why is it important to obtain both acute- and convalescent-phase specimens?

Antiviral Drugs

35

Compared with the number of drugs available to treat bacterial infections, the number of antiviral drugs is **very small.** The major reason for this difference is the difficulty in obtaining selective toxicity against viruses; their replication is intimately involved with the normal synthetic processes of the cell. Despite the difficulty, several virus-specific replication steps have been identified that are potentially useful (Table 35–1).

Another limitation of antiviral drugs is that they are relatively ineffective, because many cycles of viral replication occur during the incubation period when the patient is well. By the time the patient has a recognizable systemic viral disease, the virus has spread throughout the body and it is too late to interdict it. Furthermore, some viruses, eg, herpesviruses, become latent within cells, and no current antiviral drug can eradicate them.

Another potential limiting factor is the emergence of viral mutants that are resistant to the drug. At present, this is of little clinical significance. Mutants of herpesvirus resistant to acyclovir have been recovered from patients, but they do not interfere with recovery.

Inhibition of Early Events Amantadine (α-adamantanamine) is a tricyclic compound (Fig 35–1) that is used to prevent influenza A infections. It may inhibit uncoating of the virus; absorption and penetration occur normally, but transcription by the virion RNA polymerase does not. This drug specifically inhibits influenza A virus; influenza B and C viruses are not affected. Despite its efficacy in preventing influenza, it is not widely used in the USA because the vaccine is preferred for the high-risk population.

Table 35–1. Potential sites for antiviral chemotherapy.

Site of Action	Effective Drugs
Early events (entry or uncoating of the virus)	Amantadine
Nucleic acid synthesis by viral DNA and RNA polymerases	Acyclovir, vidarabine, idoxuridine, trifluridine, azidothymidine, ribavirin
Other virus-specific enzymes	
Protein synthesis directed by viral mRNA	Interferon, methisazone
Cleavage of precursor polypeptides	
Assembly of the particle, including the matrix protein	
Release of the particle by budding	

Inhibition of Viral DNA Synthesis

A. Acyclovir: Acyclovir (acycloguanosine, Zovirax) is a nucleoside analogue with a 3-carbon fragment in place of the normal sugar, ribose (Fig 35–1). Acyclovir is active primarily against herpes simplex virus types 1 and 2 and varicella-zoster virus. It is relatively nontoxic, because it is incorporated preferentially into virus-infected cells. This is due to the **virus-encoded thymidine kinase,** which phosphorylates acyclovir much more effectively than does the cellular thymidine kinase. Because only herpes simplex virus and varicella-zoster virus encode a kinase that efficiently phosphorylates the drug, it is active primarily against these viruses. It has no activity against cytomegalovirus. Once the drug is phosphorylated to acyclovir monophosphate within the infected cell, cellular kinases synthesize acyclovir triphosphate, which inhibits viral DNA polymerase much more effectively than it inhibits cellular DNA polymerase.

Topical acyclovir is effective in the treatment of primary genital herpes and reduces the frequency of recurrences while it is being taken. However, it has **no effect on latency** or on the rate of recurrences after treatment is stopped. Acyclovir is the treatment of choice for herpes simplex virus type 1 encephalitis and is effective in preventing systemic infection by herpes simplex virus type 1 or varicella-zoster virus in immunocompromised patients. It is not effective treatment for herpes simplex virus type 1 recurrent lesions in immunocompetent hosts. Acyclovir-resistant mutants have been isolated from herpes simplex virus type 1–infected patients.

B. Vidarabine: Vidarabine (adenosine arabinoside, ara-A) is a nucleoside analogue with arabinose in place of the normal sugar, ribose (Fig 35–1). On entering the cell, the drug is phosphorylated by cellular kinases to the triphosphate, which inhibits the herpesvirus-encoded DNA polymerase more effectively than the cellular DNA polymerase. Vidarabine is effective against herpes simplex virus type 1 infections such as encephalitis and keratitis but is used less frequently than acyclovir.

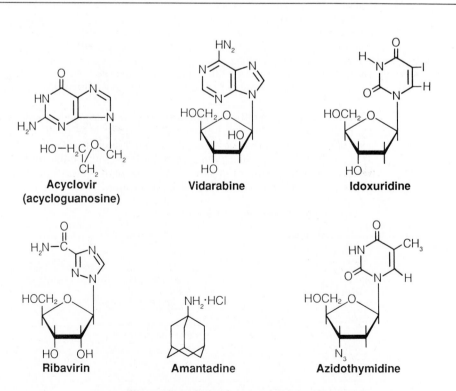

Figure 35–1. Structures of antiviral drugs.

C. Iododeoxyuridine: Iododeoxyuridine (idoxuridine, IDU, IUDR) is a nucleoside analogue in which the methyl group of thymidine is replaced by an iodine atom (Fig 35–1). The drug is phosphorylated to the triphosphate by cellular kinases and incorporated into DNA. Because IDU has a high frequency of mismatched pairing to guanine, it causes the formation of faulty progeny DNA and mRNA. However, because IDU is incorporated into normal cell DNA as well as viral DNA, it is too toxic to be used systemically. It is clinically useful in the topical treatment of herpes simplex virus keratoconjunctivitis.

D. Trifluorothymidine: Trifluorothymidine (trifluridine) is a nucleoside analogue in which the methyl group of thymidine contains 3 fluorine atoms instead of 3 hydrogen atoms. Its mechanism of action is probably similar to that of IDU. Like IDU, it is too toxic for systemic use but is clinically useful in the topical treatment of herpes simplex virus keratoconjunctivitis.

E. Azidothymidine: Azidothymidine (zidovudine, Retrovir) is a nucleoside analogue that causes chain termination during DNA synthesis; it has an azido group in place of the hydroxyl group on the ribose (Fig 35–1). It is particularly effective against DNA synthesis by the reverse transcriptase of human immunodeficiency virus and inhibits growth of the virus in cell culture. It is currently being used clinically in patients with AIDS.

F. Ribavirin: Ribavirin (Virazole) is a nucleoside analogue in which a triazole-carboxamide moiety is substituted in place of the normal purine precursor aminoimidazole-carboxamide (Fig 35-1). The drug inhibits the synthesis of guanine nucleotides, which are essential for both DNA and RNA viruses. Ribavirin aerosol is used clinically to treat pneumonitis caused by respiratory syncytial virus in infants and to treat severe influenza B infections.

G. Ganciclovir: Ganciclovir (dihydroxypropoxymethylguanine, DHPG) is a nucleoside analogue that is active against cytomegalovirus. It is effective in the treatment of retinitis caused by cytomegalovirus in AIDS in patients and may be useful in other disseminated infections caused by this virus.

Inhibition of Viral Protein Synthesis

A. Interferon: The mode of action of interferon is described in Chapter 33. Interferon is not yet clinically available to treat viral diseases.

B. Methisazone: Methisazone (N-methylisatin-β-thiosemicarbazone) specifically inhibits the protein synthesis of poxviruses, such as smallpox and vaccinia viruses, by blocking the translation of late mRNA. The drug, which was available in the USA for the treatment of certain rare, severe side effects of smallpox vaccine, is no longer used; smallpox has been eradicated, and the vaccine is no longer recommended for the general population.

Review Questions

1. Why are there fewer antiviral drugs than antibacterial drugs?
2. What is the basis of the selective action of acyclovir against herpes simplex viruses?
3. Describe amantadine, vidarabine, azidothymidine, and ganciclovir from 2 points of view: (a) mechanism of action and (b) spectrum of activity.

Because few drugs are useful against viral infections, prevention of infection by the use of vaccines is very important. There are 2 types of vaccines: those that contain **live virus** whose pathogenicity has been **attenuated*** and those that contain **killed virus**. The attributes of the 2 types of vaccines are listed in Table 36–1. In general, live vaccines are preferred to vaccines containing killed virus because their protection is **greater** and **longer-lasting.** With live vaccines, the virus multiplies in the host, producing a prolonged antigenic stimulus, and both IgA and IgG are elicited when the vaccine is administered by the natural route of infection, eg, when polio vaccine is given orally. Killed vaccines, which are usually given intramuscularly, do not stimulate a major IgA response.

There are 3 concerns about the use of live vaccines:

(1) They are composed of attenuated viral mutants, which can **revert to virulence** either during vaccine production or in the immunized person. Reversion to virulence during production can be detected by quality control testing, but there is no test to predict whether reversion will occur in the immunized individual.

(2) The live vaccine can be **excreted** by the immunized person. This is a double-edged sword. It is advantageous if the spread of the virus successfully immunizes others, as occurs with the live polio vaccine. However, it could be a problem if, eg, a virulent poliovirus revertant spreads to a susceptible person. Rare cases of paralytic polio occur in the USA each year by this route of infection.

(3) A second virus could **contaminate** the vaccine if it was present in the cell cultures used to prepare the vaccine. This concern exists for both live and killed vaccines, although, clearly, the live vaccine presents a greater problem, because the process that inactivates the virus in the killed vaccine could inactivate the contaminant as well. It is interesting, therefore, that the most striking incidence of contamination of a vaccine occurred with the *killed* polio vaccine. In 1960, it was reported that live simian vacuolating virus 40 (SV40 virus), an inapparent "passenger" virus in monkey kidney cells, had contaminated some lots of polio vaccine and was resistant to the formaldehyde used to inactivate the poliovirus. There was great concern when it was found that SV40 virus causes sarcomas in a variety of rodents. Fortunately, it has not caused cancer in the individuals inoculated with the contaminated polio vaccine.

In addition to the disadvantages of the killed vaccines already mentioned–namely that they induce a **shorter duration** of protection, are **less protective,** and **induce fewer IgA antibodies**–there is the potential problem that the inactivation process might be inadequate.

Table 36–1. Characteristics of live and killed viral vaccines.

Characteristic	Live Vaccine	Killed Vaccine
Duration of immunity	Longer	Shorter
Effectiveness of protection	Greater	Lower
Immunoglobulins produced	IgA[1] and IgG	IgG
Reversion to virulence	Possible	No
Stability at room temperature	Low	High
Excretion of virus and transmission to nonimmune contacts	Possible	No

[1]If the vaccine is given by the natural route.

---

*In this context, attenuation means that the virus is unable to cause disease but retains its antigenicity and can induce protection.

Table 36–2. Current viral vaccines (1987).

Vaccine	Availability		Efficacy[1]
	Live	Killed	
Measles	Yes	No	4+
Mumps	Yes	No	4+
Rubella	Yes	No	4+
Polio	Yes	Yes[2]	4+
Yellow fever	Yes	No	4+
Adenovirus	Yes[2]	No	3+
Smallpox[3]	Yes[2]	No	4+
Influenza	No	Yes	2+ or 3+
Hepatitis B	No	Yes[4]	3+
Rabies	No	Yes	4+

[1]Efficacy: 1+, 50–65%; 2+, 65–80%; 3+, 80–90%; 4+, more than 90%.
[2]Limited availability; it is used only in special situations.
[3]Contains vaccinia virus.
[4]Vaccine contains particles of surface antigen.

Although this is rare, it happened in the early days of the manufacture of the killed polio vaccine. However, killed vaccines do have 2 advantages; ie, they **cannot revert to virulence** and they are **more heat-stable,** so they can be used more easily in tropical climates.

The prospect for the future is that some of the disadvantages of current vaccines will be bypassed by the use of purified viral antigens produced from genes cloned in either bacteria or yeasts. The advantages of antigens produced by the cloning process are that they contain no viral nucleic acid and so cannot replicate or revert to virulence; they have no contaminating viruses from cell culture; and they can be produced in large amounts.

The viral vaccines currently in use are described in Table 36–2.

Review Questions

1. Some viral vaccines contain live virus. What attribute of the virus must be altered before it can be used in a vaccine, and what major problem can arise?
2. If you were in charge of an immunization program, would you choose a live or a killed vaccine? Why?

Part IV: Clinical Virology

Most of the clinically important viral pathogens can be categorized into groups according to their structural characteristics, ie, DNA enveloped viruses, DNA nonenveloped* viruses, RNA enveloped viruses, and RNA nonenveloped viruses (see Chapters 37–40 and Table 1). However, some viruses, eg, arboviruses, tumorviruses, and slow viruses (see Chapters 41–45), are described best in terms of their biologic features. Several clinically less prominent viruses, eg, parvoviruses and coronaviruses, are described in Chapter 46.

An overview of the viruses in the 4 structural categories follows.

DNA ENVELOPED VIRUSES

A. Herpesviruses: (See Chapter 37.)   These viruses are noted for their ability to cause latent infections. This family includes (1) herpes simplex virus types 1 and 2, which cause painful vesicles on the face and genitals, respectively; (2) varicella-zoster virus, which causes varicella (chickenpox) in children and zoster (shingles) in adults; (3) cytomegalovirus, an important cause of congenital malformations; and (4) Epstein-Barr virus, which causes infectious mononucleosis and is implicated in Burkitt's lymphoma.

B. Hepatitis B Virus: (See Chapter 41.)   This is one of the important causes of viral hepatitis. In contrast to hepatitis A virus (an RNA nucleocapsid virus), hepatitis B virus causes a more severe form of hepatitis, results more frequently in a chronic carrier state, and is implicated in the induction of hepatocellular carcinoma, the most common cancer worldwide.

C. Poxvirus: (See Chapter 37.)   Poxviruses are the largest and most complex of the viruses. The disease smallpox has been eradicated by effective use of the vaccine.

DNA NONENVELOPED VIRUSES   Adenoviruses (See Chapter 38) are best known for causing upper and lower respiratory tract infections, including pharyngitis and pneumonia.

RNA ENVELOPED VIRUSES

A. Respiratory Viruses (See Chapter 39):

(1) Influenza A and B viruses.   Influenza A virus is the major cause of recurrent epidemics of influenza.

(2) Parainfluenza viruses.   These are the leading cause of croup in young children and an important cause of common colds in adults.

(3) Respiratory syncytial virus (RSV).   This is the leading cause of bronchiolitis and pneumonia in infants.

Table 1. Major viral pathogens.

Structure	Viruses
DNA enveloped viruses	Herpesviruses (herpes simplex virus types 1 and 2, varicella-zoster virus, cytomegalovirus, Epstein-Barr virus), hepatitis B virus, smallpox virus
DNA nucleocapsid viruses	Adenovirus
RNA enveloped viruses	Influenza virus, parainfluenza virus, respiratory syncytial virus, measles virus, mumps virus, rubella virus, rabies virus
RNA nucleocapsid viruses	Enteroviruses (poliovirus, coxsackievirus, echovirus, hepatitis A virus), rhinovirus, reovirus

*Nonenveloped viruses are also called naked nucleocapsid viruses.

B. Measles, Mumps, and Rubella Viruses: (See Chapter 39). These viruses are well known for the complications associated with the diseases they cause; eg, rubella virus infection in a pregnant woman can cause congenital malformations. The incidence of these 3 diseases has been markedly reduced in the USA as a result of immunization.

C. Rabies Virus: (See Chapter 39.) This virus causes an almost invariably fatal encephalitis following the bite of a rabid animal. In the USA, wild animals such as skunks, raccoons, and bats are the major sources.

RNA NONENVELOPED VIRUSES

A. Enteroviruses: (See Chapter 40.) These viruses infect the enteric tract and are transmitted by the fecal-oral route. Poliovirus rarely causes disease in the USA because of the vaccine but remains an important cause of aseptic meningitis and paralysis in developing countries. Of more importance in the USA are coxsackieviruses, which cause aseptic meningitis, myocarditis, and pleurodynia; and echoviruses, which cause aseptic meningitis.

B. Rhinoviruses: (See Chapter 40.) These viruses are the most prominent cause of the common cold. They have a large number of antigenic types, which may account for their ability to cause disease so frequently.

C. Reoviruses: (See Chapter 40.) These viruses possess an unusual genome composed of double-stranded RNA in 10 segments. "Reo" is an acronym for *r*espiratory *e*nteric *o*rphan. They were initially called "orphan" viruses because they were not associated with any specific disease. However, one of the reoviruses, rotavirus, is an important cause of viral gastroenteritis in young children.

D. Hepatitis A Virus: (See Chapter 41.) This virus is an important cause of hepatitis. It is an enterovirus but is described in this book in conjunction with hepatitis B virus. It is structurally different from hepatitis B virus, a DNA enveloped virus. Furthermore, it is epidemiologically distinct; ie, it primarily affects children, is transmitted by the fecal-oral route, and rarely causes a prolonged carrier state.

OTHER CATEGORIES Chapter 42 describes the large and varied group of arboviruses, which have the common feature of being transmitted by an arthropod. Chapter 43 covers tumor viruses, and Chapter 44 covers the "slow viruses," which cause degenerative central nervous system diseases primarily. Chapter 45 describes the human immunodeficiency virus, the cause of acquired immunodeficiency syndrome (AIDS). The less common viral pathogens are described in Chapter 46.

Table 2 lists the frequency of the 10 most common notifiable viral diseases in the USA for 1986 (the latest year for which complete data are available). Chickenpox (varicella) is by far the most frequent, with hepatitis B and A a distant second and third, respectively. Note that the common cold, which is probably the most frequent disease, is not listed because it is not a notifiable disease.

Table 2. Notifiable viral diseases in the USA (1986).[1]

Disease	Number of Cases
Chickenpox	183,243
Hepatitis B	26,107
Hepatitis A	23,430
Acquired immunodeficiency syndrome (AIDS)	12,932
Mumps	7,790
Measles	6,282
Hepatitis, non-A, non-B (NANB)	3,634
Rubella	551
Poliomyelitis	3
Rabies, human	0

[1]The latest year for which complete data are available.

37

DNA Enveloped Viruses

Herpesviruses

The herpesvirus family contains 5 important human pathogens: herpes simplex virus types 1 and 2, varicella-zoster virus, cytomegalovirus, and Epstein-Barr virus.

All herpesviruses are structurally similar. Each has an **icosahedral** core surrounded by a lipoprotein **envelope.** The genome is linear double-stranded DNA. The virion does not contain a polymerase. They are large (120–200 nm in diameter), second in size only to poxviruses. They replicate in the nucleus and are the only viruses that obtain their envelopes by budding from the nuclear membrane.

Herpesviruses are noted for their ability to cause **latent infections.** In these infections, the acute disease is followed by an asymptomatic period during which the virus remains in a quiescent (latent) state, perhaps in the form of its genome integrated into cellular DNA. When the patient is exposed to an inciting agent or immunosuppression occurs , reactivation of virus replication and disease can occur. With some herpesviruses, eg, herpes simplex virus, the symptoms of the subsequent episodes are similar to those of the initial one; however, with others, eg, varicella-zoster virus, they are different (Table 37–1).

Certain herpesviruses are suspected of causing cancer in humans; eg, Epstein-Barr virus is associated with Burkitt's lymphoma and nasopharyngeal carcinoma. Several herpesviruses cause cancer in animals, eg, leukemia in monkeys and lymphomatosis in chickens (see tumor viruses, Chapter 43).

HERPES SIMPLEX VIRUSES (HSV) Herpes simplex virus type 1 (HSV-1) and type 2 (HSV-2) are distinguished by 2 main criteria: antigenicity and location of lesions. Lesions caused by HSV-1 are, in general, above the waist, whereas those caused by HSV-2 are below the waist.

Diseases HSV-1 causes acute gingivostomatitis, recurrent herpes labialis (cold sores), keratoconjunctivitis, and encephalitis. HSV-2 causes genital herpes, neonatal herpes, and aseptic meningitis.

Important Properties HSV-1 and HSV-2 are structurally and morphologically indistinguishable. They can, however, be differentiated by the restriction endonuclease patterns of their genome DNA and by type-specific monoclonal antisera. Humans are the natural hosts of both HSV-1 and HSV-2.

Table 37–1. Important features of common herpesvirus infections.

Virus	Primary Infection	Usual Site of Latency	Recurrent Infection	Route of Transmission
HSV-1	Gingivostomatitis.[1]	Cranial sensory ganglia	Herpes labialis;[2] encephalitis; keratitis.	Via respiratory secretions and saliva.
HSV-2	Herpes genitalis; perinatal disseminated disease.	Lumbar or sacral sensory ganglia	Herpes genitalis.	Sexual contact, perinatal infection.
VZV	Varicella.	Cranial or thoracic sensory ganglia	Zoster.[2]	Via respiratory secretions.
EBV	Infectious mononucleosis.[1]	B lymphocytes	None.[3]	Via respiratory secretions and saliva.
CMV	Congenital infection (in utero); mononucleosis.	Uncertain[4]	Asymptomatic shedding.[2]	intrauterine infection, transfusions, sexual contact, via secretions, eg, saliva and urine.

[1]Primary infection is often asymptomatic.
[2]In immunocompromised patients, dissemination is common.
[3]The relationship of EBV infection to "chronic fatigue syndrome" and B cell neoplasms is unclear.
[4]CMV may be latent within circulating lymphoid cells or epithelial cells.

Summary of Replicative Cycle   After entry into the cell, the virion is uncoated and the genome DNA enters the nucleus. Early virus messenger RNA (mRNA) is transcribed by host cell RNA polymerase and then translated into early, nonstructural proteins in the cytoplasm. Two of these early proteins, thymidine kinase and DNA polymerase, are important because they are sufficiently different from the corresponding cellular enzymes to be involved in the action of antiviral drugs e.g. Acyclovir.

The viral DNA polymerase replicates the genome DNA, at which time early protein synthesis is shut off and late protein synthesis begins. These late, structural proteins are transported to the nucleus, where virion assembly occurs. The virion obtains its envelope by budding through the nuclear membrane and exits the cell via tubules or vacuoles that communicate with the exterior.

Transmission & Epidemiology   HSV-1 is transmitted primarily by **saliva,** whereas HSV-2 is transmitted by **sexual contact.** As a result, HSV-1 infections occur mainly on the face, whereas HSV-2 lesions occur in the genital area. However, oral-genital sexual practices can result in HSV-1 infections of the genitals and HSV-2 lesions in the oral cavity (this occurs in about 10–20% of cases).

The number of HSV-2 infections has markedly increased in recent years, whereas that of HSV-1 infections has not. Roughly 80% of people in the USA are infected with HSV-1, and 40% have recurrent herpes labialis. Most primary infections by HSV-1 occur in childhood, as evidenced by the early appearance of antibody. In contrast, antibody to HSV-2 does not appear until the age of sexual activity.

Pathogenesis & Immunity   The virus replicates in the skin or mucous membrane at the initial site of infection, then migrates up the neuron and becomes latent in the sensory ganglion cells. In general, HSV-1 becomes latent in the **trigeminal** ganglia, whereas HSV-2 becomes latent in the **lumbar and sacral ganglia.** The precise nature of the virus during latency is unknown, but lysogeny in bacterial viruses can be used as a model. The virus can be reactivated from the latent state by a variety of inducers, eg, sunlight, hormonal changes, trauma, stress, and fever, at which time it migrates down the neuron and replicates in the skin, causing lesions.

The typical skin lesion is a **vesicle** that contains serous fluid filled with virus particles and cell debris. When the vesicle ruptures, virus is liberated and can be transmitted to other individuals. **Multinucleated giant cells** are typically found at the base of herpesvirus lesions.

Immunity is type-specific, but some cross-protection exists. However, immunity is incomplete, and both reinfection and reactivation occur in the presence of circulating IgG. **Cell-mediated immunity** is important in limiting herpesviruses, since its suppression often results in reactivation, spread, and severe disease.

Clinical Findings   HSV-1 causes several forms of primary and recurrent disease:

(1) Acute gingivostomatitis occurs primarily in children and is characterized by fever, irritability, and vesicular lesions in the mouth. The primary disease is more severe and lasts longer than recurrences. The lesions heal spontaneously in 2–3 weeks. Many children have asymptomatic primary infections.

(2) Herpes labialis (fever blisters or cold sores) is the milder, recurrent form and is characterized by crops of vesicles, usually at the mucocutaneous junction of the lips or nose. Recurrences frequently reappear at the same site.

(3) Keratoconjunctivitis is characterized by corneal ulcers and lesions of the conjunctival epithelium. Recurrences can lead to scarring and blindness.

(4) Encephalitis, which usually involves the temporal lobe, is associated with a high mortality rate and causes severe neurologic sequelae in those who survive.

(5) Herpetic whitlow is a pustular lesion of the skin of the finger or hand. It often occurs in medical personnel as a result of contact with patient's lesions.

(6) Disseminated infections, such as esophagitis and pneumonia, occur in immunocompromised patients with depressed T cell function.

HSV-2 causes several diseases, both primary and recurrent:

(1) Genital herpes is characterized by painful vesicular lesions of the male and female genitals and anal area. The lesions are more severe and protracted in primary disease than in recurrences. Primary infections are associated with fever and inguinal adenopathy. Asymptomatic infections occur in both men (in the prostate or urethra) and women (in the cervix) and can be a source of infection of other individuals.

(2) Neonatal herpes originates chiefly from contact with vesicular lesions within the birth canal. In some cases, there are no visible lesions. Neonatal herpes varies from a severe generalized disease or encephalitis through milder local lesions to asymptomatic infection. Neonatal disease may be prevented by performing cesarean section on women with either active lesions or positive viral cultures. Both HSV-1 and HSV-2 can cause severe neonatal infections that are acquired after birth from carriers handling the child. Despite their association with neonatal infections, neither HSV-1 nor HSV-2 causes congenital abnormalities or abortions to any significant degree, presumably because they do not cross the placenta.

(3) Aseptic meningitis caused by HSV-2 is usually a mild, self-limited disease with few sequelae.

Laboratory Diagnosis The most important diagnostic procedure is isolation of the virus from the lesion by growth in cell culture. The typical cytopathic effect occurs in 1–3 days, after which the virus is identified by fluorescent-antibody staining of the infected cells. A rapid diagnosis from skin lesions can be made by using the **Tzanck smear**, in which cells from the base of the vesicle are stained with Giemsa's stain. The presence of multinucleated giant cells suggests herpesvirus infection. A rapid diagnosis of encephalitis can be made by fluorescent-antibody staining of a brain biopsy, but virus is rarely recovered from the cerebrospinal fluid.

Serologic tests such as the neutralization test can be used in the diagnosis of primary infections, since a significant rise in antibody titer is readily observed. However, they are of no use in the diagnosis of recurrent infections, because many adults already have circulating antibodies and recurrences rarely cause a rise in antibody titer.

Treatment **Acyclovir** (acycloguanosine) is the treatment of choice for encephalitis and systemic disease caused by HSV-1. It is also the treatment for primary and recurrent genital herpes; it **shortens the duration** of the lesions and **reduces the extent of shedding** of the virus. Before acyclovir was available, a more toxic drug, vidarabine (adenine arabinoside), was the treatment of choice for HSV-1 encephalitis. For HSV-1 eye infections, other nucleoside analogues, eg, idoxuridine and trifluridine, are used topically. Note that no drug treatment of the primary infection prevents recurrences; drugs have **no effect on the latent state,** but prophylactic long-term acyclovir administration can suppress clinical recurrences.

Prevention Prevention involves avoiding contact with the vesicular lesion or ulcer. Cesarean section should be considered for women who are at term and who have genital lesions or positive viral cultures.

VARICELLA-ZOSTER VIRUS (VZV)

Disease Varicella (chickenpox) is the primary disease; zoster (shingles) is the recurrent form.

Important Properties VZV is structurally and morphologically identical to other herpesviruses but is antigenically different. It has a single serotype. The same virus causes both varicella and zoster. Humans are the natural hosts.

Summary of Replicative Cycle The cycle is similar to that of HSV (see p 157).

Transmission & Epidemiology The virus is transmitted by **respiratory droplets** and by direct contact with the lesions. Varicella is a highly contagious disease of childhood; over 90% of people in the USA have antibody by age 10 years. Varicella occurs worldwide.

Pathogenesis & Immunity VZV infects the mucosa of the upper respiratory tract, then spreads via the blood to the skin, where the typical **vesicular rash** occurs. **Multinucleated**

giant cells with intranuclear inclusions are seen in the base of the lesions. After the host has recovered, the virus becomes **latent,** probably in the **dorsal root ganglia.** Later in life, frequently at times of reduced cell-mediated immunity or local trauma, the virus is activated and causes the vesicular skin lesions and **nerve pain** of zoster.

Immunity following varicella is lifelong: a person gets varicella only once, but zoster can occur despite this immunity to varicella. Zoster usually occurs only once. The frequency of zoster increases with advancing age, perhaps as a consequence of waning immunity.

Clinical Findings

A. Varicella: After an incubation period of 14–21 days, brief prodromal symptoms of fever and malaise occur. A papulovesicular rash then appears in crops on the trunk and spreads to the head and extremities. The rash evolves from papules to vesicles, pustules, and, finally, crusts. Itching is marked. Varicella is mild in children but more severe in adults. Varicella pneumonia and encephalitis are the major rare complications. **Reye's syndrome,** characterized by encephalopathy and liver degeneration, is associated with VZV and influenza B virus infection, especially in children given aspirin. Its pathogenesis is unknown.

B. Zoster: The occurrence of painful vesicles along the course of a sensory nerve of the head or trunk is the usual picture. The pain can last for weeks, and postzoster neuralgia can be debilitating. In immunocompromised patients, life-threatening disseminated infections such as pneumonia can occur.

Laboratory Diagnosis   Although most diagnoses are made clinically, laboratory tests are available. A presumptive diagnosis can be made by using the Tzanck smear. Multinucleated giant cells are seen in VZV as well as in HSV lesions. The definitive diagnosis is made by isolation of the virus in cell culture and identification with specific antiserum. A rise in antibody titer can be used to diagnose varicella but is less useful in the diagnosis of zoster, since antibody is already present.

Treatment   No antiviral therapy is necessary for chicken pox or shingles in normal patients. Systemic disease in immunocompromised patients can be treated with acyclovir.

Prevention   **Acyclovir** is useful in preventing varicella in immunocompromised children exposed to the virus. **Varicella-zoster immune globulin** (VZIG), which contains a high titer of antibody to the virus, is also used for such prophylaxis. A vaccine has been tested successfully but is not yet available.

CYTOMEGALOVIRUS (CMV)

Diseases   These include cytomegalic inclusion disease in infants; congenital abnormalities; systemic disease, such as pneumonia (in immunocompromised patients) and heterophil-negative mononucleosis.

Important Properties   CMV is structurally and morphologically identical to other herpesviruses but is antigenically different. It has a single serotype. Humans are the natural hosts; animal CMV strains do not infect humans.

Summary of Replicative Cycle   The cycle is similar to that of HSV (see p 157).

Transmission & Epidemiology   CMV is transmitted by a **variety of modes.** Early in life it is transmitted across the placenta, within the birth canal, and in mother's milk. Its most common mode of transmission is via saliva in young children. Later in life it is transmitted sexually; it is present in both semen and cervical secretions. It can also be transmitted during blood transfusions and organ transplants. CMV infection occurs worldwide, and over 80% of adults have antibody.

Pathogenesis & Immunity   Infection of the fetus can cause **cytomegalic inclusion disease,** characterized by multinucleated giant cells with prominent intranuclear inclusions. Many organs are affected, and widespread congenital abnormalities result. Infections of children and adults are usually asymptomatic, except in immunocompromised individuals. CMV enters a **latent** state in leukocytes and can be reactivated when cell-mediated immunity is decreased. CMV can also persist in kidneys for years.

CMV infection causes an immunosuppressive effect by inhibiting T cells. Host defenses against CMV infection include both circulating antibody and cell-mediated immunity. Cellular immunity is more important, because its suppression can lead to systemic disease.

Clinical Findings Approximately 20% of infants infected with CMV during gestation show clinically apparent manifestations of cytomegalic inclusion disease such as microcephaly, seizures, deafness, jaundice, and purpura. Hepatosplenomegaly is very common. Cytomegalic inclusion disease is one of the leading causes of mental retardation in the USA. Infected infants can continue to excrete CMV, especially in the urine, for several years.

In adults, CMV can cause **"heterophil-negative" mononucleosis,** which is characterized by fever, lethargy, and the presence of abnormal lymphocytes in peripheral blood smears. Systemic CMV infections, especially interstitial pneumonitis, occur in a high proportion of immunosuppressed patients, eg, those with renal and bone marrow transplants.

Laboratory Diagnosis The virus can be recovered in cell culture, but the appearance of cytopathic effect is slow, usually taking 1–2 weeks. Most of the virus produced remains cell-associated. The virus is identified by immunofluorescence. Other diagnostic methods include fluorescent-antibody and histologic staining of inclusion bodies in giant cells in urine and in tissue. A 4-fold or greater rise in antibody titer is also diagnostic.

Treatment There is no antiviral therapy, although dihydroxypropoxymethyl guanine (DHPG; ganciclovir) is somewhat effective in the treatment of CMV retinitis and pneumonia in patients with the acquired immunodeficiency syndrome. Unlike HSV and VZV, CMV is largely resistant to acyclovir, a finding in accord with the absence of virus-induced thymidine kinase in CMV-infected cells.

Prevention There is no vaccine. Infants with cytomegalic inclusion disease who are shedding virus in their urine should be kept isolated from other infants. Blood for transfusion to newborns should be CMV antibody-negative. If possible, only organs from CMV antibody-negative donors should be transplanted to antibody-negative recipients.

EPSTEIN-BARR VIRUS (EBV)

Diseases EBV is the agent of infectious mononucleosis. It is associated with Burkitt's lymphoma, other B cell lymphomas, and nasopharyngeal carcinoma.

Important Properties

EBV is structurally and morphologically identical to other herpesviruses but is antigenically different. The most important antigen is the **viral capsid antigen** (VCA), because it is used most often in diagnostic tests. The early antigens (EA), which are produced prior to viral DNA synthesis, and nuclear antigen (EBNA), which is located in the nucleus bound to chromosomes, are sometimes diagnostically helpful as well. Two other antigens, lymphocyte-determined membrane antigen and viral membrane antigen, have been detected also. Neutralizing activity is directed against the viral membrane antigen.

Humans are the natural hosts. EBV infects mainly lymphoid cells, primarily B lymphocytes.

Summary of Replicative Cycle The cycle is similar to that of HSV (see p 157).

Transmission & Epidemiology EBV is transmitted primarily by the exchange of **saliva,** eg, during kissing. EBV infection is one of the most common infections worldwide; over 90% of adults in the USA have antibody. Infection in the first few years of life is usually asymptomatic. Early infection tends to occur in individuals in lower socioeconomic groups. The frequency of clinically apparent infectious mononucleosis, however, is highest in those who are exposed to the virus later in life, eg, college students.

Pathogenesis & Immunity The initial infection occurs in the oropharynx (?epithelium, ?lymphoid tissue), then spreads to the blood, where it infects B lymphocytes. T lymphocytes react against the infected B cells. The T cells are the "atypical lymphs" seen in the blood smear. EBV remains **latent within B lymphocytes.** A few copies of EBV DNA are integrated into the cell genome; many copies of circular EBV DNA are found in the cytoplasm.

The immune response to EBV infection consists first of IgM antibody to the VCA. IgG antibody to the VCA follows and persists for life. The IgM response is therefore useful for diagnosing acute infection, whereas the IgG response is best for revealing prior infection. Lifetime immunity against second episodes of infectious mononucleosis is based on antibody to the viral membrane antigen.

In addition to the EBV-specific antibodies, nonspecific **heterophil antibodies** also occur. The term "heterophil" refers to antibodies that are detected by tests using antigens different from the antigens that induced them. The heterophil antibodies formed in infectious mononucleosis agglutinate sheep or horse red blood cells in the laboratory. (Cross-reacting Forssman antibodies in human serum are removed by adsorption with guinea pig kidney extract prior to agglutination.) Note that these antibodies do not react with any component of EBV. It seems likely that EBV infection modifies a cell membrane constituent so that it becomes antigenic and induces the heterophil antibody. Heterophil antibodies usually disappear within 6 months after recovery. These antibodies are not specific for EBV infection and are also seen in individuals with hepatitis B and serum sickness.

Clinical Findings   Infectious mononucleosis is characterized primarily by fever, sore throat, lymphadenopathy, and splenomegaly. Anorexia and lethargy are prominent. Hepatitis is frequent; encephalitis occurs in some patients. Spontaneous recovery usually occurs in 2–3 weeks. Splenic rupture, associated with contact sports such as football, is a feared but rare complication. In certain immunosuppressed patients, a severe, often fatal EBV infection occurs.

Laboratory Diagnosis   The diagnosis of infectious mononucleosis in the clinical laboratory is based primarily on 2 approaches:

(1) In the **hematologic** approach, an absolute lymphocytosis occurs and as many as 30% abnormal lymphocytes are seen on a smear. These **"atypical lymphs"** are large and have a lobulated nucleus and a vacuolated, basophilic cytoplasm. They are modified T cells.

(2) In the **immunologic** approach, there are 2 tests. (a) The **heterophil antibody** test is useful for the early diagnosis of infectious mononucleosis because it is usually positive by week 2 of illness. However, the antibody titer declines after recovery and so is not useful for detection of prior infection. The Monospot test is often used to detect the heterophil antibody; it is more sensitive, more specific, and cheaper than the tube agglutination test. (b) The **EBV-specific antibody** test is used primarily in diagnostically difficult cases. The IgM VCA antibody response can be used to detect early illness; the IgG VCA antibody response can be used to detect prior infection. In certain instances, antibodies to EA and EBNA can be useful diagnostically. Antibody to EBNA appears 3–4 weeks after infection and persists for life.

Although EBV can be isolated from clinical samples such as saliva by morphologic transformation of cord blood lymphocytes, it is a technically difficult procedure and is not readily available. No virus is synthesized in the cord lymphocytes; its presence is detected by fluorescent-antibody staining of the nuclear antigen.

Treatment   No antiviral therapy is necessary for uncomplicated infectious mononucleosis. Acyclovir has little activity against EBV, but administration of high doses may be useful in life-threatening EBV infections.

Prevention   There is no EBV vaccine.

Association With Cancer   EBV infection is associated with cancers of lymphoid origin; **Burkitt's lymphoma** in African children, other B cell lymphomas, nasopharyngeal carcinoma in the Chinese population, and thymic carcinoma in the USA. The initial evidence of an association of EBV infection with Burkitt's lymphoma was the production of EBV by the lymphoma cells in culture. In fact, this was how EBV was discovered by Epstein and Barr in 1964. Additional evidence includes the finding of EBV DNA and EBNA in the tumor cells. EBV DNA and antigens are found in nasopharyngeal and thymic carcinoma cells also. The role of EBV in carcinogenesis is unclear.

Poxviruses

The poxvirus family includes 3 viruses of medical importance: smallpox virus, vaccinia virus, and molluscum contagiosum virus. Poxviruses are the **largest and most complex** viruses.

SMALLPOX VIRUS

Disease Smallpox virus, also called variola virus, is the agent of smallpox, the only disease that has been eradicated from the face of the earth. **Eradication** is due to the vaccine.

Important Properties Poxviruses are brick-shaped particles containing linear double-stranded DNA, a disk-shaped core within a double membrane, and a lipoprotein envelope. The virion contains a DNA-dependent RNA polymerase. This enzyme is required because the virus replicates in the cytoplasm and does not have access to the cellular RNA polymerase, which is located in the nucleus.

Smallpox virus has a single, stable serotype that is the key to the success of the vaccine. If the antigenicity varied as it does in influenza virus, eradication would not have succeeded.

Summary of Replicative Cycle Vaccinia virus, a poxvirus virtually nonpathogenic for humans, is used for studies on poxvirus replication. After penetration of the cell and uncoating, the virion DNA-dependent RNA polymerase synthesizes early mRNA, which is translated into early, nonstructural proteins, mainly enzymes required for subsequent steps in viral replication. The viral DNA is replicated in typical semiconservative fashion, after which late, structural proteins are synthesized that will form the progeny virions. The virions are assembled and acquire their envelopes by budding from the cell membrane as they are released from the cell. Note that all steps in replication occur in the cytoplasm, which is unusual for a DNA virus.

Transmission & Epidemiology Before the disease was eradicated, smallpox virus was transmitted via respiratory aerosol or by direct contact with virus either in the skin lesions or on fomites such as bedding.

Prior to the 1960s, smallpox was widespread throughout large areas of Africa, Asia, and South America, and millions of people were affected. In 1967, the World Health Organization embarked on a vaccination campaign that led to the eradication of smallpox. The last case occurred in Somalia in 1977.

Pathogenesis & Immunity Smallpox begins when the virus infects the upper respiratory tract and local lymph nodes, then enters the blood (primary viremia). Internal organs are infected; then the virus reenters the blood (secondary viremia) and spreads to the skin. These events occur during the incubation period, when the patient is still well. The rash is the result of virus replication in the skin, but there may be an immune component as well.

Immunity following smallpox disease is lifelong; immunity following vaccination lasts about 10 years.

Clinical Findings After an incubation period of 7–14 days, there is a sudden onset of prodromal symptoms such as fever and malaise. This is followed by the rash, which begins on the face and spreads over the body to include the extremities. The rash evolves through stages from macules to papules, vesicles, pustules, and, finally, crusts in 2–3 weeks.

Laboratory Diagnosis In the past, the diagnosis was made either by growing the virus in cell culture or chick embryos or by detecting viral antigens in vesicular fluid by immunofluorescence.

Prevention The disease was eradicated by global use of the **vaccine,** which contains live, attenuated vaccinia virus. The success of the vaccine is dependent upon 5 critical factors: (1) smallpox virus has a single stable serotype; (2) there is no animal reservoir, and humans are the only hosts; (3) the antibody response is prompt, so that exposed persons can be protected; (4) the disease is easily recognized clinically, so that exposed persons can be immunized promptly, and (5) there is no carrier state or subclinical infection.

The vaccine is inoculated intradermally, where virus replication occurs. The formation of a vesicle is indicative of a "take" (success). Although the vaccine was relatively safe, it became apparent in the 1970s that the incidence of side effects such as encephalitis, generalized vaccinia, and vaccinia gangrenosa exceeded the incidence of smallpox. Routine vaccination of civilians was discontinued, and it is no longer a prerequisite for international travel. Military personnel are still vaccinated.

Methisazone was used to treat the complications of vaccination. Rifampin inhibits viral DNA-dependent RNA polymerase but was not used clinically against smallpox.

MOLLUSCUM CONTAGIOSUM VIRUS   This virus is a member of the poxvirus family but is quite distinct from smallpox and vaccinia viruses. It causes small, pink, wartlike benign tumors of the skin. Note that warts are caused by papillomavirus, a member of the papovavirus family.

Hepatitis B Virus

Hepatitis B virus, a DNA-enveloped virus, is described in Chapter 41 with the other hepatitis viruses.

Review Questions

1. Herpesviruses cause latent infections. In which cells are the 5 important human herpesviruses typically latent?
2. What are the main differences between HSV-1 and HSV-2?
3. Describe the important steps in the replication of HSV.
4. What is the best way to make the diagnosis of HSV infection in the laboratory?
5. What is the characteristic appearance of HSV-infected cells?
6. Acyclovir is effective treatment for infections by certain herpesviruses. Which ones? What accounts for the selective toxicity of acyclovir?
7. What is the relationship between varicella (chickenpox) and zoster (shingles)?
8. You can get varicella only once. Why?
9. What is the predisposing factor to disseminated disease from VZV? How can the likelihood of dissemination be reduced?
10. What are the modes of transmission of CMV? To fetuses? In infants? In young children? In adults?
11. Describe the effects of CMV on fetuses and newborn infants.
12. What disease does EBV cause?
13. How is EBV transmitted, and what cells are initially infected?
14. Describe the heterophil test.
15. Antibodies against what antigen indicate prior, rather than current, EBV infection?
16. What are the laboratory findings in a typical case of infectious mononucleosis?
17. What is the relationship of EBV and cancer?
18. What attributes of smallpox virus have led to the successful eradication of the disease?
19. Smallpox and vaccinia viruses are DNA viruses that contain a virion RNA polymerase. Why do they require this enzyme in the virion?
20. In the 1970s before smallpox was eradicated, the vaccine was no longer required in the USA. Why?

38

DNA Nonenveloped Viruses

ADENOVIRUSES

Diseases   Adenoviruses cause a variety of upper and lower respiratory tract diseases such as pharyngitis, conjunctivitis, and pneumonia. Keratoconjunctivitis, hemorrhagic cystitis, and gastroenteritis also occur. Some adenoviruses cause sarcomas in rodents.

Important Properties   Adenoviruses are **nonenveloped** particles with double-stranded linear DNA and an **icosahedral** nucleocapsid. They are the only viruses with a **fiber** protruding from each of the 12 vertices of the capsid. The fiber is the organ of attachment and is a hemagglutinin. When purified free of virions, the fiber is toxic to human cells.

There are 41 known antigenic types; the fiber protein is the type-specific antigen. All adenoviruses have a common group-specific antigen located on the hexon protein.

Certain serotypes of human adenoviruses (especially 12, 18, and 31) cause **sarcomas** at the site of injection in laboratory rodents such as guinea pigs. There is no evidence that adenoviruses cause tumors in humans.

Summary of Replicative Cycle   After attachment to the cell surface via its fiber, the virus penetrates and uncoats, and the viral DNA moves to the nucleus. Host cell DNA-dependent RNA polymerase transcribes the early genes, and splicing enzymes remove the RNA representing the introns, resulting in functional mRNA (note that introns and exons, which are common in eukaryotic DNA, were first described for adenovirus DNA). Early mRNA is translated into nonstructural proteins in the cytoplasm. After viral DNA replication in the nucleus, late mRNA is transcribed and then translated into structural virion proteins. Viral assembly occurs in the nucleus, and the virus is released by lysis of the cell, not by budding.

Transmission & Epidemiology   Adenoviruses are transmitted by several mechanisms: **aerosol** droplet; the **fecal-oral** route; and **direct inoculation** of conjunctivas by tonometers, fingers, and contaminated swimming-pool water. The fecal-oral route is the most common mode of transmission among young children and their families. Many species of animals are infected by strains of adenovirus, but these strains are not pathogenic for humans.

Adenovirus infections are endemic worldwide, but outbreaks occur among military recruits, apparently as a result of the close living conditions that facilitate transmission. Certain serotypes are associated with specific syndromes; eg, types 3, 4, and 7 cause respiratory disease, especially in military recruits; types 8 and 19 cause epidemic keratoconjunctivitis; types 11 and 21 cause hemorrhagic cystitis; and types 40 and 41 cause infantile gastroenteritis.

Pathogenesis & Immunity   Adenoviruses infect the mucosal epithelium of several organs, eg, the **respiratory tract** (both upper and lower), the **gastrointestinal tract,** and **conjunctivas.** Immunity based on neutralizing antibody is type-specific and lifelong.

In addition to acute infection leading to death of the cells, adenoviruses cause a latent infection, particularly in the adenoidal and tonsillar tissues of the throat. In fact, these viruses were named for the adenoids, from which they were first isolated in 1953.

Clinical Findings   Upper respiratory tract infections such as pharyngitis, pharyngoconjunctival fever, and acute respiratory disease manifest with varying degrees of fever, sore throat, coryza, and conjunctivitis. In the lower respiratory tract, atypical pneumonia is characterized primarily by fever, cough, and patchy consolidation. Hematuria and dysuria are prominent in hemorrhagic cystitis. Gastroenteritis occurs in children under 1 year of age and is characterized by nonbloody diarrhea. Most adenoviral infections resolve spontaneously. Approximately half of all adenoviral infections are asymptomatic.

Laboratory Diagnosis   The most frequent methods of diagnosis are isolation of the virus in cell culture and detection of a 4-fold or greater rise in antibody titer. Complement fixation and hemagglutination inhibition are the most important serologic tests. Complement fixation tests detect antibody against the type-specific penton hemagglutinin.

Treatment   There is no antiviral therapy.

Prevention   A **live nonattenuated vaccine** (types 4 and 7) delivered in an enteric-coated capsule is used only in military recruits. The virus infects the gastrointestinal tract, where it causes an asymptomatic infection and induces immunity to respiratory disease. This vaccine is not available for civilian use.

Epidemic keratoconjunctivitis is an iatrogenic disease, preventable by strict asepsis and hand washing by those who examine eyes.

Review Questions

1. What are the important sites of infection for the various types of adenoviruses?
2. What is the importance of the fibers on the surface of adenoviruses?
3. What measures are available for prevention of adenovirus infection?

RNA Enveloped Viruses

39

Orthomyxoviruses

INFLUENZA VIRUSES   Influenza viruses are the only members of the orthomyxovirus family. The term ''myxo'' refers to the observation that these viruses interact with mucins (glycoproteins). The orthomyxoviruses differ from the paramyxoviruses primarily in that the former have a segmented RNA genome (usually 8 pieces), whereas the latter's RNA genome consists of a single piece.* In addition, the orthomyxoviruses are smaller (110 nm in diameter) than the paramyxoviruses (150 nm in diameter). See Table 39–1 for additional differences.

Table 39–1. Properties of orthomyxoviruses and paramyxoviruses.

Property	Orthomyxoviruses	Paramyxoviruses
Viruses	Influenza A, B, and C viruses	Measles, mumps, respiratory syncytial, and parainfluenza viruses
Genome	Segmented (8 pieces) single-stranded RNA of negative polarity	Nonsegmented single-stranded RNA of negative polarity
Virion RNA polymerase	Yes	Yes
Capsid	Helical	Helical
Envelope	Yes	Yes
Size	Smaller (110 nm)	Larger (150 nm)
Surface spikes	Hemagglutinin and neuraminidase on different spikes	Hemagglutinin and neuraminidase on the same spike[1]
Giant cell formation	No	Yes

[1]Individual viruses differ in detail. See Table 39–3.

*The total molecular weight of influenza virus RNA is approximately 2–4 x 10^6, whereas the molecular weight of paramyxovirus RNA is higher, approximately 5–8 x 10^6.

Table 39–2. Features of viruses that infect the respiratory tract.

Virus	Disease	Number of Serotypes	Lifelong Immunity to Disease	Vaccine Available	Viral Latency	Treatment
RNA viruses						
Influenza A virus	Influenza	Many	No	+	–	Amantadine
Parainfluenza virus	Croup	Many	No	–	–	None
Respiratory syncytial virus	Bronchiolitis	One	Incomplete	–	–	Ribavirin
Rubella virus	Rubella	One	Yes	+	–	None
Measles virus	Measles	One	Yes	+	–	None
Mumps virus	Parotitis, meningitis	One	Yes	+	–	None
Rhinovirus	Common cold	Many	No	–	–	None
Coronavirus	Common cold	Many	No	–	–	None
Coxsackievirus	Herpangina, pleurodynia	Many	No	–	–	None
DNA viruses						
Herpes simplex virus type 1	Gingivostomatitis	One	No	–	+	Acyclovir in immunodeficient patients
Epstein-Barr virus	Infectious mononucleosis	One	Yes	–	+	None
Varicella-zoster virus	Chickenpox, shingles	One	Yes	–	+	Acyclovir in immunodeficient patients
Adenovirus	Pharyngitis	Many	No	+[1]	+	None

[1]For military recruits only.

Table 39–2 shows a comparison of influenza virus with several other viruses that infect the respiratory tract.

Disease Influenza.

Important Properties Influenza virus is composed of a **segmented** single-stranded RNA genome, a **helical** nucleocapsid, and an outer lipoprotein **envelope.** The virion contains an RNA-dependent RNA **polymerase**, which transcribes the **negative-polarity** genome into mRNA. The genome is therefore not infectious. The envelope is covered with 2 different types of spikes, a **hemagglutinin and a neuraminidase.**[*] The former agglutinates red blood cells and the latter cleaves neuraminic acid, a component of the surface of many human cells.

Influenza viruses, especially influenza A virus, show changes in the antigenicity of their hemagglutinin and neuraminidase proteins; this property contributes to their capacity to cause devastating worldwide epidemics. These changes are attributed to the **reassortment** (high-frequency recombination) of the segments of the genome RNA. Note that in reassortment, entire segments of RNA are exchanged, each one of which codes for a single protein, eg, the hemagglutinin.

Influenza viruses have both **group-specific** and **type-specific** antigens.

(a) The internal ribonucleoprotein is the group-specific antigen that distinguishes influenza A, B, and C viruses. Influenza A viruses cause epidemics much more frequently than do influenza B viruses, whereas influenza C viruses do not cause epidemics and are associated only with minor respiratory ailments.

(b) The hemagglutinin and the neuraminidase are the type-specific antigens located on the surface and are antigenically distinct. Antibody against the hemagglutinin neutralizes the infectivity of the virus (and prevents disease), whereas antibody against the group-specific antigen does not (it is located internally). Antibody against the neuraminidase does not neutralize infectivity but does reduce disease, perhaps by decreasing the amount of virus released from the infected cell and thus reducing spread. Note that influenza A viruses change their type-specific antigens more frequently than do influenza B viruses.

---

[*]Paramyxoviruses also have a hemagglutinin and a neuraminidase, but the 2 proteins are located on the same spike.

Many species of animals have their own influenza A viruses, eg, chickens, swine, and horses. These animal viruses are probably the source of the new antigenic types that cause epidemics among humans. For example, if an equine and a human A influenza virus infect the same cell (eg, in a farmer's respiratory tract), reassortment could occur and a new variant of the human A virus, bearing the equine virus hemagglutinin, may appear.

A/Philippines/82 (H3N2) illustrates the nomenclature of influenza viruses. ''A'' refers to the group antigen. Next are the location and year the virus was isolated. H3N2 is the designation of the hemagglutinin (H) and neuraminidase (N) types.

Summary of Replicative Cycle   The virus adsorbs to the cell as the hemagglutinin interacts with glycoprotein receptors on the surface and then enters the cell in vesicles and uncoats. The virion RNA polymerase transcribes the 8 genome segments into 8 mRNAs, which are translated into virion proteins in the cytoplasm. Progeny RNA genomes are synthesized in the nucleus. The helical ribonucleoprotein assembles in the cytoplasm; matrix protein mediates the interaction of the nucleocapsid with the envelope; and the virion is released from the cell by budding from the outer cell membrane at the site where the hemagglutinin and neuraminidase have interdigitated. The neuraminidase may play a role in release of the virus by cleaving neuraminic acid on the cell surface.

Transmission & Epidemiology   The virus is transmitted by **airborne respiratory droplets.** The ability of influenza A virus to cause epidemics is dependent on antigenic changes in the hemagglutinin and neuraminidase. There are 2 types of changes: **antigenic shifts,** which are major changes based on the reassortment of genome pieces, and **antigenic drifts,** which are minor changes based on mutation. Antigenic shifts appear less frequently, about every 10 or 11 years, whereas drift variants appear virtually every year. Epidemics and pandemics (worldwide epidemics) occur when the antigenicity of the virus has changed sufficiently that the preexisting immunity of many people is no longer effective. The antigenicity of influenza B viruses also varies but not as dramatically nor as often.

Influenza occurs primarily in the winter months, when it and secondary bacterial pneumonia cause a significant number of deaths, especially in older people.

Pathogenesis & Immunity   After the virus has been inhaled, the neuraminidase degrades the protective mucus layer, allowing the virus to gain access to the cells of the upper and lower respiratory tract. The infection is limited primarily to this area, and, despite systemic symptoms, viremia rarely occurs. There is necrosis of the superficial layers of the respiratory epithelium. Influenza virus pneumonia, which can complicate influenza, is interstitial in location.

Although circulating IgG antibody against influenza virus occurs after infection, it offers little protection. Secretory IgA in the respiratory tract is protective.

Clinical Findings   After an incubation period of 24–48 hours, fever, myalgias, headache, and cough develop suddenly. Vomiting and diarrhea are infrequent. The symptoms usually resolve spontaneously in 4–7 days, but influenzal or bacterial pneumonia may complicate the course.

Reye's syndrome, characterized by encephalopathy and liver degeneration, is a rare, life-threatening complication in children following some viral infections, particularly influenza B and chickenpox. Aspirin given to reduce fever in viral infections has been implicated in the pathogenesis of Reye's syndrome.

Laboratory Diagnosis   Although most diagnoses of influenza are made on clinical grounds, 2 laboratory diagnostic approaches are available: (1) The virus can be grown in cell culture from throat washings and identified by fluorescent-antibody staining of the infected cells by using antisera to influenza A and B. This process takes several days. (2) A rise in antibody titer of at least 4-fold in paired serum samples taken early in the illness and 10 days later is sufficient for diagnosis. Either the hemagglutination inhibition or complement fixation (CF) test can be used to assay the antibody titer.

Treatment   **Amantadine** is approved for use as both treatment for and prevention of influenza A; however, it is rarely used in practice. Its main indication is in a confined, elderly, unimmunized population, such as in a retirement home, where influenza can be life-threatening. Note that amantadine is effective only against influenza A, not against influenza B.

Prevention   The main mode of protection is the **vaccine,** which consists of killed influenza A and B viruses. The vaccine is not a good immunogen, and yearly boosters are recommended. These boosters also provide an opportunity to immunize against the latest antigenic changes. The vaccine should be given to people over age 65 years and to those with chronic diseases, particularly respiratory and cardiovascular conditions.

In addition to the vaccine containing whole, killed virus, a second vaccine containing "split" (disrupted) virus is available, particularly for children; it causes fewer side effects. An experimental vaccine containing a live, temperature-sensitive mutant is effective and may become available. This virus can replicate in the cooler (33 °C) nasal passages, where it induces IgA, but not in the warmer (37 °C) lower respiratory tract. It therefore immunizes but does not cause disease.

Paramyxoviruses

The paramyxovirus family contains 4 important human pathogens: measles virus, mumps virus, respiratory syncytial virus (RSV), and parainfluenza viruses. They differ from orthomyxoviruses in that their genomes are not segmented, they have a larger diameter, and their surface spikes are different (Table 39–1).

Paramyxoviruses are composed of **one piece** of single-stranded RNA, a **helical nucleocapsid,** and an outer lipoprotein **envelope.** The virion contains an RNA-dependent RNA **polymerase,** which transcribes the **negative polarity** genome into mRNA. The genome is, therefore, not infectious. The envelope is covered with spikes, which contain either hemagglutinin, neuraminidase, or a fusion protein that causes cell fusion and, in some cases, hemolysis (Table 39–3).

MEASLES VIRUS

Disease   This virus causes measles.

Important Properties   The genome RNA and nucleocapsid of measles virus are those of a typical paramyxovirus (see above). The virion has 2 types of envelope spikes, one with hemagglutinating activity and the other with cell-fusing and hemolytic activities (Table 39–3). It has a single serotype, and the hemagglutinin is the antigen against which neutralizing antibody is directed. Humans are the natural host.

Summary of Replicative Cycle   After adsorption to the cell surface via its hemagglutinin, the virus penetrates and uncoats, and the virion RNA polymerase transcribes the negative-stranded genome into mRNA. Multiple mRNAs are synthesized, each of which is translated into the specific viral proteins; no polyprotein analogous to that synthesized by poliovirus is made. The helical nucleocapsid is assembled, the matrix protein mediates the interaction with the envelope, and the virus is released by budding from the cell membrane.

Transmission & Epidemiology   Measles virus is transmitted via **respiratory droplets** produced by coughing and sneezing both during the prodromal period and for a few days after the rash appears. Measles occurs worldwide, usually in outbreaks every 2–3 years, when the number of susceptible children reaches a high level. The attack rate is one of the highest of

Table 39–3. Envelope spikes of paramyxoviruses.

Virus	Hemagglutinin	Neuraminidase	Fusion Protein[1]
Measles virus	+	−	+
Mumps virus[2]	+	+	+
Respiratory syncytial virus	−	−	+
Parainfluenza virus[2]	+	+	+

[1]The measles and mumps fusion proteins are hemolysins also.
[2]In mumps and parainfluenza viruses, the hemagglutinin and neuraminidase are on the same spike and the fusion protein is on a different spike.

viral diseases; most children contract the clinical disease on exposure. When this virus is introduced into a population that has not experienced measles, such as the inhabitants of the Hawaiian Islands in the 1800s, devastating epidemics occur. In malnourished children, especially in developing countries, measles is a much more serious disease than in well-nourished children.

Pathogenesis & Immunity   After infecting the cells lining the upper respiratory tract, the virus enters the blood and infects reticuloendothelial cells, where it replicates again. It then spreads via the blood to the skin. The **rash** is due to a vasculitis coupled with necrosis of the epithelial cells. **Multinucleated giant cells,** which form as a result of the fusion protein in the spikes, are characteristic of the lesions.

   Lifetime immunity occurs in individuals who have had the disease. Although IgG antibody may play a role in neutralizing the virus during the viremic stage, cell-mediated immunity is also important; agammaglobulinemic children have a normal course of disease, are subsequently immune, and are protected by immunization. Maternal antibody passes the placenta, and infants are protected during the first 6 months of life.

Clinical Findings   After an incubation period of 10–14 days, a prodromal phase characterized by fever, conjunctivitis (causing photophobia), running nose, and coughing occurs. Koplik's spots are bright red lesions with a white, central dot that are located on the buccal mucosa and are virtually diagnostic. A few days later, a maculopapular rash appears on the face and proceeds gradually down the body to the lower extremities. The rash develops a brownish hue several days later.

   The complications of measles can be quite severe. Encephalitis occurs once in 1000 cases; the mortality rate is 10%, and there are permanent sequelae in 40% of cases. In addition, both primary measles (giant-cell) pneumonia and secondary bacterial pneumonia occur. Bacterial otitis media is quite common. Although very rare, subacute sclerosing panencephalitis (SSPE) is a fatal disease of the central nervous system that occurs several years after measles (see Chapter 44).

   Atypical measles occurs in some people who were given the killed vaccine and were subsequently infected with measles virus. It is characterized by an atypical rash without Koplik's spots. Because the killed vaccine has not been used for many years, atypical measles occurs only in adults and is infrequent.

Laboratory Diagnosis   Most diagnoses are made on clinical grounds, but the virus can be isolated in cell culture; a rise in antibody titer of greater than 4-fold can be used to diagnose difficult cases.

Treatment   There is no antiviral therapy available.

Prevention   Prevention rests on immunization with the live, attenuated **vaccine.** The vaccine is effective and causes few side effects. It is given subcutaneously to children at 15 months of age, usually in combination with rubella and mumps vaccines. Since immunity can wane, a booster dose is recommended. Because it is a live vaccine, it should not be given to immunocompromised persons or pregnant women. No booster dose is necessary. The vaccine has decreased the number of cases of measles markedly in the USA. However, outbreaks still occur among unimmunized individuals, eg, children in the inner cities and in developing countries.

   The killed vaccine should not be used. Immune globulin can be used to modify the disease if given to unimmunized individuals early in the incubation period.

MUMPS VIRUS

Disease   This virus causes mumps.

Important Properties   The genome RNA and nucleocapsid are those of a typical paramyxovirus. The virion has 2 types of envelope spikes, one with both hemagglutinin and neuraminidase activities and the other with cell-fusing and hemolytic activities (Table 39–3).

   The virus has a single serotype. Neutralizing antibody is directed against the hemagglutinin. The internal nucleocapsid protein is the "S" (soluble) antigen detected in the complement fixation test used for diagnosis. Humans are the natural host.

Summary of Replicative Cycle   Replication is similar to that of measles virus (see p 168).

Transmission & Epidemiology   Mumps virus is transmitted via **respiratory droplets**. Mumps occurs worldwide, with a peak incidence in the winter. About 30% of children have a subclinical (inapparent) infection, which provides them with immunity.

Pathogenesis & Immunity   The virus infects the upper respiratory tract and then spreads throughout the blood to infect the parotid glands, testes, ovaries, pancreas, and, in some cases, meninges. Alternatively, the virus may ascend from the buccal mucosa up Stensen's duct to the parotid gland.

   Lifelong immunity occurs in persons who have had the disease. There is a popular misconception that unilateral mumps can be followed by mumps on the other side. Mumps occurs only once; subsequent cases of parotitis can be caused by other viruses such as parainfluenza viruses, by bacteria, and by duct stones. Maternal antibody passes the placenta and provides protection during the first 6 months of life.

Clinical Findings   After an incubation period of 18–21 days, a prodromal stage of fever, malaise, and anorexia is followed by tender swelling of the parotid glands, either unilateral or bilateral. There is a characteristic increase in parotid pain when drinking citrus juices. The disease is typically benign and resolves spontaneously within a week.

   Two complications are of significance. One is orchitis in postpubertal males, which, if bilateral, can result in sterility. Postpubertal males have a fibrous tunica albuginea, which resists expansion, thereby causing pressure necrosis of the spermatocytes. Unilateral orchitis, although quite painful, does not lead to sterility. The other complication is meningitis, which is usually benign, self-limited, and without sequelae. Mumps virus, coxsackievirus, and echovirus are the 3 most frequent causes of viral (aseptic) meningitis.

Laboratory Diagnosis   The diagnosis of mumps is usually made clinically, but laboratory tests are available for confirmation. The virus can be isolated in cell culture from saliva, spinal fluid, or urine. In addition, a 4-fold rise in antibody titer in either the hemagglutination inhibition or the complement fixation (CF) test is diagnostic. A single CF test that assays both the S and the V (viral) antigen can also be used. Because antibody to S antigen appears early and is short-lived, it indicates current infection. If only V antibody is found, the patient has had mumps in the past.

   A mumps skin test based on delayed hypersensitivity can be used to detect previous infection, but serologic tests are preferred. The mumps skin test is widely used to determine whether a patient's cell-mediated immunity is competent.

Treatment   There is no antiviral therapy for mumps.

Prevention   Prevention consists of immunization with the live, attenuated **vaccine.** The vaccine is effective and long-lasting (at least 10 years) and causes few side effects. It is given subcutaneously to children at 15 months of age, usually in combination with measles and rubella vaccines. Because it is a live vaccine, it should not be given to immunocompromised persons or pregnant women. Immune globulin is not useful for preventing or mitigating mumps orchitis.

RESPIRATORY SYNCYTIAL VIRUS (RSV)

Diseases   This virus is the most important cause of pneumonia and bronchiolitis in infants.

Important Properties   The genome RNA and nucleocapsid are those of a typical paramyxovirus (Table 39–1). Its surface spikes are **fusion proteins,** not hemagglutinins or neuraminidases (Table 39–3). The fusion protein causes cells to fuse, forming syncytia which give rise to the name of the virus.

   Humans and chimpanzees are the natural hosts of RSV. It has one antigenic type. Antibody against the fusion protein neutralizes infectivity.

Summary of Replicative Cycle   Replication is similar to that of measles virus (see p 168).

Transmission & Epidemiology Transmission occurs via **respiratory droplets** and the hands. RSV causes **outbreaks** of respiratory infections **every winter,** in contrast to many other "cold" viruses, which reenter the community every few years. It occurs worldwide, and virtually everyone has been infected by the age of 3 years. RSV also causes **outbreaks** of respiratory infections in **hospitalized infants;** these outbreaks can be controlled by hand washing and use of gloves.

Pathogenesis & Immunity RSV infection in **infants is more severe** and more often involves the lower respiratory tract than in older children and adults, in whom it causes mild upper respiratory tract infections. The infection is localized to the respiratory tract; viremia does not occur.

The severe disease in infants may have an **immunopathogenetic** mechanism. Maternal antibody passed to the infant may react with the virus and damage the respiratory tract cells. Immune complexes (IgG plus virus), as well as IgE antibody and histamine, may be involved. Trials with a killed vaccine resulted in more severe disease, an unexpected finding that supports such a mechanism.

Most individuals have multiple infections due to RSV, indicating that immunity is incomplete. The reason for this is unknown, but it is not due to antigenic variation of the virus. IgA respiratory antibody reduces the frequency of RSV infection as a person ages.

Clinical Findings In infants, lower respiratory tract disease such as bronchiolitis and pneumonia predominates. Surprisingly, secondary bacterial pneumonia is rare. In older children and adults, upper respiratory tract infections resemble the common cold.

Laboratory Diagnosis The presence of the virus can be detected rapidly by immunofluorescence on smears of respiratory epithelium or by isolation in cell culture. A rise in antibody titer of at least 4-fold is also diagnostic.

Treatment Aerosolized ribavirin is recommended for severely ill hospitalized infants, but there is uncertainty regarding its effectiveness.

Prevention There is **no vaccine.** Previous attempts to protect with a killed vaccine resulted in an increase in severity of symptoms. Nosocomial outbreaks can be limited by hand washing and use of gloves.

PARAINFLUENZA VIRUSES

Diseases These viruses cause croup and pneumonia in children and a disease resembling the common cold in adults.

Important Properties The genome RNA and nucleocapsid are those of a typical paramyxovirus (Table 39–1). The surface spikes consist of hemagglutinin, neuraminidase, and fusion proteins (Table 39–3). The fusion protein mediates the formation of multinucleated giant cells. The H and N proteins are on the same spike; the F protein is on a separate spike. Both humans and animals are infected by parainfluenza viruses, but the animal strains do not infect humans. There are 4 types which are distinguished by antigenicity, cytopathic effect, and pathogenicity (see below). Antibody to either the H or the F protein neutralizes infectivity.

Summary of Replicative Cycle Replication is similar to that of measles virus (see p 168).

Transmission & Epidemiology These viruses are transmitted via **respiratory droplets**. They cause disease worldwide, primarily in the winter months.

Pathogenesis & Immunity These viruses cause upper and lower respiratory tract disease without viremia. A large proportion of infections are subclinical. Parainfluenza viruses 1 and 2 are **major causes of croup** but cause pharyngitis as well. Parainfluenza virus 3 causes disease less frequently, and parainfluenza virus 4 rarely causes disease, except for the common cold.

Clinical Findings   Parainfluenza viruses are best known as the cause of croup (acute laryngotracheobronchitis) in children under 5 years of age. Croup is characterized by a harsh cough and hoarseness. In addition to croup, these viruses cause a variety of respiratory diseases such as the common cold, pharyngitis, bronchitis, and pneumonia.

Laboratory Diagnosis   Most infections are diagnosed clinically. The diagnosis can be made in the laboratory either by isolation of the virus in cell culture or by observing a 4-fold or greater rise in antibody titer.

Treatment & Prevention   There is neither antiviral therapy nor a vaccine available.

Togaviruses

RUBELLA VIRUS

Diseases   This virus causes rubella (German measles) and congenital rubella syndrome.

Important Properties   Rubella virus is a member of the togavirus family. It is composed of one piece of **single-stranded** RNA, an **icosahedral** nucleocapsid, and a lipoprotein **envelope.** However, unlike the paramyxoviruses, such as measles and mumps viruses, it has a **positive-strand** RNA and therefore has no virion polymerase. Its surface spikes contain hemagglutinin. The virus has a single antigenic type. Antibody against hemagglutinin neutralizes infectivity. Humans are the natural host.

Summary of Replicative Cycle   Because knowledge of rubella virus replication is incomplete, the following cycle is based on the replication of other togaviruses. After penetration of the cell and uncoating, the plus-strand RNA genome is translated into several nonstructural and structural proteins. Note the difference between togaviruses and poliovirus, which also has a plus-strand RNA genome but translates its RNA into a single large polyprotein, which is subsequently cleaved. One of the nonstructural rubella proteins is an RNA-dependent RNA polymerase, which replicates the genome first by making a minus-strand template and then, from that, plus-strand progeny. Both replication and assembly occur in the cytoplasm, and the envelope is acquired from the outer membrane as the virion exits the cell.

Transmission & Epidemiology   The virus is transmitted via **respiratory droplets.** The disease occurs worldwide. In areas where the vaccine is not used, epidemics occur every 6–9 years. In the USA, approximately 10% of young adult women are susceptible and are therefore at risk of giving birth to children with congenital malformations.

Pathogenesis & Immunity   Initial replication of the virus occurs in the nasopharynx and local lymph nodes. From there it spreads via the blood to the internal organs and skin.
   Natural infection leads to **lifelong immunity.** Second cases of rubella do not occur; similar rashes are caused by other viruses, such as coxsackieviruses and echoviruses. Antibody crosses the placenta and protects the newborn.

Clinical Findings

A. Rubella: Rubella is a milder, shorter disease than measles. After an incubation period of 14–21 days, a brief prodromal period with fever and malaise is followed by a maculopapular rash, which starts on the face and progresses downward to involve the extremities. Posterior auricular lymphadenopathy is characteristic. The rash typically lasts for 3 days. When rubella occurs in adults, especially women, polyarthritis due to immune complexes often occurs.

B. Congenital Rubella Syndrome: The significance of rubella virus is not as a cause of mild childhood disease but as a **teratogen.** When a pregnant woman is infected during the first trimester, especially the first month, significant congenital malformations can occur as a result of maternal viremia and fetal infection. The increased rate of abnormalities during the early weeks of pregnancy is attributed to the very sensitive organ development that occurs at that time. The malformations are widespread and include primarily the heart (eg, patent ductus arteriosus), the eyes (eg, cataracts), and the brain (eg, deafness and mental retardation).

In addition, children infected in utero can **continue to excrete** rubella virus for months following birth, which is a significant public health hazard because the virus can be transmitted to pregnant women. Some congenital shedders are asymptomatic and without malformations and hence can be diagnosed only if the virus is isolated. Congenitally infected infants also have significant IgM titers and persistent IgG titers long after maternal antibody has disappeared.

Laboratory Diagnosis Rubella virus can be grown in cell culture, but is produces little cytopathic effect (CPE). It is therefore usually identified by its ability to interfere with echovirus CPE. If rubella virus is present, no CPE will appear when the cultures are superinfected with an echovirus. The diagnosis can also be made by observing a 4-fold or greater rise in antibody titer between acute-phase and convalescent-phase sera in the hemagglutination inhibition test or ELISA or by observing the presence of IgM antibody in a single acute-phase serum sample. In a pregnant woman exposed to rubella virus, the presence of **IgM antibody indicates recent infection,** whereas a 1:8 or greater titer of IgG antibody indicates immunity and consequent protection of the fetus. If recent infection has occurred, an **amniocentesis** can reveal whether there is rubella virus in the amniotic fluid, which indicates definite fetal infection.

Treatment There is no antiviral therapy.

Prevention Prevention involves immunization with the live, attenuated **vaccine.** The vaccine is effective and long-lasting (at least 10 years) and causes few side effects, except for transient arthralgias in some women. It is given subcutaneously to children at 15 months of age (usually in combination with measles and mumps vaccine) and to unimmunized young adult women if they are not pregnant and will use contraception for the next 3 months. To date, there is no evidence that the vaccine virus causes malformations. Because it is a live vaccine, it should not be given to immunocompromised patients.

The vaccine has caused a marked reduction in the incidence of both rubella and congenital rubella syndrome. It induces some respiratory IgA, thereby interrupting the spread of virulent virus by nasal carriage. Administration of immune globulin does not prevent fetal infection in pregnant women who have been exposed to rubella virus.

To protect pregnant women from exposure to rubella virus, many hospitals require their personnel to demonstrate immunity, either by serologic testing or by proof of immunization.

OTHER TOGAVIRUSES Several other medically important togaviruses are described in the chapter on arboviruses (see Chapter 42).

Rhabdoviruses

RABIES VIRUS

Disease This virus causes rabies.

Important Properties Rabies virus is the medically important member of the rhabdovirus family. It has a **single-stranded** RNA enclosed within a **bullet-shaped capsid** surrounded by a lipoprotein **envelope.** Because the genome RNA has **negative polarity,** the virion contains an RNA-dependent RNA **polymerase.** Rabies virus has a single antigenic type. The antigenicity resides in the envelope glycoprotein spikes.

Rabies virus has a **broad host range:** it can infect all mammals. Virus isolated directly from infected animals is called ''street'' virus, whereas virus continuously passaged in rabbit brains is ''fixed.'' The fixed virus was used in the original Pasteur type of the vaccine.

Summary of Replicative Cycle   After entry into the cell, the virion RNA polymerase synthesizes 5 mRNAs that code for viral proteins. After replication of the genome viral RNA by a virus-encoded RNA polymerase, progeny RNA is assembled with virion proteins to form the nucleocapsid, and the envelope is acquired as the virion buds through the cell membrane.

Transmission & Epidemiology   The virus is transmitted by the **bite** of a rabid animal. In the USA, this is usually due to the bite of **wild animals** such as skunks, raccoons, and bats; dogs and cats are frequently immunized. Bats are unusual because they can transmit the virus while remaining healthy, whereas in other animals the ability to transmit is associated with aberrant behavior caused by viral encephalitis. Rodents and rabbits do not transmit rabies. In the USA, fewer than 10 cases of rabies occur each year (mostly imported), whereas in developing countries there are hundreds of cases, mostly due to rabid dogs.

Pathogenesis & Immunity   The virus multiplies locally at the bite site and then infects the sensory neurons and **moves by axonal transport to the central nervous system.** It multiplies in the central nervous system and then travels down the peripheral nerves to the salivary glands and other organs. From the salivary glands, it enters the saliva to be transmitted by the bite. There is no viremic stage.

Within the central nervous system, an **encephalitis** develops, with the death of neurons and demyelination. Infected neurons contain an eosinophilic cytoplasmic inclusion called a **Negri body,** which is important in laboratory diagnosis of rabies. Because so few individuals have survived rabies, there is no information regarding immunity to disease upon being bitten again.

Clinical Findings   The incubation period varies according to the location of the bite from as short as 2 weeks to 16 weeks or longer. It is shorter when bites are sustained on the head rather than on the leg, because the virus has a shorter distance to travel to reach the central nervous system.

Clinically, the patient exhibits a prodrome of nonspecific symptoms such as fever, anorexia, and changes in sensation at the site. Within a few days, signs such as confusion, lethargy, and increased salivation develop. Most notable is the painful spasm of the throat muscles on swallowing. This results in **hydrophobia,** an aversion to swallowing water because it is so painful. Within several days, the disease progresses to seizures, paralysis, and coma. Death almost invariably ensues, but with the advent of life support systems a few individuals have survived.

Laboratory Diagnosis   Rapid diagnosis of rabies infection in the animal is usually done by examination of brain tissue by using either fluorescent antibody to rabies virus or histologic staining of Negri bodies in the cytoplasm of hippocampal neurons. The virus can be isolated from the animal brain by growth in cell culture, but this takes too long to be useful in the decision of whether to give the vaccine.

Rabies in humans can be diagnosed either by isolation of the virus or by a rise in titer of antibody to the virus. Negri bodies can be demonstrated in corneal scrapings and in autopsy specimens of the brain.

Treatment   There is no antiviral therapy for a patient with rabies. Only supportive treatment is available.

Prevention   There are 2 approaches to prevention of rabies in humans: **preexposure and postexposure.** Preexposure immunization with rabies vaccine should be given to individuals in high-risk groups, such as veterinarians, zoo keepers, and travelers to hyperendemic areas, eg, Peace Corps members.

In the USA, the **rabies vaccine** (HDCV) contains inactivated "fixed" virus grown in human diploid cells. In other countries, the duck embryo vaccine or various nerve tissue vaccines are available as well. Duck embryo vaccine has low immunogenicity, and the nerve tissue vaccines can cause an allergic encephalomyelitis as a result of a cross-reaction with human myelin; for these reasons, the human cell vaccine is preferred.

Postexposure immunization involves the use of both the vaccine and **human rabies immune globulin** (RIG, obtained from hyperimmunized persons) plus immediate cleaning of the wound. Tetanus immunization should also be considered.

The decision to give postexposure immunization depends on a variety of factors, such as (1) the type of animal (all wild-animal attacks demand immunization); (2) whether an attack by a domestic animal was provoked, whether the animal was immunized adequately, and whether the animal is available to be observed; (3) the severity of the bite and its location; and (4) whether rabies is endemic in the area. The advice of local public health officials should be sought.

If the decision is to immunize, both HDCV and RIG are recommended. Five doses of HDCV are given, but RIG is given only once with the first dose of HDCV (at a different site). If the animal has been captured, it should be observed for 10 days and sacrificed if symptoms develop. The brain of the sacrificed animal should be examined by immunofluorescence.

The vaccine for immunization of dogs and cats consists of live, attenuated rabies virus grown in chick embryos. Vaccination must be repeated at intervals.

Review Questions

1. Describe the genome and proteins of influenza virus.
2. What is the origin of the changing antigenicity of the influenza virus surface proteins?
3. What is the basis on which influenza virus is divided into A, B, and C viruses?
4. Antibody against which proteins protects against influenza virus infection?
5. What is the function of the virion polymerase?
6. Distinguish between antigenic shift and antigenic drift. What is the impact of each on disease occurrence?
7. What is the mode of action of amantadine? What is its clinical use?
8. Describe influenza vaccine (the nature of the antigen, the number of virus types, its effectiveness, and its target population).
9. What are the main differences between orthomyxoviruses and paramyxoviruses?
10. Why do paramyxoviruses have a virion RNA polymerase?
11. You get measles only once. What factors contribute to this?
12. What is the pathogenesis of measles?
13. What is the relationship between measles and subacute sclerosing panencephalitis?
14. What is the nature of the measles vaccine? How effective is it?
15. What is the pathogenesis of mumps?
16. What is the nature of the mumps vaccine? How effective is it?
17. Why is mumps of concern in a man but less so in a young boy?
18. Respiratory syncytial virus is a major cause of which disease in which age group?
19. Why is the term "syncytial" in the name "respiratory syncytial virus"? What causes syncytia?
20. What is the major disease caused by parainfluenza viruses in children?
21. How does the rubella virus genome differ from the orthomyxovirus and paramyxovirus genomes?
22. What is the most important complication of rubella infection in young women?
23. What is congenital rubella syndrome?
24. What is the nature of rubella vaccine? How effective is it?
25. What is the host range of rabies virus?
26. What are the main reservoirs of rabies virus in the USA and in developing countries?
27. What is the pathogenesis of rabies?
28. Trace the path of rabies virus from its entry into the normal animal to its appearance in the saliva of the rabid animal.
29. What are the laboratory procedures for the diagnosis of rabies in animals and in humans?
30. Discuss the criteria that determine whether postexposure rabies prophylaxis should be given.
31. What is the nature of the rabies vaccine? In what cells is it made? Why?

40

RNA Nonenveloped Viruses

Picornaviruses

Picornaviruses are small (20–30 nm) **nonenveloped** viruses composed of an **icosahedral nucleocapsid** and **a single-stranded** RNA genome. The genome RNA has **positive polarity;** ie, on entering the cell, it functions as the viral mRNA. The genome RNA is unusual because it has a protein on the 5′ end that serves as a primer for transcription by RNA polymerase. Picornaviruses replicate in the cytoplasm of cells. They are not inactivated by lipid solvents, such as ether, because they do not have an envelope.

The picornavirus family includes 2 groups of medical importance: the **enteroviruses** and the **rhinoviruses.** Among the major enteroviruses are poliovirus, coxsackieviruses, echoviruses, and hepatitis A virus (which is described in Chapter 41). Enteroviruses infect primarily the enteric tract, whereas rhinoviruses are found in the nose and throat (hence their name). Important features of viruses that commonly infect the intestinal tract are summarized in Table 40–1. Enteroviruses replicate optimally at 37 °C, whereas rhinoviruses grow better at 33 °C, in accordance with the lower temperature of the nose. Enteroviruses are stable under acid conditions (pH 3–5), which enables them to survive exposure to gastric acid, whereas rhinoviruses are acid-labile. This may explain why rhinoviruses are restricted to the nose and throat.

ENTEROVIRUSES

1. Poliovirus

Disease This virus causes poliomyelitis.

Important Properties The host range is limited to **primates,** ie, humans and nonhuman primates such as apes and monkeys. This limitation is due to the binding of the viral capsid protein to a receptor found only on primate cell membranes. However, note that purified viral RNA (without the capsid protein) can enter and replicate in many nonprimate cells; the RNA can bypass the cell membrane receptor, ie, it is "infectious RNA."

There are **3 serologic (antigenic) types** based on different antigenic determinants on the outer capsid proteins. Because there is little cross reaction, protection from disease requires the presence of antibody against each of the 3 types.

Summary of Replicative Cycle The virion interacts with specific cell receptors on the cell membrane and then enters the cell. The capsid proteins are then removed. After coating, the genome RNA functions as mRNA and is translated into one very large polypeptide called

Table 40–1. Features of viruses commonly infecting the intestinal tract.

Virus	Nucleic Acid	Disease	Number of Serotypes	Lifelong Immunity to Disease	Vaccine Available	Antiviral Therapy
Poliovirus	RNA	Poliomyelitis	3	Yes (type-specific)	+	−
Echoviruses	RNA	Meningitis, etc	Many	No	−	−
Coxsackieviruses	RNA	Meningitis, carditis, etc	Many	No	−	−
Hepatitis A virus (enterovirus 72)	RNA	Hepatitis	1	Yes	−	−
Rotavirus	RNA	Diarrhea	Several[1]	No	−	−
Norwalk-like viruses	RNA	Diarrhea	Unknown	Unknown	−	−
Adenovirus	DNA	Diarrhea	2 of 41[2]	Unknown	−	−

[1]Exact number uncertain.
[2]Two of the 41 serotypes of adenovirus are known to cause diarrhea.

noncapsid viral protein 00. This polypeptide is cleaved by proteases in multiple steps to form both the capsid proteins of the progeny virions and several noncapsid proteins including the RNA polymerase that synthesizes the progeny RNA genomes. Replication of the genome occurs by synthesis of a complementary negative strand, which then serves as the template for the positive strands. Some of these positive strands function as mRNA to make more viral proteins, and the remainder become progeny virion genome RNA. Assembly of the progeny virions occurs by coating of the genome RNA with capsid proteins. Virions accumulate in the cell cytoplasm and are released upon death of the cell. They do not bud from the cell membrane.

Transmission & Epidemiology   Poliovirus is transmitted by the **fecal-oral** route. It replicates in the oropharynx and intestinal tract. Humans are the only natural hosts.

As a result of the success of the vaccine, there have been very few cases of poliomyelitis (less than 20 per year) in the USA during recent years. The rare cases in the USA occur mainly in (1) people exposed to virulent revertants of the attenuated virus in the live vaccine and (2) unimmunized people exposed to virulent poliovirus while traveling abroad. Before the vaccine was available, epidemics occurred in the summer and fall.

Poliomyelitis occurs worldwide with varying frequency. In developing countries, particularly in areas where hygiene and sanitation are poor, children are exposed at an early age and experience mostly asymptomatic infections. In more developed countries, exposure is frequently delayed, with a consequent increase in the frequency of symptomatic infection among the unimmunized.

Pathogenesis & Immunity   After replicating in the oropharynx and small intestine, especially in lymphoid tissue, the virus spreads through the bloodstream to the central nervous system. It can also spread retrograde along nerve axons.

In the central nervous system, poliovirus preferentially replicates in the **motor neurons** located in the **anterior horn** of the spinal cord. Death of these cells results in paralysis of the muscles innervated by those neurons. Paralysis is not due to virus infection of muscle cells. The virus also affects the brain stem, leading to ''bulbar'' poliomyelitis (with respiratory paralysis), but rarely damages the cerebral cortex.

In infected individuals, the immune response consists of both intestinal IgA and humoral IgG to the specific serotype. Infection provides lifelong type-specific immunity.

Clinical Findings   The range of responses to poliovirus infection includes (1) inapparent, asymptomatic infection; (2) abortive poliomyelitis; (3) nonparalytic poliomyelitis; and (4) paralytic poliomyelitis. Asymptomatic infection is quite common. Roughly 1% of infections are clinically apparent. The incubation period is usually 10–14 days.

The most common clinical form is abortive poliomyelitis, which is a mild, febrile illness characterized by headache, sore throat, nausea, and vomiting. Most patients recover spontaneously. Nonparalytic poliomyelitis manifests as an aseptic meningitis with fever, headache, and a stiff neck. This also usually resolves spontaneously. In paralytic poliomyelitis, flaccid paralysis is the predominant finding but brain stem involvement can lead to life-threatening respiratory paralysis. Painful muscle spasms also occur. The motor nerve damage is permanent, but some recovery of muscle function occurs as other nerve cells take over.

A postparalytic syndrome that occurs many years after the acute illness has been described recently. Marked deterioration of the residual function of the affected muscles occurs many years after the acute phase. The cause of this deterioration is unknown.

No permanent carrier state occurs following infection by poliovirus, but virus excretion in the feces can occur for several months.

Laboratory Diagnosis   The diagnosis is made either by isolation of the virus or by a rise in antibody titer. Virus can be recovered from the throat, stool, or spinal fluid by inoculation of cell cultures. The virus causes a cytopathic effect (CPE) and can be identified by neutralization of the CPE with specific antisera.

Treatment   There is no antiviral therapy. Treatment is limited to symptomatic relief and respiratory support, if needed. Physiotherapy for the affected muscles is important.

Prevention Poliomyelitis can be prevented by both the **killed** (Salk) and the **live, attenuated** (Sabin) vaccines (Table 40–2). Both vaccines induce humoral antibodies, which neutralize virus entering the blood and hence prevent central nervous system infection and disease. The **live vaccine is currently preferred** in the USA for 2 main reasons: (1) It interrupts fecal-oral transmission by inducing secretory IgA in the gastrointestinal tract. IgA is induced by the live virus because it replicates in the gastrointestinal tract, whereas the killed vaccine does not. (2) It is given orally and so is more readily accepted than the killed vaccine, which must be injected.

The live vaccine has 4 disadvantages: (1) Rarely, **reversion** of the attenuated virus to virulence will occur, and disease may ensue (especially for the type 3 virus); (2) it can cause disease in immunodeficient persons and therefore should not be given to them; (3) infection of the gastrointestinal tract by other enteroviruses can limit replication of the vaccine virus and reduce protection; and (4) it must be kept refrigerated to prevent heat inactivation of the live virus.

The duration of immunity is thought to be longer with the live than with the killed vaccine, but booster doses are recommended with both.

The killed vaccine is used in the USA in 2 special instances: (1) initial vaccination of unimmunized adults, because the risk of disease from the live vaccine is higher in adults than in children; and (2) vaccination of immunodeficient individuals.

Both the killed and the live vaccines contain all 3 serologic types. The live vaccine should be given at 2, 4, 6, and 18 months of age, with a booster when the child enters school.

In the past, some lots of poliovirus vaccines were contaminated with a papovavirus, SV40 virus, which causes sarcomas in rodents. SV40 virus was a "passenger" virus in the monkey kidney cells used to grow the poliovirus for the vaccine. Fortunately, no increase in cancer occurred in persons inoculated with the SV40 virus-containing polio vaccine. At present, cell cultures used for vaccine purposes are carefully screened to exclude the presence of adventitious viruses.

Passive immunization with immune serum globulin is available for protection of unimmunized individuals known to have been exposed. Passive immunization of newborns as a result of passage of maternal IgG antibodies across the placenta also occurs.

Quarantine of patients with disease is not effective, because fecal excretion of the virus occurs in infected individuals prior to the onset of symptoms and in those who remain asymptomatic.

2. Coxsackieviruses Coxsackieviruses are named for the town of Coxsackie, NY, where they were first isolated.

Diseases Coxsackieviruses cause a variety of diseases. Group A viruses cause, for example, herpangina and hand-foot-and-mouth disease, whereas group B viruses cause

Table 40–2. Important features of poliovirus vaccines.

Attribute	Killed (Salk)	Live (Sabin)
Prevents disease	Yes	Yes
Interrupts transmission	No	Yes
Induces humoral IgG	Yes	Yes
Induces intestinal IgA	No	Yes
Affords secondary protection by spread to others	No	Yes
Interferes with replication of virulent virus in gut	No	Yes
Reverts to virulence	No	Yes (rarely)
Coinfection with other enteroviruses impairs immunization	No	Yes
Can cause disease in the immunocompromised	No	Yes
Route of administration	Injection	Oral
Requires refrigeration	No	Yes
Duration of immunity	Shorter	Longer

pleurodynia, myocarditis, and pericarditis. Both types cause nonspecific upper respiratory tract disease, febrile rashes, and aseptic meningitis.

Important Properties   Group classification is based on pathogenicity in mice. Group A viruses cause widespread myositis and flaccid paralysis, which is rapidly fatal, whereas group B viruses cause generalized, less severe lesions of the heart, pancreas, and central nervous system and a focal myositis. Currently, 23 serotypes of coxsackievirus A and 6 serotypes of coxsackievirus B are recognized.

The size and structure of the virion and the nature of the genome RNA are similar to those of poliovirus. Unlike poliovirus, they can infect mammals other than primates.

Summary of Replicative Cycle   Replication is similar to that of poliovirus.

Transmission & Epidemiology   Coxsackieviruses are transmitted primarily by the **fecal-oral** route, but respiratory **aerosols** also play a role. They replicate in the oropharynx and the intestinal tract. Humans are the only natural hosts. Coxsackievirus infections occur worldwide, primarily in the summer and fall.

Pathogenesis & Immunity   Group A viruses have a predilection for skin and mucous membranes, whereas group B viruses cause disease in various organs such as the heart, pleura, pancreas, and liver. Both group A and B viruses can affect the meninges and the motor neurons (anterior horn cells) to cause paralysis. From their original site of replication in the oropharynx and gastrointestinal tract, they disseminate via the bloodstream.

Immunity following infection is provided by type-specific IgG antibody.

Clinical Findings

A. Group A-Specific Diseases: **Herpangina** is characterized by fever, sore throat, and tender vesicles in the oropharynx. Hand-foot-and-mouth disease is characterized by a vesicular rash on the hands and feet and ulcerations in the mouth, mainly in children.

B. Group B-Specific Diseases: **Pleurodynia** (Bornholm disease, epidemic myalgia, "devil's grip") is characterized by fever and severe pleuritic-type chest pain. **Myocarditis** and pericarditis are characterized by fever, chest pain, and signs of congestive failure. Diabetes in mice can be caused by pancreatic damage as a result of infection with coxsackievirus B4. This virus is suspected to have a similar role in juvenile diabetes in humans.

C. Diseases Caused by Both Groups: Both groups of viruses can cause **aseptic meningitis,** mild paresis, and transient paralysis, Upper respiratory infections and minor febrile illnesses with or without rash can occur also.

Laboratory Diagnosis   The diagnosis is made either by isolating the virus in cell culture or suckling mice or by observing a rise in titer of neutralizing antibodies.

Treatment & Prevention   There is neither antiviral drug therapy nor a vaccine available against these viruses. No passive immunization is recommended.

3. Echoviruses   The prefix ECHO is an acronym for *e*nteric *c*ytopathic *h*uman *o*rphan. Although called "orphans" because they were not initially associated with any disease, they are now known to cause a variety of diseases such as aseptic meningitis, upper respiratory infection, febrile illness with and without rash, infantile diarrhea, and hemorrhagic conjunctivitis.

The structure of echoviruses is similar to that of other enteroviruses. More than 30 serotypes have been isolated. In contrast to coxsackieviruses, they are not pathogenic for mice. Unlike polioviruses, they do not cause disease in monkeys. They are transmitted by the fecal-oral route and occur worldwide. Pathogenesis is similar to that of the other enteroviruses.

Along with coxsackieviruses, echoviruses are one of the **leading causes of aseptic (viral) meningitis.** The diagnosis is made by isolation of the virus in cell culture. Serologic tests are of little value, because there are a large number of serotypes and no common antigen. There is no antiviral therapy or vaccine available.

4. Other Enteroviruses   In view of the difficulty in classifying many enteroviruses, all new isolates have been given a simple numerical designation since 1969.

Enterovirus 70 is the main cause of acute hemorrhagic conjunctivitis, characterized by petechial hemorrhages on the bulbar conjunctivas. Complete recovery usually occurs, and there is no therapy. Enterovirus 71 is one of the leading causes of viral central nervous system disease, including meningitis, encephalitis, and paralysis. Enterovirus 72 is hepatitis A virus, which is described in Chapter 41.

RHINOVIRUSES

Disease   These viruses cause the common cold.

Important Properties   There are **more than 100 serologic types.** They **replicate better at 33 °C** than at 37 °C, which explains why they affect primarily the nose and conjunctiva rather than the lower respiratory tract. They are **acid-labile** and so are killed by gastric acid when swallowed. This explains why they do not infect the gastrointestinal tract, unlike the enteroviruses. The host range is limited to humans and chimpanzees.

Summary of Replicative Cycle   Replication is similar to that of poliovirus.

Transmission & Epidemiology   There are **2 modes** of transmission for these viruses. In the past, it was accepted that they were transmitted directly from person to person via aerosols of respiratory droplets. However, now it appears that an indirect mode, in which respiratory droplets are deposited on the hands or on a surface such as a table and then transported by fingers to the nose or eyes, is also important.

The common cold is reputed to be the most common human infection, although data are difficult to obtain because it is not a well-defined or notifiable disease. Millions of days of work and school are lost each year as a result of "colds." Rhinoviruses occur worldwide, causing disease particularly in the fall and winter. The reason for this seasonal variation is unclear. Low temperatures per se do not predispose to the common cold, but the crowding that occurs at schools, for example, may enhance transmission during fall and winter. The frequency of colds is high in childhood and tapers off during adulthood, presumably owing to the acquisition of immunity.

A few serotypes of rhinoviruses are prevalent during one season, only to be replaced by other serotypes during the following season. It appears that the population builds up immunity to the prevalent serotypes but remains susceptible to the others.

Pathogenesis & Immunity   The portal of entry is the upper respiratory tract, and the infection is limited to that region. Rhinoviruses rarely cause lower respiratory tract disease, probably because they grow poorly at 37 °C.

Immunity is serotype-specific and is a function of nasal secretory antibody rather than humoral antibody.

Clinical Findings   After an incubation period of 2–4 days, sneezing, nasal discharge, sore throat, cough, and headache are common. A chilly sensation may occur, but there are few other systemic symptoms. The illness lasts about 1 week. Note that other viruses such as coronaviruses, adenoviruses, influenza C virus, and coxsackieviruses also cause the common cold syndrome.

Laboratory Diagnosis   Diagnosis can be made by isolation of the virus from nasal secretions in cell culture, but this is rarely attempted. Serologic tests are not done.

Treatment & Prevention   No specific antiviral therapy is available. Vaccines appear impractical because of the large number of serotypes. Paper tissues impregnated with disinfectants, such as iodine, appear to limit transmission when used to remove rhinoviruses from contaminated fingers.

Reoviruses

REO is an acronym for *r*espiratory *e*nteric *o*rphan; when the virus was discovered, it was isolated from the respiratory and enteric tracts and was not associated with any disease. Rotaviruses are the most important human pathogens in the reovirus family.

ROTAVIRUSES

Disease   Rotaviruses are the most common cause of gastroenteritis in young children.

Important Properties   Reoviruses, including rotaviruses, are composed of a **segmented,* double-stranded RNA genome** surrounded by a double-layered icosahedral capsid without an envelope. The virion contains an **RNA-dependent RNA polymerase.**

Many domestic animals are infected with their own strains of rotaviruses, but these are not a source of human disease. There are at least 4 serotypes of human rotavirus. The viral hemagglutinin is the type-specific antigen.

Summary of Replicative Cycle   After entry of the virion into the cell, the RNA-dependent RNA polymerase synthesizes mRNA from each of the 10 or 11 segments within the cytoplasm. The 10 or 11 mRNAs are translated into the corresponding number of structural and nonstructural proteins. One of these, an RNA polymerase, synthesizes minus strands that will become part of the genome of the progeny virus. Capsid proteins form an incomplete capsid around the minus strands, and then the plus strands of the progeny genome segments are synthesized. The virus is released from the cytoplasm by lysis of the cell, not by budding.

Transmission & Epidemiology   Rotaviruses are transmitted by the **fecal-oral** route. Infection occurs worldwide, and by age 6 years the majority of children have antibodies to at least one serotype.

Pathogenesis & Immunity   Rotaviruses replicate in the mucosal cells of the small intestine, damaging the transport mechanisms. The consequent loss of salt, glucose, and water leads to diarrhea. No inflammation occurs, and the diarrhea is nonbloody.

The virulence of certain reoviruses in mice has been localized to the proteins encoded by several specific genome segments. For example, one gene governs tissue tropism, whereas another controls the inhibition of cell RNA and protein synthesis.

Immunity to rotavirus infection is unclear. It is likely that intestinal IgA directed against specific serotypes protects against reinfection and that colostrum IgA protects newborns up to the age of 6 months.

Clinical Findings   Rotavirus infection is characterized by nausea, vomiting, and watery, nonbloody diarrhea. **Gastroenteritis** is most serious in **young children,** in whom dehydration and electrolyte imbalance are a major concern. Adults usually have minor symptoms.

Laboratory Diagnosis   Although the diagnosis of most cases of viral gastroenteritis does not involve the laboratory, a diagnosis can be made by **detection of rotavirus in the stool** by using radioimmunoassay or ELISA. This approach is feasible because there are large numbers of virus particles in the stool. The original demonstration of rotavirus in the stool was done by immune electron microscopy in which antibody aggregated the virions, allowing them to be visualized in the electron microscope. This technique is not feasible for routine clinical use. In addition to antigen detection, the diagnosis can be made by observation of a 4-fold or greater rise in antibody titer. The virus can be cultured, but it is too difficult to do on a routine basis.

Treatment & Prevention   There is neither antiviral therapy nor a vaccine available. Prevention rests on sanitation.

---

*Rotaviruses have 11 segments; other reoviruses have 10.

Review Questions

1. What are the differences between enteroviruses and rhinoviruses?
2. What is the nature of the picornavirus genome?
3. Why does poliovirus infect only primate cells?
4. Poliovirus has 3 serotypes. What is the importance of this for the prevention of poliomyelitis?
5. What is the nature of the translation product of the poliovirus RNA? How are viral capsid proteins formed?
6. How is poliovirus transmitted?
7. What is the pathogenesis of paralytic poliomyelitis?
8. Compare the advantages and disadvantages of the killed and live poliovirus vaccines.
9. How did SV40 virus get into some lots of poliovirus vaccine? Why is this of concern?
10. On what basis are coxsackievirus groups A and B distinguished?
11. What clinical entities do coxsackievirus groups A and B specifically cause? What disease do both groups A and B cause?
12. What is the significance of the fact that there are more than 100 serotypes of rhinoviruses?
13. What are 2 modes of transmission of rhinoviruses?
14. What is the nature of the reovirus genome? Why is there a virion polymerase?
15. Rotaviruses are clinically important reoviruses. What disease do they cause? In what population?
16. How is rotavirus infection diagnosed in the laboratory?

41

Hepatitis Viruses

Many viruses cause hepatitis. Of these, 4 are commonly described as "hepatitis viruses," ie, hepatitis A virus (HAV); hepatitis B virus (HBV); non-A, non-B viruses (NANB); and delta agent (Table 41–1). The other viruses, such as Epstein-Barr virus (the cause of infectious mononucleosis), cytomegalovirus, and yellow fever virus, cause inflammation of the liver but are not called hepatitis viruses per se. They are discussed elsewhere.

HEPATITIS A VIRUS

Disease   HAV causes hepatitis A.

Important Properties   HAV is a typical **enterovirus** classified in the picornavirus family. It has a single-stranded RNA genome and a nonenveloped icosahedral nucleocapsid and replicates in the cytoplasm of the cell. It is also known as enterovirus 72.

It has one serotype, and there is no antigenic relationship to HBV or other hepatitis viruses. Humans and chimpanzees are the only natural hosts.

Summary of Replicative Cycle   HAV has a replicative cycle similar to that of other enteroviruses (the replicative cycle of poliovirus is discussed in Chapter 40).

Transmission & Epidemiology   HAV is transmitted by the **fecal-oral** route. Virus appears in the feces roughly 2 weeks before the appearance of symptoms, so quarantine of patients is ineffective. **Children are the most frequently infected** group, and outbreaks occur in special living situations such as summer camps and boarding schools. Common-source outbreaks arise

Table 41–1. Glossary of hepatitis viruses and their serologic markers.

Abbreviation	Name and Description
HAV	Hepatitis A virus (enterovirus 72), a picornavirus (nonenveloped RNA virus).
IgM HAVAb	IgM antibody to HAV; best test to detect active hepatitis A.
HBV	Hepatitis B virus, a hepadnavirus (enveloped, partially double-stranded DNA virus); also known as Dane particle.
HBsAg	Antigen found on surface of HBV, also found on spheres and filaments in patient's blood; positive during acute disease; continued presence indicates carrier state.
HBsAb	Antibody to HBsAg; provides immunity to hepatitis B.
HBcAg	Antigen associated with core of HBV.
HBcAb	Antibody to HBcAg; positive during window phase. IgM HBcAb is an indicator of recent disease.
HBeAg	A second, different antigenic determinant on the HBV core. Important indicator of transmissibility.
HBeAb	Antibody to e antigen; indicates low transmissibility.
NANB	Hepatitis viruses that are neither HAV nor HBV; no serologic tests are available.
Delta agent	Small RNA virus with HBsAg envelope; defective virus that replicates only in HBV-infected cells.

from fecally contaminated water or food such as oysters grown in polluted water and eaten raw. Unlike HBV, HAV is **rarely transmitted via the blood,** because the level of viremia is low and chronic infection does not occur. About 50% of adults in the USA have been infected, as evidenced by IgG antibody.

Pathogenesis & Immunity   The pathogenesis of HAV infection is not completely understood. The virus probably replicates in the gastrointestinal tract and spreads to the liver via the blood. Hepatocytes are infected, but the mechanism by which cell damage occurs is unclear. HAV infection of cultured cells produces no cytopathic effect. Unlike HBV, there is no evidence that immune attack on the hepatocytes plays a role in pathogenesis, and there is no chronic infection. Hepatitis caused by the different viruses cannot be distinguished pathologically.

The immune response consists initially of IgM antibody, which is detectable at the time jaundice appears. It is therefore important in the laboratory diagnosis of hepatitis A. The appearance of IgM is followed 1–3 weeks later by the production of IgG antibody, which provides lifelong protection.

Clinical Findings   The clinical manifestations of hepatitis are virtually the same, regardless of which hepatitis virus is the cause. Fever, anorexia, nausea, vomiting, and jaundice are typical. Most cases resolve spontaneously in 2–4 weeks. Hepatitis A has a short incubation period (3–4 weeks), in contrast to that of hepatitis B, which is 10–12 weeks.

Laboratory Diagnosis   The detection of **IgM antibody** is the most important test. A 4-fold rise in IgG antibody titer can also be used. Isolation of the virus in cell culture is possible but not available in the clinical laboratory.

Treatment & Prevention   No antiviral therapy or vaccine is available. **Passive immunization** with immune serum globulin early in the incubation period can prevent or mitigate the disease. Observation of proper hygiene, eg, sewage disposal and hand washing after bowel movements, is of prime importance.

HEPATITIS B VIRUS

Disease   HBV causes hepatitis B.

Important Properties   HBV is a member of the hepadnavirus family. It is a 42-nm **enveloped** virion,* with an icosahedral nucleocapsid core containing a **partially double-stranded circular** DNA genome (Table 41–1). The envelope contains a protein called the **surface antigen** (HBsAg), which is important for laboratory diagnosis and immunization.** Within the core is a **DNA-dependent DNA polymerase.**

Electron microscopy of a patient's serum reveals 3 particles: a few 42-nm virions and many 22-nm **spheres** and long **filaments** 22 nm wide, which are composed of surface antigen. These spheres and filaments are the immunogen in one form of the vaccine.

In addition to HBsAg, there are 2 other important antigens: the **core antigen** (HBcAg) and the **e antigen** (HBeAg), both of which are located in the core but have different antigenicities. HBeAg is an important indicator of **transmissibility.** HBsAg has a group-specific antigen, "a," and 2 sets of mutually exclusive epitopes, d or y and w or r. This leads to 4 serotypes–adw, adr, ayw, and ayr—which are useful in epidemiologic studies because they are concentrated in certain geographic areas.

Humans are the only natural hosts of HBV.

Summary of Replicative Cycle   After entry of the virion into the cell and its uncoating, the DNA polymerase synthesizes the missing portion of DNA and a double-stranded closed-circular DNA is formed in the nucleus. Some of this DNA integrates into hepatocyte DNA, and some serves as a template for mRNA synthesis. mRNA not only functions in protein synthesis but is the template for the minus strand of the progeny DNA. The minus strand then serves as the template for the plus strand of the genome DNA. This RNA-dependent DNA synthesis takes place within the newly assembled virion core in the cytoplasm. (Note that this type of RNA-dependent DNA synthesis is similar to but different from the process in retroviruses, in which the genome RNA is transcribed into a circular DNA intermediate.) Progeny HBV with its HBsAg-containing envelope is released from the cell by budding through the cell membrane.

Transmission & Epidemiology   The most important mode of transmission is via **blood** and blood products. The observation that needle-stick injuries can transmit the virus indicates that only very small amounts of blood are necessary. Screening of blood for the presence of HBsAg has greatly decreased the number of transfusion-associated cases of hepatitis B. However, because blood transfusion is a modern procedure, there must be another, natural route of transmission. It is likely that **sexual** transmission and transmission from **mother to child** during birth or breast feeding are the natural routes.

Hepatitis B is found worldwide but is particularly prevalent in the Orient. In that region, there is a high incidence of **hepatoma,** a finding that may be related to the integration of HBV DNA into the cell DNA.

Pathogenesis & Immunity   After entering the blood, the virus infects hepatocytes, causing necrosis and inflammation. **Immune attack** against viral antigens on infected hepatocytes may play an important role in pathogenesis. Immune complexes cause some of the symptoms, eg, arthralgias.

Unlike hepatitis A patients, about 10% of patients with hepatitis B become **chronic carriers** of HBV. This is attributed to a persistent infection of the hepatocytes mediated by HBV DNA integrated into cell DNA, which results in the prolonged presence of HBV and HBsAg in the blood. A high rate of hepatocellular carcinoma occurs in chronic carriers.

Lifelong immunity is mediated by humoral antibody against HBsAg.

Clinical Findings   The mean incubation period for hepatitis B is 10–12 weeks, which is much longer than that of hepatitis A (3–4 weeks). The clinical appearance of acute hepatitis B is similar to that of hepatitis A. However, with hepatitis B, symptoms tend to be more severe and life-threatening hepatitis can occur. Most chronic carriers are asymptomatic, but some have chronic active hepatitis, which can lead to cirrhosis and death.

---

*Also known as a Dane particle (named for the scientist who first published electron micrographs of the virion).
**HBsAg is also known as Australia antigen, because it was first found in the serum of an Australian aborigine.

Laboratory Diagnosis The most important laboratory test for the detection of HBV infection is the immunoassay for **HBsAg.** HBsAg appears during the incubation period and is detectable in most patients during the prodrome and acute disease (Fig 41–1). It falls to undetectable levels during convalescence in most cases; its prolonged presence indicates the carrier state and the risk of chronic hepatitis. Note that there is a period of several weeks when HBsAg has disappeared but HBsAb is not yet detectable. This is the **"window phase."** At this time, the HBcAb is always positive and can be used to make the diagnosis. The test for HBcAg is not readily available.

HBeAg arises during the incubation period and is present during the prodrome and early acute disease. Its presence is an important indicator of transmissibility, and, conversely, the finding of HBeAb indicates low transmissibility. DNA polymerase activity is detectable during the incubation period and early in the disease, but the assay is not available in most clinical laboratories.

Treatment & Prevention No antiviral therapy is available. Prevention involves the use of either the **vaccine** or **hyperimmune globulin,** or both.

(a) One form of the vaccine consists of HBsAg from the spherical particles purified from the sera of infected individuals. The preparation is treated with pepsin, urea, and formaldehyde to kill any viruses that may be present. A second form contains HBsAg manufactured by using genetic engineering techniques with yeast. Both vaccines are highly effective in preventing hepatitis B and have few side effects. No diseases are known to be transmitted by the vaccine. It is indicated for people who are frequently exposed to blood or blood products, such as certain health care personnel (eg, surgeons and dentists), patients receiving multiple transfusions or dialysis, patients with frequent sexually transmitted disease, and abusers of illicit intravenous drugs.

(b) Hepatitis B immune globulin (HBIG) contains a high titer of HBsAb, because it is prepared from sera of patients who have recovered from hepatitis B. It is used to provide

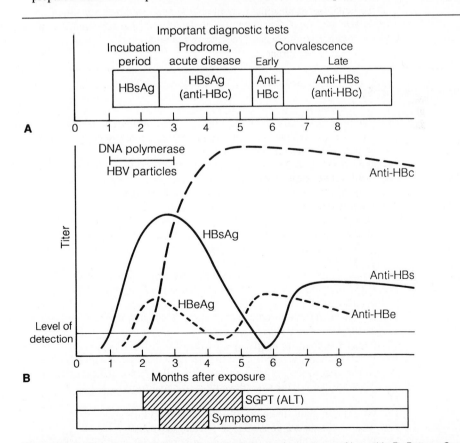

Figure 41–1. *Top:* Important diagnostic tests during various stages of hepatitis B. *Bottom:* Serologic findings in a patient with hepatitis B. (Modified and reproduced, with permission, from Hollinger FB, Dienstag JL: *Manual of Clinical Microbiology,* 4th ed. American Society for Microbiology, 1985.)

immediate, passive protection to individuals known to be exposed to HBsAg-positive blood, eg, after an accidental needle stick.

Precise recommendations for use of the vaccine and HBIG are beyond the scope of this book. However, the recommendation regarding one common concern of medical students, the needle-stick injury from a patient with HBsAg-positive blood, is that both the vaccine and HBIG be given (at separate sites). This is a good example of "passive-active" immunization, in which both immediate and long-term protection are provided.

All blood for transfusion should be screened for HBsAg. No one with a history of hepatitis (of any type) should donate blood, because NANB viruses may be present.

NON-A, NON-B HEPATITIS VIRUSES   Because there are cases of hepatitis for which serologic tests have ruled out all known viral causes, it is presumed that additional agents are involved. However, no serologic tests are available and the nature of these viruses is unknown. Cross-protection studies indicate that at least 2 other viruses are involved.

NANB hepatitis is transmitted primarily via blood and resembles hepatitis B in its course and severity. A chronic carrier state can occur. Most cases of posttransfusion hepatitis in the USA are now due to NANB viruses. One major cause of NANB hepatitis is hepatitis C virus, an enveloped, single-stranded RNA virus resembling yellow fever virus, a flavivirus.

DELTA AGENT (HEPATITIS DELTA VIRUS)   This virus is unusual in that it has a **small RNA genome** surrounded by an **envelope composed of HBsAg.** Its genome RNA is a **single-stranded circle** with no sequence homology to hepatitis B DNA. Delta agent is a **defective** virus, because its genome does not code for its own envelope protein. This implies that delta hepatitis can occur only in patients previously infected by HBV since the virus can replicate only in HBV-infected cells. The name "delta" is derived from the **delta antigen,** a distinctive determinant present in this virus but not in HBV.

Delta hepatitis is transmitted via the blood and resembles hepatitis B in severity. A chronic carrier state can occur. Infection can be detected by the appearance of IgM antibody to delta antigen. Neither treatment nor vaccine is available.

Review Questions

1. Compare HAV and HBV according to the following criteria: classification, genome, presence of envelope, number of serotypes, and existence of animal reservoir.
2. How is HAV transmitted?
3. How is the diagnosis of acute hepatitis A made in the laboratory?
4. How can hepatitis A be prevented?
5. What are the 3 important antigens in the HBV particle?
6. What is the function of the DNA polymerase in the virion?
7. In the replication of HBV, there is a step in which RNA is transcribed into DNA, analogous to reverse transcription in retroviruses. When does this step occur in HBV replication?
8. HBV is transmitted by blood transfusion. What are thought to be the natural modes of transmission?
9. What is the role of the immune response in the pathogenesis of hepatitis B?
10. HBV infection is associated with hepatoma. What step in HBV replication might explain this relationship?
11. HBV can cause a chronic carrier state. What step in HBV replication might explain the persistence of the virus?
12. Is there lifelong immunity against (a) HAV? (b) HBV?
13. What laboratory test is used (a) to detect acute infection with HBV? (b) as the best indicator of transmissibility? (c) to indicate immunity? (d) to indicate the chronic carrier state?
14. What are the 2 modes of prevention of hepatitis B?
15. What is the antigen in the vaccine?
16. Why do we think there are NANB hepatitis viruses?
17. What is the nature of the agent of delta hepatitis?
18. Why is the delta agent found only in persons infected with HBV?
19. How is delta agent transmitted?
20. Clinically, does delta hepatitis resemble hepatitis A or hepatitis B more closely?

Arboviruses

42

The term "arbovirus" is an acronym for *ar*thropod-*bo*rne virus and highlights the fact that these viruses are transmitted by **arthropods,** primarily mosquitoes and ticks. It is a collective name for a large group of diverse viruses, more than 400 at last count. In general, they are named either for the diseases they cause,. eg, yellow fever virus, or for the place where they were first isolated, eg, St. Louis encephalitis virus.

IMPORTANT PROPERTIES Most arboviruses are classified in 2 families,* namely **togaviruses** and **bunyaviruses** (Table 42–1).

(a) Togaviruses[†] are characterized by an icosahedral nucleocapsid surrounded by an envelope and a single-stranded, positive-polarity RNA genome. This family is subdivided into 4 genera on the basis of size and antigenic relationships: the alphaviruses and rubiviruses are 60–70 nm, whereas the flaviviruses and pestiviruses are 45–55 nm. Only alphaviruses and flaviviruses are considered here. The only rubivirus is rubella virus, which is discussed in Chapter 39, and pestiviruses do not cause human disease.

(b) Bunyaviruses[††] have a helical nucleocapsid surrounded by an envelope and a genome consisting of 3 segments of negative-polarity RNA that are hydrogen-bonded together.

TRANSMISSION The life cycle of the arboviruses is based on the ability of these viruses to multiply in **both** the vertebrate host and the bloodsucking vector. For effective transmission to occur, the virus must be present in the bloodstream of the vertebrate host (viremia) in sufficiently high titer to be taken up in the small volume of blood ingested during an insect bite. After ingestion, the virus replicates in the gut of the arthropod and then spreads to other organs, including the salivary glands. Only the female of the species serves as the vector of the virus, because only she requires a blood meal in order for progeny to be produced. An obligatory length of time, called the **extrinsic incubation period,**** must pass for the virus to replicate sufficiently for the saliva of the vector to contain enough virus to transmit an infectious dose. For most viruses, the extrinsic incubation period ranges from 7 to 14 days.

Table 42–1. Classification of the major arboviruses.

Family	Genus	Viruses of Medical Interest in the Americas
Togavirus	Alphavirus[1]	Eastern equine encephalitis virus, western equine encephalitis virus
Togavirus	Flavivirus[2]	St. Louis encephalitis virus, yellow fever virus, dengue virus
Bunyavirus	Bunyavirus[3]	California encephalitis virus
Reovirus	Orbivirus	Colorado tick fever virus

[1]Alphaviruses of other regions include Chikungunya, Mayaro, O'Nyong-Nyong, Ross River, and Semliki Forest viruses.
[2]Flaviviruses of other regions include Japanese encephalitis, Kyasanur Forest, Murray Valley encephalitis, Omsk hemorrhagic fever, Powassan encephalitis, and West Nile fever viruses.
[3]Bunyaviruses of other regions include the Bunyamwera complex of viruses and Oropouche virus.

---

*A few arboviruses belong to 2 other families. For example, Colorado tick virus is a reovirus; Kern Canyon virus and vesicular stomatitis virus are rhabdoviruses.

†Toga means cloak.

††"Bunya" is short for Bunyamwera, the town in Africa in which the prototype virus was isolated.

**The intrinsic incubation period is the interval between the time of the bite and the appearance of symptoms in the human host.

In addition to transmission through vertebrates, some arboviruses are transmitted by vertical "transovarian" passage from the mother tick to her offspring. Vertical transmission has important survival value for the virus if a vertebrate host is unavailable.

Humans are involved in the transmission cycle of arboviruses in 2 different ways. Usually, humans are **"dead-end" hosts,** because the concentration of virus in human blood is too low and the duration of viremia too brief for the next bite to transmit the virus. However, in some diseases, eg, yellow fever and dengue, humans have a high-level viremia and act as reservoirs of the virus.

Infection by arboviruses usually does not result in disease either in the arthropod vector or in the vertebrate animal that serves as the natural host. Disease occurs primarily when the virus infect dead-end hosts. For example, yellow fever virus cycles harmlessly among the jungle monkeys in South America but when the virus infects a human, yellow fever can occur.

CLINICAL FINDINGS & EPIDEMIOLOGY   The diseases caused by arboviruses range in severity from mild to rapidly fatal. The clinical picture usually fits one of 3 categories: (1) **encephalitis;** (2) **hemorrhagic fever;** or (3) fever with myalgias, arthralgias, and nonhemorrhagic rash. The pathogenesis of these diseases involves not only the cytocidal effect of the virus but also, in some, a prominent immunopathologic component. Following recovery from the disease, immunity is usually lifelong.

The arboviral diseases occur primarily in the **tropics** but are also found in temperate zones such as the USA and as far north as Alaska and Siberia. They have a tendency to cause sudden outbreaks of disease, generally at the interface between human communities and jungle or forest areas.

Arboviruses That Cause Disease in the USA

EASTERN EQUINE ENCEPHALITIS VIRUS   Of the 4 encephalitis viruses listed in Table 42–2, eastern equine encephalitis (EEE) virus causes the **most severe** disease and is associated with the highest fatality rate (approximately 50%). In its natural habitat, the virus is transmitted primarily by the swamp **mosquito,** *Culiseta,* among the small wild birds of the Atlantic and Gulf Coast states. Species of *Aedes* mosquitoes are suspected of carrying the virus from its **wild-bird reservoir** to the 2 principal dead-end hosts, **horses and humans.** The number of cases of human encephalitis caused by EEE virus in the USA usually ranges from zero to 4 per year, but outbreaks involving hundreds of cases also occur.

The encephalitis is characterized by the sudden onset of severe headache, nausea, vomiting, and fever. Changes in mental status, such as confusion and stupor, ensue. A rapidly progressive downhill course with nuchal rigidity, seizures, and coma occurs. If the patient survives, the central nervous system sequelae are severe. Immunity following the infection is lifelong.

The diagnosis is made by either isolating the virus or demonstrating a rise in antibody titer. Clinicians should have a high index of suspicion in the summer months in the appropriate geographic areas. The disease does not occur in the winter, because mosquitoes are not active. It is not known how the virus survives the winter—in birds, mosquitoes, or perhaps some other animal.

No antiviral therapy is available. A killed vaccine is available to protect horses but not humans. The disease is too rare for production of a human vaccine to be economically feasible.

WESTERN EQUINE ENCEPHALITIS VIRUS   Western equine encephalitis (WEE) virus causes disease more frequently than does EEE virus, but the illness is less severe. Inapparent infections outnumber the apparent by at least 100:1, and the fatality rate is roughly 2%. The number of cases in the USA usually ranges between 5 and 20 per year.

The virus is transmitted primarily by *Culex* **mosquitoes** among the **wild-bird** population of the western states, especially in areas with irrigated farmland.

The clinical picture of WEE virus infection is similar to but less severe than that caused by EEE virus. Sequelae are less common. The diagnosis is made by isolating the virus or observing a rise in antibody titer. There is no antiviral therapy. There is a killed vaccine for horses but not for humans.

ST. LOUIS ENCEPHALITIS VIRUS Of the 3 encephalitis viruses belonging to the togavirus family, St. Louis encephalitis (SLE) virus causes disease over the widest geographic area. It is found in the southern, central, and western states and causes 10–30 cases of encephalitis per year in the USA.

The virus is transmitted by several species of *Culex* **mosquitoes** that vary depending upon location. Again, small **wild birds**, especially English sparrows, are the reservoir and humans are dead-end hosts. Although EEE and WEE viruses are predominantly rural, SLE virus occurs in **urban areas** because these mosquitoes prefer to breed in stagnant wastewater.

SLE virus causes a moderately severe encephalitis associated with a fatality rate that approaches 10%. Most infections are inapparent; the ratio of inapparent to apparent infections is roughly 60:1. Sequelae are uncommon.

The diagnosis is usually made serologically, because the virus is difficult to isolate. No antiviral therapy or vaccine is available.

CALIFORNIA ENCEPHALITIS VIRUS California encephalitis (CE) virus was first isolated from mosquitoes in California in 1952, but its name is something of a misnomer because most human disease occurs in the north-central states. The most frequent strain of the 11 CE viruses to cause encephalitis is called La Crosse for the city in Wisconsin where it was isolated. CE virus is the only one of the 4 major encephalitis viruses in the USA that is a member of the **bunyavirus** family.

The La Crosse strain of CE virus is transmitted by the **mosquito** *Aedes triseriatus* among forest **rodents.** The virus is passed transovarially in mosquitoes and thus survives the winter when mosquitoes are not active.

The clinical picture varies from mild to severe, but fatalities are rare. Diagnosis is usually made serologically rather than by isolation of the virus. No antiviral therapy or vaccine is available.

COLORADO TICK FEVER VIRUS Of the 5 diseases described in Table 42–2, Colorado tick fever (CTF) is the most easily distinguished from the others, both biologically and clinically. CTF virus is a **reovirus** transmitted by the wood **tick** *Dermacentor andersoni* among the small **rodents,** eg, chipmunks and squirrels, of the Rocky Mountains. There are approximately 100–300 cases per year in the USA.

The disease occurs primarily in people hiking or camping in the Rocky Mountains and is characterized by fever, headache, retro-orbital pain, and severe myalgia. The diagnosis is made either by isolating the virus from the blood or by detecting a rise in antibody titer. No antiviral therapy or vaccine is available. Prevention involves wearing protective clothing and inspecting the skin for ticks.

Table 42–2. Epidemiology of important arbovirus diseases in the USA.

Disease[1]	Vector	Animal Reservoir	Geographic Distribution	Approximate Incidence per Year[2]
EEE	Mosquito	Wild birds[3]	Atlantic and Gulf states	0–4
WEE	Mosquito	Wild birds[3]	West of Mississippi	5–20[4]
SLE	Mosquito	Wild birds	Widespread in southern, central, and western states	10–30[4]
CE	Mosquito	Small mammals	North-central states	40–80
CTF	Tick	Small mammals	Rocky Mountains	100–300

[1]Venezuelan equine encephalitis virus causes disease in the USA too rarely to be included.
[2]Human cases.
[3]Horses are dead-end hosts, not reservoirs.
[4]Hundreds of cases during an outbreak.

Important Arboviruses that Cause Disease Outside the USA

Although yellow fever and dengue are not endemic in the USA, extensive travel by Americans to tropical areas means that imported cases occur. It is reasonable, therefore, that physicians in the USA be acquainted with these 2 diseases. Japanese encephalitis, an important cause of epidemic encephalitis in Asia, is described in Chapter 46.

YELLOW FEVER VIRUS As the name implies, yellow fever is characterized by jaundice and fever. It is a severe, life-threatening disease that begins with the sudden onset of fever, headache, myalgias, and photophobia. After this prodome, the symptoms progress to involve the liver, kidneys, and heart. Prostration and shock, accompanied by upper gastrointestinal tract hemorrhage with hematemesis, follow. Diagnosis in the laboratory can be made either by isolating the virus or by detecting a rise in antibody titer. No antiviral therapy is available, and the mortality rate is high. If the patient recovers, no chronic infection ensues and lifelong immunity is conferred.

In the epidemiology of yellow fever, **2 distinct cycles** exist in nature, with different reservoirs and vectors.

(a) Jungle yellow fever is a disease of **monkeys** in Africa and South America that is transmitted primarily by the treetop mosquitoes of the *Haemagogus* species. Monkeys are the permanent reservoir, whereas humans are accidental hosts. Humans (eg, tree cutters) are infected when they enter the jungle occupationally.

(b) In contrast, urban yellow fever is a disease of **humans** that is transmitted by the mosquito *Aedes aegypti,* which breeds in stagnant water. In the urban form of the disease, humans are the reservoir. For effective transmission to occur, the virus must replicate in the mosquito during the 12- to 14-day extrinsic incubation period. After the infected mosquito bites the person, the intrinsic incubation period is 3–6 days.

Prevention of yellow fever involves mosquito control and immunization with the **vaccine** containing live, attenuated yellow fever virus. Travelers to and residents of endemic areas should be immunized. Protection lasts up to 10 years. Epidemics still occur in parts of Africa and South America.

DENGUE VIRUS Although dengue is **not endemic** in the USA, some tourists to the Caribbean and other tropical areas return with this disease. In recent years, there were 100–200 cases per year in the USA, mostly in the southern and eastern states. No indigenous transmission occurred within the USA.

Classic dengue (**"breakbone fever"**) begins suddenly with an influenzalike syndrome consisting of fever, malaise, cough, and headache. Severe pains in muscles and joints (breakbone) occur. Enlarged lymph nodes, a maculopapular rash, and leukopenia are common. After a week or so, the symptoms regress but weakness may persist. Although unpleasant, this typical form of dengue is rarely fatal and has few sequelae.

In contrast, **dengue hemorrhagic fever** is a much more severe disease and is associated with a fatality rate that approaches 10%. The initial picture is the same as classic dengue, but then shock and hemorrhage, especially into the gastrointestinal tract and skin, develop. Dengue hemorrhagic fever occurs particularly in southern Asia, whereas the classic form is found in tropical areas worldwide.

Hemorrhagic shock syndrome is due to the production of large amounts of **cross-reacting antibody** at the time of a second dengue infection. The pathogenesis is as follows: The patient recovers from classic dengue caused by one of the 4 serotypes, and antibody against that serotype is produced. When the patient is infected with another serotype of dengue virus, an anamnestic, heterotypic response occurs and large amounts of cross-reacting antibody to the first serotype are produced. Immune complexes composed of virus and antibody are formed that activate complement, causing increased vascular permeability and thrombocytopenia. Shock and hemorrhage result.

Dengue virus is transmitted by the *A aegypti* **mosquito,** which is also the vector of yellow fever virus. Humans are the reservoir for dengue virus, but a jungle cycle involving monkeys as the reservoir and other *Aedes* species as vectors is suspected.

No antiviral therapy or vaccine for dengue is available. Outbreaks are controlled by using insecticides and draining stagnant water that serves as the breeding place for the mosquitoes.

Review Questions

1. What does the term "arbovirus" mean?
2. Contrast the structure and genomes of togaviruses and bunyaviruses.
3. Distinguish between extrinsic and intrinsic incubation periods.
4. Humans are frequently dead-end hosts for arboviruses. What does this mean, and why does it occur?
5. Regarding EEE, WEE, and SLE, (a) what is the vector? (b) what is the reservoir? (c) which one is the most severe? (d) which one is most likely to occur in an urban setting?
6. Describe the 2 epidemiologic cycles of yellow fever.
7. How can yellow fever be prevented?
8. What is the pathogenesis of dengue hemorrhagic shock?

Tumor Viruses

43

OVERVIEW Viruses can cause benign or malignant tumors in many species of animals, eg, frogs, fishes, birds, and mammals. Despite the common occurrence of tumor viruses in animals, the number of viruses associated with **human** tumors is few and evidence that they are truly the causative agents exists for very few.

Tumor viruses have no characteristic size, shape, or chemical composition. Some are large, and some are small; some are enveloped, and others are "naked"; some have DNA as their genetic material, and others have RNA. The factor that unites all of them is their common ability to cause tumors.

Tumor viruses are at the forefront of cancer research for 2 main reasons:

(1) They are more rapid, reliable, and efficient tumor producers than either chemicals or radiation. For example, many of these viruses can cause tumors in all susceptible animals in 1 or 2 weeks and can produce malignant transformation in cultured cells in just a few days.

(2) They have a small number of genes compared with a human cell (only 3, 4, or 5 for many retroviruses), and hence their role in the production of cancer can be readily analyzed and understood. To date, the genomes of many tumor viruses have been cloned and sequenced and the number of genes and their functions have been determined; all of this has provided important information.

MALIGNANT TRANSFORMATION OF CELLS The term "malignant transformation" refers to changes in the growth properties, shape, and other features of the tumor cell (Table 43–1). Malignant transformation can be induced by tumor viruses not only in animals but also in cultured cells. In culture, the following changes occur when cells become malignantly transformed.

Altered Morphology Malignant cells lose their characteristic differentiated shape and appear rounded and more refractile when visualized under a microscope. The rounding may be due to the disaggregation of actin filaments, and the reduced adherence of the cell to the surface of the culture dish may be due to changes in the surface charge of the cell.

Altered Growth Control
(1) Malignant cells grow in a disorganized, piled-up pattern in contrast to normal cells, which have an organized, flat appearance. The term applied to this change in growth pattern in malignant cells is **loss of contact inhibition.** Contact inhibition is a property of normal cells

Table 43–1. Features of malignant transformation.

Feature	Description
Altered morphology	Loss of differentiated shape Rounded as a result of disaggregation of actin filaments and decreased adhesion to surface More refractile
Altered growth control	Loss of contact inhibition of growth Loss of contact inhibition of movement Reduced requirement for serum growth factors Increased ability to be cloned from a single cell Increased ability to grow in suspension Increased ability to continue growing ("immortalization")
Altered cellular properties	Induction of DNA synthesis Chromosomal changes Appearance of new antigens Increased agglutination by lectins
Altered biochemical properties	Reduced level of cyclic AMP Enhanced secretion of plasminogen activator Increased anaerobic glycolysis Loss of fibronectin Changes in glycoproteins and glycolipids

that refers to their ability to stop their growth and movement upon contact with another cell. Malignant cells have lost this ability and consequently move on top of one another, continue to grow to large numbers, and form a random array of cells.

(2) Malignant cells are able to grow in vitro at a much lower concentration of serum than are normal cells.

(3) Malignant cells grow well in suspension, whereas normal cells grow well only when they are attached to a surface, eg, a culture dish.

(4) Malignant cells are easily cloned; ie, they can grow into a colony of cells starting with a single cell, whereas normal cells cannot do this effectively.

(5) Infection of a cell by a tumor virus "immortalizes" that cell by enabling it to continue growing long past the time when its normal counterpart would have died. Normal cells in culture have a lifetime of about 50 generations, but malignantly transformed cells grow indefinitely.

Altered Cellular Properties

(1) DNA synthesis is induced. If cells resting in the G1 phase are infected with a tumor virus, they will promptly enter S phase, ie, synthesize DNA and go on to divide.

(2) The karyotype becomes altered; ie, there are changes in the number and shape of the chromosomes as a result of deletions, duplications, and translocations.

(3) Antigens different from those in normal cells appear. These new antigens can be either virus-encoded proteins, preexisting cellular proteins that have been modified, or previously repressed cellular proteins that are now being synthesized. Some new antigens are on the cell surface and elicit either circulating antibodies or a cell-mediated response that can kill the tumor cell. These new antigens are the recognition sites for immune surveillance against tumor cells.

(4) Agglutination by lectins is enhanced. Lectins are glycoproteins isolated from plants that bind specifically to certain sugars on the plasma membrane surface, eg, wheat germ agglutinin. The increased agglutination of malignant cells may be due to the clustering of existing receptor sites rather than to the synthesis of new ones.

Altered Biochemical Properties

(1) Reduced levels of cyclic AMP (cAMP) occur in malignant cells. Addition of cAMP will cause the malignant cells to revert to the appearance and growth properties of normal cells.

(2) Malignant cells secrete more plasminogen activator than do normal cells. This activator is a protease that converts plasminogen to plasmin, the enzyme that dissolves the fibrin clot.

(3) Increased anaerobic glycolysis leads to increased lactic acid production (Warburg effect). The mechanism for this change is unknown and so is its implication.

(4) There is a loss of high-molecular-weight glycoprotein called fibronectin. The effect of this loss is unknown.

(5) There are changes in the sugar components of glycoproteins and glycolipids in the membranes of malignant cells.

ROLE OF TUMOR VIRUSES IN MALIGNANT TRANSFORMATION Malignant transformation is a permanent change in the behavior of the cell. Must the viral genetic material be present and functioning at all times, or can it alter some cell component and not be required subsequently? The answer to this question was obtained by using a temperature-sensitive mutant of Rous sarcoma virus (RSV). This mutant has an altered transforming gene that is functional at the low, permissive temperature (35 °C) but not at the high, restrictive temperature (39 °C). When chicken cells were infected at 35 °C, they transformed as expected, but when placed at 39 °C they regained their normal morphology and behavior within a few hours. Days or weeks later, when these cells were returned to 35 °C, they recovered their transformed phenotype. Thus, continued production of some functional virus-encoded protein is required for the maintenance of the transformed state.

Although malignant transformation is a permanent change, revertants to normality do appear, albeit rarely. In the revertants studied, the viral genetic material remains integrated in cellular DNA but changes in the quality and quantity of the virus-specific RNA occur.

PROVIRUSES & ONCOGENES The 2 major concepts of the way in which viral tumorigenesis occurs are expressed in the terms "**provirus**" and "**oncogene**." These contrasting ideas address the fundamental question of the source of the genes for malignancy.

(a) In the provirus model, the genes enter the cell at the time of infection by the tumor virus.
(b) In the oncogene model, the genes for malignancy are already present in all cells of the body by virtue of being present in the initial sperm and egg. These oncogenes may serve some normal function during development but are nonfunctional in the normal differentiated cell. In the oncogene model, carcinogens such as chemicals, radiation, and tumor viruses activate oncogenes to produce proteins that initiate malignant transformation.

Both proviruses and oncogenes may play a role in malignant transformation. Evidence for the provirus mode consists of finding copies of viral DNA integrated into cell DNA only in cells that have been infected with the tumor virus. The corresponding uninfected cells have no copies of the viral DNA.

The first direct evidence that oncogenes exist in normal cells was based on results of experiments in which a DNA copy of the *onc* gene of the chicken retrovirus RSV was used as a probe. DNA in normal embryonic cells hybridized to the probe, indicating that the cells contain a gene homologous to the viral gene. It is hypothesized that the **cellular oncogenes** (proto-oncogenes) may be the precursors of viral oncogenes. Although cellular oncogenes and viral oncogenes are similar, they are not identical. They differ in base sequence at various points; and cellular oncogenes have exons and introns, whereas viral oncogenes do not. It seems likely that viral oncogenes were acquired by incorporation of cellular oncogenes into retroviruses lacking these genes. Retroviruses can be thought of as **transducing agents,** carrying oncogenes from one cell to another.

Since this initial observation, more than 20 cellular oncogenes have been identified by using either the RSV DNA probe or probes made from other viral oncogenes. Many cells contain several different cellular oncogenes. In addition, the same cellular oncogenes have been found in species as diverse as fruit flies, rodents, and humans. Such conservation through evolution suggests a normal physiologic function for these genes. Some are known to be expressed during normal embryonic development.

A marked diversity of viral oncogene function has been found. Some encode a **protein kinase** that specifically phosphorylates the amino acid tyrosine,* in contrast to the commonly

*The cellular protein(s) phosphorylated by this kinase are unknown.

found protein kinase of cells which preferentially phosphorylates serine. Other oncogenes have a base sequence almost identical to the gene for certain cellular **growth factors,** eg, epidermal growth factor. Several proteins encoded by oncogenes have their effect at the cell membrane, but some act in the nucleus by binding to DNA. These observations suggest that growth control is a multistep process and that carcinogenesis can be induced by affecting one or more of several steps.

Not all tumor viruses of the retrovirus family contain *onc* genes. How do these viruses cause malignant transformation? It appears that the DNA copy of the viral RNA integrates near a cellular oncogene, causing a marked increase in its expression. **Overexpression** of the cellular oncogene may play a key role in malignant transformation by these viruses.

Although it has been demonstrated that viral oncogenes can cause malignant transformation, it has not been directly shown that cellular oncogenes can do so. However, as described in Table 43–2, evidence suggests that they do:

Table 43–2. Evidence that cellular oncogenes (c-*onc*) can cause tumors.

Evidence	Description
Mutation of c-*onc* gene	DNA isolated from tumor cells can transform normal cells. This DNA has a c-*onc* gene with a mutation consisting of single base change.
Translocation of c-*onc* gene	Movement of c-*onc* gene to a new site on a different chromosome results in malignancy accompanied by increased expression of the gene.
Amplification of c-*onc* gene	The number of copies of c-*onc* genes is increased, resulting in enhanced expression of their mRNA and proteins.
Insertion of retrovirus near c-*onc* gene	Proviral DNA inserts near c-*onc* gene, which alters its expression and causes tumors.
Overexpression of c-*onc* gene by modification in the laboratory	Addition of an active promoter site enhances expression of the c-*onc* gene, and malignant transformation occurs.

(1) DNA containing cellular oncogenes isolated from certain tumor cells can transform normal cells in culture. When the base sequence of these "transforming" cellular oncogenes was analyzed, it was found to have a **single base change** from the normal cellular oncogene. In several tumor cell isolates, the altered sites in the gene are the same.

(2) In certain tumors, characteristic **translocations** of chromosomal segments can be seen. In Burkitt's lymphoma cells, a translocation occurs that moves a cellular oncogene (*c-myc*) from its normal site on chromosome 8 to a new site adjacent to an immunoglobulin heavychain gene on chromosome 14. This shift enhances expression of the *c-myc* gene.

(3) Some tumors have multiple copies of the cellular oncogenes, either on the same chromosome or on multiple tiny chromosomes. The **amplification** of these genes results in overexpression of their mRNA and proteins.

(4) Insertion of the DNA copy of the retroviral RNA (proviral DNA) near a cellular oncogene stimulates expression of the c-*onc* gene.

(5) Certain cellular oncogenes isolated from normal cells can cause malignant transformation if they have been modified to be overexpressed within the recipient cell.

In summary, 2 different mechanisms—**mutation** and **increased expression**—appear to be able to activate the quiescent "proto-oncogene" into a functioning oncogene capable of transforming a cell. Cellular oncogenes provide a rationale for carcinogenesis by chemicals and radiation; eg, a chemical carcinogen might act by enhancing the expression of a cellular oncogene. Furthermore, DNA isolated from cells treated with a chemical carcinogen can malignantly transform other normal cells. The resulting tumor cells contain cellular oncogenes from the chemically treated cells, and these genes are expressed with high efficiency.

OUTCOME OF TUMOR VIRUS INFECTION The outcome of tumor virus infection is dependent on the virus and the type of cell. Some tumor viruses go through their entire replicative cycle with the production of progeny virus, whereas others undergo an interrupted cycle, analogous to lysogeny, in which the **proviral DNA is integrated** into cellular DNA and limited expression of proviral genes occurs. It is not necessary, therefore, for progeny virus to be produced for malignant transformation to occur. Rather, all that is required is the expression of one or, at most, a few viral genes. Note, however, that some tumor viruses transform by inserting their proviral DNA in a manner that activates a cellular oncogene.

In most cases, the DNA tumor viruses such as the papovaviruses transform only cells in which they do not replicate. These cells are called "nonpermissive" because they do not permit viral replication. Cells of the species from which the DNA tumor virus was initially isolated are "permissive"; ie, the virus replicates and usually kills the cells, and no tumors are formed. For example, SV40 virus replicates in the cells of the African green monkey (its species of origin) and causes a cytopathic effect but no tumors. However, in rodent cells the virus does not replicate, expresses only its early genes, and causes malignant transformation. In the "nonproductive" transformed cell, the viral DNA is integrated into the host chromosome and remains there through subsequent cell divisions. The underlying concept applicable to both DNA and RNA tumor viruses is that **only viral gene expression,** not replication of the viral genome or production of progeny virus, is required for transformation.

The essential step required for a DNA tumor virus, eg, SV40 virus, to cause malignant transformation is expression of the **"early" genes** of the virus (Table 43–3). (The early genes are those expressed prior to the replication of the viral genetic material.) These required early genes produce a set of proteins called **T antigens.*** The large T antigen, which is both necessary and sufficient to induce transformation, binds to SV40 DNA at the site of initiation of viral DNA synthesis. This is compatible with the finding that the large T antigen is required for the initiation of cellular DNA synthesis in the virus-infected cell. Biochemically, large T antigen has protein kinase and adenosine triphosphatase (ATPase) activity. Almost all of the large T antigen is located in the cell nucleus, but some of it is in the outer cell membrane. In that location, it can be detected as a transplantation antigen called **tumor-specific transplantation antigen (TSTA).** TSTA is the antigen that induces the immune response against the transplantation of virally transformed cells. Relatively little is known about the SV40 virus small T antigen, except that if it is not synthesized the efficiency of transformation decreases. In polyomavirus-infected cells, the middle T antigen plays the same role as the SV40 virus large T antigen.

In RNA tumor virus-infected cells, this required gene has one of several different functions depending on the retrovirus. The oncogene of RSV and several other viruses codes for a protein kinase that phosphorylates tyrosine. Some viruses have a gene for a factor that regulates cell growth (eg, epidermal growth factor or platelet-derived growth factor), and still others have a gene that codes for a protein that binds to DNA. The conclusion is that normal growth control is a multistep process that can be affected at any one of several levels. The addition of a viral oncogene perturbs the growth control process, and a tumor cell results.

Table 43–3. Viral oncogenes.

Characteristic	DNA Virus	RNA Virus
Prototype virus	SV40	Rous sarcoma virus
Name of gene	Early-region A gene	*src* gene
Name of protein	T antigen	Protein kinase[1]
Function of protein	Protein kinase, ATPase activity, binding to DNA, and stimulation of DNA synthesis	Phosphorylation of tyrosine[1]
Location of protein	Primarily nuclear, but some in plasma membrane	Plasma membrane
Required for viral replication	Yes	No
Required for cell transformation	Yes	Yes
Gene has cellular homolog	No	Yes

[1]Some retroviruses have *onc* genes that code for other proteins such as platelet-derived growth factor and epidermal growth factor.

*In SV40-infected cells, 2 T antigens are produced, a large (MW 100,000) and a small (MW 17,000); whereas in polyomavirus-infected cells, 3 T antigens, a large (MW 90,000), middle (MW 60,000), and small (MW 22,000), are made. Other tumor viruses such as adenoviruses also induce T antigens that are immunologically distinct from those of the 2 papoviruses.

Table 43–4. Lysogeny as a model for the integration of tumor viruses.

Type of Virus	Name	Genome[1]	Circular dsDNA Within Cell	Integration	Viral Repressor	Limited Transcription of Viral Genes
Temperate phage	Lambda phage	Linear dsDNA	+	+	+	+[2]
DNA tumor virus	Simian virus 40	Circular dsDNA	+	+	NI[3]	+[2]
RNA tumor virus	Rous sarcoma virus	Linear ssRNA	+	+	NI[3]	+[2]

[1]Abbreviations: ds, double-stranded; ss, single-stranded.
[2]Limited transcription in some cells or under certain conditions but full transcription with viral replication in others.
[3]Not identified at present.

The viral genetic material remains stably integrated in host cell DNA by a process similar to lysogeny. In the lysogenic cycle, bacteriophage DNA becomes stably integrated into the bacterial genome. The linear DNA genome of the temperate phage, lambda, forms a double-stranded circle within the infected cell and then covalently integrates into bacterial DNA (Table 43–4). A repressor is synthesized that prevents transcription of most of the other lambda genes. Similarly, the double-stranded circular DNA of the DNA tumor virus covalently integrates into eukaryotic-cell DNA and only early genes are transcribed. Thus far, no repressor has been identified in any DNA tumor virus-infected cell. With RNA tumor viruses (retroviruses), the single-stranded linear RNA genome is transcribed into a double-stranded circular DNA that integrates into cellular DNA. In summary, despite the differences in their genomes and in the nature of the host cells, these viruses go through the common pathway of a double-stranded DNA intermediate followed by covalent integration into cellular DNA and subsequent expression of certain genes.

Just as a lysogenic bacteriophage can be induced to enter the replicative cycle by ultraviolet radiation and certain chemicals, tumor viruses can be induced by several mechanisms. Induction is one of the approaches used to determine whether tumor viruses are present in human cancer cells; eg, human T-cell leukemia virus was discovered by inducing the virus from leukemic cells with iododeoxyuridine.

Three techniques have been used to induce tumor viruses to replicate in the transformed cells.

(a) The most frequently used method is the addition of nucleoside analogues, eg, iodo-deoxyuridine. The mechanism of induction by these analogues is uncertain.
(b) The second method involves fusion with "helper" cells; ie, the transformed, nonpermissive cell is fused with a permissive cell, in which the virus undergoes a normal replicative cycle. Within the heterokaryon (a cell with 2 or more nuclei that is formed by the fusion of 2 different cell types), the tumor virus is induced and infectious virus is produced. The mechanism of induction is unknown.
(c) In the third method, helper viruses provide a missing function to complement the integrated tumor virus. Infection with the helper virus results in the production of both the integrated tumor virus and the helper virus.

The process of rescuing tumor viruses from cells revealed the existence of **"endogenous"** viruses. Treatment of *normal, uninfected* embryonic cells with nucleoside analogues resulted in the production of retroviruses. Retroviral DNA is integrated within the chromosomal DNA of all cells and serves as the template for viral replication. This proviral DNA probably arose by retroviral infection of the germ cells of some prehistoric ancestor.

Endogenous retroviruses, which have been rescued from the cells of many species (including humans), differ depending upon the species of origin. Endogenous viruses are xenotropic (**xeno** means foreign; **tropism** means to be attracted to); ie, they infect cells of other species more efficiently than they infect the cells of the species of origin. Entry of the endogenous virus into the cell of origin is limited as a result of defective viral envelope-cell receptor interaction. Although they are retroviruses, most endogenous viruses are not tumor viruses; ie, only a few cause leukemia.

TRANSMISSION OF TUMOR VIRUSES

Tumor virus transmission in experimental animals can occur by 2 processes, vertical and horizontal. **Vertical transmission** indicates movement of the virus from mother to newborn offspring, whereas **horizontal transmission** describes the passage of virus between animals that do not have a mother-offspring relationship. Vertical transmission occurs by 3 methods: (1) The viral genetic material is in the sperm and the egg; (2) the virus is passed across the placenta; and (3) the virus is transmitted in the breast milk.

When vertical transmission occurs, exposure to the virus early in life can result in tolerance to viral antigens, and the immune system will not recognize the virus. Large amounts of virus are produced, and a high frequency of cancer occurs. In contrast, when horizontal transmission occurs the immunocompetent animal produces antibody against the virus, and the frequency of cancer is low. If an immunocompetent animal is experimentally made immunodeficient, the frequency of cancer increases markedly.

Horizontal transmission probably does not occur in humans; those in close contact with cancer patients, eg, family members and medical personnel, do not have an increased frequency of cancer. There have been "outbreaks" of leukemia in several children at the same school, but these have been interpreted statistically as random, rare events that happen to coincide.

EVIDENCE FOR HUMAN TUMOR VIRUSES   At present, no virus is known definitely to cause malignant tumors in humans. However, several candidate viruses are implicated by epidemiologic correlation, by serologic relationship, or by recovery of virus from tumor cells.

Human T-Cell Leukemia Virus   There are 2 human T-cell leukemia virus (HTLV) isolates so far, HTLV-I and HTLV-II, both of which are associated with leukemias and lymphomas. HTLV-I was isolated in 1980 from the cells of a patient with a cutaneous T cell lymphoma. It was induced from the tumor cells by exposure to iododeoxyuridine. Its RNA and proteins are different from those of all other retroviruses. Its closest relative is a retrovirus that causes lymphoma in cattle.

HTLV-I may cause cancer by a mechanism different from that of other retroviruses. It has **no viral oncogene,** and it does not directly activate a cellular oncogene. Rather, its **tat* gene** encodes a protein that stimulates transcription of the cellular genes controlling cell division.

HTLV-I is not an endogenous virus ie proviral DNA corresponding to its RNA genome is not found in normal human cell DNA. It is an **exogenously acquired** virus, because its proviral DNA is found only in the DNA of the malignant lymphoma cells. Some (but not all) patients with T cell lymphomas have antibodies against the virus, indicating that it may not be the cause of all T cell lymphomas. Antibodies against the virus are not found in the general population, indicating that infection is not widespread.

At about the same time that HTLV-I was found, a similar virus was isolated from malignant T cells in Japan. In that country, a clustering of cases in the rural areas of the west coast of Kyushu was found. Antibodies in the sera of leukemic individuals and in the sera of 25% of the normal population of Kyushu react with the Japanese isolate and with HTLV-I. In addition, HTLV-I is endemic in some areas of Africa and on several Caribbean islands, as shown by the high frequency of antibodies. The number of people with positive antibody titers in the USA is quite small, except in certain parts of the southeastern states.

HTLV-II, also a retrovirus, was recovered from a T cell variant of hairy-cell leukemia in 1982. It is similar to HTLV-I in the antigenicity and molecular weight of its proteins.

Epstein-Barr Virus   Epstein-Barr virus (EBV; also discussed in Chapter 37) is a herpesvirus that was isolated from the cells of an east African individual with **Burkitt's lymphoma.** EBV, the cause of infectious mononucleosis, transforms B lymphocytes in culture and causes lymphomas in marmoset monkeys. It is also associated with **nasopharyngeal carcinoma,** a tumor that occurs primarily in China, and with thymic carcinoma in the USA. However, cells from Burkitt's lymphoma patients in the USA show no evidence of EBV infection.

Cells isolated from east African individuals with Burkitt's lymphoma contain EBV DNA and EBV nuclear antigen. Only a small fraction of the many copies of EBV DNA is integrated; most viral DNA is in the form of closed circles in the cytoplasm.

The difficulty in proving that EBV is a human tumor virus is that infection by the virus is widespread, but the tumor is rare. The current hypothesis is that EBV infection induces B cells to proliferate, thus increasing the likelihood that a second event (such as activation of a cellular oncogene) will occur. In Burkitt's lymphoma cells, a cellular oncogene, c-*myc*, which is

---

*tat = transactivation of transcription.

normally located on chromosome 8, is **translocated** to chromosome 14 at the site of immunoglobulin heavy-chain genes. This translocation brings the c-*myc* gene in juxtaposition to an active promoter, and large amounts of c-*myc* RNA are synthesized.

Herpes Simplex Virus Type 2   Herpes simplex virus type 2 (HSV-2) is included as a possible human tumor virus on the basis of 2 main lines of evidence: (1) epidemiologic; ie, women with HSV-2 genital infections have a higher incidence of **carcinoma of the cervix** than do matched controls, and women with carcinoma of the cervix have antibody to HSV-2 more frequently than matched controls; and (2) molecular; ie, HSV-2 DNA and proteins are located in cervical carcinoma cells, and HSV-2 can malignantly transform certain cells in vitro.

Despite this evidence, HSV-2 is not considered to be a human tumor virus; most of these findings can be explained by the alternative hypothesis that HSV-2 causes latent genital infections in patients who began sexual activity at an early age. Certain serotypes of human papillomavirus are also associated with cervical carcinoma (see below).

Hepatitis B Virus   Hepatitis B virus (HBV) infection is significantly more common in patients with primary hepatocellular carcinoma (**hepatoma**) than in controls. This relationship is striking in areas of Africa and Asia where the incidence of both HBV infection and hepatoma is high. HBV-induced cirrhosis predisposes to hepatoma. However, some hepatoma patients have no evidence of HBV infection. HBV DNA and surface antigen can be found in malignant cells. The integration of HBV DNA may cause insertional mutagenesis, resulting in the activation of a cellular oncogene.

Human Papillomavirus   Human papillomavirus (HPV) is the only virus definitely known to cause tumors (warts) in humans. Warts are benign but can progress to form carcinomas, albeit rarely.

Papillomaviruses are members of the family of papovaviruses, an acronym of *pa*pilloma, *po*lyoma, and *va*cuolating (eg, SV40 virus) viruses. They are DNA nucleocapsid viruses with double-stranded, circular, supercoiled DNA and an icosahedral nucleocapsid. The papillomaviruses have a somewhat larger genome and diameter than do viruses in the other 2 groups.* Unlike the case with SV40 virus and polyoma virus, most of the papilloma virus DNA in infected cells occurs as an episome rather than being integrated into the cellular DNA.

There are at least 15 different serotypes of HPV, many of which cause distinct clinical entities. For example, HPV 1 and HPV 4 cause plantar warts on the soles of the feet, whereas HPV 6 and HPV 11 cause anogenital warts (condylomata acuminata) and laryngeal papillomas. Certain serotypes of HPV, especially 16 and 18, are implicated as the cause of carcinoma of the cervix. Papillomaviruses also cause warts in a wide variety of animals; one of these viruses, bovine papillomavirus, is the cause of significant economic loss in cattle.

DO ANIMAL TUMOR VIRUSES CAUSE CANCER IN HUMANS?

There is no evidence that animal tumor viruses cause tumors in humans. In fact, the only available information suggests that they do not, because (1) people who were inoculated with poliovirus vaccine contaminated with SV40 have no greater incidence of cancers than do uninoculated controls, (2) soldiers inoculated with yellow fever vaccine contaminated with avian leukemia virus do not have a high incidence of tumors, and (3) members of families whose cats have died of leukemia caused by feline leukemia virus show no increase in the occurrence of leukemia over control families.

ANIMAL TUMOR VIRUSES

1. DNA Tumor Viruses   The important DNA tumor viruses are listed in Table 43–5.

Papovaviruses   The 2 best-characterized oncogenic papovaviruses are **polyomavirus** and **SV40.** Polyomavirus (*poly* means many; *oma* means tumor) causes a wide variety of histologically different tumors when inoculated into newborn rodents. Its natural host is the

---

*Papillomaviruses are 55 nm in diameter with a DNA molecular weight of 5×10^6, in contrast to the others, which have a diameter of 45 nm and a DNA molecular weight of 3×10^6.

Table 43–5. Varieties of tumor viruses.

Nucleic Acid	Virus
DNA	Papovaviruses, eg, polyomavirus, SV40, papillomaviruses; adenoviruses, especially types 12, 18, and 31; herpesviruses, eg, herpesvirus saimiri; poxviruses, eg, fibroma-myxoma virus.
RNA	Avian sarcoma viruses, eg, Rous sarcoma virus; avian leukemia viruses; murine sarcoma viruses; murine leukemia viruses; mouse mammary tumor virus; feline sarcoma virus; feline leukemia virus; simian sarcoma virus; human T-cell leukemia virus.

mouse. SV40 virus, which was isolated from normal rhesus monkey kidney cells, causes sarcomas in newborn hamsters.

Polyomavirus and SV40 virus share many chemical and biologic features, eg, double-stranded, circular, supercoiled DNA of molecular weight 3×10^6 and a 45-nm icosahedral nucleocapsid. However, the sequence of their DNA and the antigenicity of their proteins are quite distinct. Both undergo a lytic (permissive) cycle in the cells of their natural hosts, with the production of progeny virus. However, when they infect the cells of a heterologous species, the nonpermissive cycle ensues, no virus is produced, and the cell is malignantly transformed.* In the transformed cell, the viral DNA integrates into the cell DNA and only early proteins are synthesized. Some of these proteins, eg, the T antigens described on p 195, are required for induction and maintenance of the transformed state.

JC virus, a human papovavirus, is the cause of progressive multifocal leukoencephalopathy (see Chapter 44). It also causes brain tumors in monkeys and hamsters. There is no evidence that it causes human cancer.

Adenoviruses Some human adenoviruses, especially serotypes 12, 18, and 31, induce sarcomas in newborn hamsters and transform rodent cells in culture. There is no evidence that these viruses cause tumors in humans, and no adenoviral DNA has been detected in the DNA of any human tumor cells.

Adenoviruses undergo both a permissive cycle in some cells and a nonpermissive, transforming cycle in others. The linear genome DNA (MW 23×10^6) circularizes within the infected cell, but—in contrast to the papovaviruses, whose entire genome integrates—only a small region (10%) of the adenovirus genome does so; yet transformation still occurs. This region codes for several proteins, one of which is the T (tumor) antigen. Adenovirus T antigen is required for transformation and is antigenically distinct from the polyomavirus and SV40 virus T antigens.

Herpesviruses Several animal herpesviruses are known to cause tumors. Four species of herpesviruses cause **lymphomas** in nonhuman primates. Herpesviruses saimiri and ateles induce T cell lymphomas in New World monkeys, and herpesviruses pan and papio transform B lymphocytes in chimpanzees and baboons, respectively.

A herpesvirus of chickens causes Marek's disease, a contagious, rapidly fatal neuro-lymphomatosis. Immunization of chickens with a live, attenuated vaccine has resulted in a marked decrease in the number of cases. A herpesvirus is implicated as the cause of kidney carcinomas in frogs.

Poxviruses Two poxviruses cause tumors in animals; these are the fibroma-myxoma virus, which causes fibromas or myxomas in rabbits and other animals, and Yaba monkey tumor virus, which causes benign histiocytomas in animals and human volunteers. Little is known about either of these viruses.

---

*The ability of polyomavirus to transform mouse cells is an exception to the generalization that cells of the natural host do not become malignant. Polyomavirus not only causes a cytopathic effect in most mouse cells but also can induce a rare transformed cell.

2. RNA Tumor Viruses (Retroviruses)   RNA tumor viruses have been isolated from a large number of species: snakes, birds, and mammals including nonhuman primates. The important RNA tumor viruses are listed in Table 43–5. They are important because of their ubiquity, their ability to cause tumors in the host of origin, their small number of genes, and the relationship of their genes to cellular oncogenes (see p 193).

These viruses belong to the retrovirus family (the prefix "retro" means reverse), so named because a **"reverse transcriptase"** is located in the virion. This enzyme transcribes the genome RNA into double-stranded proviral DNA and is essential to their replication. The viral genome consists of 2 identical molecules of positive-strand RNA. Each molecule has a molecular weight of approximately 2×10^6 (these are the only viruses that are diploid, ie, have 2 copies of their genome in the virion). The 2 molecules are hydrogen-bonded together by complementary bases located near the 5' end of both RNA molecules. Also bound near the 5' end of each RNA is a transfer RNA (tRNA) that serves as the primer* for the transcription of the RNA into DNA. The icosahedral capsid is surrounded by an envelope with glycoprotein spikes. Some internal capsid proteins are group-specific antigens, which are common to retroviruses within a species. There are 3 important morphologic types of retroviruses, labeled B, C, and D, depending primarily on the location of the capsid or core. Most of the retroviruses are C-type particles, but mouse mammary tumor virus is a B-type particle, and HTLV-III, the cause of AIDS, is a D-type particle.

The gene sequence of the RNA of a typical avian sarcoma virus is *gag, pol, env,* and *src.* The nontransforming retroviruses have 3 genes; they are missing *src.* The *gag* region codes for the group-specific *a*ntigens, the *pol* gene codes for the reverse transcriptase, the *env* gene codes for the 2 envelope spike proteins, and the *src* gene codes for the protein kinase. In other retroviruses, such as human T-cell leukemia virus type I (HTLV-I), there is a fifth coding region (the *tat* gene) near the 3' end, which codes for a protein that may activate cellular oncogenes.

The sequences at the 5' and 3' end function in the integration of the proviral DNA and in the transcription of mRNA from the integrated proviral DNA by host cell RNA polymerase II. At each end is a sequence† called a long terminal repeat (LTR) that is composed of several regions, one of which, near the 5' end, is the binding site for the primer tRNA.

After infection of the cell by a retrovirus, the following events occur. Using the genome RNA as the template, the reverse transcriptase (RNA-dependent DNA polymerase) synthesizes double-stranded proviral DNA. The DNA forms a closed circle and integrates into cellular DNA. There is no specific site of integration. Insertion of the viral LTR can enhance the transcription of adjacent host cell genes. If this host gene is a cellular oncogene, malignant transformation may result. This explains how retroviruses without viral oncogenes can cause transformation.

Review Questions

1. Describe some of the changes that occur when cells undergo malignant transformation.
2. Distinguish between a provirus and an oncogene.
3. What is the relationship between viral and cellular oncogenes?
4. What are some of the functions of oncogenes?
5. What is the fate of viral DNA when a DNA tumor virus infects a nonpermissive cell? What typically happens to the cell?
6. Describe the importance of the T antigen of papovaviruses.
7. Describe the similarities between the temperate bacteriophages, the papovaviruses, and the retroviruses.
8. What are 3 techniques to recover viruses from the integrated state?
9. What are endogenous viruses?
10. Describe the vertical transmission of viruses. What is its consequence for the immune system?

---

*The purpose of the primer tRNA is to act as the point of attachment for the first deoxynucleotide at the start of DNA synthesis. The primers are normal-cell tRNAs that are characteristic for each retrovirus.

†The length of the sequence varies from 250 to 1200 bases, depending on the virus.

11. Describe HTLV-I: (a) the nature of the virus, (b) its *tat* gene, (c) how it was first isolated, (d) the locations where it is endemic.

12. What is the relationship of the following viruses to human cancers? (a) EBV, (b) HSV-2, (c) HBV, (d) HPV, (e) adenoviruses.

13. What is the nature of papovaviruses, eg, SV40, and their relationship to cancer?

14. What is the nature of retroviruses and their relationship to cancer?

Slow Viruses

44

This is a heterogeneous group of agents containing both conventional viruses and unconventional agents, eg, prions. **Prions** are **protein-containing particles** with **no detectable nucleic acid** that are highly resistant to inactivation by heat, formaldehyde, and nucleases but are killed by protein-and lipid-disrupting agents such as phenol, ether, and hypochlorite.

In humans, the ''slow'' agents cause **central nervous system** diseases characterized by a gradual onset and a progressive, invariably fatal course. Note that the term ''slow'' refers to the disease, not to the rate of replication of the causative viruses. The replication rate of these viruses is similar to that of most other viruses.

DISEASES CAUSED BY CONVENTIONAL VIRUSES

Progressive Multifocal Leukoencephalopathy Progressive multifocal leukoencephalopathy (PML) is a demyelinating disease of the white matter and involves multiple areas of the brain. It occurs primarily in **immunocompromised** individuals. PML is caused by JC virus, a papovavirus antigenically distinct from other papovaviruses such as SV40 and polyomavirus. Antibodies to JC virus are found in approximately 75% of normal human sera, showing that infection is widespread.

Subacute Sclerosing Panencephalitis Subacute sclerosing panencephalitis (SSPE) is a slowly progressive disease characterized by inflammatory lesions in many areas of the brain. It is a rare disease of **children** who have been infected by **measles virus** several years earlier. SSPE begins with mild changes in personality and ends with dementia and death.

SSPE is a persistent infection by a variant of measles virus that cannot complete its replication. The evidence for this is as follows:

(1) Inclusion bodies containing helical nucleocapsids, which react with antibody to measles virus, are seen in the affected neurons.

(2) A virus very similar to measles virus can be induced from these cells by co-cultivation with permissive cells in culture. The induced virus has a different matrix protein; this protein is important in viral assembly.

(3) Patients have high titers of measles antibody in the blood and spinal fluid.

(4) SSPE has virtually disappeared in the USA since the onset of widespread immunization with measles vaccine.

A progressive panencephalitis can also occur in patients with congenital rubella.

DISEASES CAUSED BY UNCONVENTIONAL AGENTS

Kuru In contrast to the agents of PML and SSPE, no conventional virus is associated with kuru. This fatal disease is characterized by progressive tremors and ataxia but not dementia.

It occurs **only** among the **Fore tribes in New Guinea.** It was transmitted during a ritual in which the skulls of the dead were opened and the brains eaten. It is suspected that transmission occurred through cuts in the skin during preparation rather than by eating the brain, because the women who prepared the brains were affected more frequently than the men who ate them. Since the practice has stopped, kuru has almost disappeared. The agents of kuru and Creutzfeldt-Jakob disease (see below) have been transmitted serially in primates.

CREUTZFELDT-JAKOB DISEASE   Pathologic examination of the brains of patients with Creutzfeldt-Jakob disease (CJD) and kuru reveals a **spongiform** (sponge or swiss-cheese) appearance similar to that associated with scrapie in sheep (see below). **Prions** cause scrapie and have been found in the brains of CJD patients; they may cause CJD and kuru as well.

In contrast to kuru, CJD is **found sporadically worldwide** and affects both sexes. This rare disease is characterized by presenile dementia and ataxia, progressing to coma and death. It is not highly transmissible; an increased incidence within families does not occur. It has been transmitted **iatrogenically,** eg, in a corneal transplant, via intracerebral electrodes, and in hormones extracted from human pituitaries. Proper sterilization of CJD agent-contaminated material consists of either autoclaving or sodium hypochlorite treatment.

SLOW VIRUS DISEASES OF ANIMALS   There are 2 slow virus diseases of animals, scrapie and visna, that are important models for human diseases.

Scrapie   Scrapie is a disease of sheep, characterized by tremors, ataxia, and itching, in which the sheep scrape off their wool against fence posts. It has an incubation period of many months. Spongiform degeneration without inflammation is seen in the brain tissue of affected animals. It has been transmitted to mice and other animals via a brain extract that contained no recognizable virus particles. Studies of mice revealed that the infectivity is associated with a 27,000-molecular-weight protein known as a prion (see p. 128).

Visna   Visna is a disease of sheep that is characterized by pneumonia and demyelinating lesions in the brain. It is caused by visna virus, a member of the lentivirus subgroup of retroviruses. As such, it has a single-stranded, diploid RNA genome and an RNA-dependent DNA polymerase in the virion. It is thought that integration of the DNA provirus into the host cell DNA may be important in the persistence of the virus within the host and, consequently, in its long incubation period and prolonged, progressive course.

Review Questions

1. To what does the term ''slow virus'' refer?
2. Contrast the etiology and pathogenesis of PML and SSPE.
3. What are prions, and what is the evidence that they may be involved in human disease?
4. Contrast the transmission of Kuru and Creutzfeldt-Jakob disease.
5. Contrast the causative agents of scrapie and visna.

Human Immunodeficiency Virus

45

Disease   Human immunodeficiency virus (HIV)* is the agent of acquired immunodeficiency syndrome (AIDS).

Important Properties   HIV is one of the human T-cell lymphotrophic retroviruses (human T-cell leukemia virus is another). HIV preferentially infects and **kills helper (CD4†) T lymphocytes,** resulting in the loss of cell-mediated immunity and a high probability that the host will develop **opportunistic infections.** Other cells, eg, macrophages and monocytes, that have CD4 proteins on their surfaces can be infected also.

HIV belongs to the lentivirus subgroup of retroviruses, which cause "slow" infections with long incubation periods (see Chapter 44). HIV has a bar-shaped (type D) nucleoid surrounded by an envelope containing virus-specific glycoproteins (gp120 and gp 41). In addition to the 3 typical retroviral genes *gag, pol,* and *env,* which encode the structural proteins, the genome RNA has at least 5 other genes. There is evidence that these are regulatory genes. One important example of a regulatory gene is the **tat** (transactivation of transcription)† **gene,** which encodes a protein that enhances viral (and perhaps cellular) gene transcription. It may also enhance viral translation.

The important antigens of HIV are as follows:

(1) gp120 and gp 41 are the **type-specific envelope glycoproteins.** While gp120 protrudes from the surface and interacts with the CD4 receptor on the cell surface, gp 41 is embedded in the envelope and mediates the fusion of the viral envelope and the cell membrane at the time of infection. The gene that encodes gp120 mutates rapidly, resulting in many **antigenic variants.** Antibody against gp120 neutralizes the infectivity of HIV, but the rapid appearance of gp120 variants will make production of an effective vaccine difficult. The high mutation rate may be due to lack of an editing function in the reverse transcriptase.

(2) The group-specific antigen, p24, is located in the core and is not known to vary. Antibodies against p24 do not neutralize HIV infectivity but serve as important serologic markers of infection.

The natural host range of HIV is limited to humans, although certain primates can be infected in the laboratory. HIV is **not an endogenous virus** of humans; ie, no HIV sequences are found in normal human cell DNA.

Viruses similar to HIV continue to be isolated.

(1) Human immunodeficiency virus type 2 (HIV-2) was isolated from AIDS patients in west Africa in 1986. The proteins of HIV-2 are only about 40% identical to those of the original HIV isolates.

(2) Simian immunodeficiency virus (SIV) was isolated from monkeys with an AIDS-like illness. Antibodies in some African women cross-react with SIV. The proteins of SIV resemble those of HIV-2 more closely than they resemble those of the original HIV isolates.

(3) HTLV-IV infects T cells but does not kill them and is not associated with any disease. These isolates (and others) differ significantly from one another in restriction map analysis, particularly in the envelope gene region.

Summary of Replicative Cycle   At this time, the details of the replicative cycle are incomplete, but it is thought to follow the typical retroviral cycle. After entering the helper T

---

*Also known as human T-lymphotropic virus type 3 (HTLV-III), lymphadenopathy-associated virus (LAV), and AIDS-related virus (ARV).

†Transactivation refers to activation of transcription of genes distant from the gene, ie, other genes on the same proviral DNA or on cellular DNA. One site of action of the *tat* protein is the long terminal repeat at the 5′ end of the viral genome.

lymphocyte by binding to the cell surface receptor (the CD4 antigen), the virion RNA-dependent DNA polymerase transcribes the genome RNA into double-stranded circular DNA, which integrates into the host cell DNA. The viral DNA can integrate at different sites in the host cell DNA, and multiple copies of viral DNA can integrate. Integration is mediated by a virus-encoded endonuclease (integrase). Viral mRNA is transcribed by host cell RNA polymerase and translated into several large polyproteins, which are then cleaved to form the virion structural proteins, namely the reverse transcriptase, the core proteins, and the 2 envelope glycoproteins. The virions assemble in the cytoplasm and are released from the cell by budding. Much of the virus remains cell-associated and may be difficult to neutralize with antibody.

Transmission & Epidemiology Transmission occurs by the **transfer of body fluids,** primarily blood and semen. Transmission to neonates may occur trans-placentally and via breast milk. Although small amounts of virus have been found in other fluids, eg, saliva and tears, there is no evidence that they play a role in infection. In general, transmission of HIV follows the pattern of hepatitis B virus, except that HIV infection is much less efficiently transferred; ie, the dose of HIV required to cause infection is much higher than that of HBV.

In the USA and Europe, HIV infection and AIDS occur primarily in promiscuous homosexual men, intravenous drug abusers, and hemophiliacs. Offspring of infected mothers are often infected. Heterosexual transmission occurs infrequently in these regions but is an important mode in African countries. Very few health care personnel have been infected despite prolonged exposure and needle-stick injuries, supporting the concept that the infectious dose of HIV must be high.

Pathogenesis & Immunity HIV infects helper T cells and kills them, resulting in **suppression of cell-mediated immunity.** This predisposes the host to various opportunistic infections and certain cancers such as Kaposi's sarcoma and lymphoma. However, viral genes are not found in these cancer cells, so HIV does not directly cause these tumors. HIV also infects brain monocytes and macrophages, producing multinucleated giant cells and significant central nervous system symptoms. The fusion of HIV-infected cells in the brain and elsewhere is one of the main pathologic findings.

Persistent noncytopathic infection of T lymphocytes also occurs. Persistently infected cells continue to produce HIV, which may help to sustain the infection in vivo. A person infected with HIV is considered to be infected for life. This seems likely to be the result of viral DNA integrated into the DNA of infected cells.

Approximately 90% of AIDS patients have antibodies against HIV. However, these antibodies, which are detected by ELISA in the laboratory, **neutralize** the infectivity of the virus **poorly.** This indicates that immunity is incomplete and that infectious virus and antibodies can coexist.

In addition to the detrimental effects on T cells, abnormalities of B cells occur. Polyclonal activation of B cells is seen, with resultant high immunoglobulin levels. Autoimmune diseases, such as thrombocytopenia, occur.

One aspect of pathogenesis that has yet to be explained is the finding that **less** than one in 10,000 helper T lymphocytes contains viral DNA. If so few cells are infected, it is difficult to account for such profound immunosuppression. However, there is evidence that about 15% of macrophages are infected, which may explain the loss of immunity.

Clinical Findings The 2 most characteristic manifestations of AIDS are *Pneumocystis carinii* pneumonia and Kaposi's sarcoma. However, many other opportunistic infections occur with some frequency. These include viral infections such as disseminated herpes simplex, herpes zoster, and cytomegalovirus infections and progressive multifocal leukoencephalopathy; fungal infections such as thrush (caused by *Candida albicans*), cryptococcal meningitis, and disseminated histoplasmosis; protozoal infections such as toxoplasmosis and cryptosporidiosis; and bacterial infections such as disseminated *Mycobacterium avium-intracellulare* and *Mycobacterium tuberculosis* infections. Many AIDS patients have severe neurologic problems, eg, dementia and neuropathy, which can be due either to HIV infection of the brain or to many of these opportunistic organisms. The mortality rate of AIDS approaches 50% at 2 years after the diagnosis is made.

A syndrome called AIDS-related complex (ARC) also occurs. In ARC patients, persistent fevers, fatigue, weight loss, and lymphadenopathy are the most frequent manifestations. ARC often progresses to AIDS.

Laboratory Diagnosis The presumptive diagnosis of HIV infection is made by the detection of antibodies by **ELISA.** Because there are some false-positives with this test, the definitive diagnosis is made by **"Western blot"** analysis, in which the viral proteins are displayed by acrylamide gel electrophoresis, transferred to nitrocellulose paper, and reacted with the patient's serum. If antibodies are present, they will bind to the viral proteins (predominantly to the gp41 or p24 protein). Radioactively labeled antibody to human IgG is then added. Autoradiography reveals the presence of the HIV antibody in the infected patient's serum.

HIV can be grown in culture from clinical specimens, but this procedure is available only at a few medical centers.

Treatment & Prevention No vaccine is available. **Azidothymidine** (AZT), an inhibitor of HIV replication, results in temporary clinical remissions but does not eliminate the virus. AZT inhibits proviral DNA synthesis by chain termination but cannot cure an infected cell of an already integrated copy of the proviral DNA. The main approach to the treatment of AIDS is treatment of the opportunistic infections and tumors. Prevention consists of taking measures to avoid exposure to the virus, eg, using condoms and discarding blood and blood products that may be contaminated with HIV.

Review Questions

1. What are the important structural and chemical characteristics of HIV?
2. What is the unusual characteristic of the envelope glycoprotein of HIV that may impede development of a vaccine?
3. What are the 2 important modes of transmission?
4. What population groups are mainly infected?
5. What is the pathogenesis of AIDS?
6. Which 2 tests for what components of the virus are used to determine whether HIV infection has occurred?
7. Which antiviral drug is clinically effective against HIV, and what is its mode of action?
8. How can HIV infection be prevented?

Minor Viral Pathogens

46

These viruses are presented in alphabetical order. They are listed in Table 46–1 in terms of their nucleic acid and presence of envelope.

Table 46–1. Minor viral pathogens.

Characteristics	Representative Virus(es)
DNA enveloped viruses	Herpes B virus, molluscum contagiosum virus, cowpox virus, monkeypox virus
DNA nonenveloped viruses	Parvovirus B19
RNA enveloped viruses	Coronaviruses, Ebola virus, Japanese encephalitis virus, Lassa fever virus, lymphocytic choriomeningitis virus, Marburg virus, Tacaribe complex of viruses, eg, Junin and Machupo viruses
RNA nonenveloped viruses	Encephalomyocarditis virus, Norwalk virus

Coronaviruses Coronaviruses are enveloped, single-stranded, positive-polarity RNA viruses with club-shaped surface spikes that resemble a "corona." They cause **upper respiratory tract infection** (colds) in adults. Although the incidence varies from year to year, approximately 20% of colds are caused by these viruses. Laboratory diagnosis is rarely done. No antiviral drugs or preventive measures are available.

Ebola Virus Ebola virus is named for the river in Zaire that was the site of an outbreak of **"hemorrhagic fever"** in 1976. The disease begins with fever, headache, vomiting, and diarrhea. Later, bleeding into the gastrointestinal tract occurs, followed by shock and disseminated intravascular coagulation. The mortality rate associated with this virus approaches 100%. Most cases arise by secondary transmission from contact with the patient's blood or secretions, eg, in hospital staff.

Structurally, Ebola virus resembles a rhabdovirus. The natural cycle of this virus is uncertain. Diagnosis is made by isolating the virus or by detecting a rise in antibody titer. (Extreme care must be taken when handling specimens in the laboratory.) No antiviral therapy is available. Prevention centers on limiting secondary spread by proper handling of patient's secretions and blood.

Encephalomyocarditis Virus This virus, a rare agent of human disease, causes either encephalitis or mild febrile illness. It is a member of the picornavirus family and derives its name from the central nervous system and cardiac muscle lesions it causes in mice. Infection can be diagnosed either by virus isolation or by detecting a rise in antibody titer. No antiviral therapy or vaccine is available.

Herpes B Virus This virus (monkey B virus or herpesvirus simiae) causes a rare, often fatal **encephalitis** in persons in close contact with monkeys or their tissues, eg, zookeepers or cell culture technicians. The virus causes a latent infection in monkeys that is similar to HSV-1 in humans.

Herpes B virus and HSV-1 cross-react antigenically, but antibody to HSV-1 does not protect from herpes B encephalitis. The presence of HSV-1 antibody can, however, confuse serologic diagnosis by making the interpretation of a rise in antibody titer difficult. The diagnosis, therefore, can be made only by recovering the virus. No antiviral therapy is available. Prevention consists of using protective clothing and masks to prevent exposure to the virus. Immune globulin containing antibody to herpes B virus should be given after a monkey bite.

Japanese Encephalitis Virus This virus is the most common cause of **epidemic encephalitis.** The disease is characterized by fever, headache, nuchal rigidity, altered states of consciousness, tremors, incoordination, and convulsions. The mortality rate is high, and neurologic sequelae are severe and can be detected in the majority of survivors. The disease occurs throughout Asia but is most prevalent in Southeast Asia. The rare cases seen in the USA have occurred in travelers returning from that continent. American military personnel in Asia have been affected.

Japanese encephalitis virus is a member of the flavivirus genus in the togavirus family. It is transmitted to humans by certain species of *Culex* mosquitoes endemic to Asian rice fields. There are 2 main reservoir hosts, birds and pigs. The diagnosis can be made by isolating the virus, by detecting IgM antibody in serum or spinal fluid, or by staining brain tissue with fluorescent antibody. There is no antiviral therapy. Prevention consists of an inactivated vaccine and pesticides to control the mosquito vector. Immunization is recommended for individuals living in endemic areas for several months or longer.

Lassa Fever Virus Lassa fever virus was first seen in 1969 in the Nigerian town of that name. It is a severe, often fatal **hemorrhagic fever** characterized by multiple organ involvement. It begins slowly with fever, headache, vomiting, and diarrhea and progresses to involve the lungs, heart, kidneys, and brain. A petechial rash and gastrointestinal tract hemorrhage ensue, and death is from vascular collapse.

Lassa fever virus is a member of the arenavirus family, which includes other infrequent human pathogens such as lymphocytic choriomeningitis virus and certain members of the Tacaribe group. Arenaviruses ("arena" means sand) are united by their unusual appearance in the electron microscope. Their most striking feature is the "sandlike" particles on their surface, which are ribosomes. The function, if any, of these ribosomes is unknown.

Arenaviruses are enveloped viruses with surface spikes, a helical nucleocapsid, and single-stranded RNA with negative polarity.

The natural host for Lassa fever virus is the small rodent *Mastomys,* which undergoes a chronic, lifelong infection. The virus is transmitted to humans by contamination of food or water with animal excrement. Secondary transmission among hospital personnel occurs also. Asymptomatic infection is widespread in endemic areas.

The diagnosis is made either by isolating the virus or by detecting a rise in antibody titer. Ribavirin reduces mortality if given early, and hyperimmune serum, obtained from persons who have recovered from the disease, has been beneficial in some cases. No vaccine is available, and prevention centers around proper infection control practices and rodent control.

Lymphocytic Choriomeningitis Virus Lymphocytic choriomeningitis virus is a rare cause of aseptic meningitis and cannot be distinguished clinically from the more frequent viral causes, eg, echovirus, coxsackievirus, or mumps virus. The usual picture consists of fever, headache, vomiting, stiff neck, and changes in mental status. Spinal fluid shows an increased number of cells, mostly lymphocytes, with an elevated protein level and a normal or low sugar level.

The virus is endemic in the mouse population, in which chronic infection occurs. Animals infected transplacentally become healthy lifelong carriers. The virus is transmitted to humans via food or water contaminated by mouse urine or feces. There is no human-to-human spread; ie, humans are accidental dead-end hosts. Diagnosis is made by isolating the virus from the spinal fluid or by detecting an increase in antibody titer. No antiviral therapy or vaccine is available.

This disease is the prototype used to illustrate **immunopathogenesis** and immune complex disease. If immunocompetent adult mice are inoculated, meningitis and death ensue. If, however, newborn mice or x-irradiated immunodeficient adults are inoculated, no meningitis occurs despite extensive viral replication. If sensitized T cells are transplanted to the immunodeficient adults, meningitis and death occur. The immunodeficient adult mice, who are apparently well, slowly develop immune complex glomerulonephritis. It appears that the mice are partially tolerant to the virus in that their cell-mediated immunity is inactive but sufficient antibody is produced to cause immune complex disease.

Marburg Virus Marburg virus and Ebola virus are similar in that they both cause **hemorrhagic fevers** and have a rhabdoviruslike morphology; however, they are antigenically distinct. Marburg virus was first recognized as a cause of human disease in 1967 in Marburg, Germany. The common feature of the infected individuals was their exposure to African green monkeys that had recently arrived from Uganda. The role of the monkey in the natural cycle of the virus is unclear, because monkeys in Uganda do not have antibody to the virus.

The clinical picture of this hemorrhagic fever is as described for Ebola virus (see p 206). No cases of disease caused by either Ebola or Marburg virus have occurred in the USA. The diagnosis is made by isolating the virus or detecting a rise in antibody titer. No antiviral therapy or vaccine is available. As with Ebola virus, secondary cases among medical personnel have occurred; therefore, stringent infection control practices must be instituted to prevent nosocomial spread.

Molluscum Contagiosum Virus This virus is one of the 2 causes of **warts** in the adult genital region, the other being the human papillomavirus (see p 198). The lesions are a few millimeters long and soft, pink, and rounded. In children the warts are most often found on the face and body. The virus is transmitted by direct skin contact. Transmission during sexual intercourse accounts for the frequency of genital lesions.

Molluscum contagiosum virus is classified as a member of the poxvirus family on the basis of its morphology when visualized in the electron microscope. Typical cytoplasmic inclusion bodies are seen in the cells of the malpighian layer. The virus has not been grown in cell culture, and little is known about its life cycle.

Lesions are usually removed by surgery, electrocautery, or cryotherapy. Even if untreated, the lesions will resolve spontaneously in a few years.

Norwalk Virus Norwalk virus is one cause of outbreaks of **gastroenteritis,** usually in settings such as schools, camps, cruise ships, and similar confined populations. It is named for an outbreak in a school in Norwalk, Ohio, in 1969. The virus was first identified in the stool by immune electron microscopy; antibody from a patient who had recovered from the disease was used to aggregate the virus into clumps that contained particles of small (27 nm) icosahedral viruses without envelopes. Subsequent study showed that the genome was RNA and that the capsid contained only one protein. This description is sufficient to tentatively classify it as a member of the calicivirus family.

The clinical picture consists of nausea, vomiting, and diarrhea that resolve spontaneously in 12–24 hours. The virus is transmitted by the fecal-oral route and occurs worldwide. In contrast to most viruses transmitted by the fecal-oral route, it is uncommon in children, and antibody response peaks in young adulthood.

Immunity following infection is relatively brief, ie, less than 2 years. Laboratory diagnosis is not done for this disease. If, for epidemiologic reasons, a specific viral diagnosis is required, either immunoelectron microscopy or radioimmunoassay can be used. No antiviral therapy is indicated, and no preventive measures other than hand washing are available.

Parvovirus B19 The B19 virus is the first parvovirus to be confirmed as a cause of human disease. Pavoviruses are very small (22 nm) naked icosahedral viruses with a single-stranded DNA genome. The common disease caused by B19 virus is **erythema infectiosum,** a self-limited disease of children that is characterized by a "slapped-cheek" rash. A less common, more severe manifestation is aplastic crisis in patients with sickle cell anemia. B19 virus preferentially infects the immature red blood cell precursors and kills them. Parvoviruses cause birth defects in animals and may do so in humans.

Poxviruses of Animal Origin Four poxviruses cause disease in animals and also cause poxlike lesions in humans on rare occasions. They are transmitted by contact with the infected animals, usually in an occupational setting.

Cowpox virus causes vesicular lesions on the udders of cows and can cause similar lesions on the skin of persons who milk cows. Pseudocowpox virus causes a similar picture but is antigenically distinct. Orf virus is the cause of contagious pustular dermatitis in sheep and of vesicular lesions on the hands of sheepshearers.

Monkeypox virus is different from the other 3; it causes a human disease that resembles smallpox. Any new case of smallpoxlike disease must be precisely diagnosed to ensure that it is not due to smallpox virus. There has not been a case of smallpox in the world since 1972* and smallpox immunization has been allowed to lapse, so it is important to ensure that new cases are due to monkeypox virus. Monkeypox virus can be distinguished from smallpox virus in the laboratory both antigenically and by the distinctive lesions it causes on the chorioallantoic membrane of chicken eggs.

Tacaribe Complex of Viruses The Tacaribe** complex contains 2 human pathogens both of which cause **hemorrhagic fever,** namely Junin virus in Argentina and Machupo virus in Bolivia. Hemorrhagic fevers, as the name implies, are characterized by fever and bleeding into the gastrointestinal tract, skin, and other organs. The bleeding is due to thrombocytopenia. Death occurs in up to 20% of cases, and outbreaks can involve thousands of people. Agricultural workers are particularly at risk.

Similar to other arenaviruses such as Lassa fever virus and lymphocytic choriomeningitis virus, these viruses are endemic in the rodent population and are transmitted to humans by accidental contamination of food and water by rodent excreta. The diagnosis can be made either by isolating the virus or by detecting a rise in antibody titer. No antiviral therapy or vaccine is available.

---

*With the exception of 2 laboratory-acquired cases in 1978.

**Tacaribe virus was isolated from bats in Trinidad in 1956. It does not cause human disease.

Part V: Mycology

Basic Mycology

47

STRUCTURE & GROWTH Because fungi (yeasts and molds) are **eukaryotic** organisms whereas bacteria are prokaryotic, they differ in several fundamental respects (Table 47–1). Two fungal cell structures are important medically:

(1) The fungal cell wall consists primarily of chitin* (not peptidoglycan as in bacteria); thus, fungi are insensitive to antibiotics such as penicillin that inhibit peptidoglycan synthesis.

(2) The fungal cell membrane contains ergosterol and zymosterol, in contrast to human cell membranes which contain cholesterol. The selective action of amphotericin B on fungi is based on this difference in membrane sterols.

Yeasts grow as **single cells** that reproduce by asexual budding. **Molds** grow as **long filaments (hyphae)** and form a mat **(mycelium).** Some hyphae form transverse walls **(septate hyphae),** whereas others do not **(nonseptate hyphae).** Nonseptate hyphae are multinucleated (coencytic).

Several important fungi are thermally **dimorphic;** ie, they form different structures at different temperatures. They exist as molds in the saprophytic, free-living state at ambient temperature and as yeasts in host tissues at body temperature.

Most fungi are obligate aerobes; some are facultative anaerobes; but none are obligate anaerobes. All fungi require a preformed organic source of carbon, hence their frequent association with decaying matter. The natural habitat of most fungi is, therefore, the **environment.** An important exception is *Candida albicans,* which is part of the human normal flora.

Some fungi reproduce sexually by mating and forming sexual spores, eg, **zygospores, ascospores,** and **basidiospores.** Zygospores are single large spores with thick walls; ascospores are formed in a sac called an ascus; and basidiospores are formed externally on the tip of a pedestal called a basidium. The classification of these fungi is based on their sexual spores. Fungi that do not form sexual spores are termed ''imperfect'' and are classified as **Fungi imperfecti.** Many human pathogens are classified as Fungi imperfecti.

Table 47–1. Comparison of fungi and bacteria.

Feature	Fungi	Bacteria
Diameter	Approximately 4 μm (Candida)	Approximately 1 μm (Staphylococcus)
Nucleus	Eukaryotic	Prokaryotic
Cytoplasm	Mitochondria and endoplasmic reticulum present	Mitochondria and endoplasmic reticulum absent
Cell membrane	Sterols present	Sterols absent (except Mycoplasma)
Cell wall content	Chitin	Peptidoglycan
Spores	Sexual and asexual spores for reproduction	Endospores for survival, not for reproduction
Thermal dimorphism	Yes (some)	No
Metabolism	Require organic carbon; no obligate anaerobes.	Many do not require organic carbon; many obligate anaerobes.

*Chitin is a homopolymer of N-acetylglucosamine.

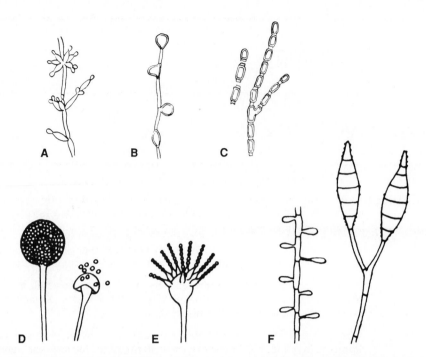

Figure 47–1. Asexual spores. *A:* Blastoconidia and pseudohyphae (*Candida*). *B:* Chlamydospores (*Candida*). *C:* Arthrospores (*Coccidioides*). *D:* Sporangia and sporangiospores (*Mucor*). *E:* Micro-conidia (*Aspergillus*). *F:* Microconidia and macroconidia (*Microsporum*). (Modified and reproduced, with permission, from Conant NF et al: *Manual of Clinical Mycology,* 3rd ed. Saunders, 1971.)

Most fungi of medical interest propagate asexually by forming **conidia** (asexual spores) from the sides or ends of specialized structures (Fig 47–1). The shape, color, and arrangement of conidia aid in the identification of fungi. Some important conidia are (1) **arthrospores,*** which arise by fragmentation of the ends of hyphae and are the mode of transmission of *Coccidioides immitis;* (2) **chlamydospores,** which are rounded, thick-walled, and quite resistant (the terminal chlamydospores of *C albicans* aid in identification); (3) **blastospores,** which are formed by the budding process by which yeasts reproduce asexually (some yeasts, eg, *C albicans,* can form multiple buds that do not detach, thus producing sausagelike chains called pseudohyphae, which can be used for identification); and (4) **sporangiospores,** which are formed within a sac (sporangium) on a stalk by molds such as *Rhizopus* and *Mucor*.

Although this book focuses on the fungi that are human pathogens, it should be remembered that fungi are used in the production of important foods, eg, bread, cheese, wine, and beer. Fungi are also responsible for the spoilage of certain foods. Because molds can grow in a drier, more acidic, and higher-osmotic-pressure environment than bacteria, they tend to be involved in the spoilage of fruits, grains, vegetables, and jams.

PATHOGENESIS   The response to infection with many fungi is the formation of **granulomas.** Granulomas are produced in the major systemic fungal diseases, eg, coccidioidomycosis, histoplasmosis, and blastomycosis, as well as several others. The cell-mediated immune response is involved in granuloma formation. Acute suppuration, characterized by the presence of neutrophils in the exudate, also occurs in certain fungal diseases such as aspergillosis and sporotrichosis. Fungi do not have endotoxin in their cell walls and do not produce exotoxins.

Activation of the cell-mediated immune system results in a **delayed hypersensitivity skin test** response to certain fungal antigens injected intradermally. A positive skin test indicates exposure to the fungal antigen. It does not imply current infection, because the exposure may have occurred in the past. A negative skin test makes the diagnosis unlikely unless the patient is immunocompromised. Because most people carry *Candida* as part of the normal flora, skin

*The term ''spores'' can be replaced by ''conidia,'' eg, arthroconidia.

Table 47–2. Transmission and location of some important fungi.

Genus	Habitat	Form of Organism Transmitted	Portal of Entry	Endemic Geographic Location
Coccidioides	Soil	Arthrospores	Inhalation into lungs	Southwestern USA and Latin America
Histoplasma	Soil (associated with bird feces)	Microconidia	Inhalation into lungs	Mississippi and Ohio River valleys
Blastomyces	Soil	Microconidia	Inhalation into lungs	States east of Mississippi River
Paracoccidioides	Soil	Uncertain	Inhalation into lungs	Latin America
Cryptococcus	Soil (associated with pigeon feces)	Yeast	Inhalation into lungs	Worldwide
Aspergillus	Soil and vegetation	Conidia	Inhalation into lungs	Worldwide
Candida	Human body	Yeast	Normal flora of skin, mouth, gastrointestinal tract, and vagina	Worldwide

testing with *Candida* antigens can be used to determine whether cell-mediated immunity is normal.

The transmission and geographic locations of some important fungi are described in Table 47–2.

Intact skin is an effective host defense against fungi, but if the skin is damaged, organisms can become established. Fatty acids in the skin inhibit dermatophyte growth, and hormone-associated skin changes at puberty limit ringworm of the scalp caused by *Trichophyton*. The normal flora of the skin and mucous membranes suppresses fungi. When the normal flora in inhibited, eg, by antibiotics, overgrowth of fungi such as *C albicans* can occur.

In the respiratory tract, the important host defenses are the mucous membranes of the nasopharynx, which trap inhaled fungal spores, and alveolar macrophages. Circulating IgG and IgM are produced in response to fungal infection, but their role in protection from disease is uncertain. The cell-mediated immune response is protective; its suppression can lead to reactivation and dissemination of asymptomatic fungal infections and to disease caused by opportunistic fungi.

FUNGAL TOXINS & ALLERGIES In addition to mycotic infections, there are 2 other kinds of fungal disease: (1) **mycotoxicoses** caused by ingested toxins and (2) **allergies** to fungal spores. The best-known mycotoxicosis occurs after eating *Amanita* mushrooms. These fungi produce 5 toxins, 2 of which—amanitin and phalloidin—are among the most potent hepatotoxins. Another mycotoxicosis, ergotism, is caused by the mold *Claviceps purpura,* which infects grains and produces alkaloids (eg, ergotamine and lysergic acid diethylamide [LSD]) that cause pronounced vascular and neurologic effects. Other ingested toxins, **aflatoxins,** are coumarin derivatives produced by *Aspergillus flavus* that cause liver damage and tumors in animals and are suspected of causing hepatic carcinoma in humans. Aflatoxins are ingested with spoiled grains and peanuts and are metabolized by the liver to epoxide, a potent carcinogen. Allergies to fungal spores, particularly those of *Aspergillus,* are manifested primarily by an asthmatic reaction (rapid bronchoconstriction mediated by IgE), eosinophilia, and a "wheal and flare" immediate skin test reaction.

LABORATORY DIAGNOSIS There are 3 approaches to the laboratory diagnosis of fungal diseases: (1) direct microscopic examination, (2) culture of the organism, and (3) serologic tests. Direct microscopic examination of clinical specimens such as sputum, lung biopsy material, and skin scrapings depends on finding characteristic asexual spores, hyphae, or yeasts in the light microscope. The specimen is either treated with 10% KOH to dissolve tissue material, leaving the alkali-resistant fungi intact, or stained with special fungal stains. Some examples of diagnostically important findings made by direct examination are (1) the spherules of *C immitis* and (2) the wide capsule of *Cryptococcus neoformans* seen in India ink preparations of spinal fluid.

Fungi are frequently cultured on Sabouraud's agar, which facilitates the appearance of the slow-growing fungi by inhibiting the growth of bacteria in the specimen. Inhibition of bacterial growth is due to the low pH of the medium and to the chloramphenicol and cycloheximide that are frequently added. The appearance of the mycelium (seen from the top and bottom of the agar) and the nature of the asexual spores are frequently sufficient to identify the organism.

Tests for the presence of antibodies in the patient's serum or spinal fluid are useful in diagnosing the systemic mycoses but less so in diagnosing other fungal infections. As is the case for bacterial and viral serologic testing, a significant rise in the antibody titer must be observed to confirm a diagnosis. The complement fixation test is most frequently used in suspected cases of coccidioidomycosis, histoplasmosis, and blastomycosis. In cryptococcal meningitis, the presence of the polysaccharide capsular antigens of *C neoformans* in the spinal fluid can be detected by the latex agglutination test.

ANTIFUNGAL THERAPY   See page 48 for a description of the action of antifungal drugs.

Review Questions

1. How do fungal and bacterial cell walls differ?
2. How do fungal and human cell membranes differ?
3. Describe dimorphism.
4. In general, what is the natural habitat of fungi? How does *Candida albicans* differ?
5. Contrast sexual and asexual reproduction of fungi.
6. Describe budding in yeasts.
7. What type of lesions are formed in most of the systemic fungal diseases? What is the pathogenesis of these lesions?
8. In the laboratory diagnosis of fungi, why is Sabouraud's agar used?
9. Why is amphotericin B selectively toxic for fungi?

48

Cutaneous & Subcutaneous Mycoses

Medical mycoses can be divided into 4 categories: (1) **cutaneous,** (2) **subcutaneous,** (3) **systemic,** and (4) **opportunistic.** Some features of the important fungal diseases are described in Table 48–1. Cutaneous and subcutaneous mycoses are discussed below; systemic and opportunistic mycoses are discussed in later chapters.

CUTANEOUS MYCOSES

(1) Dermatophytoses are caused by fungi **(dermatophytes)** that infect only superficial keratinized structures (skin, hair, and nails), not deeper tissues. The most important dermatophytes are classified in 3 genera: *Epidermophyton, Trichophyton,* and *Microsporum.* They are spread from infected persons, cats, and dogs by direct contact.

Dermatophytoses (tinea, ringworm) are chronic infections favored by heat and humidity, eg, athlete's foot and jock itch.* They are characterized by pruritic papules and vesicles, broken hairs, and thickened, broken nails. In some infected persons, hypersensitivity causes

---

*These infections are also known as tinea pedis and tinea cruris, respectively.

Table 48–1. Features of important fungal diseases.

Type	Anatomic Location	Representative Disease	Genus of Causative Organism(s)	Seriousness of Illness
Cutaneous	Hair shaft and dead layer of skin	Tinea versicolor	*Malassezia*	1+
	Epidermis, hair, nails	Dermatophytosis (ringworm)	*Microsporum, Trichophyton, Epidermophyton*	2+
Subcutaneous	Subcutis	Sporotrichosis	*Sporothrix*	2+
		Mycetoma	Several genera	2+
Systemic	Internal organs	Coccidioidomycosis	*Coccidioides*	4+
		Histoplasmosis	*Histoplasma*	4+
		Blastomycosis	*Blastomyces*	4+
		Paracoccidioidomycosis	*Paracoccidioides*	4+
Opportunistic	Internal organs	Cryptococcosis	*Cryptococcus*	4+
		Candidiasis	*Candida*	2+–4+
		Aspergillosis	*Aspergillus*	4+

dermatophytid ("id") reactions, eg, vesicles on the fingers. Id lesions are a response to circulating fungal antigens; the lesions do not contain hyphae. Patients with tinea infections show positive skin tests with fungal extracts, eg, trichophytin.

Scrapings of skin or nail placed in 10% KOH on a glass slide show hyphae under microscopy. Cultures on Sabouraud's medium at room temperature develop typical hyphae and conidia. Treatment uses local antifungal creams (undecylenic acid, miconazole, tolnaftate, etc) or oral griseofulvin. Prevention centers on keeping skin dry and cool.

(2) Tinea versicolor (pityriasis versicolor), a superficial skin infection of cosmetic importance only, is caused by *Malassezia furfur*. The lesions are usually noticed as hypopigmented areas, especially on tanned skin in the summer. There may be slight scaling or itching, but usually the infection is asymptomatic. It occurs more frequently in hot, humid weather. The lesions contain both budding yeast cells and hyphae. Diagnosis is usually made by observing this mixture in KOH preparations of skin scrapings. Culture is not usually done. The treatment of choice is topical miconazole, but the lesions have a tendency to recur and a permanent cure is difficult to achieve.

(3) Tinea nigra is an infection of the keratinized layers of the skin. It appears as a brownish spot due to the melaninlike pigment in the hyphae. The causative organism, *Cladosporium werneckii*, is found in the soil and transmitted during injury. In the USA, the disease is seen in the southern states. Diagnosis is made by microscopic examination and culture of skin scrapings. The infection is treated with a topical keratolytic agent, eg, salicylic acid.

SUBCUTANEOUS MYCOSES These are caused by fungi that grow in soil and on vegetation and are introduced into subcutaneous tissue through **trauma**.

Sporotrichosis *Sporothrix schenckii* is a **dimorphic** fungus that lives on vegetation. When introduced into the skin, typically by a thorn, it causes a local pustule or ulcer with nodules along the draining lymphatics. There is little systemic illness. Lesions may be chronic.

In the clinical laboratory, round or cigar-shaped budding cells are seen in tissue specimens. In culture, oval conidia in clusters occur at the tip of slender conidiophores (resembling a daisy). The disease is treated with oral potassium iodide or ketoconazole. It can be prevented by protecting skin when touching plants, moss, and wood.

Chromomycosis This is a slowly progressive granulomatous infection that is caused by several soil fungi (*Phialophora, Cladosporium,* etc) when introduced into the skin through trauma. Wartlike lesions with crusting abscesses extend along the lymphatics. The disease occurs mainly in the tropics and is found on bare feet and legs. In the clinical laboratory, dark brown, round fungal cells are seen in leukocytes or giant cells. The disease is treated with oral flucytosine or thiabendazole, plus local surgery.

Mycetoma Soil organisms (*Petriellidium, Madurella*) enter through wounds on feet, hands, or back and cause abscesses, with pus discharged through sinuses. The pus contains compact colored granules. Actinomycetes such as *Nocardia* can cause similar lesions (actinomycotic mycetoma). Sulfonamides may help the actinomycotic form. There is no effective drug against the fungal form; surgical excision is recommended.

Review Questions

1. What part of the skin do the dermatophytes infect?
2. How are dermatophytes spread?
3. Describe the typical tinea lesion.
4. How is the diagnosis of tinea infections usually made?
5. What is the "id" reaction?
6. How is sporotrichosis acquired?

49

Systemic Mycoses

These infections result from **inhalation** of the spores of **dimorphic** fungi that have their saprophytic **mold** forms in the **soil.** Within the **lungs,** the spores differentiate into **yeasts** or other specialized forms. Most lung infections are asymptomatic and self-limited. However, some persons develop disseminated disease in which the organisms grow in other organs, cause destructive lesions, and may result in death. Infected persons do not communicate these diseases to others.

COCCIDIOIDES

Disease *Coccidioides immitis* causes coccidioidomycosis.

Properties, Transmission, & Epidemiology *C immitis* is a **dimorphic** fungus that exists as a **mold** in soil and as a **spherule** in tissue (Fig 49–1). It is **endemic** in arid regions of the **southwestern USA** and **Latin America.** In soil, it forms hyphae with alternating **arthrospores** and empty cells. Arthrospores are very light and are carried by the wind. They can be **inhaled** and infect the lungs.

Pathogenesis & Immunity In the lungs, arthrospores form spherules that are 30 μm in diameter, have a thick, doubly refractive wall, and are filled with **endospores.** Upon rupture of the wall, endospores are released and enlarge to form new spherules. The organism can spread by direct extension or via the bloodstream. Granulomatous lesions can occur in virtually any organ but are found primarily in bones and the central nervous system (meningitis). **Dissemination** indicates some host defense defect in the ability to localize and control the infection. Most persons who develop a positive skin test to infection develop immunity to spread and to reinfection. However, if their cellular immunity is suppressed by drugs or disease, dissemination can occur at any time.

Clinical Findings Infection of the lungs is often asymptomatic and is evident only by a positive skin test and the presence of antibodies. Some infected persons have an influenzalike illness with fever and cough. About 50% have changes in the lungs as seen in x-rays, and 10% develop erythema nodosum as a hypersensitivity reaction. This syndrome is called "valley

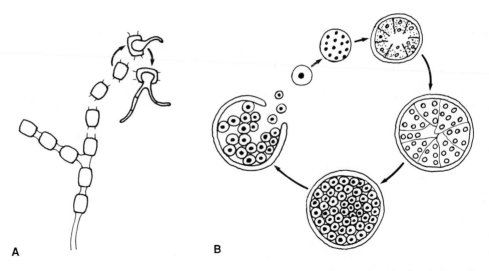

Figure 49–1. Stages of *Coccidioides immitis.* **A:** Arthrospores form at the ends of hyphae in the soil. They germinate in the soil to form new hyphae. If inhaled, the arthrospores differentiate into spherules. **B:** Endospores form within spherules in tissue. When spherules rupture, endospores disseminate and form new spherules. (Modified and reproduced, with permission, from Jawetz E et al: *Review of Medical Microbiology,* 18th ed. Appleton & Lange, 1989.)

fever'' (in the San Joaquin Valley of California) or ''desert rheumatism'' (in Arizona); it tends to subside spontaneously. The overall incidence of dissemination in persons infected with *C immitis* is 1%, although the incidence in Filipinos and blacks is 10 times higher.

Laboratory Diagnosis In tissue specimens, spherules are seen microscopically. Cultures on Sabouraud's agar show hyphae with arthrospores. (*Caution:* Cultures are highly infectious; precautions against inhaling arthrospores must be taken.) In infected persons, **skin tests** with fungal extracts (coccidioidin or spherulin) cause at least a 5-mm induration 48 hours after injection (delayed hypersensitivity reaction). Skin tests become positive within 2–4 weeks of infection and remain so for years but are often negative (anergy) in patients with disseminated disease. In serologic tests, IgM and IgG precipitins appear within 2–4 weeks of infection and then decline in subsequent months. Complement-fixing antibodies occur at low titer initially, but the titer rises greatly if dissemination occurs.

Treatment & Prevention No treatment is needed in asymptomatic or mild primary infection. Amphotericin B is used for persisting lung lesions or disseminated disease. Ketoconazole is also effective in lung disease. If meningitis occurs, amphotericin B intravenously and intrathecally may induce remission but long-term results are often poor. There are no means of prevention except avoiding travel to endemic areas.

HISTOPLASMA

Disease *Histoplasma capsulatum* causes histoplasmosis.

Properties *H capsulatum* is a **dimorphic** fungus that exists as a **mold** in soil and as a **yeast** in tissue. It forms 2 types of asexual spores (Fig 49–2): (1) **tuberculate macroconidia,** with typical thick walls and fingerlike projections that are important in laboratory identification, and (2) **microconidia,** which are smaller, thin, smooth-walled spores that, if inhaled, transmit the infection.

Transmission & Epidemiology This fungus occurs in many parts of the world. In the USA it is **endemic** in central and eastern states, especially in the **Ohio and Mississippi River valleys.** It grows in soil, particularly if the soil is heavily contaminated with **bird droppings.**

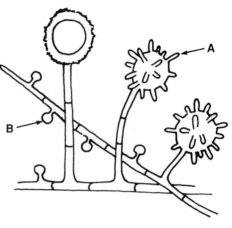

Figure 49–2. Asexual spores of *Histoplasma capsulatum*. *A:* Tuberculate macroconidia. *B:* Microconidia. (Reproduced, with permission, from Jawetz E et al: *Review of Medical Microbiology*, 18th ed. Appleton & Lange, 1989.)

Pathogenesis & Clinical Findings   Inhaled **spores** are engulfed by **macrophages** and develop into yeast forms. In tissues, *H capsulatum* occurs as an **oval budding yeast inside macrophages** (Fig 49–3). The organisms spread widely throughout the body, but most infections remain asymptomatic because the small granulomatous foci heal by calcification. With intense exposure (eg, in a chicken house or bat-infested cave), pneumonia may become clinically manifest. Severe disseminated histoplasmosis develops in a small minority of infected persons, especially infants and elderly or immunocompromised individuals.

Laboratory Diagnosis   In tissue biopsies or bone marrow aspirates, oval yeast cells within macrophages are seen microscopically. Cultures on Sabouraud's agar shows typical structures, eg, tuberculate macroconidia.

   A **skin test** with fungal extract (histoplasmin) becomes positive (induration) within 2–3 weeks of infection and remains so for years. It may be negative in disseminated disease. Repeated skin testing stimulates antibody formation and therefore should be avoided. In serologic tests, precipitating antibodies appear within 4–6 weeks of infection. Complement-fixing antibody levels rise later and fall sharply if the disease is inactive. However, in disseminated disease the complement fixation titer remains high, and *Histoplasma* antigen is detectable in urine and serum by radioimmunoassay. Some cross reactions with other fungi may occur.

Treatment & Prevention   No therapy is needed in asymptomatic or mild primary infections. With progressive lung lesions, oral ketoconazole is beneficial. In disseminated disease, amphotericin B is the treatment of choice. There are no means of prevention except avoiding exposure in endemic areas.

BLASTOMYCES

Disease   *Blastomyces dermatitidis* causes blastomycosis.

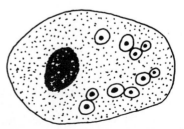

Figure 49-3. *Histoplasma capsulatum.* Yeasts are located within the macrophage. (Reproduced, with permission, from Jawetz E et al: *Review of Medical Microbiology*, 18th ed. Appleton & Lange, 1989.)

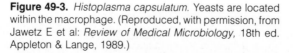

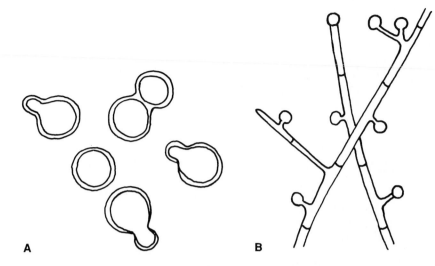

Figure 49–4. *Blastomyces dermatitidis. A:* Yeast with a broad-based bud at 37 °C. *B:* Mold with microconidia at 20 °C. (Reproduced, with permission, from Jawetz E et al: *Review of Medical Microbiology,* 18th ed. Appleton & Lange, 1989.)

Properties   *B dermatitidis* is a **dimorphic** fungus that exists as a mold in soil and as a yeast in tissue. The yeast is round with a doubly refractive wall and a single **broad-based bud** (Fig 49–4).

Transmission & Epidemiology   This fungus is **endemic** in **North and Central America** and in Africa. It grows in moist soil rich in organic material, forming hyphae with small pear-shaped conidia. Inhalation of the conidia causes human infection.

Pathogenesis & Clinical Findings   Infection occurs mainly via the respiratory tract. Asymptomatic or mild cases are rarely recognized. Dissemination may result in ulcerated granulomas of skin, bone, or other sites.

Laboratory Diagnosis   In tissue biopsies, thick-walled yeast cells with single broad-based buds are seen microscopically. Hyphae with small pear-shaped conidia are visible on culture. The skin test lacks specificity and has little value. Serology shows that yeast-phase antigens are precipitated by sera of infected persons in immunodiffusion tests, but cross reactions occur.

Treatment & Prevention   Ketoconazole is the drug of choice in persons with lesions. Surgical excision may be helpful. There are no means of prevention.

PARACOCCIDIOIDES

Disease   *Paracoccidioides brasiliensis* causes paracoccidioidomycosis.

Properties   *P brasiliensis* is a **dimorphic** fungus that exists as a mold in soil and as a yeast in tissue. The yeast is thick-walled with **multiple buds** in contrast to *B dermatitidis*, which has a single bud.

Transmission & Epidemiology   This fungus grows in the soil and is endemic in rural Latin America. Disease occurs only in that region.

Pathogenesis & Clinical Findings   The spores are **inhaled,** and early lesions occur in the lungs. Asymptomatic infection is common. Alternatively, oral mucous membrane lesions, lymph node enlargement, and sometimes dissemination to many organs may develop.

Laboratory Diagnosis   In pus or tissues, yeast cells with multiple buds are seen microscopically. A specimen cultured for 2–4 weeks may grow typical organisms. Skin tests are rarely helpful. Serology shows that when significant antibody titers (by immunodiffusion or complement fixation) are found, active disease is present.

Treatment & Prevention   The drug of choice is ketoconazole taken orally for several months. There are no means of prevention.

Review Questions

In regard to coccidioidomycosis, histoplasmosis, and blastomycosis:
1. Which of the causative organisms are dimorphic?
2. What is the geographic distribution of the disease?
3. How are the infections acquired? What is the site of the initial lesions?
4. What is the morphology of the organism in the body?
5. What is the role of skin tests?
6. What is the role of complement-fixing antibodies?
7. What is the treatment for mild primary disease? for disseminated disease?

50

Opportunistic Mycoses

Opportunistic fungi fail to induce disease in most normal persons but may do so in those with **impaired** host defenses.

CANDIDA

Diseases   *Candida albicans,* the most important species, causes thrush, vaginitis, and chronic mucocutaneous candidiasis as well as other diseases.

Properties   *C albicans* is an **oval yeast with a single bud.** It is part of the **normal flora** of mucous membranes of the upper respiratory, gastrointestinal, and female genital tracts. In tissues it may appear as budding yeasts or as elongated budding "**pseudohyphae**" (Fig 50–1). Carbohydrate fermentation reactions differentiate it from other species, eg, *Candida tropicalis, Candida parapsilosis, Candida krusei,* or *torulopsis glabrata.*

Transmission   As a member of the normal flora, it is not transmitted.

Pathogenesis & Clinical Findings   When local or systemic host defenses are impaired, disease may result. Overgrowth of *Candida* in the mouth produces white patches (thrush). Vulvovaginitis with itching and discharge is favored by high pH, diabetes, or use of antibiotics. Skin invasion occurs in warm, moist areas, which become red and weeping. Fingers and nails become involved when repeatedly immersed in water; persons employed as dishwashers in restaurants and institutions are commonly affected. Thickening or loss of the nail can occur. In immunosuppressed individuals, *Candida* may disseminate to many organs or cause chronic mucocutaneous candidiasis. Intravenous drug abuse also predisposes to disseminated candidiasis.

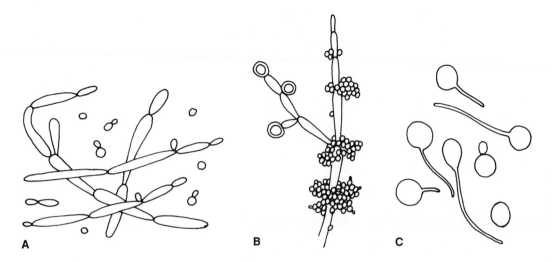

Figure 50–1. *Candida albicans.* *A:* Budding yeasts and pseudohyphae in tissues or exudate. *B:* Pseudohyphae and chlamydospores in culture at 20 °C. *C:* Germ tubes at 37 °C. (Reproduced, with permission, from Jawetz E et al: *Review of Medical Microbiology,* 18th ed. Appleton & Lange, 1989.)

Laboratory Diagnosis   In exudates or tissues, budding yeasts and pseudohyphae are seen microscopically. Such specimens grow typical yeasts when cultured. **Germ tubes** form in serum at 37 °C, which serves to distinguish *C albicans* from most other *Candida* species (Fig 50–1). **Chlamydospores** are typically formed by *C albicans* but not by other species of *Candida.* Serology is rarely helpful. **Skin tests** with *Candida* antigens are uniformly positive in normal adults. Such tests are used as an indicator of competent cellular immunity.

Treatment & Prevention   For local infection, removal of the cause (eg, moisture) and administration of antimicrobial agents are effective. Topical creams, eg, nystatin and miconazole, may be used. For systemic infection, oral ketoconazole can control mucocutaneous candidiasis. For disseminated candidiasis, intravenous amphotericin B, oral flucytosine, or oral ketoconazole can be effective if cellular immunity improves.

CRYPTOCOCCUS

Disease   *Cryptococcus neoformans* causes cryptococcosis, especially cryptococcal meningitis.

Properties   *C neoformans* is an **oval, budding yeast** surrounded by a **wide polysaccharide capsule** (Fig 50–2). It is not dimorphic.

Transmission   This yeast occurs widely in nature and grows abundantly in **soil containing bird (especially pigeon) droppings.** Human infection results from **inhalation** of the organism.

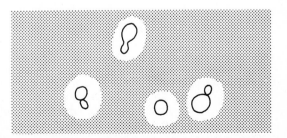

Figure 50–2. *Cryptococcus neoformans.* India ink preparation shows a wide capsule. (Reproduced, with permission, from Jawetz E et al: *Review of Medical Microbiology,* 18th ed. Appleton & Lange, 1989.)

Pathogenesis & Clinical Findings   Lung infection is often asymptomatic or may produce pneumonia. Disease occurs mainly in immunocompromised persons, in whom the organism disseminates to the central nervous system (meningitis) and other organs. However, roughly half of patients with cryptococcal meningitis fail to show evidence of immunosuppression.

Laboratory Diagnosis   In spinal fluid mixed with **India ink,** the yeast cell is seen microscopically surrounded by a wide, unstained capsule. The organism can be cultured from spinal fluid and other specimens. Serologic tests can be done for both antibody and antigen. In infected spinal fluid, **capsular antigen** occurs in high titer.

Treatment & Prevention   Combined treatment with amphotericin B and flucytosine is effective against meningitis or other disseminated disease. There are no specific means of prevention.

ASPERGILLUS

Disease   *Aspergillus* species cause aspergillosis.

Properties   *Aspergillus* species exist **only as molds;** they are not dimorphic. They have septate hyphae.

Transmission   These molds are widely distributed in nature. They grow on decaying vegetation, producing chains of conidia. Transmission is by **airborne conidia.**

Pathogenesis & Clinical Findings   *Aspergillus fumigatus,* the most important pathogen, can colonize and later invade abraded skin, wounds, burns, the cornea, the external ear, or paranasal sinuses. In immunocompromised persons, it can invade the lungs and other organs, producing hemoptysis and granulomas. Aspergilli can grow in pulmonary cavities (eg, those due to tuberculosis) and produce a **"fungus ball,"** which can be seen on x-ray. They can cause allergic asthma. *Aspergillus flavus* growing on cereals or nuts produces aflatoxins that may be carcinogenic or acutely toxic.

Laboratory Diagnosis   Biopsy specimens show **septate, branching hyphae** invading tissue. Cultures show colonies with characteristic radiating chains of conidia. However, positive cultures do not prove disease because colonization is common. Serology shows that in persons with allergic asthma, high levels of IgE are present. In persons with invasive aspergillosis, there may be high titers of galactomannan antigen in serum.

Treatment & Prevention   Invasive aspergillosis is treated with amphotericin B, but results may be poor. A fungus ball growing in a sinus or in a pulmonary cavity can be surgically removed. There are no specific means of prevention.

MUCOR & RHIZOPUS   Mucormycosis (zygomycosis and phycomycosis) is a disease caused by saprophytic **molds** (eg, *Mucor* and *Rhizopus*) found widely in the environment. They invade tissues of immunocompromised hosts. These and similar organisms proliferate in the walls of blood vessels, particularly of the paranasal sinuses, lungs, or gut, and result in tissue necrosis. Patients with diabetic ketoacidosis, burns, or leukemias are particularly susceptible. In biopsies, organisms are seen microscopically as **nonseptate, broad hyphae.** These molds can be grown on laboratory media, but cultures of biopsies are typically negative. If diagnosed early, treatment of the underlying disorder, plus administration of amphotericin B and surgical removal of necrotic infected tissue, has resulted in some remissions and cures.

Review Questions

1. Where is *Candida albicans* usually found as part of the normal flora?
2. What factors predispose to candidal invasion or infection?

3. Contrast the appearance of *C albicans* as part of the normal flora and as the cause of invasive disease.
4. What is the role of serology and skin tests in the diagnosis of candidiasis?
5. What is the most striking structural feature of *Cryptococcus neoformans?*
6. What are the natural habitat and mode of transmission of *C neoformans?*
7. What is the main predisposing factor to cryptococcal meningitis?
8. What are 2 tests used in the diagnosis of cryptococcal meningitis?
9. Contrast the appearance of the hyphae of *Aspergillus* and *Mucor*.
10. What are the predisposing factors to aspergillosis? To mucormycosis?

Part VI: Parasitology

Parasites occur in 2 distinct forms: single-celled **protozoa** and multicellular metazoa called **helminths** or worms. For medical purposes, protozoa can be subdivided into 4 groups: Sarcodina (amebas), Sporozoa (sporozoa), Mastigophora (flagellates), and Ciliata (ciliates). Metazoa are subdivided into 2 phyla: the Platyhelminthes (flatworms) and the Nemathelminthes (roundworms or nematodes). The phylum Platyhelminthes contains 2 medically important classes: Cestoda (tapeworms) and Trematoda (flukes). This classification is diagrammed in Figure 1.

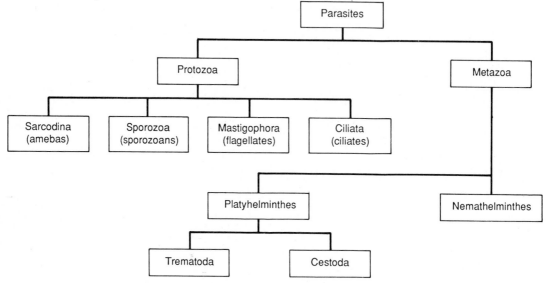

Figure 1. Relationships of the medically important parasites.

51 Intestinal & Urogenital Protozoa

In this book, the major protozoan pathogens are grouped according to the primary location in the body where they most frequently cause disease.

(a) Within the intestinal tract, 3 organisms—the ameba *Entamoeba histolytica,* the flagellate *Giardia lamblia,* and the sporozoan *Cryptosporidium* species—are the most important.

(b) In the urogenital tract, the flagellate *Trichomonas vaginalis* occurs commonly.

(c) The blood and tissue protozoa are a varied group consisting of the flagellates *Trypanosoma* and *Leishmania* and the sporozoans *Plasmodium* and *Toxoplasma.* The important opportunistic lung pathogen *Pneumocystis* will be discussed in this group, although there is recent molecular evidence that it should be classified as a fungus.

The major and minor pathogenic protozoa are listed in Table 51–1.

Although immigrants and Americans returning from abroad can present to physicians in the USA with any parasitic disease, certain parasites are much more likely to occur outside the USA. The features of the medically important protozoa, including their occurrence in the USA, are described in Table 51–2.

Table 51–1. Major and minor pathogenic protozoa.

Type and Location	Species	Disease
Major protozoa Intestinal tract	*Entamoeba histolytica* *Giardia lamblia* *Cryptosporidium* species	Ambiasis Giardiasis Cryptosporidiosis
Urogenital tract	*Trichomonas vaginalis*	Trichomoniasis
Blood and tissue	*Trypanosoma* species *T cruzi* *T gambiense*[1] *T rhodesiense*[1] *Leishmania* species *L donovani* *L tropica* *L mexicana* *L braziliensis* *Plasmodium* species *Toxoplasma gondii* *Pneumocystis carinii*	Trypanosomiasis Chagas' disease Sleeping sickness Sleeping sickness Leishmaniasis Kala-azar Cutaneous leishmaniasis[2] Cutaneous leishmaniasis[2] Mucocutaneous leishmaniasis Malaria Toxoplasmosis Pneumonia
Minor protozoa Intestinal tract	*Balantidium coli* *Isospora belli*	Dysentery Isosporosis
Blood and tissue	*Naegleria* species *Acanthamoeba* species *Babesia microti*	Meningitis Meningitis Babesiosis

[1]Also known as *T brucei* subspecies *gambiense* and *T brucei* subspecies *rhodesiense.*
[2]*L tropica* and *L mexicana* cause Old World and New World cutaneous leishmaniasis, respectively.

Table 51–2. Features of medically important protozoa.

Genus	Mode of Transmission	Occurrence in USA	Diagnosis	Treatment
Entamoeba	Ingestion of cysts in food.	Yes	Trophozoites or cysts in stool; serology.	Metronidazole plus iodoquinol.
Giardia	Ingestion of cysts in food.	Yes	Trophozoites or cysts in stools.	Metronidazole.
Cryptosporidium	Ingestion of cysts in food.	Yes	Cysts on acid-fast stain.	None.
Trichomonas	Sexual.	Yes	Trophozoites in wet mount.	Metronidazole.
Trypanosoma *T cruzi*	Reduviid bug.	Rare	Blood smear, bone marrow, xenodiagnosis.	Nifurtimox.
T gambiense, *T rhodesiense*	Tsetse fly.	No	Blood smear.	Suramin[1]
Leishmania *L donovani*	Sand fly.	No	Bone marrow, spleen, or lymph node.	Stibogluconate.
L tropica, L mexicana, *L braziliensis*	Sand fly.	No	Fluid from lesion.	Stibogluconate.
Plasmodium *P vivax, P ovale,* *P malariae*	*Anopheles* mosquito.	Rare	Blood smear.	Chloroquine; also primaquine for *P vivax* and *P ovale.*
P falciparum	*Anopheles* mosquito.	No	Blood smear.	Chloroquine; quinine, sulfadoxine, and pyrimethamine if resistant.
Toxoplasma	Ingestion of cysts in raw meat; contact with soil contaminated by cat feces.	Yes	Serology; microscopic examination of tissue; mouse inoculation.	Sulfonamide and pyrimethamine for congenital disease and immunocompromised patients.
Pneumocystis	Inhalation.	Yes	Lung biopsy or lavage.	Trimethoprim-sulfamethoxazole or pentamidine.

[1]Melarsoprol is used if the central nervous system is involved.

Intestinal Protozoa

ENTAMOEBA

Diseases *Entamoeba histolytica* causes amebic dysentery and liver abscess.

Important Properties The life cycle of *E histolytica* has 2 stages: the motile **ameba (trophozoite)** and the nonmotile **cyst.** The trophozoite is found within the intestinal and extraintestinal lesions and in diarrheal stools. The cyst predominates in nondiarrheal stools. These cysts are not highly resistant and are readily killed by heat and dehydration but not by chlorination of water supplies.

The cyst has **4 nuclei,** an important diagnostic criterion. Upon excystation in the intestinal tract, an ameba with 4 nuclei emerges and then divides to form 8 trophozoites. The mature trophozoite has a single nucleus with an even lining of peripheral chromatin and a prominent central nucleolus (karyosome).

Antibodies are formed against trophozoite antigens in invasive amebiasis, but they are not protective; prior infection does not prevent reinfection. The antibodies are useful, however, for serologic diagnosis.

Pathogenesis & Epidemiology The cysts are transmitted primarily by the **fecal-oral** route in contaminated food and water. Anal-oral transmission, eg, among male homosexuals, also occurs. There is **no animal reservoir.** The ingested cysts differentiate into trophozoites in the ileum but tend to colonize the cecum and colon.

The trophozoites invade the colonic epithelium and secrete enzymes that cause localized necrosis. Little inflammation occurs at the site. As the lesion reaches the muscularis layer, a typical **"teardrop" ulcer** forms that can undermine and destroy large areas of the intestinal epithelium. Progression into the submucosa leads to invasion of the portal circulation by the trophozoites. By far the most frequent site of systemic disease is the **liver.**

Infection by *E histolytica* is found worldwide but occurs most frequently in tropical countries, especially in areas with poor sanitation. About 1–2% of people in the USA are affected. The disease is widely prevalent in male homosexuals.

Clinical Findings Acute intestinal amebiasis presents as dysentery (ie, bloody, mucus-containing diarrhea) accompanied by lower abdominal discomfort, flatulence, and tenesmus. Chronic amebiasis with low-grade symptoms such as occasional diarrhea, weight loss, and fatigue also occurs. Roughly 90% of those infected are asymptomatic carriers, who pass cysts in their feces that can be transmitted to others.

Amebic abscess of the liver is characterized by right-upper-quadrant pain, weight loss, fever, and a tender, enlarged liver. Right-lobe abscesses can penetrate the diaphragm and cause lung disease. Most cases of amebic liver abscess occur in patients who have not had overt intestinal amebiasis.

Laboratory Diagnosis Diagnosis of intestinal amebiasis rests on finding either trophozoites in diarrheal stools or cysts in formed stools. Diarrheal stools should be examined within 1 hour to see the ameboid motility of the trophozoite. Trophozoites characteristically contain ingested red blood cells. The most common error is to mistake fecal leukocytes for trophozoites. Because cysts are passed intermittently, at least 3 specimens should be examined. About half of patients with extraintestinal amebiasis have negative stool examinations.

E histolytica can be distinguished from other amebas by 2 major criteria: (1) The nature of the **nucleus** of the trophozoite. The *E histolytica* nucleus has a small central nucleolus and fine chromatin granules along the border of the nuclear membrane. The nuclei of other amebas are quite different. (2) The **cyst size and number of its nuclei.** Mature cysts of *E histolytica* are smaller than those of *Entamoeba coli* and contain 4 nuclei, whereas *Entamoeba coli* cysts have 8 nuclei.

A complete examination for cysts includes a wet mount in saline, an iodine-stained wet mount, and a fixed, trichrome-stained preparation, each of which brings out different aspects of cyst morphology. These preparations are also helpful in distinguishing amebic from bacillary dysentery. In the latter, many inflammatory cells such as polymorphonuclear leukocytes are seen, whereas in amebic dysentery they are not.

Serologic testing is useful. For most patients with invasive amebiasis, the indirect hemagglutination test will be positive. The test is frequently negative for asymptomatic individuals who are passing cysts.

Treatment The treatment of choice for symptomatic intestinal amebiasis or hepatic abscesses is metronidazole plus iodoquinol. Hepatic abscesses need not be drained. Asymptomatic cyst carriers should be treated with iodoquinol.

Prevention Prevention involves avoiding fecal contamination of food and water and observing good personal hygiene such as hand washing. Purification of municipal water supplies is usually effective, but outbreaks of amebiasis in city dwellers still occur when contamination is heavy. The use of "night soil" (human feces) for fertilization of crops should be discouraged. In endemic areas, vegetables should be cooked.

GIARDIA

Disease *Giardia lamblia* causes giardiasis.

Important Properties The life cycle consists of 2 stages, the **trophozoite** and the **cyst.** The trophozoite is pear-shaped with 2 nuclei, 4 pairs of flagella, and a suction disk with which it attaches to the intestinal wall. The oval cyst is thick-walled with 4 nuclei and several internal fibers. Each cyst gives rise to 2 trophozoites during excystation in the intestinal tract.

Pathogenesis & Epidemiology Transmission occurs by ingestion of the cyst in **fecally contaminated** food and water. Excystation takes place in the duodenum, where the trophozoite attaches to the gut wall but does not invade. The trophozoite causes inflammation of the duodenal mucosa, leading to **malabsorption** of protein and fat.

The organism is found worldwide; about 5% of stool specimens in the USA contain *Giardia* cysts. Approximately half of those infected are asymptomatic carriers, who continue to excrete the cysts for years. IgA deficiency greatly predisposes to symptomatic infection.

In addition to being endemic, giardiasis occurs in outbreaks related to contaminated water supplies. Chlorination does not kill the cysts, but filtration removes them. Hikers who drink untreated stream water are frequently infected. Animals as well as humans may pass the cysts and contaminate water sources. Giardiasis is frequent in male homosexuals as a result of oral-anal contact. The incidence is high among children in day-care centers and among patients in mental hospitals.

Clinical Findings Nonbloody, foul-smelling diarrhea is accompanied by nausea, anorexia, flatulence, and abdominal cramps persisting for weeks or months. There is no fever.

Laboratory Diagnosis Diagnosis is made by finding trophozoites or cysts or both in diarrheal stools. In formed stools, eg, in asymptomatic carriers, only cysts are seen.

If microscopic examination of the stool is negative, the **string test,** which consists of swallowing a weighted piece of string until it reaches the duodenum, should be performed. The trophozoites adhere to the string and can be visualized after withdrawal of the string. No serologic test is available.

Treatment The treatment of choice is metronidazole or quinacrine hydrochloride.

Prevention Prevention involves drinking boiled or iodine-treated water in endemic areas and while hiking. No prophylactic drug or vaccine is available.

CRYPTOSPORIDIUM

Disease *Cryptosporidium* species cause diarrhea, mainly in **immunocompromised** patients, eg, those with AIDS, but also in **immunocompetent** individuals.

Important Properties   Some aspects of the life cycle remain uncertain, but the following stages have been identified. Oocysts release sporozoites, which form trophozoites. Several stages ensue, involving the formation of schizonts and merozoites. Eventually microgametes and macrogametes form; these unite to produce a zygote, which differentiates into an oocyst. This cycle has several features in common with other sporozoa, eg, *Isospora*. Taxonomically, *Cryptosporidium* is in the subclass Coccidia.

Pathogenesis & Epidemiology   The organism is acquired by **fecal-oral** transmission of oocysts from either human or animal sources. The oocysts excyst in the small intestine, where the trophozoites (and other forms) attach to the gut wall. Invasion does not occur. The jejunum is the site most heavily infested.

Clinical Findings   The disease in immunocompromised patients presents primarily as a watery, nonbloody diarrhea causing large fluid loss. The pathogenesis of the diarrhea is unclear; no toxin has been identified. Symptoms persist for long periods in immunocompromised patients, whereas they are self-limited in immunocompetent patients.

Laboratory Diagnosis   Diagnosis is made by finding oocysts in fecal smears when using a modified Kinyoun **acid-fast** stain. Serologic tests are not available.

Treatment & Prevention   There is no effective drug therapy, and no means of prevention are available. Although immunocompromised patients usually do not die from cryptosporidiosis, the fluid loss and malnutrition are severely debilitating.

Urogenital Protozoa

TRICHOMONAS

Disease   *Trichomonas vaginalis* causes trichomoniasis.

Important Properties   *T vaginalis* is a pear-shaped organism with a central nucleus and 4 anterior flagella. It has an undulating membrane that extends about two-thirds of its length. It exists **only as a trophozoite;** there is no cyst form.

Pathogenesis & Epidemiology   The primary mode of transmission is **sexual contact;** the trophozoites require a warm, moist environment to remain viable. The primary locations of the organism are the vagina and the prostate. An important predisposing factor to symptomatic infection is loss of the normal acidity of the vagina.

Trichomoniasis is one of the most common infections worldwide. Roughly 25–50% of women in the USA harbor the organism. The frequency of symptomatic disease is highest among sexually active women in their 30s and lowest in postmenopausal women.

Clinical Findings   In women, a watery, foul-smelling, greenish discharge accompanied by itching and burning occurs. Infection in men is usually asymptomatic, but about 10% of infected men have urethritis.

Laboratory Diagnosis   In a wet mount of vaginal (or prostatic) secretions, the pear-shaped trophozoites have a typical jerky motion. There is no serologic test.

Treatment & Prevention   The drug of choice is metronidazole for both partners to prevent reinfection. Maintenance of the low pH of the vagina is helpful. Condoms limit transmission. No prophylactic drug or vaccine is available.

Review Questions

1. What are the 3 important protozoa that cause intestinal tract disease?
2. What are the 2 stages in the life cycle of *Entamoeba histolytica*? of *Giardia lamblia*?
3. How is *E histolytica* transmitted? *G lamblia*? Is there an animal reservoir for either?
4. How is the laboratory diagnosis made for *E histolytica*? for *G lamblia*? How is *E histolytica* distinguished from *Entamoeba coli*?
5. How is *Cryptosporidium* transmitted? Is there an animal reservoir?
6. How is the laboratory diagnosis of cryptosporidiosis made?
7. What is the life cycle of *Trichomonas vaginalis?*
8. How is *T vaginalis* transmitted?
9. How is the laboratory diagnosis of trichomoniasis made?

Blood & Tissue Protozoa 52

The medically important organisms in this category of protozoa consist of the sporozoans *Plasmodium* and *Toxoplasma* and the flagellates *Trypanosoma* and *Leishmania. Pneumocystis* is discussed in this book as a protozoan, but molecular data published in 1988 indicate that it should be reclassified as a fungus related to yeasts such as *Saccharomyces cerevisiae*.

PLASMODIUM

Disease Malaria is caused by 4 plasmodia: *Plasmodium vivax, Plasmodium ovale, Plasmodium malariae,* and *Plasmodium falciparum*.

Important Properties The vector and definitive host for plasmodia is the **female *Anopheles* mosquito** (only the female takes a blood meal). There are 2 phases in the life cycle: the sexual cycle, which occurs primarily in mosquitoes, and the asexual cycle, which occurs in humans, the intermediate hosts.* The sexual cycle is called **sporogony** because sporozoites are produced, and the asexual cycle is called **schizogony** because schizonts are made.

The life cycle in humans begins with the introduction of sporozoites into the blood from the saliva of the biting mosquito. The sporozoites are taken up by hepatocytes within 30 minutes. This "exoerythrocytic" phase consists of cell multiplication and differentiation into **merozoites.** *P vivax* and *P ovale* produce a latent form **(hypnozoite)** in the liver; this form is the cause of relapses seen with vivax and ovale malaria.

Merozoites are released from the liver cells and infect red blood cells. During the erythrocytic phase, the organism differentiates into a ring-shaped trophozoite. The ring form grows into an ameboid form and then differentiates into a schizont filled with merozoites. After release, the merozoites infect other erythrocytes. This cycle in the red cell repeats at regular intervals typical for each species. The periodic release of merozoites causes the typical recurrent symptoms of chills, fever, and sweats seen in malaria patients.

The sexual cycle begins in the human erythrocyte when some merozoites develop into male and others into female gametocytes. The gametocyte-containing red blood cells are ingested by the female *Anopheles* mosquito and, within her gut, produce a female macrogamete and 8 spermlike male microgametes. After fertilization, the diploid zygote differentiates into a

---

*The sexual cycle is initiated in humans with the formation of gametocytes within red blood cells (gametogony) and completed in mosquitoes with the fusion of the male and female gametes, oocyst formation, and production of many sporozoites (sporogony).

motile ookinete that burrows into the gut wall, where it grows into an oocyst within which many haploid sporozoites are produced. The sporozoites are released and migrate to the salivary glands, ready to complete the cycle when the mosquito takes her next blood meal.

Pathogenesis & Epidemiology   Most of the pathology of malaria is due to the **destruction of red blood cells.** Not only does the parasite rupture erythrocytes upon release of the merozoites, but the spleen sequesters and destroys many red cells also. The enlarged spleen characteristic of malaria is due to congestion of sinusoids with erythrocytes, coupled with hyperplasia of lymphocytes and macrophages.

Malaria caused by *P falciparum* is **more severe** than that caused by the other plasmodia. It is characterized by infection of far more red cells than the other malarial species and by occlusion of the capillaries with aggregates of parasitized red cells. This leads to life-threatening hemorrhage and necrosis, particularly in the brain. Furthermore, extensive hemolysis and kidney damage occur, with resulting hemoglobinuria. The dark color of the patient's urine has given rise to the term "blackwater fever."

The timing of the fever cycle is 72 hours for *P malariae* and 48 hours for the other plasmodia. Disease caused by *P malariae* is called quartan malaria because it recurs every fourth day, whereas malaria caused by the others is called tertian because it recurs every third day. Tertian malaria is subdivided into malignant malaria, caused by *P falciparum*, and benign malaria, caused by *P vivax* and *P ovale*.

P falciparum causes a high level of parasitemia, because it can infect red cells of all ages. In contrast, *P vivax* infects only reticulocytes and *P malariae* infects only mature red cells; thus they produce much lower levels of parasites in the blood. Individuals with sickle cell trait (heterozygotes) are protected against malaria because their red cells have too little ATPase activity and cannot produce sufficient energy to support the growth of the parasite. People with homozygous sickle cell anemia are also protected but rarely live long enough to obtain much benefit.

Malaria is transmitted primarily by mosquito bites, but transmission across the placenta, in blood transfusions, and by intravenous drug abuse also occurs.

Partial immunity based on humoral antibodies that block merozoites from invading the red cells occurs in infected individuals. A low level of parasitemia and low-grade symptoms result; this condition is known as premunition.

More than 200 million people worldwide have malaria, and more than 1 million die from it each year, making it the most common lethal disease. It occurs primarily in tropical and subtropical areas, especially in Asia, Africa, and Central and South America. Malaria in the USA is seen in Americans who travel to endemic areas without adequate chemoprophylaxis and in immigrants from endemic areas. It is not endemic in the USA. Certain regions in Southeast Asia, South America, and east Africa are particularly affected by chloroquine-resistant strains of *P falciparum*.

Clinical Properties   Malaria presents with abrupt onset of fever and chills, accompanied by headache, myalgias, and arthralgias, about 2 weeks after the mosquito bite. Fever may be continuous early in the disease; the typical periodic cycle does not develop for several days after onset. The fever spike, which can reach 41 °C, is frequently accompanied by nausea, vomiting, and abdominal pain. The fever is followed by drenching sweats. Splenomegaly is seen in most patients, and hepatomegaly occurs in roughly one-third. Anemia is prominent.

Untreated malaria caused by *P falciparum* is potentially life-threatening as a result of extensive brain and kidney damage. Malaria caused by the other 3 plasmodia is usually self-limited, with a low mortality rate. However, relapses of *P vivax* and *P ovale* malaria can occur up to several years after the initial illness as a result of hypnozoites latent in the liver.

Laboratory Diagnosis   Diagnosis rests on microscopic examination of blood, using both **thick and thin** Giemsa-stained smears. The thick smear is used to screen for the presence of organisms, and the thin smear is used for species identification. It is important to identify the species, because the treatment of different species can differ. The indirect fluorescent-antibody test is useful for epidemiologic studies but not for diagnosis.

Treatment   Chloroquine is the drug of choice for acute malaria caused by sensitive strains. Chloroquine kills the merozoites, thereby reducing the parasitemia, but does not affect the hypnozoites of *P vivax* and *P ovale* in the liver. These are killed by primaquine, which must be used to prevent relapses. For chloroquine-resistant strains of *P falciparum,* a combination of quinine and Fansidar (sulfadoxine and pyrimethamine) is used.

Prevention **Chemoprophylaxis** of malaria for travelers to areas where *P falciparum* is endemic consists of chloroquine plus Fansidar, although the possibility of serious side effects resulting from the prolonged use of Fansidar limits its use as a prophylactic drug. Travelers to areas where the other plasmodia are found should take chloroquine starting 2 weeks before arrival and continuing for 6 weeks after departure. This should be followed by a 2-week course of primaquine if exposure was high.

Other preventive measures include the use of mosquito netting, window screens, protective clothing, and insect repellents. Communal preventive measures are directed against reducing the mosquito population. Many insecticide sprays, such as DDT, are no longer effective because the mosquitoes have developed resistance. Drainage of stagnant water in swamps and ditches reduces the breeding areas. There is no vaccine, although several are under development.

TOXOPLASMA

Disease   *Toxoplasma gondii* causes toxoplasmosis.

Important Properties   The definitive host is the **domestic cat** and other felines; humans and other mammals are intermediate hosts. Infection of humans begins with the **ingestion of cysts** in undercooked meat or from contact with cat feces. In the small intestine, the cysts rupture and release forms that invade the gut wall, where they are ingested by macrophages and differentiate into rapidly multiplying trophozoites (**tachyzoites**), which kill the cells and infect other cells. Cell-mediated immunity usually limits the spread of tachyzoites, and the parasites enter host cells in the brain, muscle, and other tissues, where they develop into cysts in which the parasites multiply slowly. These forms are called **bradyzoites.** These tissue cysts are both an important diagnostic feature and a source of organisms when the tissue cyst breaks in an immunocompromised patient.

The cycle within the cat begins with the ingestion of cysts in raw meat, eg, mice. Bradyzoites are released from the cysts in the small intestine, infect the mucosal cells, and differentiate into male and female gametocytes, whose gametes fuse to form oocysts that are excreted in cat feces. The cycle is completed when soil contaminated with cat feces is accidentally ingested. Human infection usually occurs from eating undercooked meat, eg, lamb and pork, from animals that grazed in soil contaminated with infected cat feces.

Pathogenesis & Epidemiology   *T gondii* is usually acquired by **ingestion; transplacental transmission** from an infected mother to the fetus occurs also.

Following infection of the intestinal epithelium, the organisms spread to other organs, especially the brain, lungs, liver, and eyes. Progression of the infection is usually limited by a competent immune system. **Cell-mediated immunity** plays the major role, but circulating antibody enhances killing of the organism. Most initial infections are asymptomatic. When contained, the organisms persist as cysts within tissues. There is no inflammation, and the individual remains well unless immunosuppression allows activation of organisms in the cysts.

Congenital infection of the fetus occurs **only** when the mother is infected during pregnancy. If she is infected before the pregnancy, there will be no circulating organisms to pass the placenta. The mother who is reinfected during pregnancy but who has immunity from a previous infection will not transmit the organism to her child. Roughly one-third of mothers infected during pregnancy give birth to infected infants, but only 10% of those infants are symptomatic.

Infection by *T gondii* occurs worldwide. Serologic surveys reveal that in the USA antibodies are found in 5–50% of people in various regions. Infection is usually sporadic, but outbreaks due to ingestion of raw meat or contaminated water occur. Approximately 1% of domestic cats in the USA shed *Toxoplasma* cysts.

Clinical Findings   Primary infection in immunocompetent adults resembles infectious mononucleosis, except that the heterophil antibody test is negative. Congenital infection can result in abortion, stillbirth, or neonatal disease with encephalitis, chorioretinitis, and hepatosplenomegaly. Fever, jaundice, and intracranial calcifications are also seen. Most infected newborns are asymptomatic, but some will develop chorioretinitis or mental retardation months or years later. In immunosuppressed patients, life-threatening disseminated disease occurs, primarily encephalitis.

Laboratory Diagnosis   For the diagnosis of acute and congenital infections, an immuno-fluorescence assay for **IgM antibody** is used. IgM is used to diagnose congenital infection, because IgG can be maternal in origin. Tests of IgG antibody can be used to diagnose acute infections if a significant rise in antibody titer in paired sera is observed.

Microscopic examination of Giemsa-stained preparations shows crescent-shaped tropho-zoites during acute infections. Cysts may be seen in the tissue. The organism can be grown in cell culture. Inoculation into mice can confirm the diagnosis.

Treatment   Congenital toxoplasmosis, whether symptomatic or asymptomatic, should be treated with a combination of a sulfonamide and pyrimethamine. These drugs also constitute the treatment of choice for disseminated disease in immunocompromised patients. Acute toxoplasmosis in an immunocompetent individual is usually self-limited, but any patient with chorioretinitis should be treated.

Prevention   The most effective means of preventing toxoplasmosis is to cook meat thoroughly to kill the cysts. Pregnant women should be especially careful to avoid under-cooked meat and contact with cats. They should refrain from emptying cat litter boxes. Cats should not be fed raw meat.

PNEUMOCYSTIS

Disease   *Pneumocystis carinii* is an important cause of pneumonia in immunocompromised individuals.

Important Properties   The classification and life cycle of *Pneumocystis* are unclear. An analysis of rRNA sequences published in 1988 indicates that *Pneumocystis* should be classified as a **fungus** related to yeasts such as *Saccharomyces cerevisiae*. The organism has been found in domestic animals such as horses and sheep and in a variety of rodents, but it is not known whether these animals form a reservoir for human infection.

Pathogenesis & Epidemiology   Transmission occurs by **inhalation,** and infection is prominent in the lungs. The presence of cysts in the alveoli induces an inflammatory response, resulting in a frothy exudate that blocks oxygen exchange. Pneumonia occurs when host defenses, eg, the number of helper T cells, are reduced. This accounts for the prominence of *Pneumocystis* pneumonia in patients with AIDS and in premature or debilitated infants.

P carinii is distributed worldwide; perhaps 70% of people have been infected. Asymptomatic infection is therefore quite common. Prior to the advent of immunosuppressive therapy, *Pneumocystis* pneumonia was rarely seen in the USA. Its incidence has paralleled the increase in immunosuppression and the rise of AIDS cases.

Clinical Findings   The sudden onset of fever, cough, dyspnea, and tachypnea is typical of *Pneumocystis* pneumonia. Bilateral rales and rhonchi are heard, and the chest x-ray shows a diffuse interstitial pneumonia. In infants, the disease usually has a more gradual onset. The mortality rate of untreated *Pneumocystis* pneumonia approaches 100%, but with treatment about half survive the first episode.

Laboratory Diagnosis   Diagnosis is made by examination of lung tissue obtained by bronchoscopy, bronchial lavage, or open lung biopsy. Sputum is usually less suitable. Cysts containing sporozoites are seen in silver-stained preparations. There is no serologic test, and the organism has not been grown in culture.

Treatment   The treatment of choice is a combination of trimethoprim and sulfamethoxazole. Pentamidine is an alternative drug.

Prevention   Trimethoprim-sulfamethoxazole can be used as **chemoprophylaxis** in immuno-suppressed patients.

TRYPANOSOMA   The genus *Trypanosoma* includes 3 major pathogens: *Trypanosoma cruzi, Trypanosoma gambiense,* and *Trypanosoma rhodesiense.**

1. Trypanosoma cruzi

Disease   *T cruzi* is the cause of Chagas' disease (American trypanosomiasis).

Important Properties   The life cycle involves the **reduviid bug** (*Triatoma,* cone-nose or kissing bug) as the vector and both humans and animals as reservoir hosts. The animal reservoirs include domestic cats and dogs and wild species such as the armadillo, raccoon, and rat as hosts. The cycle in the reduviid bug begins with ingestion of trypomastigotes in the blood of the human or reservoir host. In the insect's gut, they multiply and differentiate first into epimastigotes and then into trypomastigotes. When the bug bites again, the site is contaminated with feces containing trypomastigotes, which enter the blood of the person (or other reservoir) and form nonflagellated amastigotes within host cells. Many cells can be affected, but myocardial, glial, and reticuloendothelial cells are the most frequent sites. To complete the cycle, amastigotes differentiate into trypomastigotes, which enter the blood and are taken up by the reduviid bug.

Pathogenesis & Epidemiology   Chagas' disease occurs primarily in rural Central and South America and rarely in the southern USA. The reduviid bug lives in the walls of rural huts and feeds at night. It bites preferentially around the mouth or eyes, hence the name "kissing bug."

  The amastigotes can kill cells and cause inflammation, consisting mainly of mononuclear cells. **Cardiac muscle** is the most frequently and severely affected tissue. In addition, neuronal damage leads to cardiac arrhythmias and loss of tone in the colon (megacolon) and esophagus (megaesophagus). During the acute phase, there are both trypomastigotes in the blood and amastigotes intracellularly in the tissues. In the chronic phase, amastigotes predominate in the tissue.

Clinical Findings   The acute phase of Chagas' disease consists of facial edema and a nodule (chagoma) near the bite, coupled with fever, lymphadenopathy, and hepatosplenomegaly. The acute phase resolves in about 2 months. Most individuals then remain asymptomatic, but some progress to the chronic form with myocarditis and megacolon. Death from chronic Chagas' disease is usually due to cardiac arrhythmias and failure.

Laboratory Diagnosis   Acute disease is diagnosed by demonstrating the presence of trypomastigotes in thick or thin films of the patient's blood. Both stained and wet preparations should be examined, the latter for motile organisms. Because the trypomastigotes are not numerous in the blood, other diagnostic methods may be required, namely (1) a stained preparation of a bone marrow aspirate or muscle biopsy (which may reveal amastigotes); (2) culture of the organism on special medium; and (3) "**xenodiagnosis**," which consists of allowing an uninfected, laboratory-raised reduviid bug to feed on the patient and, after several weeks, examining the intestinal contents of the bug for the organism.

  Serologic tests can be helpful also. The indirect fluorescent-antibody test is the earliest to become positive. Indirect hemagglutination and complement fixation tests are also available. Diagnosis of chronic disease is difficult, because there are few trypomastigotes in the blood. Xenodiagnosis and serologic tests are used.

Treatment   The drug of choice for the acute phase is nifurtimox, which kills trypomastigotes in the blood but is much less effective against amastigotes in tissue. There is no drug effective against the chronic form.

---

*Taxonomically, the last 2 organisms are morphologically identical species called *T brucei* subspecies *gambiense* and *T brucei* subspecies *rhodesiense,* but the shortened names are used here.

Prevention Prevention involves protection from the reduviid bite, improved housing, and insect control. No prophylactic drug or vaccine is available.

2. Trypanosoma gambiense & Trypanosoma rhodesiense

Disease These pathogens cause sleeping sickness (African trypanosomiasis).

Important Properties The morphology and life cycle of the 2 species are similar. The vector for both is the **tsetse fly**, *Glossina*, but different species of fly are involved for each. Humans are the reservoir for *T gambiense*, whereas *T rhodesiense* has reservoirs both in domestic animals, especially cattle, and wild animals, eg, antelopes.

The 3-week life cycle in the tsetse fly begins with ingestion of trypomastigotes in a blood meal from the reservoir host. They multiply in the insect's gut and then migrate to the salivary glands, where they transform into epimastigotes, multiply further, and then form metacyclic trypomastigotes, which are transmitted by the tsetse fly bite. The organisms in the saliva are injected into the skin, where they enter the bloodstream, differentiate into blood-form trypomastigotes, and multiply, thereby completing the cycle.

These trypanosomes exhibit remarkable **antigenic variation** of their surface glycoproteins, with hundreds of antigenic types found. One antigenic type will coat the surface of the parasites for approximately 10 days, followed by other types in sequence in the new progeny. This variation is due to sequential movement of the glycoprotein genes to a preferential location on the chromosome, where only that specific gene is transcribed into mRNA. These antigenic variations allow the organism to continually evade the host's immune response.

Pathogenesis & Epidemiology The trypomastigotes spread from the skin through the blood to the lymph nodes and the brain. The typical somnolence (**sleeping sickness**) progresses to coma as a result of a demyelinating encephalitis.

In the acute form, a cyclical fever spike (approximately every 2 weeks) occurs that is related to antigenic variation. As antibody-mediated agglutination and lysis of the trypomastigotes occur, the fever subsides. However, a few antigenic variants survive, multiply, and cause a new fever spike. This cycle repeats itself over a long period. The lytic antibody is directed against the surface glycoprotein.

The disease is endemic in sub-Saharan Africa, the natural habitat of the tsetse fly. Both sexes of fly take blood meals and can transmit the disease. The fly is infectious throughout its 2- to 3-month lifetime. *T gambiense* is the species that causes the disease along water courses in west Africa, whereas *T rhodesiense* is found in the arid regions of east Africa. Both species are found in central Africa.

Clinical Findings Although both species cause sleeping sickness, the progress of the disease differs. *T gambiense*-induced disease runs a low-grade chronic course over a few years, whereas *T rhodesiense* causes a more acute, rapidly progressive disease that is usually fatal within several months.

The initial lesion is an indurated skin ulcer (''trypanosomal chancre'') at the site of the fly bite. After the organisms enter the blood, intermittent weekly fever and lymphadenopathy develop. The encephalitis is characterized initially by headache, insomnia, and mood changes, followed by muscle tremors, slurred speech, and apathy that progress to somnolence and coma. Untreated disease is usually fatal as a result of pneumonia.

Laboratory Diagnosis During the early stages, microscopic examination of the blood (either wet films or thick or thin smears) reveals trypomastigotes. An aspirate of the chancre or enlarged lymph node can also demonstrate the parasites. The presence of trypanosomes in the spinal fluid, coupled with an elevated protein level and pleocytosis, indicates that the patient has entered the late, encephalitic stage. Serologic tests can be helpful, especially the ELISA for IgM antibody.

Treatment Treatment must be initiated before the development of encephalitis, because suramin, the most effective drug, does not pass the blood-brain barrier well. Suramin will effect a cure if given early. Pentamidine is an alternative drug. If central nervous system symptoms are present, suramin (to clear the parasitemia) followed by melarsoprol should be given.

Prevention   The most important preventive measure is protection against the fly bite by the use of netting and protective clothing. Clearing the forest around villages and using insecticides are helpful. No vaccine is available.

LEISHMANIA   The genus *Leishmania* includes 4 major pathogens: *Leishmania donovani, Leishmania tropica, Leishmania mexicana,* and *Leishmania braziliensis.*

1. Leishmania donovani

Disease   *L donovani* is the cause of kala-azar (visceral leishmaniasis).

Important Properties   The life cycle involves the **sandfly*** as the vector and a variety of mammals such as dogs, foxes, and rodents as reservoirs. Only female flies are vectors because only they take blood meals (a requirement for egg maturation). When the sandfly sucks blood from an infected host, it ingests **macrophages containing amastigotes.**[†] After dissolution of the macrophages, the freed amastigotes differentiate into promastigotes in the gut. They multiply and then migrate to the pharynx, where they can be transmitted during the next bite. The cycle in the sandfly takes approximately 10 days.

Shortly after an infected sandfly bites a human, the promastigotes are engulfed by macrophages, where they transform into amastigotes. The infected cells die and release progeny amastigotes that infect other macrophages and reticuloendothelial cells. The cycle is completed when the fly ingests macrophages containing the amastigotes.

Pathogenesis & Epidemiology   In visceral leishmaniasis, the organs of the **reticulo-endothelial** system (liver, spleen, and bone marrow) are the most severely affected. Reduced bone marrow activity, coupled with cellular destruction in the spleen, results in anemia, leukopenia, and thrombocytopenia. This leads to secondary infections and a tendency to bleed. The striking **enlargement of the spleen** is due to a combination of proliferating macrophages and sequestered blood cells. The marked increase in IgG is neither specific nor protective.

Kala-azar occurs in 3 distinct epidemiologic patterns. In one area, which includes the Mediterranean basin, the Middle East, southern Russia, and parts of China, the reservoir hosts are primarily dogs and foxes. In sub-Saharan Africa, rats and small carnivores, eg, civets, are the main reservoirs. A third pattern is seen in India and neighboring countries (and Kenya), in which humans appear to be the only reservoir and the disease is transmitted by various domesticated species of sandfly.

Clinical Findings   Symptoms begin with intermittent fever, weakness, and weight loss. Massive enlargement of the spleen is characteristic. Hyperpigmentation of the skin is seen in light-skinned patients (kala-azar means ''**black sickness**''). The course of the disease runs for months to years. Initially, patients feel reasonably well despite persistent fever. As anemia, leukopenia, and thrombocytopenia become more profound, weakness, infection, and gastrointestinal bleeding occur. Untreated severe disease is nearly always fatal as a result of secondary infection.

Laboratory Diagnosis   Diagnosis is usually made by detecting amastigotes in a bone marrow, spleen, or lymph node biopsy or ''touch'' preparation. The organisms can also be cultured. Serologic (indirect immunofluorescence) tests are positive in most patients. Although not diagnostic, a very high concentration of IgG is indicative of infection. A skin test using a crude homogenate of promastigotes (leishmanin) as the antigen is available. The skin test is negative during active disease but positive in patients who have recovered.

---

*Phlebotomus species in the Old World; *Lutzomyia* species in South America.

[†]Amastigotes are nonflagellated, in contrast to promastigotes, which have a flagellum with a characteristic anterior kinetoplast.

Treatment The treatment is sodium stibogluconate, a pentavalent antimony compound. With proper therapy, the mortality rate is near 5%. Recovery results in permanent immunity.

Prevention Prevention involves protection from sandfly bites (use of netting, protective clothing, and insect repellents) and insecticide spraying.

2. Leishmania tropica, Leishmania mexicana, & Leishmania braziliensis

Disease *L tropica* and *L mexicana* both cause cutaneous leishmaniasis; the former organism is found in the Old World, whereas the latter is found only in the Americas. *L braziliensis* causes mucocutaneous leishmaniasis (espundia), which occurs only in Central and South America.

Important Properties The vectors for these 3 parasites are **sandflies,** ie, *Phlebotomus* species in the Old World and *Lutzomyia* species in the New World. The main reservoirs for these organisms are forest rodents. The life cycle of these parasites is essentially the same as that of *L donovani.*

Pathogenesis & Epidemiology The lesions are confined to the skin in cutaneous leishmaniasis and to the mucous membranes, cartilage, and skin in mucocutaneous leishmaniasis. A granulomatous response occurs, and a necrotic ulcer forms at the bite site. The lesions tend to become superinfected with bacteria.

Old World cutaneous leishmaniasis (Oriental sore, Delhi boil), caused by *L tropica,* is endemic in the Middle East, Africa, and India. New World cutaneous leishmaniasis (chicle ulcer, bay sore), caused by *L mexicana,* is found in Central and South America. Mucocutaneous leishmaniasis, caused by *L braziliensis,* occurs mostly in Brazil and Central America, primarily in forestry and construction workers.

Clinical Findings The initial lesion of cutaneous leishmaniasis is a red papule at the bite site, usually on an exposed extremity. This enlarges slowly to form multiple satellite nodules that coalesce and ulcerate. There is usually a single lesion that heals spontaneously in patients with a competent immune system. However, in certain individuals, if cell-mediated immunity does not develop, the lesions can spread to involve large areas of skin and contain enormous numbers of organisms. (Compare tuberculoid and lepromatous leprosy, Chapter 21.)

Mucocutaneous leishmaniasis begins with a papule at the bite site, but then metastatic lesions form, usually at the mucocutaneous junction of the nose and mouth. Disfiguring granulomatous, ulcerating lesions destroy nasal cartilage but not adjacent bone. These lesions heal slowly, if at all. Death can occur from secondary infection.

Laboratory Diagnosis Diagnosis is usually made microscopically by demonstrating the presence of **amastigotes** in a smear taken from the skin lesion. The leishmanin skin test becomes positive when the skin ulcer appears and can be used to diagnose cases outside the endemic area.

Treatment The drug of choice is sodium stibogluconate, but results are frequently unsatisfactory.

Prevention Prevention involves protection from sandfly bites by the use of netting, window screens, protective clothing, and insect repellents.

Review Questions

1. Distinguish between sporogony and schizogony in the life cycle of plasmodia.
2. What happens to the plasmodia during the (a) exoerythrocytic and (b) erythrocytic stages?
3. Where does the sexual cycle of plasmodia occur?
4. What is the main mode of transmission of plasmodia? their typical pathogenetic feature?
5. What is "blackwater fever"? What *Plasmodium* species causes it? Why?
6. What causes the recurrent fever pattern seen in malaria?

7. How is the laboratory diagnosis of malaria made?
8. Describe the chemoprophylaxis of malaria and the problem of resistant strains.
9. What animal is the reservoir for *Toxoplasma gondii*? How is it transmitted from animals to humans? What is the other important mode of transmission?
10. What are the differences between *Toxoplasma* infection in an immunocompetent adult and a newborn?
11. How is the laboratory diagnosis of toxoplasmosis made?
12. How can toxoplasmosis be prevented?
13. What is the mode of transmission of *Pneumocystis*?
14. What is the predisposing factor to Pneumocystis pneumonia?
15. How is the laboratory diagnosis of *Pneumocystis* pneumonia made?
16. What diseases are caused by *Trypanosoma cruzi*? *Trypanosoma gambiense*?
17. What is the vector for *T cruzi*? *T gambiense*?
18. In what geographic area does Chagas' disease primarily occur?
19. What is the pathogenesis of Chagas' disease? of sleeping sickness?
20. How is the laboratory diagnosis of these diseases made?
21. How do trypanosomes evade the host immune system?
22. What diseases are caused by *Leishmania donovani*? *Leishmania tropica*?
23. What is the vector for the *Leishmania* species?
24. In what geographic areas does kala-azar occur?
25. What types of cells are primarily affected in kala-azar? What is its pathogenesis?
26. How is the laboratory diagnosis of kala-azar made?

Minor Protozoan Pathogens

53

ACANTHAMOEBA & NAEGLERIA   *Acanthamoeba* and *Naegleria* species are 2 free-living **amebas** that cause **meningoencephalitis.** The organisms are found in warm freshwater lakes and in soil. Their life cycle involves trophozoite and cyst stages. Cysts are quite resistant and are not killed by chlorination.

Naegleria trophozoites usually enter the body through mucous membranes while an individual is **swimming.** They can penetrate the nasal mucosa and cribriform plate to produce a purulent meningitis and encephalitis that are usually rapidly fatal. *Acanthamoeba* is carried into the skin or eyes during trauma. *Acanthamoeba* infections occur primarily in immuno-compromised individuals, whereas *Naegleria* infections occur in otherwise healthy persons, usually children. In the USA, these rare infections occur mainly in the southern states and California.

Diagnosis is made by finding amebas in the spinal fluid. The prognosis is poor even in treated cases. There is no effective therapy; occasionally, amphotericin B has resulted in recovery.

BABESIA   *Babesia microti* causes babesiosis, a zoonosis acquired chiefly in the coastal areas and islands off the northeastern coast of the USA, eg, Nantucket Island. The sporozoan organism is endemic in rodents and is transmitted by the bite of the **tick** *Ixodes dammini*. *Babesia* infects red blood cells, causing them to lyse, but, unlike plasmodia, it has no exoerythrocytic phase. Asplenic patients are affected more severely.

The influenzalike symptoms begin gradually and may last for several weeks. Hepatospleno-megaly and anemia occur. Diagnosis is made by seeing intraerythrocytic ring-shaped parasites on Giemsa-stained blood smears. Unlike the case with plasmodia, there is no pigment in the erythrocytes. Combined therapy with quinine and clindamycin may be effective. Prevention involves protection from tick bites and, if a person is bitten, prompt removal of the tick.

BALANTIDIUM Balantidium coli is the **only ciliated protozoan** that causes human disease, ie, **diarrhea.** It is found worldwide but only infrequently in the USA. Domestic animals, especially pigs, are the main reservoir for the organism, and humans are infected after ingesting the cysts in food or water contaminated with animal or human feces. The trophozoites excyst in the small intestine, travel to the colon, and, by burrowing into the wall, cause an ulcer similar to that of *Entamoeba histolytica.* However, unlike the case with *E histolytica,* extraintestinal lesions do not occur.

Most infected individuals are asymptomatic; diarrhea rarely occurs. Diagnosis is made by finding large ciliated trophozoites or large cysts with a characteristic V-shaped nucleus in the stool. There are no serologic tests. The treatment of choice is tetracycline. Prevention consists of avoiding contamination of food and water by domestic-animal feces.

ISOSPORA *Isospora belli* is an intestinal protozoan that can cause **diarrhea,** especially in **immunocompromised patients,** eg, those with AIDS. Its life cycle parallels that of other members of the Coccidia* with sexual and asexual cycles. The organism is acquired by fecal-oral transmission of oocysts from either human or animal sources. The oocysts excyst in the upper small intestine and can invade the mucosa, causing destruction of the brush border.

The disease in immunocompromised patients presents as a chronic, profuse, watery diarrhea. The pathogenesis of the diarrhea is unknown. Diagnosis is made by finding the typical oocysts in fecal specimens. Serologic tests are not available. The treatment of choice is trimethoprim-sulfamethoxazole.

54

Cestodes

Platyhelminthes (platy means flat; helminth means worm) are divided into 2 classes: Cestoda (tapeworms) and Trematoda (flukes). Tapeworms consist of a rounded head, called a **scolex,** and a flat body of multiple segments called **proglottids.** The scolex has specialized means of attaching to the intestinal wall, namely suckers, hooks, or sucking grooves. The worm grows by adding new proglottids from its germinal center next to the scolex. The oldest proglottids at the distal end are gravid and produce many eggs, which are excreted in the feces and transmitted to various intermediate hosts such as cattle, pigs, and fish. Humans usually acquire the infection when undercooked flesh containing the larvae is ingested. In certain instances, eg, cysticercosis and hydatid disease, the eggs are ingested and the resulting larvae cause the disease.

There are 4 medically important cestodes: *Taenia solium, Taenia saginata, Diphyllobothrium latum,* and *Echinococcus granulosus.* Their features are summarized in Table 54–1. Two cestodes of lesser importance, *Echinococcus multilocularis* and *Hymenolepis nana,* are described on p. 240.

TAENIA There are 2 important human pathogens in the genus *Taenia: T solium* (the pork tapeworm) and *T saginata* (the beef tapeworm).

1. *Taenia solium*

Diseases The adult form of *Taenia solium* causes taeniasis. *T solium* larvae cause cysticercosis.

---

*Coccidia is a subclass of Sporozoa.

Table 54–1. Features of medically important cestodes (tapeworms).

Cestode	Mode of Transmission	Intermediate Host(s)	Main Sites Affected in Human Body	Diagnosis	Treatment
Taenia solium	(A) Ingest larvae in undercooked pork	Pigs	Intestine	Proglottids in stool	Praziquantel (adult worm)
	(B) Ingest eggs in food or water contaminated with human feces		Cysticerci in brain and eyes	Biopsy, CT scan	Praziquantel or surgery if necessary (cysticerci)
Taenia saginata	Ingest larvae in undercooked beef	Cattle	Intestine	Proglottids in stool	Praziquantel
Diphyllobothrium latum	Ingest larvae in undercooked fish	Copepods and fish	Intestine	Operculated eggs in stool	Praziquantel
Echinococcus granulosus	Ingest eggs in food contaminated with dog feces	Sheep	Hydatid cyst in liver, lung, brain	Biopsy, CT scan, serology	Surgical removal of cyst

Important Properties *T solium* can be identified by its scolex with 4 **suckers and circle of hooks** and by its gravid proglottids, which have 5–10 primary uterine branches. The eggs appear the same microscopically as those of *T saginata* and *Echinococcus* species.

Humans are infected by eating raw or undercooked **pork** containing the larvae, called **cysticerci.** (A cysticercus consists of a pea-sized fluid-filled bladder with an invaginated scolex.) In the small intestine, the larvae attach to the gut wall and take about 3 months to grow into adult worms measuring up to 5 m. The gravid terminal proglottids detach daily, are passed in the feces, and are eaten by pigs. A 6-hooked embryo (oncosphere) emerges from each egg in the pig's intestine. The embryos burrow into a blood vessel and are carried to skeletal muscle. They develop into cysticerci in the muscle, where they remain until eaten by a human. Humans are the definitive hosts, and pigs are the intermediate hosts.

A different and far more dangerous sequence occurs when a person **ingests the eggs** in food or water that has been fecally contaminated. The eggs hatch in the small intestine, and the oncospheres burrow through the wall into a blood vessel. They can disseminate to many organs, especially the eyes and brain, where they encyst to form cysticerci.

Pathogenesis & Epidemiology The adult tapeworm attached to the intestinal wall causes little damage. The **cysticerci,** on the other hand, can become very large, especially in the **brain,** where they manifest as a **space-occupying lesion.** Living cysticerci do not cause inflammation, but when they die they can release substances that provoke an inflammatory response. Eventually, the cysticerci calcify and can be seen on x-ray.

The epidemiology of taeniasis and cysticercosis is related to the access of pigs to human feces and to consumption of raw or undercooked pork. The disease occurs worldwide but is endemic in areas of Asia, South America, and eastern Europe. Most cases in the USA are imported.

Clinical Findings Most patients with adult tapeworms are asymptomatic, but anorexia and diarrhea can occur. Some may notice proglottids in the stools. Cysticercosis in the brain causes headache, vomiting, and seizures. Cysticercosis in the eyes can appear as uveitis or retinitis, or the larvae can be visualized floating in the vitreous.

Laboratory Diagnosis Identification of *T solium* consists of finding gravid proglottids with 5–10 primary uterine branches in the stools. In contrast, *T saginata* proglottids have 15–20 primary uterine branches. Eggs are found in the stools less often than are proglottids. Diagnosis of cysticercosis depends on demonstrating the presence of the cyst in tissue by x-ray or computerized tomography (CT) scan.

Treatment The treatment of choice for the intestinal worms is praziquantel. Although asymptomatic, patients should be treated to prevent autoinfection with the eggs, leading to cysticercosis. Surgical excision of the cysticercus may be necessary, but a massive dosage of praziquantel should be tried first.

Prevention   Prevention of taeniasis involves cooking pork adequately and preventing pigs from ingesting human feces by disposing of waste properly. Prevention of cysticercosis consists of treatment of patients with taeniasis to prevent autoinfection plus observation of proper hygiene, including hand washing, to prevent contamination of food with the eggs.

2. *Taenia saginata*

Disease   *Taenia saginata* causes taeniasis. *T saginata* larvae do not cause cysticercosis.

Important Properties   *T saginata* has a scolex with 4 suckers but, in contrast to *T solium*, **no hooklets.** Its gravid proglottids have 15–25 primary uterine branches, in contrast to *T solium* proglottids, which have 5–10. The eggs are morphologically indistinguishable from those of *T solium*.

Humans are infected by eating raw or undercooked **beef** containing larvae (cysticerci). In the small intestine, the larvae attach to the gut wall and take about 3 months to grow into adult worms measuring up to 10 m. The gravid proglottids detach, are passed in the feces, and are eaten by cattle. The embryos **(oncospheres)** emerge from the eggs in the cow's intestine and burrow into a blood vessel, where they are carried to skeletal muscle. In the muscle, they develop into cysticerci. The cycle is completed when the cysticerci are ingested. Humans are the definitive hosts and cattle the intermediate hosts. Unlike *T solium*, *T saginata* **does not cause cysticercosis** in humans.

Pathogenesis & Epidemiology   Little damage results from the presence of the adult worm in the small intestine. The epidemiology of taeniasis caused by *T saginata* is related to the access of cattle to human feces and to the consumption of raw or undercooked beef. The disease occurs worldwide but is endemic in Africa, South America, and eastern Europe. In the USA, most cases are imported.

Clinical Findings   Most patients with adult tapeworms are asymptomatic. In some, proglottids appear in the stools and may even protrude from the anus.

Laboratory Diagnosis   Identification of *T saginata* consists of finding gravid proglottids with 15–20 uterine branches in the stools. Eggs are found in the stools less often than are the proglottids.

Treatment   The treatment of choice is praziquantel.

Prevention   Prevention involves cooking beef adequately and preventing cattle from consuming human feces by disposing of waste properly.

DIPHYLLOBOTHRIUM

Disease   *Diphyllobothrium latum,* the fish tapeworm, causes diphyllobothriasis.

Important Properties   In contrast to the other cestodes, which have suckers, the scolex of *D latum* has 2 elongated **sucking grooves** by which the worm attaches to the intestinal wall. The scolex has no hooks, unlike *T solium* and *Echinococcus*. The proglottids are wider than they are long, and the gravid uterus is in the form of a rosette. Unlike other tapeworm eggs, which are round, *D latum* eggs are oval and have a lidlike opening **(operculum)** at one end. *D latum* is the longest of the tapeworms, measuring up to 13 m.

Humans are infected by ingesting raw or undercooked **fish** containing larvae (called plerocercoid or sparganum larvae). In the small intestine, the larvae attach to the gut wall and develop into adult worms. Gravid proglottids release fertilized eggs through a genital pore, and the eggs are then passed in the stools. The immature eggs must be deposited in fresh water for the life cycle to continue. The embryos emerge from the eggs and are eaten by tiny copepod crustacea (first intermediate hosts). There, the embryos differentiate and form procercoid larvae in the body cavity. When the copepod is eaten by freshwater fish, eg, pike, trout, and perch, the larvae differentiate into plerocercoids in the muscle of the fish (second intermediate host). The cycle is completed when raw or undercooked fish is eaten by humans (definitive hosts).

Pathogenesis & Epidemiology   Infection by *D latum* causes little damage in the small intestine. In some individuals, megaloblastic anemia occurs as a result of vitamin B_{12} deficiency caused by preferential uptake of the vitamin by the worm.

The epidemiology of *D latum* infection is related to the ingestion of raw or inadequately cooked fish and to contamination of bodies of fresh water with human feces. The disease is found worldwide but is endemic in areas where eating raw fish is the custom, such as Scandinavia, northern Russia, Japan, Canada, and certain north-central states of the USA.

Clinical Findings   Most patients are asymptomatic, but abdominal discomfort and diarrhea can occur.

Laboratory Diagnosis   Diagnosis depends on finding the typical eggs, ie, oval, yellow-brown eggs with an operculum at one end, in the stools. There is no serologic test.

Treatment   The treatment of choice is praziquantel.

Prevention   Prevention involves adequate cooking of fish and proper disposal of human feces.

ECHINOCOCCUS

Disease   The larva of *Echinococcus granulosus* (dog tapeworm) causes unilocular hydatid cyst disease. Multilocular hydatid disease is caused by *E multilocularis,* which is a minor pathogen and is discussed below.

Important Properties   *E granulosus* is composed of a scolex and only 3 proglottids, making it **one of the smallest tapeworms. Dogs** are the most important definitive hosts. The intermediate hosts are usually **sheep.** Humans are almost always dead-end intermediate hosts.

In the typical life cycle, worms in the dog's intestine liberate thousands of eggs, which are ingested by sheep (or humans). The oncosphere embryos emerge in the small intestine and migrate primarily to the liver but also to the lungs, bones, and brain. The embryos develop into large fluid-filled **hydatid cysts,** the inner germinal layer of which generates many protoscoleces within ''brood capsules.'' The life cycle is completed when the entrails (eg, liver containing hydatid cysts) of slaughtered sheep are eaten by dogs.

Pathogenesis & Epidemiology   *E granulosus* usually forms one large fluid-filled cyst (unilocular) that contains thousands of individual scoleces as well as many daughter cysts. The cyst acts as a space-occupying lesion, putting pressure on adjacent tissue. The outer layer of the cyst is thick, fibrous tissue produced by the host. The cyst fluid contains parasite antigens, which can sensitize the host. Later, if the cyst ruptures spontaneously or during trauma or surgical removal, life-threatening **anaphylaxis can** occur. Rupture of a cyst can also spread protoscoleces widely.

The disease is found primarily in shepherds living in the Mediterranean region, the Middle East, and Australia. In the USA, the western states report the largest number of cases.

Clinical Findings   Many individuals with hydatid cysts are asymptomatic, but **liver cysts** may cause hepatic dysfunction. Cysts in the lungs can erode into a bronchus, causing bloody sputum, and cerebral cysts can present with headache and focal neurologic signs. Rupture of the cyst can cause fatal anaphylactic shock.

Laboratory Diagnosis   Diagnosis is based either on microscopic examination demonstrating the presence of brood capsules containing multiple protoscoleces or on serologic tests, eg, the indirect hemagglutination test.

Treatment   Treatment involves surgical removal of the cyst. Extreme care must be exercised to prevent release of the protoscoleces during surgery. A protoscolicidal agent, eg, hypertonic saline, should be injected into the cyst to kill the organisms and prevent accidental dissemination. Mebendazole can be given in inoperable cases.

Prevention   Prevention of human disease involves not feeding the entrails of slaughtered sheep to dogs.

CESTODES OF MINOR IMPORTANCE

Echinococcus multilocularis   Many of the features of this organism are the same as those of *E granulosus,* but the definitive hosts are mainly foxes and the intermediate hosts are various rodents. Humans are infected by accidental ingestion of food contaminated with fox feces. The disease occurs primarily in hunters and trappers and is endemic in northern Europe, Siberia, and the western provinces of Canada. In the USA, it occurs in North and South Dakota, Minnesota, and Alaska.

Within the human liver, the larvae form multiloculated cysts with few protoscoleces. No outer fibrous capsule forms, so the cysts continue to proliferate, producing a honeycomb effect of hundreds of small vesicles. The clinical picture usually involves jaundice and weight loss. The prognosis is poor. Mebendazole treatment may be successful in some cases. Surgical removal is rarely feasible.

Hymenolepis nana   *H nana* (dwarf tapeworm) is the **most frequently** found tapeworm in the USA. It is only 3–5 cm in length and is different from other tapeworms, because its eggs are **directly infectious** for humans; ie, ingested eggs can develop into adult worms without an intermediate host. Within the duodenum, the eggs hatch and differentiate into cysticercoid larvae and then into adult worms. Gravid proglottids detach, disintegrate, and release fertilized eggs. The eggs either pass in the stool or can reinfect the small intestine (autoinfection). In contrast to infection by other tapeworms, where only one adult worm is present, many *H nana* worms (sometimes hundreds) are found.

Infection causes little damage, and most patients are asymptomatic. The organism is found worldwide, commonly in the tropics. In the USA, it is most prevalent in the southeastern states, usually in children. Diagnosis is based on finding eggs in stools. The characteristic feature of *H nana* eggs is the 8–10 polar filaments lying between the membrane of the 6-hooked larva and the outer shell. The treatment is praziquantel. Prevention consists of good personal hygiene and avoidance of fecal contamination of food and water.

Review Questions

1. Which cestode causes cysticercosis?
2. What is the pathogenesis of cysticercosis?
3. How is *Taenia solium* transmitted? *Taenia saginata? Diphyllobothrium latum?*
4. What is the difference in appearance of the scoleces of *T, solium, T saginata,* and *D latum?*
5. How is the laboratory diagnosis of these 3 cestodes made?
6. How can (a) taeniasis, (b) cysticercosis, and (c) diphyllobothriasis be prevented?
7. What is the treatment for these 3 diseases?
8. Which cestode causes unilocular hydatid cyst disease?
9. How is the agent of unilocular hydatid cyst disease acquired by humans? In what population is the disease endemic? Why? What animal is the definitive host?
10. What is inside the hydatid cyst? Why is this important during surgical removal of the cyst? What is done to minimize risk during removal?

Trematodes

55

Trematoda (flukes) and Cestoda (tapeworms) are the 2 large classes of parasites in the phylum Platyhelminthes. The most important trematodes are *Schistosoma* species (blood flukes), *Clonorchis sinensis* (liver fluke), and *Paragonimus westermani* (lung fluke). Schistosomes have by far the greatest impact in terms of the number of people infected, morbidity, and mortality. Features of the medically important trematodes are summarized in Table 55–1. Three trematodes of lesser importance, *Fasciola hepatica, Fasciolopsis buski,* and *Heterophyes heterophyes,* are described later in the chapter.

The life cycle of the medically important trematodes involves a sexual cycle in humans and asexual reproduction in **freshwater snails** (intermediate hosts). Transmission to humans takes place either via penetration of the skin by the **free-swimming cercariae** of the schistosomes or via **ingestion of cysts** in undercooked (raw) fish or crabs in *Clonorchis* and *Paragonimus* infection, respectively.

Trematodes that cause human disease are not endemic in the USA. However, immigrants from tropical areas, especially Southeast Asia, are frequently infected.

SCHISTOSOMA

Disease *Schistosoma* causes schistosomiasis. *Schistosoma mansoni* and *Schistosoma japonicum* affect the gastrointestinal tract* whereas *Schistosoma hematobium* affects the urinary tract.

Important Properties In contrast to the other trematodes, which are hermaphrodites, adult schistosomes exist as **separate sexes** but live attached to each other. The female resides in a groove in the male, the "schist," where he continuously fertilizes her eggs. The 3 species can be distinguished by the appearance of their eggs in the microscope: *S mansoni* eggs have a **prominent lateral spine,** whereas *S japonicum* eggs have a very small lateral spine and *S hematobium* eggs have a **terminal spine.** *S mansoni* and *S japonicum* adults live in the **mesenteric veins,** whereas *S hematobium* lives in the veins draining the **urinary bladder.** Schistosomes are therefore known as "**blood flukes.**"

Humans are infected when the free-swimming, fork-tailed **cercariae** penetrate the skin. They differentiate to larvae (schistosomula), enter the blood, and are carried via the veins into the arterial circulation. Those that enter the superior mesenteric artery pass into the portal circulation and reach the liver, where they mature into adult flukes. *S mansoni* and *S japonicum* adults migrate against the portal flow to reside in the mesenteric venules.

Table 55–1. Features of medically important trematodes (flukes).

Trematode	Mode of Transmission	Main Sites Affected	Intermediate Host(s)	Diagnostic Features of Eggs	Endemic Area(s)	Treatment
Schistosoma mansoni	Penetrate skin	Veins of colon	Snail	Large lateral spine	Africa, Latin America (Caribbean)	Praziquantel
Schistosoma japonicum	Penetrate skin	Veins of small intestine, liver	Snail	Small lateral spine	Orient	Praziquantel
Schistosoma hematobium	Penetrate skin	Urinary bladder	Snail	Large terminal spine	Africa, Middle East	Praziquantel
Clonorchis sinensis	Ingested with raw fish	Liver	Snail and fish	Operculated	Orient	Praziquantel
Paragonimus westermani	Ingested with raw crab	Lung	Snail and crab	Operculated	Orient, India	Praziquantel

*as does Schistosoma mekongi

S hematobium adults reach the bladder veins through the venous plexus between the rectum and the bladder.

In their definitive venous site, the female lays fertilized eggs, which penetrate the vascular endothelium and enter the gut or bladder lumen, respectively. The eggs are excreted in the stools or urine and must enter fresh water to hatch. Once hatched, the ciliated larvae (miracidia) penetrate **snails** and undergo further development and multiplication to produce many cercariae. (The 3 schistosomes use different species of snails as intermediate hosts.) Cercariae leave the snails, enter fresh water, and complete the cycle by penetrating human skin.

Pathogenesis & Epidemiology Most of the pathology is due to the presence of eggs in the liver, spleen, or wall of the gut or bladder. Eggs in the liver induce granulomas, which lead to fibrosis, hepatomegaly, and portal hypertension. The granulomas are formed in response to antigens secreted by the eggs. Hepatocytes are usually undamaged, and liver function tests remain normal. Portal hypertension leads to **splenomegaly.**

S mansoni eggs damage the wall of the distal colon (inferior mesenteric venules), whereas *S japonicum* eggs damage the walls of both the small and large intestines (superior and inferior mesenteric venules). The damage is due both to digestion of tissue by proteolytic enzymes produced by the egg and to the host's inflammatory response. The eggs of *S hematobium* in the wall of the bladder induce granulomas and fibrosis, which can lead to **carcinoma of the bladder.**

Schistosomes have evolved a remarkable process for **evading the host defenses.** There is evidence that their surface becomes coated with host antigens, thereby limiting the ability of the immune system to recognize them as foreign.

The epidemiology of schistosomiasis depends on the presence of the specific freshwater snails that serve as intermediate hosts. *S mansoni* is found in Africa and Latin America (including Puerto Rico), whereas *S hematobium* is found in Africa and the Middle East. *S japonicum* is found only in the Orient and is the only one for which domestic animals, eg, water buffalo and pigs, act as important reservoirs. More than 150 million people in the tropical areas of Africa, Asia, and Latin America are affected.

Clinical Findings Most patients are asymptomatic, but chronic infections may become symptomatic. The acute stage, which begins shortly after cercarial penetration, consists of itching and dermatitis followed 2–3 weeks later by fever, chills, diarrhea, lymphadenopathy, and hepatosplenomegaly. Eosinophilia is seen in response to the migrating larvae. This stage usually resolves spontaneously.

The chronic stage causes significant morbidity and mortality. In patients with *S mansoni* and *S japonicum* infections, gastrointestinal hemorrhage, hepatomegaly, and massive splenomegaly develop. The most common cause of death is exsanguination from ruptured esophageal varices. Patients infected with *S hematobium* have hematuria as their chief early complaint. Superimposed bacterial urinary tract infections occur frequently.

"Swimmer's itch," a frequent problem in many lakes in the USA, is due to penetration of the skin by the cercariae of nonhuman schistosomes which are incapable of replicating in humans.

Laboratory Diagnosis Diagnosis depends on finding the characteristic ova in the feces or urine. The large lateral spine of *S mansoni* and the rudimentary spine of *S japonicum* are typical, as is the large terminal spine of *S hematobium*. Serologic tests are not useful.

Treatment Praziquantel is the treatment choice for all 3 species.

Prevention Prevention involves proper disposal of human waste and eradication of the snail host when possible. Swimming in endemic areas should be avoided.

CLONORCHIS

Disease *Clonorchis sinensis* causes clonorchiasis (Oriental liver fluke infection).

Important Properties Humans are infected by eating raw or undercooked **fish** containing the encysted larvae (metacercariae). Following excystation in the duodenum, immature flukes enter the **biliary ducts** and differentiate into adults. The hermaphroditic adults produce eggs, which are excreted in the feces. Upon reaching fresh water, the eggs are ingested by snails,* which are the first intermediate hosts. The eggs hatch within the gut and differentiate first to form larvae (rediae), then into many free-swimming cercariae. Cercariae encyst under the scales of certain freshwater fish (second intermediate hosts), which are then eaten by humans.

Pathogenesis & Epidemiology In some infections, the inflammatory response can cause hyperplasia and fibrosis of the biliary tract, but often there are no lesions. Clonorchiasis is endemic to China, Japan, Korea, and Indochina, where it affects about 20 million people. It is seen in the USA among immigrants from these endemic areas.

Clinical Findings Most infections are asymptomatic. In patients with a heavy worm burden, upper abdominal pain, anorexia, hepatomegaly, and eosinophilia can occur.

Laboratory Diagnosis Diagnosis is made by finding the typical small, brownish, operculated eggs in the stool. Serologic tests are not useful.

Treatment Praziquantel is an effective drug.

Prevention Prevention centers on adequate cooking of fish and proper disposal of human waste.

PARAGONIMUS

Disease *Paragonimus westermani,* the lung fluke, causes paragonimiasis.

Important Properties Humans are infected by eating raw **crab meat** containing the encysted larvae (metacercariae). Following excystation in the small intestine, immature flukes penetrate the intestinal wall and migrate through the diaphragm into the **lung** parenchyma. They differentiate into hermaphroditic adults and produce eggs that enter the bronchioles and are coughed up or swallowed. Eggs in either sputum or feces that reach fresh water hatch into miracidia, which enter snails (first intermediate hosts). There, they differentiate first into larvae (rediae) and then into many free-swimming cercariae. The cercariae infect and encyst in freshwater crabs (second intermediate hosts). The cycle is completed when undercooked infected crabs are eaten by humans.

Pathogenesis & Epidemiology Within the lung, the worms exist in a fibrous capsule that communicates with a bronchiole. Secondary bacterial infection frequently occurs, resulting in bloody sputum. Paragonimiasis is endemic in the Orient and India. In the USA, it occurs in immigrants from endemic areas.

Clinical Findings The main symptom is a chronic cough with bloody sputum. Dyspnea, pleuritic chest pain, and recurrent attacks of bacterial pneumonia occur. The disease can resemble tuberculosis.

Laboratory Diagnosis Diagnosis is made by finding the typical operculated eggs in sputum or feces. Serologic tests are not useful.

Treatment Praziquantel is the treatment of choice.

Prevention Cooking crabs properly is the best method of prevention.

TREMATODES OF MINOR IMPORTANCE

Fasciola *F hepatica,* the sheep liver fluke, causes disease primarily in sheep and other domestic animals in Latin America, Africa, Europe, and China. Humans are infected by

---

*The genus of snail varies with location.

eating watercress (or other aquatic plants) contaminated by larvae (metacercariae) that excyst in the duodenum, penetrate the gut wall, and reach the liver, where they mature into adults. Hermaphroditic adults in the bile ducts produce eggs that are excreted in the feces. The eggs hatch in fresh water, and miracidia enter the snails. Miracidia develop into cercariae, which then encyst on aquatic vegetation. Sheep and humans eat the plants, thus completing the life cycle. Humans can also acquire the organism by eating raw sheep liver, in which case adult flukes attach to the pharynx and larynx. This disease (halzoun) is confined to the Middle East.

Symptoms are due primarily to the presence of the adult worm in the biliary tract. In early infection, right-upper-quadrant pain, fever, and hepatomegaly can occur, but most infections are asymptomatic. Months or years later, obstructive jaundice can occur. Halzoun is a painful pharyngitis caused by the presence of adult flukes on the posterior pharyngeal wall.

Diagnosis is made by identification of eggs in the feces. There is no serologic test. Praziquantel and bithional are effective drugs. Adult flukes in the pharynx and larynx can be removed surgically. Prevention involves not eating wild aquatic vegetables or raw sheep liver.

Fasciolopsis   *F buski* is an intestinal parasite of humans and pigs that is endemic to Asia and India. Humans are infected by **eating aquatic vegetation** that carries the cysts. After excysting in the small intestine, they attach to the mucosa and differentiate into adults. Eggs are passed in the feces; on reaching fresh water, they differentiate into miracidia. The ciliated miracidia penetrate snails and, after several stages, develop into cercariae that encyst on aquatic vegetation. The cycle is completed when plants carrying the cysts are eaten.

Pathology is due to damage of the intestinal mucosa by the adult fluke. Most infections are asymptomatic, but ulceration, abscess formation, and hemorrhage can occur. Diagnosis is based on finding typical eggs in the feces. Praziquantel is the treatment of choice. Prevention consists of proper disposal of human sewage.

Heterophyes   *H heterophyes* is an intestinal parasite of people living in Africa, the Middle East, and Asia who are infected by **eating raw fish** containing cysts. Larvae excyst in the small intestine, attach to the mucosa, and develop into adults. Eggs are passed in the feces and, on reaching brackish water, are ingested by snails. After several developmental stages, cercariae are produced that encyst under the scales of certain fish. The cycle is completed when fish carrying the infectious cysts are eaten.

Pathology is due to inflammation of the intestinal epithelium as a result of the presence of the adult flukes. Most infections are asymptomatic, but abdominal pain and nonbloody diarrhea can occur. Diagnosis is based on finding the typical eggs in the feces. Praziquantel is the treatment of choice. Prevention consists of proper disposal of human sewage.

Review Questions

1. The life cycle of *Schistosoma, Clonorchis,* and *Paragonimus* involves asexual reproduction in which animal?
2. What is the difference in the mode of transmission between *Schistosoma, Clonorchis,* and *Paragonimus?*
3. How do the 3 species of *Schistosoma* differ in (a) location of adults in the human body and (b) appearance of eggs?
4. What is the cause of swimmer's itch?
5. How is the laboratory diagnosis of (a) the 3 *Schistosoma* species, (b) *Clonorchis,* and (c) *Paragonimus* made?
6. What is the treatment of choice for (a) *Schistosoma,* (b) *Clonorchis,* and (c) *Paragonimus?* How can infection by these trematodes be prevented?
7. In general, which of the trematodes are found in (a) Latin America, (b) Africa, and (c) the Orient?

Nematodes

56

Nematodes (also known as Nemathelminthes) are nonsegmented roundworms with a cylindrical body and a complete digestive tract including mouth and anus. The body is covered with a noncellular, highly resistant coating called a cuticle. Nematodes have separate sexes; the female is usually larger than the male. The male typically has a coiled tail.

The medically important nematodes can be divided into 2 categories according to their primary location in the body, namely **intestinal** and **tissue** nematodes.

(1) The intestinal nematodes include *Enterobius* (pinworm), *Trichuris* (whipworm), *Ascaris* (giant roundworm), *Necator* and *Ancylostoma* (the 2 hookworms), *Strongyloides* (small roundworm), and *Trichinella*. *Enterobius, Trichuris,* and *Ascaris* are transmitted by ingestion of eggs; the others are transmitted as larvae. There are 2 larval forms: the first- and second-stage **(rhabditiform)** larvae are noninfectious, feeding forms; the third-stage **(filariform)** larvae are the infectious, nonfeeding forms. As adults, these nematodes live within the human body except for *Strongyloides,* which can also exist as adults in the soil.

(2) The important tissue nematodes *Wuchereria, Loa,* and *Onchocerca* are called the "filarial worms," because they produce motile embryos called **microfilariae** in blood and tissue fluids. These organisms are transmitted from person to person by bloodsucking mosquitoes or flies. A fourth species is the guinea worm, *Dracunculus,* whose larvae inhabit tiny crustaceans (copepods) and are ingested in drinking water.

The nematodes described above cause disease as a result of the presence of adult worms within the body. In addition, several species cannot mature to adults in human tissue but their larvae can cause disease. The most serious of these diseases is visceral larva migrans, caused primarily by the larvae of the dog ascarid, *Toxocara canis.* Cutaneous larva migrans, caused mainly by the larvae of the dog and cat hookworm, *Ancylostoma caninum,* is less serious. A third disease, anisakiasis, is caused by the ingestion of *Anisakis* larvae in raw seafood.

Features of the medically important nematodes are summarized in Table 56–1.

Intestinal Nematodes

ENTEROBIUS

Disease *Enterobius vermicularis* causes pinworm infection.

Important Properties The life cycle is **confined to humans.** The adult male and female worms live in the colon, where mating occurs. At night, the female migrates from the anus and releases thousands of fertilized eggs on the perianal skin and into the environment. Within 6 hours, the eggs develop into larvae and become infectious. Reinfection can occur if they are carried to the mouth by fingers after scratching the itching skin. The ingested eggs hatch in the small intestine, where the larvae differentiate into adults and migrate to the colon.

Pathogenesis & Clinical Findings **Perianal pruritus** is the most prominent symptom. Scratching predisposes to secondary bacterial infection.

Epidemiology *Enterobius* is found worldwide and is the **most common** helminth in the USA. Children under 12 years of age are usually affected.

Laboratory Diagnosis The eggs are recovered from perianal skin by using the **"Scotch tape"** technique and can be observed microscopically. Unlike those of other intestinal

Table 56–1. Features of medically important nematodes.

Primary Location	Species	Common Name or Disease	Mode of Transmission	Endemic Areas	Diagnosis	Treatment
Intestines	*Enterobius*	Pinworm	Ingestion of eggs	Worldwide	Eggs on skin.	Mebendazole or pyrantel pamoate
	Trichuris	Whipworm	Ingestion of eggs	Worldwide, especially tropics	Eggs in stools.	Mebendazole
	Ascaris	Ascariasis	Ingestion of eggs	Worldwide, especially tropics	Eggs in stools.	Mebendazole
	Ancylostoma and *Necator*	Hookworm	Larval penetration of skin	Worldwide, especially tropics; *Necator* in USA	Eggs in stools.	Mebendazole
	Strongyloides	Strongyloidiasis	Larval penetration of skin, also autoinfection	Tropics primarily	Larvae in stools.	Thiabendazole
	Trichinella	Trichinosis	Larvae in undercooked meat	Worldwide	Larvae encysted in muscle; serology.	Thiabendazole against adult worm
	Anisakis	Anisakiasis	Larvae in undercooked seafood	Japan, USA, Netherlands	Clinical.	No drug available
Tissue	*Wuchereria*	Filariasis	Mosquito bite	Tropics primarily	Blood smear.	Diethylcarbamazine
	Onchocerca	Onchocerciasis (river blindness)	Blackfly bite	Africa, Central America	Skin biopsy.	Ivermectin
	Loa	Loiasis	Deer fly bite	Tropical Africa	Blood smear.	Diethylcarbamazine
	Dracunculus	Guinea worm	Ingestion of copepods in water	Tropical Africa and Asia	Clinical.	Niridazole prior to extracting worm
	Toxocara larvae	Visceral larva migrans	Ingestion of eggs	Worldwide	Clinical and serologic.	Diethylcarbamazine or thiabendazole
	Ancylostoma larvae	Cutaneous larva migrans	Penetration of skin	Worldwide	Clinical.	Thiabendazole

nematodes, these **eggs are not found in the stools.** The small, whitish adult worms can be found in the stools or near the anus of diapered children. No serologic tests are available.

Treatment Both mebendazole and pyrantel pamoate are effective. They kill the adult worm in the colon but not the eggs, so that retreatment in 2 weeks is suggested. Reinfection is very common.

Prevention There are no means of prevention.

TRICHURIS

Disease *Trichuris trichiura* causes whipworm infection.

Important Properties Humans are **infected by eating eggs in soil** contaminated with human feces. The eggs hatch in the small intestine, where the larvae differentiate into immature adults. These forms migrate to the colon, where they mature, mate, and produce thousands of fertilized eggs daily, which are passed in the feces. Eggs deposited in warm, moist soil form embryos. When the embryonated eggs are ingested, the cycle is completed.

Pathogenesis & Clinical Findings Although adult *Trichuris* worms burrow their hairlike anterior ends into the intestinal mucosa, they do not cause a significant anemia, unlike the hookworms. *Trichuris* may cause diarrhea, but most infections are asymptomatic.

Epidemiology Whipworm infection occurs worldwide, especially in the tropics; more than 500 million people are affected. In the USA, it occurs mainly in the southern states.

Laboratory Diagnosis   Diagnosis is based on finding the typical eggs, ie, barrel-shaped with a plug at each end, in the stool.

Treatment   Mebendazole is the drug of choice.

Prevention   Proper disposal of feces prevents transmission.

ASCARIS

Disease   *Ascaris lumbricoides* causes ascariasis.

Important Properties   Humans are infected by **eating eggs in contaminated soil.** The eggs hatch in the small intestine, and the larvae migrate through the gut wall into the bloodstream and then to the lungs. They enter the alveoli, pass up the bronchi and trachea, and are swallowed. Within the small intestine, they become adults. They live in the lumen, do not attach to the wall, and derive their sustenance from ingested food. The adults are the **largest intestinal nematodes,** often growing to 25 cm or more. Thousands of eggs are laid daily, are passed in the feces, and form embryos in warm, moist soil. Ingestion of the embryonated eggs completes the cycle.

Pathogenesis & Clinical Findings   The major damage occurs during larval migration rather than from the presence of the adult worm in the intestine. The principal sites of tissue reaction are the **lungs,** where inflammation with an **eosinophilic exudate** occurs in response to larval antigens. Because the adults derive their nourishment from ingested food, a heavy worm burden may contribute to malnutrition, especially in children in developing countries.

Most infections are asymptomatic. **Ascaris pneumonia** with fever, cough, and eosinophilia can occur with a heavy larval burden. Abdominal pain and even obstruction can result from the presence of adult worms in the intestine.

Epidemiology   *Ascaris* infection is very common, especially in the tropics; hundreds of millions of people are infected. In the USA, most cases occur in the southern states.

Laboratory Diagnosis   Diagnosis is usually made microscopically by detecting eggs in the stools. The egg is oval with an irregular surface. Occasionally, adult worms are seen in the stools by the patient.

Treatment   Mebendazole is the drug of choice.

Prevention   Proper disposal of feces can prevent ascariasis.

ANCYLOSTOMA & NECATOR

Disease   *Ancylostoma duodenale* (Old World hookworm) and *Necator americanus* (New World hookworm) cause hookworm infection.

Important Properties   Humans are infected when **larvae in moist soil penetrate the skin,** usually of the feet or legs. They are carried by the blood to the lungs, migrate into the alveoli and up the bronchi and trachea, and then are swallowed. They develop into adults in the small intestine, attaching to the wall with either cutting plates *(Necator)* or teeth *(Ancylostoma).* They feed on blood from the capillaries of the intestinal villi. Thousands of eggs per day are passed in the feces. Eggs develop first into noninfectious, feeding (rhabditiform) larvae and then into third-stage, infectious, nonfeeding (filariform) larvae, which penetrate the skin to complete the cycle.

Pathogenesis & Clinical Findings   The major damage is due to the **loss of blood** at the site of attachment in the small intestine. Up to 0.1–0.3 mL per worm can be lost per day. Blood is consumed by the worm and oozes from the site in response to an anticoagulant made by the worm. Weakness and pallor accompany the microcytic anemia caused by blood loss. These symptoms occur in patients whose nutrition cannot compensate for the blood loss. "Ground itch," a pruritic papule or vesicle, can occur at the site of entry of the larvae into the skin. Pneumonia with eosinophilia can be seen during larval migration through the lung.

Epidemiology Hookworm is found worldwide, especially in tropical areas. In the USA, *Necator* is endemic in the rural southern states.

Laboratory Diagnosis Diagnosis is made microscopically by observing the eggs in the stools. Occult blood in the stools is frequent. Eosinophilia is typical.

Treatment Mebendazole is the drug of choice.

Prevention Disposing of sewage properly and wearing shoes are effective means of prevention.

STRONGYLOIDES

Disease *Strongyloides stercoralis* causes strongyloidiasis.

Important Properties *S stercoralis* has **2 distinct life cycles,** one within the human body and the other free-living in the soil. The life cycle in the human body begins with the **penetration of the skin** by infectious (filariform) larvae and their migration to the lungs. They enter the alveoli, pass up the bronchi and trachea, and then are swallowed. In the small intestine, the larvae molt into adults that enter the mucosa and produce eggs.

The eggs usually hatch within the mucosa, forming rhabditiform larvae that are passed in the feces. Some larvae molt to form filarial larvae, which penetrate the intestinal wall directly without leaving the host and migrate to the lungs (**autoinfection).** In immunocompetent patients, this is an infrequent, clinically unimportant event but in T cell-deficient or malnourished patients, this can lead to **massive reinfection,** with larvae passing to many organs and severe, sometimes fatal consequences.

If larvae are passed in the feces and enter warm, moist soil, they molt through successive stages to form adult male and female worms. After mating, the entire life cycle of egg, larva, and adult can occur in the soil. After several free-living cycles, filarial larvae are formed. When they contact skin, they penetrate and again initiate the parasitic cycle within humans.

Pathogenesis & Clinical Findings Most patients are asymptomatic, especially those with a low worm burden. Adult female worms in the wall of the small intestine can cause inflammation resulting in watery diarrhea. In autoinfection, the penetrating larvae may cause sufficient damage to the intestinal mucosa that sepsis due to enteric bacteria can occur. Larvae in the lung can produce a pneumonitis similar to that caused by *Ascaris.* Pruritus (ground itch) can occur at the site of larval penetration of the skin, as with hookworm.

Epidemiology Strongyloidiasis occurs primarily in the tropics, especially in Southeast Asia. Its geographic pattern is similar to that of hookworm because the same type of soil is required. In the USA, *Strongyloides* is endemic in the southeastern states.

Laboratory Diagnosis Diagnosis depends on finding larvae in the stool. As with all migratory nematode infections, **eosinophilia can be striking.** Serologic tests are not useful.

Treatment Thiabendazole is the drug of choice.

Prevention Prevention involves disposing of sewage properly and wearing shoes.

TRICHINELLA

Disease *Trichinella spiralis* causes trichinosis.

Important Properties Any mammal can be infected, but **pigs** are the most important reservoirs of human disease in the USA (except in Alaska, where bears constitute the reservoir). Humans are infected by **eating raw** or **undercooked meat** containing larvae encysted in the muscle. The larvae excyst and mature into adults within the mucosa of the small intestine. Eggs hatch within the adult females, and larvae are released and distributed via the bloodstream to many organs; however, they develop only in **striated muscle cells.** Within these "nurse cells," they encyst within a fibrous capsule and can remain viable for several years but eventually calcify.

The parasite is maintained in nature by cycles within reservoir hosts, primarily swine and rats. Humans are **end-stage hosts,** because the infected flesh is not consumed by other animals.

Pathogenesis & Clinical Findings A few days after eating undercooked meat, usually pork, the patient experiences gastroenteritis followed by 1–2 weeks later by fever, **muscle pain, periorbital edema, and eosinophilia.** Signs of cardiac and central nervous system disease are frequent, because the larvae migrate to these tissues as well. Death, which is rare, is usually due to congestive heart failure or respiratory paralysis.

Epidemiology Trichinosis occurs worldwide, especially in eastern Europe and west Africa. In the USA, it is related to eating home-prepared sausage, usually on farms where the pigs are fed uncooked garbage. Bear and seal meat also are sources.

Laboratory Diagnosis Muscle biopsy reveals **larvae within striated muscle.** Serologic tests, especially the bentonite flocculation test, become positive 3 weeks after infection.

Treatment There is no treatment for trichinosis, although thiabendazole is effective against the adult intestinal worms early in infection.

Prevention The disease can be prevented by properly cooking pork and by feeding pigs only cooked garbage.

Tissue Nematodes

WUCHERERIA

Disease *Wuchereria bancrofti* causes filariasis.*

Important Properties Humans are infected when the **female mosquito** (especially *Anopheles* and *Culex* species) deposits infective larvae on the skin while biting. The larvae penetrate the skin, enter a lymph node, and, after a year, mature to adults that produce **microfilariae.** These circulate in the blood, chiefly at night, and are ingested by biting mosquitoes. Within the mosquito, the microfilariae produce infective larvae that are transferred with the next bite. Humans are the only definitive hosts.

Pathogenesis & Clinical Findings Adult worms in the lymph nodes cause inflammation that eventually obstructs the lymphatic vessels, causing edema. Microfilariae do not cause symptoms. Early infections are asymptomatic. Later, fever, lymphangitis, and cellulitis develop. Gradually, the obstruction leads to edema of the legs and genitalia. **Elephantiasis** occurs mainly in patients who have been repeatedly infected over a long period.

Epidemiology This disease occurs in the tropics. The species of mosquito that acts as the vector varies from area to area. Altogether, 200–300 million people are infected.

Laboratory Diagnosis Thick blood smears taken from the patient at night reveal the microfilariae. Serologic tests are not useful.

Brugia malayi causes filariasis in Malaysia.

Treatment   Diethylcarbamazine is effective only against microfilariae; no drug therapy for adult worms is available.

Prevention   Prevention involves mosquito control with insecticides and the use of protective clothing, mosquito netting, and repellents.

ONCHOCERCA

Disease   *Onchocerca volvulus* causes onchocerciasis.

Important Properties   Humans are infected when the **female blackfly** *Simulium* deposits infective larvae while biting. The larvae enter the wound and migrate into the subcutaneous tissue, where they differentiate into adults, usually within **dermal nodules.** The female produces microfilariae that are ingested when another blackfly bites. The microfilariae develop into infective larvae in the fly to complete the cycle. Humans are the only definitive hosts.

Pathogenesis & Clinical Findings   Inflammation occurs in subcutaneous tissue, and pruritic papules and nodules form in response to the adult worm proteins. Microfilariae migrate through subcutaneous tissue, ultimately concentrating in the eyes. There they can cause lesions that can lead to blindness.

Epidemiology   Millions of people are affected in Africa and Central America. The disease is a major cause of blindness. It is called **"river blindness,"** because the blackflies develop in rivers and people who live along those rivers are affected. Infection rates are often over 80% in endemic areas.

Laboratory Diagnosis   Biopsy of the affected skin reveals microfilariae. Examination of the blood is not useful, because microfilariae do not circulate in the blood. Serologic tests are also not helpful.

Treatment   Ivermectin is effective against microfilariae but not adults. Suramin kills adults but is quite toxic and is used particularly in those with eye disease. Skin nodules can be removed surgically, but new nodules can develop; therefore, a surgical cure is unlikely in endemic areas.

Prevention   Prevention involves control of the blackfly with insecticides such as temefos. Ivermectin prevents the disease.

LOA

Disease   *Loa loa* causes loiasis.

Important Properties   Humans are infected by the bite of the **deer fly** (mango fly), *Chrysops,* which deposits infective larvae on the skin. The larvae enter the bite wound, wander in the body, and develop into adults. The females release microfilariae that enter the blood, particularly during the day. The microfilariae are taken up by the fly during a blood meal and differentiate into infective larvae that continue the cycle when the fly bites the next person.

Pathogenesis & Clinical Findings   There is no inflammatory response to the microfilariae or adults, but a hypersensitivity reaction causes transient, localized, non-Erythematous, sub-cutaneous edema (Calabar swellings). The most dramatic finding is an adult worm **crawling across the conjunctiva** of the eye, a harmless but disconcerting event.

Epidemiology   The disease is found only in tropical central and west Africa, the habitat of the vector *Chrysops.*

Laboratory Diagnosis   Diagnosis is made by visualization of the microfilariae in a blood smear. There are no useful serologic tests.

Treatment   Diethylcarbamazine eliminates the microfilariae and may kill the adults. Worms in the eyes may require surgical excision.

Prevention   Control of the fly by insecticides can prevent the disease.

DRACUNCULUS

Disease   *Dracunculus medinensis* (guinea fire worm) causes dracunculiasis.

Important Properties   Humans are infected when tiny **crustaceans** (copepods) containing infective larvae **are swallowed in drinking water.** The larvae are released in the small intestine and migrate into the body, where they develop into adults. Meter-long adult females cause the skin to ulcerate and then release motile larvae into fresh water. Copepods eat the larvae, which molt to form infective larvae. The cycle is completed when these are ingested into the water.

Pathogenesis & Clinical Findings   The adult female produces a substance that causes inflammation, blistering, and ulceration of the skin, usually of the lower extremities. The inflamed papule **burns and itches,** and the ulcer can become secondarily infected. Diagnosis is usually made clinically by finding the **head of the worm in the skin ulcer.**

Epidemiology   The disease occurs over large areas of tropical Africa, the Middle East, and India. Tens of millions of people are infected.

Laboratory Diagnosis   The laboratory usually does not play a role in diagnosis.

Treatment   The time-honored treatment consists of gradually extracting the worm by winding it up on a stick over a period of days. Niridazole makes the worm easier to extract.

Prevention   Prevention consists of filtering or boiling drinking water.

Diseases Caused By Nematode Larvae

TOXOCARA

Disease   *T canis* is the major cause of visceral larva migrans. *T. cati* and several other related nematodes also cause this disease.

Important Properties   The definitive host for *T canis* is the dog. The adult *Toxocara* female in the dog intestine produces eggs that are passed in the feces into the soil. Humans ingest soil containing the eggs, which hatch into larvae in the small intestine. The larvae migrate to many organs, especially the liver, brain, and eyes. The larvae eventually are encapsulated and die. The life cycle is not completed in humans; humans are therefore accidental, dead-end hosts.

Pathogenesis & Clinical Findings   Pathology is related to the granulomas that form around the dead larvae as a result of a delayed hypersensitivity response to larval proteins. The most serious clinical finding is blindness due to retinal involvement. Fever, hepatomegaly, and eosinophilia are common.

Epidemiology   Young children are primarily affected, because they are likely to ingest soil containing the eggs. *T canis* is a common parasite of dogs in the USA.

Laboratory Diagnosis   Serologic tests are commonly used, but the definitive diagnosis depends on visualizing the larvae in tissue. The presence of hypergammaglobulinemia and eosinophilia support the diagnosis.

Treatment   No drug has been shown to be entirely effective.

Prevention   Dogs should be dewormed, and children should be prevented from eating dirt.

ANCYLOSTOMA   Cutaneous larva migrans is caused by the filariform larvae of *A caninum* (dog hookworm) and *Ancylostoma braziliense* (cat hookworm), as well as other nematodes. The organism cannot complete its life cycle in humans. The larvae penetrate the skin and **migrate through subcutaneous tissue,** causing an inflammatory response. The lesions (''creeping eruption'') are extremely pruritic. The disease occurs primarily in the southern USA, in children and construction workers who are exposed to infected soil. The diagnosis is made clinically; the laboratory is of little value. Oral or topical thiabendazole is usually effective.

ANISAKIS   In addition to visceral larva migrans and cutaneous larva migrans, there is a third human disease caused by the larvae of a nematode, namely anisakiasis. *Anisakis* larvae are **ingested in raw seafood** and can penetrate the submucosa of the stomach or intestine. Gastroenteritis, eosinophilia, and occult blood in the stool typically occur. Acute infection can resemble appendicitis, and chronic infection can resemble gastrointestinal cancer.

   Most cases in the USA have been traced to eating sushi and sashimi (especially salmon and red snapper) in Japanese restaurants. The diagnosis is typically made endoscopically or on laparotomy. Microbiologic and serologic tests are not helpful in diagnosis. There are no effective drugs. Prevention consists of cooking seafood adequately or freezing it for 24 hours before eating.

Review Questions

1. Which of the intestinal nematodes are transmitted by ingestion of eggs?
2. Distinguish between rhabditiform and filariform larvae.
3. Which of the tissue nematodes are transmitted by mosquitoes or flies?
4. In pinworm infection, how do the *Enterobius* eggs reach the environment?
5. How is the laboratory diagnosis of pinworms made?
6. In (a) whipworm infection, and (b) ascaris infection, how is the disease transmitted and how is the laboratory diagnosis made?
7. What is the pathogenesis of *Ascaris* pneumonia?
8. In hookworm infection, what is the mode of transmission and how is the laboratory diagnosis made?
9. What is the pathogenesis of anemia caused by hookworms?
10. Contrast the free-living and the non-free-living life cycles of *Strongyloides.*
11. In strongyloidiasis, what is the mode of transmission and how is the laboratory diagnosis made?
12. What is the pathogenesis of the severe clinical consequences of strongyloidiasis in a T cell-deficient, eg, AIDS, patient?
13. In trichinosis, what is the mode of transmission, how is the laboratory diagnosis usually made, and how can the disease be prevented?
14. Why are humans end-stage hosts for *Trichinella?*
15. Contrast visceral with cutaneous larva migrans regarding (a) the organism, (b) transmission, (c) location of lesions, and (d) laboratory diagnosis.
16. In filariasis, what is the mode of transmission and how is the laboratory diagnosis made?
17. What is the pathogenesis of elephantiasis?
18. In onchocerciasis, what is the mode of transmission and how is the laboratory diagnosis made?
19. What is the pathogenesis of ''river blindness''? Why is the term ''river'' used?
20. Contrast *Loa* and *Dracunculus* regarding (a) mode of transmission, (b) laboratory diagnosis, and (c) location of the adult worms.
21. Which nematodes are found worldwide? For those that are not found worldwide, where do they primarily occur?
22. For which nematodes is (a) mebendazole, (b) thiabendazole, (c) diethylcarbamazine or (d) ivermectin the appropriate treatment?

Part VII: Immunology

Immunity

57

INTRODUCTION The main function of the immune system is to **prevent or limit infections** by microorganisms such as bacteria, viruses, fungi, and parasites. Protection is provided primarily by the **cell-mediated** and **antibody-mediated** arms of the immune system. (Complement and phagocytes are essential also.) Cell-mediated immunity and antibody are both highly specific for the invading organism. How do these specific protective mechanisms originate? The following examples briefly describe how immunity to microorganisms occurs.

CELL-MEDIATED IMMUNITY In this example, a bacterium, eg, *Mycobacterium tuberculosis*, enters the body and is ingested by a macrophage. The bacterium is broken down, and fragments of it (antigen) appear on the surface of the macrophage in association with **class II major histocompatibility complex** (MHC) proteins. The antigen-class II protein complex interacts with antigen-specific receptors on the surface of a **helper T lymphocyte.** Activation and clonal proliferation of this antigen-specific helper T cell occur as a result of the production of **lymphokines,** the most important of which are interleukin-1 (produced by macrophages) and interleukin-2 (produced by lymphocytes). These activated helper T cells can mediate one component of cellular immunity, eg, a **delayed hypersensitivity** reaction against *M tuberculosis.*

Cytotoxic T cells mediate another important component of the cellular immune response. In this example, a virus, eg, influenza virus, is inhaled and infects a cell of the respiratory tract. Viral envelope glycoproteins appear on the surface of the infected cell in association with **class I MHC** proteins. A cytotoxic T cell recognizes and binds to the viral antigen-class I protein complex and is stimulated to grow into a clone of cells by interleukin-2 produced by helper T cells. These cytotoxic T cells can specifically kill influenza virus-infected cells by recognizing viral antigen-class I protein complexes on the cell surface.

ANTIBODY-MEDIATED IMMUNITY Antibody synthesis typically involves the cooperation of 3 cells: **macrophages, helper T cells,** and **B cells.** After processing by a macrophage, fragments of bacterial antigen appear on the surface of the macrophage in association with **class II MHC** proteins. These molecules bind to specific receptors on the surface of a helper T cell, which then produces **lymphokines** such as interleukin-2, B-cell growth factor, and B-cell differentiation factor. These factors activate the antigen-specific B cell, which has also bound to the antigen-class II protein complex. The activated B cell proliferates and differentiates to form many plasma cells that secrete large amounts of **immunoglobulins** (antibodies). Although antibody formation usually involves helper T cells, certain antigens, eg, bacterial polysaccharides, can activate B cells directly, without the help of T cells, and are called T cell-independent antigens.

In general, **antibodies neutralize** toxins and viruses and **opsonize** bacteria, making them easier to phagocytize. **Cell-mediated** immunity, on the other hand, limits the growth of many **intracellular organisms** such as fungi, parasites, and certain bacteria, as well as killing **virus-infected cells and tumor cells.**

NATURAL & ACQUIRED IMMUNITY Immunity may be **natural (innate)** or **acquired (adaptive).**

(a) Natural immunity is resistance not acquired through contact with an antigen. It is **nonspecific** and includes host defenses such as barriers to infectious agents (eg, skin and mucous membranes), certain cells (eg, natural killer cells), certain proteins (eg, the

Table 57–1. Natural immunity.

Mechanism	Factor
Entry of microorganism limited	Keratin layer of intact skin (mechanical barrier) Lysozyme in tears and other secretions (degrades peptidoglycan in bacterial cell wall) Fatty acids of the skin (inhibit growth of microorganisms) Respiratory cilia (elevate mucus containing trapped organisms) Normal flora of throat, colon, and vagina (inhibit colonization by pathogens) Low pH of vagina and stomach Surface phagocytes, eg, alveolar macrophages
Growth of microorganism in body limited	Natural killer cells Phagocytes, eg, neutrophils Interferons (inhibit virus replication) Transferrin and lactoferrin (sequester iron required for bacterial growth) Complement Elevated body temperature Inflammatory response

complement cascade and interferons), and other factors such as phagocytosis and inflammation (Table 57–1).

(b) Acquired immunity occurs after exposure to an agent, is **specific,** and is mediated by antibody and by lymphoid cells. It can be active or passive.

ACTIVE & PASSIVE IMMUNITY   **Active** immunity is resistance induced after **contact** with foreign antigens, eg, microorganisms or transplanted cells. This contact may consist of clinical or subclinical infection, immunization with live or killed infectious agents or their antigens, exposure to microbial products (eg, toxins and toxoids), or transplantation of foreign cells. In all these instances, the host actively produces antibodies and lymphoid cells acquire the ability to respond to the antigens.

The main advantage of active immunity is that resistance is **long-term.** Its major disadvantage is its **slow onset**, especially the primary response (see p 270).

Passive immunity is resistance based on antibodies **preformed** in another host. Administration of antibody against diphtheria, tetanus, botulism, etc, makes large amounts of antitoxin immediately available to neutralize the toxins. Likewise, preformed antibodies to certain viruses (eg, rabies and hepatitis A and B viruses) can be injected during the incubation period to limit viral multiplication.

The main advantage of passive immunization is the **prompt availability** of large amounts of antibody; disadvantages are the **short life** span of these antibodies and possible hypersensitivity reactions if globulins from another species are used.

ANTIGENS   Antigens are molecules that react with antibodies, whereas immunogens are molecules that induce an immune response. In most cases, antigens are immunogens and the terms are used interchangeably. However, there are certain important exceptions, eg, haptens. A **hapten** is a molecule that is not immunogenic by itself but can react with specific antibody. Haptens are usually small, but some high-molecular-weight nucleic acids are haptens as well.

The interaction of antigen and antibody is highly specific, and this characteristic is frequently used in the diagnostic laboratory to identify microorganisms. Antigen and antibody bind by **weak forces** such as hydrogen bonds and van der Waals' forces rather than by covalent bonds. The strength of the binding (the affinity) is proportionate to the fit of the antigen with its antibody-combining site, ie, its ability to form more of these bonds. Another term, avidity, is also used to express certain aspects of binding. It need not concern us here.

The features of molecules that determine immunogenicity are as follows:

(A) Foreignness: In general, molecules recognized as ''self'' are not immunogenic. To be immunogenic, molecules must be recognized as ''nonself,'' ie, foreign.

(B) Molecular Size: The most potent immunogens are proteins with molecular weight above 100,000. Generally, molecules with molecular weight below 10,000 are weakly immunogenic, and very small ones, eg, an amino acid, are nonimmunogenic. Certain small molecules, eg, haptens, become immunogenic only when linked to a carrier protein.

(C) Chemical-Structural Complexity: A certain amount of chemical complexity is required, eg, amino acid homopolymers are less immunogenic than heteropolymers containing 2 or 3 different amino acids.

(D) Antigenic Determinants (Epitopes): Epitopes are small chemical groups on the antigen molecule that can elicit and react with antibody. An antigen can have one or more determinants. Most antigens have many determinants, ie, they are multivalent. In general, a determinant is roughly 5 amino acids or sugars in size. The overall 3-dimensional structure is the main criterion of antigenic specificity.

(E) Dosage, Route, and Timing of Antigen Administration: These also affect immunogenicity. In addition, the genetic constitution of the host determines whether a molecule is immunogenic. Different strains of the same species of animal may respond differently to the same antigen.

Adjuvants enhance the immune response to an immunogen. They are chemically unrelated to the immunogen and may act by nonspecifically stimulating the immunoreactive cells or by releasing the immunogen slowly. Some human vaccines contain adjuvants such as aluminum hydroxide or lipids.

AGE & THE IMMUNE RESPONSE Immunity is **less than optimal** on both ends of life, ie, in the **newborn** and the **elderly.** The reason for the relatively poor immune response in newborns is unclear, but they appear to have inadequate T cell function. In newborns, antibodies are provided primarily by the transfer of maternal IgG across the placenta. Maternal antibody decays so that little remains by 3–6 months of age, and the risk of infection in the child is high. The fetus can mount an IgM response to certain (probably T cell-independent) antigens, eg, to *Treponema pallidum,* the cause of syphilis, which can be acquired congenitally. IgG and IgA begin to be made shortly after birth. The response to certain protein antigens is good; hence, poliovirus immunization can begin at 2 months of age. However, young children respond poorly to certain polysaccharide antigens; therefore, vaccines for protection from infections caused by *Streptococcus pneumoniae* and *Haemophilus influenzae* cannot be given until 2 years of age.

In the elderly, immunity generally declines. There is a reduced IgG response to certain antigens, fewer T cells, and a reduced delayed hypersensitivity response. As with the very young, the frequency and severity of infections are high.

Review Questions

1. What are the major protective functions of (a) antibodies and (b) cell-mediated immunity?
2. Describe how (a) antibodies and (b) cellular immunity specific for a certain antigen arise.
3. What are the mediators of natural and acquired immunity?
4. Distinguish between active and passive immunity. What are the advantages and disadvantages of both?
5. What are the main attributes that make a substance a good antigen?
6. What is (a) a hapten, (b) an epitope, (c) an adjuvant?
7. What is the nature of the interaction between antigen and antibody?
8. What are the features of the immune system in the newborn?

58

Cellular Basis
of the Immune Response

ORIGIN OF IMMUNE CELLS The capability of responding to immunologic stimuli rests mainly with lymphoid cells. During embryonic development, blood cell precursors occur in the fetal liver, yolk sac, and elsewhere; in postnatal life, the stem cells reside in the bone marrow. Stem cells differentiate into cells of the erythroid, myeloid, or lymphoid series. The latter evolve into 2 main lymphocyte populations: T cells and B cells (Fig 58–1 and Table 58–1).

  T cell precursors differentiate into immunocompetent T cells within the thymus. Stem cells lack CD3, CD4, and CD8 molecules on their surface, but during passage through the thymus they differentiate into T cells that can express these glycoproteins. B cells do not pass through the thymus. Precursors of B cells mature elsewhere, probably in "gut-associated lymphoid tissue," eg, Peyer's patches. Gut-associated lymphoid tissue is the mammalian equivalent of the bursa of Fabricius in birds. B cells are named for the **bursa,** T cells for the **thymus.** Two other important cell types, macrophages and natural killer (NK) cells, arise from myeloid precursors.

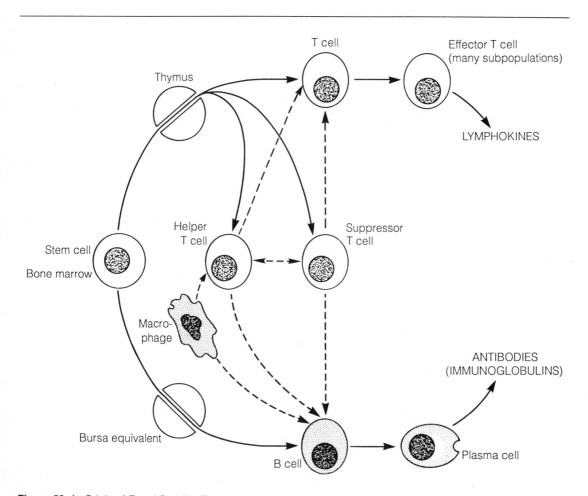

Figure 58–1. Origin of T and B cells. (Reproduced, with permission, from Jawetz E et al: *Review of Medical Microbiology,* 18th ed. Appleton & Lange, 1989.)

Table 58–1. Comparison of T cells and B cells.

Feature	T Cells	B Cells
Antigen receptors on surface	Yes	Yes
IgM on surface	No	Yes
CD3 proteins on surface	Yes	No
Clonal expansion after contact with specific antigen	Yes	Yes
Immunoglobulin synthesis	No	Yes
Helper/suppressor regulator of antibody synthesis	Yes	No
Mediator of cellular immunity and delayed hypersensitivity	Yes	No
Maturation in thymus	Yes	No
Maturation in bursa or its equivalent	No	Yes

T CELLS

CD4 & CD8 Cells* Within the thymus, perhaps within the outer cortical epithelial cells (nurse cells), T cell progenitors differentiate under the influence of thymic hormones (thymosins and thymopoietins) into T cell subpopulations. These cells are characterized by surface glycoproteins, eg, CD3, CD4, and CD8, that are distinguished by their reaction with specific monoclonal antibodies. **All T cells have CD3** molecules on their surface in association with antigen receptors. CD3 molecules are involved with transmitting, from the outside of the cell to the inside, the information that the **antigen receptor is occupied.** This results in transcription of lymphokine genes via a membrane inositol-diacylglycerol-protein kinase C pathway.

T cells are subdivided into 2 major categories on the basis of whether they have CD4 or CD8 proteins on their surface. Mature T cells have either CD4 or CD8 proteins but not both.

CD4 lymphocytes manifest the following **helper** and **effector** functions: (1) they help B cells develop into antibody-producing plasma cells; (2) they help T cells to exhibit cytotoxic effects; (3) they help T cells to become suppressor cells; and (4) they effect delayed hypersensitivity. CD4 cells make up about 65% of peripheral T cells and predominate in the thymic medulla, tonsils, and blood.

CD8 lymphocytes manifest both **cytotoxic** and **suppressor** functions:** (1) they are cytotoxic for virus-infected, tumor, and allograft cells; (2) they suppress immunoglobulin production by B cells; and (3) they suppress delayed hypersensitivity reactions and cellular immunity. CD8 cells predominate in human bone marrow and gut lymphoid tissue and constitute about 35% of peripheral T cells.

Activation The activation of helper T cells requires that they recognize a complex on the surface of antigen-presenting cells, eg, macrophages† consisting of **both** the antigen **and** a class II MHC protein product (Fig 58–2).

Helper T cells recognize **class II** MHC proteins, whereas **cytotoxic T cells** recognize **class I** MHC proteins. For activation to occur, the MHC proteins on the antigen-presenting cell and the T cell must be the same. If they are not, no activation occurs. This is called **MHC restriction.** Note that T cells bind antigen only in the context of MHC proteins, whereas the immunoglobulins on the B cell surface can bind free antigen (see Chapter 62).

This complex on the antigen-presenting cell interacts with receptors on the surface of the helper T cell, thus activating the T cell to produce various **lymphokines,** eg, interleukin–2.

---

*CD4 is the currently accepted terminology, replacing T4 and OKT4. CD8 replaces T8 and OKT8. CD is the abbreviation for "clustered determinant."

**At present (1988), many immunologists doubt that a population of CD8 lymphocytes with suppressor functions actually exists. Experiments designed to demonstrate the presence of these cells have not succeeded.

†Macrophages are the most important antigen-presenting cells, but B cells, dendritic cells in the spleen, and Langerhans cells on the skin also present antigen, ie, have class II proteins on their surface.

Figure 58–2. Activation of T cells. Helper T cells bearing CD4 surface proteins are activated by antigen-presenting cells with complexes of antigen and class II MHC proteins on their surfaces. Cytotoxic T cells bearing CD8 surface proteins are activated differently. In this example, they are activated by virus-infected cells with complexes of viral antigen and class I MHC proteins on their surfaces. (Reproduced, with permission, from Stites DP, Stobo JD, Wells JV [editors]: *Basic & Clinical Immunology,* 6th ed. Appleton & Lange, 1987.) page 259

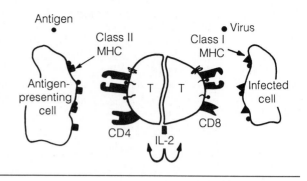

The macrophage releases **interleukin-1**, which plays an essential role in activating the T cell. The helper T cell then produces **interleukin-2** (T-cell growth factor), which induces it to multiply into a clone of antigen-specific helper T cells. Most cells of this clone perform effector and regulatory functions, but some become "**memory**" cells that are capable of being rapidly activated upon exposure to antigen at a later time. (B cells also form memory cells.)

T Cell Receptor   The T cell receptor for antigen consists of 2 polypeptides, alpha and beta, which are associated with CD3 proteins. T-cell receptor proteins are **similar** to immunoglobulin heavy chains in that (1) the genes that code for them are formed by rearrangement of multiple regions of DNA (see Chapter 59); (2) there are V (variable), D (diversity), J (joining), and C (constant) segments that rearrange to provide diversity, giving rise to an estimated number of more than 10^7 different receptor proteins; (3) each T cell has unique receptor proteins on its surface; and (4) activated T cells, like activated B cells, clonally expand to yield large numbers of cells specific for that antigen.

Although analogous to immunoglobulins in that both T cell receptors and immunoglobulins interact with antigen in a highly specific manner, the T cell receptor is different in 2 important ways: (1) it has 2 chains rather than 4; and (2) it recognizes antigen only in conjunction with MHC proteins, whereas immunoglobulins recognize free antigen.

Features of T Cells   T cells constitute 65–80% of the recirculating pool of small lymphocytes. Within lymph nodes, they are located in the inner, subcortical region, not in the germinal centers. Their life span is long: months or years. They can be stimulated to divide when exposed to certain mitogens, eg, phytohemagglutinin or concanavalin A (endotoxin, a lipopolysaccharide found on the surface of gram-negative bacteria, is a mitogen for B cells but not T cells). Many T cells have surface receptors for the Fc fragment of IgG and monomeric IgM immunoglobulins. Most human T cells have receptors for sheep erythrocytes on their surface and can form "rosettes" with them; this finding serves as a means of identifying T cells in a mixed population of cells.

Effector Functions

A. Delayed Hypersensitivity: Delayed hypersensitivity reactions are produced particularly against antigens of **intracellular microorganisms** including various viruses, fungi, protozoa, and bacteria, eg, mycobacteria. They are mediated by CD4 cells. Important lymphokines for these reactions include macrophage activation factor, migration inhibition factor for macrophages, interleukin-1, interferons, and others. A deficiency of cell-mediated immunity manifests itself as a marked susceptibility to infection by such microorganisms and to certain tumors.

B. Cytotoxicity: The **cytotoxic response** is concerned primarily with **graft rejection** and with destroying **virus-infected cells and tumor cells.** In response to allografts, cytotoxic (CD8) cells recognize the class I MHC molecules on the surface of the foreign cells. Helper (CD4) cells recognize the foreign class II molecules on certain cells in the graft, eg, macrophages and lymphocytes. The activated helper cells secrete IL-2, which stimulates the cytotoxic cell to form a clone of cells. These class I-specific cytotoxic cells kill the allograft.

In response to virus-infected cells, the CD8 lymphocytes must recognize both viral antigens and class I molecules on the surface of infected cells. Helper (CD4) lymphocytes recognize viral antigens bound to class II molecules either on the virus-infected cell or on an antigen-presenting cell, eg, macrophage displaying viral antigens. The helper cells secrete IL-2, which stimulates the cytotoxic cell to form a clone of cells. These virus-infected cytotoxic cells kill the infected cells. In addition to direct killing by cytotoxic T cells, virus-infected cells can be destroyed by a combination of antibody and phagocytic cells. In this process, called **antibody-dependent cellular cytotoxicity,** antibody bound to the surface of the infected cell is recognized by the phagocytic cell, eg, macrophage, and the infected cell is killed.

Many tumor cells develop new antigens on their surface. These antigens bound to class I proteins are recognized by cytotoxic T cells, which are stimulated to proliferate by IL-2. The resultant clone of cytotoxic T cells can kill the tumor cells, a phenomenon called **immune surveillance.**

Regulatory Functions   T cells play a central role in regulating both the humoral (antibody) and cell-mediated arms of the immune system.

A. Antibody Production: Antibody production by B cells usually requires the participation of helper T cells **(T cell-dependent response),** but antibodies to some antigens, eg, polymerized (multivalent) macromolecules such as bacterial capsular polysaccharide, are T cell-independent. In the following example illustrating the T cell-dependent response, B cells are used as the antigen-presenting cell, although macrophages commonly perform this function. In this instance, antigen bound to surface IgM or IgD is internalized within the B cell and fragmented. Some of the fragments return to the surface in association with class II MHC molecules (Fig 58–3).* These interact with the receptor on the helper T cell, which is then stimulated to produce lymphokines, eg, B-cell growth factors. These factors enhance cell division and differentiation of the B cell to form many antibody-producing plasma cells.

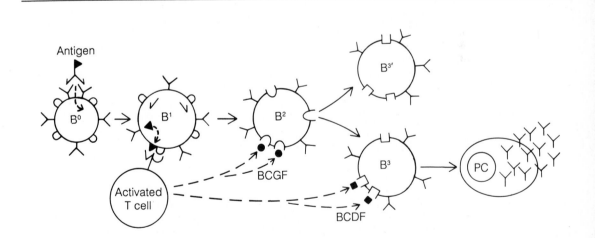

Figure 58–3. B cell activation by helper T cells. B^0 is a resting B cell to which a multivalent antigen ($\curlywedge$) is attaching to IgM receptors (Y). The antigen is internalized, and a fragment (▲) is returned to the surface in conjunction with a class II molecule (△). A receptor on an activated T cell recognizes the complex on the B cell surface and produces B-cell growth factor (BCGF; ●) and B-cell differentiation factor (BCDF; ■). These factors cause the progression of the B^1 cell to form B^2 and B^3 cells, which differentiate into antibody-producing plasma cells (PC). (Reproduced, with permission, from Stites DP, Stobo JD, Wells JV [editors]: *Basic & Clinical Immunology,* 6th ed. Appleton & Lange, 1987.)

*Note that one important difference between B cells and T cells is that B cells recognize antigen itself, whereas T cells recognize antigen only in association with MHC proteins.

For the T cell-dependent response to occur, antigen-presenting cells, T cells, and B cells must have the same class II MHC specificity. The response to haptens is usually T cell-dependent, in which case the B cells are specific for the hapten and the T cells are specific for the carrier protein. In the T cell-independent response, certain antigens can stimulate B cells to differentiate and grow directly, although B-cell growth factors from macrophages seem likely to play a role.

B. Cell-Mediated Immunity: In the cell-mediated response, the initial events are similar to those described above for antibody production. The antigen is processed by macrophages and fragments presented in conjunction with class II MHC molecules on the surface. These interact with the receptor on the helper T cell, which is then stimulated to produce lymphokines such as IL-2 (T-cell growth factor), which stimulates the specific helper T cells to grow.

C. Suppression of Certain Immune Responses: A subpopulation of CD8 suppressor T cells regulates B cell responses to antigens. Failure of such regulation may lead to unrestrained antibody production to "self" antigens and autoimmune diseases. Some CD8 cells regulate the cell-mediated responses of CD4 cells. When there is an imbalance in numbers or activity between CD4 and CD8 cells, cellular immune mechanisms are greatly impaired. For example, in lepromatous leprosy there is unrestrained multiplication of *Mycobacterium leprae,* a lack of delayed hypersensitivity to *M leprae* antigens, a lack of cellular immunity to that organism, and an excess of CD8 cells in lesions. Removal of some CD8 cells can restore cellular immunity in such patients and limit *M leprae* multiplication. In acquired immunodeficiency syndrome (AIDS), the normal ratio of CD4:CD8 cells (> 1.5) is greatly reduced. Some CD4 cells are destroyed by the human immunodeficiency virus (HIV), and other CD4 cells are thought to act as helpers to CD8 (suppressor) cells. This imbalance, ie, a loss of helper activity and an increase in suppressor activity, results in a susceptibility to opportunistic infections and certain tumors.

B CELLS

Origin During embryogenesis, B cell precursors are recognized first in the fetal liver. From there they migrate to the bone marrow, which is their main location during adult life.* Unlike T cells, they do not require the thymus for maturation. Pre-B cells lack surface immunoglobulins, but B cells display surface IgM (and commonly IgD) that serve as receptors for antigens. B cells have approximately 10^5 IgM molecules per cell. They also have receptors for the Fc portion of immunoglobulins and for several complement components.

B cells constitute about 30% of the recirculating pool of small lymphocytes, and their life span is short, ie, days or weeks. Approximately 10^9 B cells are produced each day. Within lymph nodes, they are located in germinal centers; within the spleen, they are found in the white pulp. They are also found in the gut-associated lymphoid tissue, eg, Peyer's patches.

Clonal Selection How do antibodies arise? Does the antigen "instruct" the B cell to make an antibody, or does the antigen "select" a B cell endowed with the preexisting capacity to make the antibody?

It appears that the latter alternative, ie, **clonal selection,** accounts for antibody formation. Each individual has a large pool of B lymphocytes (about 10^7). Each immunologically responsive B cell bears a surface receptor (immunoglobulin) that can react with one antigen (or closely related group of antigens); ie, there are about 10^7 different specificities. An antigen interacts with the B lymphocyte that shows the best "fit" with its immunoglobulin surface receptor (typically IgM). After the antigen binds, the B cell is stimulated to proliferate and form a clone of cells. These selected B cells soon become plasma cells and secrete antibody specific for the antigen. Plasma cells synthesize the immunoglobulins with the same antigenic specificity (ie, they have the same H chain and the same type L chain) as those carried by the selected B cell. Antigenic specificity does not change when heavy-chain class switching occurs (see Chapter 59).

Activation In the following example, the B cell is the antigen-presenting cell. Multivalent antigen binds to surface IgM (or IgD) and cross-links adjacent immunoglobulin molecules.

---

*In birds, they originate in the bursa of Fabricius.

The immunoglobulins aggregate to form "patches" and eventually migrate to one pole of the cell to form a cap. Endocytosis of the capped material follows, the antigen is processed, and epitopes appear on the surface in conjunction with class II MHC proteins. This complex is recognized by a helper T cell with a receptor for the antigen on its surface.* (There is also a requirement for the MHC protein on the T cell to be the same as that on the B cell, but, of course, in any individual this is the case.) The T cell now produces various lymphokines that stimulate the growth and differentiation of the B cell. Many **plasma cells** that produce large amounts of immunoglobulins specific for the epitope are the end result. Plasma cells secrete thousands of antibody molecules per second for a few days and then die. Some activated B cells form **memory cells**, which remain quiescent for long periods but are capable of being activated rapidly upon reexposure to antigen. The presence of these cells explains the rapid appearance of antibody in the secondary response (see Chapter 60).

MACROPHAGES The main function of macrophages is **phagocytosis.**

(a) Macrophages have surface Fc receptors that interact with the Fc portion of immunoglobulins, thereby enhancing the uptake of opsonized organisms.[†]

(b) Foreign material is ingested, degraded and fragments of antigen are presented on the macrophage cell surface (in conjunction with MHC molecules) for interaction with the T cell receptor.

(c) Macrophages also produce interleukin-1, which activates T cells to proliferate.

Macrophages are derived from bone marrow histiocytes and exist both free, eg, monocytes, and fixed in tissues, eg, Kupffer cells of the liver. Macrophages migrate to the site of inflammation, attracted by certain mediators, especially C5a, an anaphylatoxin released in the complement cascade.

NATURAL KILLER CELLS In contrast to macrophages, natural killer (NK) cells do not phagocytize foreign material. Rather, they are **cytotoxic;** ie, they specialize in killing tumor cells and virus-infected cells and do so without the need for antibody. Killing does **not** require recognition of MHC antigens on the cell surface, unlike the case with T cells, and does not require prior sensitization. NK cells are lymphocytes with some T cell markers but are not required to pass through the thymus in order to mature. The activity of NK cells is markedly enhanced by gamma interferon.

IMPORTANT CYTOKINES

Mediators Affecting Lymphocytes (Lymphokines)

(1) **Interleukin-1** is a protein produced mainly by macrophages. It activates a wide variety of target cells, eg, T and B lymphocytes, neutrophils, epithelial cells, and fibroblasts, to grow, differentiate, or synthesize specific products. For example, interleukin-1 (IL-1) stimulates T lymphocytes to differentiate and produce IL-2 (see below). In addition IL-1 is **endogenous pyrogen,** which acts on the hypothalamus to cause the fever associated with infections and other inflammatory reactions.

(2) **Interleukin-2 (T-cell growth factor)** is a protein produced mainly by helper T cells that stimulates T cells to grow. Resting T cells are stimulated by antigen (or other stimulators) both to produce IL-2 and to form IL-2 receptors on their surface, thereby acquiring the capacity to respond to IL-2. Interaction of IL-2 with its receptor triggers a series of intracellular signals involving inositol diphosphate, protein kinase C, and calcium, leading to the stimulation of DNA synthesis. Other interleukins (interleukin-3 through interleukin-6) have been reported.

(3) B-cell growth factors are proteins that are produced by helper T cells; they promote the growth and differentiation of B cells. Interleukins 4 and 5 are B-cell stimulating factors.

(4) Blastogenic or mitogenic factor causes some lymphocytes to differentiate into large, rapidly dividing blast cells with greatly increased synthesis of DNA.

---

*Macrophages bearing antigen bound to class II proteins can also present antigen to the T cell, resulting in antibody formation.

†Macrophages have receptors for complement also.

(5) Transfer factor is a dialyzable extract of lymphocytes (MW 2000) that can transfer specific delayed-type hypersensitivity to a nonreactive recipient and may temporarily restore competent cellular immunity to immunocompromised individuals.

Mediators Affecting Macrophages & Monocytes (Monokines)

(1) Chemotactic factor attracts monocytes, which then become macrophages.

(2) Migration-inhibitory factor inhibits the migration of normal macrophages in vitro and may act to retain macrophages at the site of a delayed hypersensitivity reaction in vivo.

(3) Macrophage-activating factor, like migration-inhibitory factor, is produced by lymphocytes and can activate macrophages to phagocytize certain organisms, eg, *M tuberculosis*.

Mediators Affecting Polymorphonuclear Leukocytes

(1) Leukocyte-inhibitory factor inhibits migration of neutrophils, analogous to migration-inhibitory factor (above).

(2) Chemotactic factors for neutrophils, basophils, and eosinophils selectively attract each cell type.

Mediators Affecting Stem Cells
Interleukin-3 is made by activated helper T cells and supports the growth of bone marrow stem cells.

Mediators With Other Effects

(1) **Interferons** are glycoproteins that block virus replication and exert many immuno-modulating functions. Alpha interferon (from leukocytes) and beta interferon (from fibroblasts) are induced by viruses (or double-stranded RNA) and have antiviral activity (see Chapter 33). Gamma interferon is a lymphokine produced by activated T lymphocytes; it can be induced by either antigen or certain mitogens. Interferons (alpha, beta, and gamma, but especially gamma) can activate macrophages and NK cells, thereby enhancing their ability to kill tumor cells and microorganisms. Gamma interferon can also increase antibody production (by enhancing B cell-stimulating lymphokines) and increase the synthesis of class II MHC proteins.

(2) **Lymphotoxins** are proteins produced by cytotoxic T lymphocytes; they play an important role in damaging or lysing target cells, eg, virus-infected cells.

(3) **Tumor necrosis factor** (TNF) is an inflammatory mediator released primarily by macrophages. It activates neutrophils and is cytotoxic to certain tumor cells. It also mediates endotoxin-induced septic shocki. TNF is also known as cachectin because it inhibits lipoprotein lipase thereby preventing the uptake of triglycerides. This results in cachexia.

Review Questions

1. Describe the origin of T cells and B cells.
2. T cells can be divided into subpopulations, eg, CD4 and CD8. How is this determined?
3. CD4 and CD8 subpopulations have different functions. What are they?
4. To activate T cells, 2 molecules must be recognized. One is the antigen. What is the other?
5. What contribute to cell-mediated immunity?
6. What cells have a cytotoxic effect on foreign grafts?
7. How do T cells (CD4 and CD8) regulate antibody production?
8. How do T cells (CD4 and CD8) regulate cell-mediated immune response?
9. Contrast the antigen receptor on the surface of B cells with that on T cells.
10. Describe the clonal selection model of antibody synthesis.
11. What are the main functions of (a) macrophages and (b) NK cells?
12. Distinguish between interleukin-1 and interleukin-2.
13. How does gamma interferon differ from the alpha and beta forms?

Antibodies

Antibodies are immunoglobulins that react specifically with the antigen that stimulated their production. They make up about 20% of the protein in blood plasma.

Antibodies that arise in an animal in response to typical antigens are heterogeneous, because they are formed by several different clones of cells; ie, they are **polyclonal.** Antibodies that arise from a single clone of cells, eg, in a plasma cell tumor (myeloma),* are homogeneous; ie, they are **monoclonal**. Monoclonal antibodies also can be made in the laboratory by fusing a myeloma cell with an antibody-producing cell. Such **hybridomas** produce virtually unlimited quantities of monoclonal antibodies that are useful in diagnostic tests and in research (see box).

Hybridomas & Monoclonal Antibodies

One of the most important scientific advances of this century is the hybridoma cell, which has the remarkable ability to produce large quantities of a single molecular species of immunoglobulin. These immunoglobulins, which are known as monoclonal antibodies, are called ''monoclonal'' because they are made by a clone of cells that arose from a single cell. Note, however, that this single cell is, in fact, formed by the fusion of 2 different cells; ie, it is a hybrid, hence the term ''hybridoma.''

Hybridoma cells are made in the following manner: (1) An animal, eg, a mouse, is immunized with the antigen of interest. (2) Spleen cells from this animal are grown in a culture dish in the presence of mouse myeloma cells. The strain of myeloma cells chosen has 2 important attributes: it grows indefinitely in culture, and it does not produce immunoglobulins. (3) Fusion of the cells is encouraged by adding certain chemicals, eg, polyethylene glycol. (4) The cells are grown in a special culture medium (HAT medium) that supports the growth of the fused, hybrid cells but not of the ''parental'' cells. (5) The resulting clones of cells are screened for the production of antibody to the antigen of interest.

IMMUNOGLOBULIN STRUCTURE   Immunoglobulins are glycoproteins made up of **light** (L) and **heavy** (H) polypeptide chains. The terms ''light'' and ''heavy'' refer to molecular weight; ie, light chains have a molecular weight of about 25,000, whereas heavy chains have a molecular weight of 50,000–70,000. The simplest antibody molecule has a Y shape (Fig 59–1) and consists of 4 polypeptide chains: 2 H chains and 2 L chains. The 4 chains are linked by covalent disulfide bonds. An individual antibody molecule always consists of identical H chains and identical L chains. This is primarily the result of 2 phenomena: allelic exclusion (see p 269) and regulation within the B cell, which ensure the synthesis of either kappa or lambda L chains but not both.

L and H chains are subdivided into **variable** and **constant** regions. The regions are composed of 3-dimensionally folded, repeating segments called domains. An L chain consists of one variable (VL) and one constant (CL) domain. Most H chains consist of one variable (VH) and 3 constant (CH) domains. (IgG and IgA have 3 CH domains, whereas IgM and IgE have 4.) Each domain is approximately 110 amino acids long. The **variable** regions are responsible for **antigen binding**, whereas the **constant** regions are responsible for **various biologic functions**, eg, complement activation and binding to cell surface receptors.

---

*Multiple myeloma is a malignant disease characterized by an overproduction of plasma cells (B cells). All the myeloma cells in a patient produce the same type of immunoglobulin molecule (M protein), which indicates that all the cells arose from a single progenitor. Excess kappa or lambda light chains are synthesized and appear as dimers in the urine. These are known as Bence Jones proteins and have the unusual attribute of precipitating at 50–60 °C but dissolving when the temperature is raised to the boiling point.

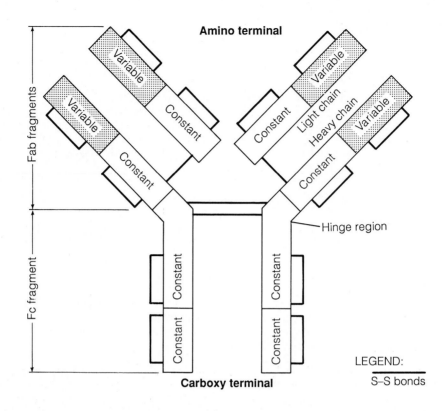

Figure 59–1. Structure of IgG. (Reproduced, with permission, from Jawetz E et al: *Review of Medical Microbiology,* 18th ed. Appleton & Lange, 1989.)

The variable regions of both L and H chains have 3 extremely variable ("**hypervariable**") amino acid sequences at the amino-terminal end that form the antigen-binding site (Fig 59–2). Only 5–10 amino acids in each hypervariable region form the antigen-binding site. Antigen-antibody binding involves electrostatic and van de Waals' forces and hydrogen and hydrophobic bonds. The remarkable specificity of antibodies is due to these hypervariable regions. (See idiotypes p 268.)

L chains belong to one of 2 types, κ (**kappa**) or λ (**lambda**), on the basis of amino acid differences in their constant regions. Both types occur in all classes of immunoglobulins (IgG, IgM, etc), but any one immunoglobulin molecule contains only one type of L chain.* The amino-terminal portion of each L chain contains part of the antigen-binding site. H chains are distinct for each of the 5 immunoglobulin classes and are designated γ, α, μ, ε, and δ (Table 59–1). The amino-terminal portion of each H chain participates in the antigen-binding site; the carboxy terminal forms the Fc fragment, which has the biologic activities described above and in Table 59–1.

If an antibody molecule is treated with a proteolytic enzyme such as papain, peptide bonds in the "hinge" region are broken, producing 2 identical **Fab fragments**, which carry the antigen-binding sites, and one **Fc fragment**, which is involved in placental transfer, complement fixation, attachment for various cells, and other biologic activities (Fig 59–1).

IMMUNOGLOBULIN CLASSES

IgG Each IgG molecule consists of 2 L chains and 2 H chains linked by disulfide bonds (molecular formula H2L2). Because it has 2 identical antigen-binding sites, it is said to be divalent. There are 4 subclasses, IgG1–IgG4, based on antigenic differences in the H chains and on the number and location of disulfide bonds. IgG1 makes up most (65%) of the total

*In humans, the ratio of immunoglobulins containing κ chains to those containing λ chains is approximately 2:1.

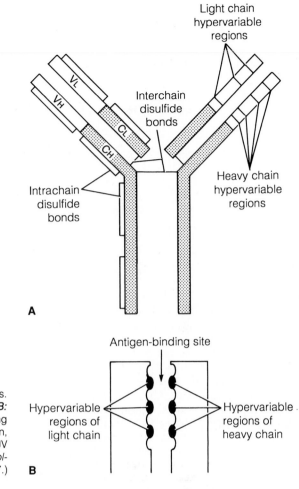

Figure 59–2. Hypervariable regions. *A:* Hypervariable regions on IgG. *B:* Magnified view of antigen-binding site. (Reproduced, with permission, from Stites DP, Stobo JD, Wells JV [editors]: *Basic & Clinical Immunology,* 6th ed. Appleton & Lange, 1987.)

IgG. IgG2 antibody is directed against polysaccharide antigens and is an important host defense against encapsulated bacteria.

IgG is the predominant antibody in the **secondary response** and constitutes an important defense against bacteria and viruses (Table 59–2). IgG is the only antibody to **cross the placenta**; only its Fc portion binds to receptors on the surface of placental cells. It is therefore the most abundant immunoglobulin in newborns.

Table 59–1. Properties of human immunoglobulins.

Property	IgG	IgA	IgM	IgD	IgE
Percentage of total immunoglobulin in serum (approx)	75	15	9	0.2	0.004
Serum concentration (mg/dL) (approx)	1000	200	120	3	0.05
Sedimentation coefficient	7S	7S or 11S[1]	19S	7S	8S
Molecular weight ($\times$ 1000)	150	170 or 400[1]	900	180	190
Structure	Monomer	Monomer or dimer	Pentamer	Monomer	Monomer
H-chain symbol	γ	α	μ	δ	ϵ
Complement fixation	+	–	+	–	–
Transplacental passage	+	–	–	?	–
Mediation of allergic responses	–	–	–	–	+

[1]The 11S form is found in secretions (eg, saliva, milk, and tears) and fluids of the respiratory, intestinal, and genital tracts.

Table 59–2. Important functions of immunoglobulins.

Immunoglobulin	Major Functions
IgG	Opsonizes bacteria, making them easier to phagocytize. Fixes complement, which enhances bacterial killing. Neutralizes bacterial toxins and viruses. Crosses the placenta.
IgA	Secretory IgA prevents attachment of bacteria and viruses to mucous membranes. Does not fix complement.
IgM	Produced in the primary response to an antigen. Functions like IgG. Fixes complement but does not cross the placenta. Found on the surface of B cells as well as in serum.
IgD	Uncertain. Found on the surface of many B cells as well as in serum.
IgE	Mediates immediate hypersensitivity by causing release of mediators from mast cells and basophils upon exposure to allergen.

IgA IgA is the main immunoglobulin in **secretions** such as colostrum, saliva, and tears and in respiratory, intestinal, and genital tract secretions. It protects mucous membranes from attack by bacteria and viruses. Each secretory IgA molecule (MW 400,000) consists of 2 H2L2 units plus one molecule each of J (joining) chain* and secretory component (Fig 59–3). The secretory component is a polypeptide synthesized by epithelial cells that provides for IgA passage to the mucosal surface. In serum, some IgA exists as a monomer H2L2 (MW 170,000).

IgM IgM is the main immunoglobulin produced early in the **primary response**. It is present as a monomer on the surface of virtually all B cells. In serum, it is a **pentamer** composed of 5 H2L2 units plus one molecule of J (joining) chain (Fig 59–3). The pentamer (MW 900,000) has a total of 10 antigen-binding sites and a valence of 5–10. It is the **most efficient** immunoglobulin in agglutination, complement fixation, and other antibody reactions and is important in defense against bacteria and viruses. It can be produced by the fetus in infections. It has the **highest avidity** of the immunoglobulins; its interaction with antigen can involve all 10 of its binding sites.

IgD This immunoglobulin has no known antibody function but may function as an antigen receptor; it is present on the surface of some B lymphocytes in cord blood (also on cells in certain lymphatic leukemias). It is present in small amounts in serum.

IgE The Fc region of IgE binds to the surface of mast cells and basophils. Bound IgE serves as a receptor for antigen (allergen), and this antigen-antibody complex triggers **allergic** responses of the **immediate (anaphylactic)** type through the release of mediators (see Chapter 65). Although IgE is present in **trace** amounts in normal serum (approximately 0.004%), persons with allergic reactivity have greatly increased amounts, and IgE may appear in external secretions. The serum IgE concentration also is typically increased during helminth (worm) infections. IgE does not fix complement and does not cross the placenta.

ISOTYPES, ALLOTYPES, & IDIOTYPES Because immunoglobulins are proteins, they are antigenic and that property allows them to be subdivided into various isotypes, allotypes, and idiotypes.

(1) Isotypes are immunoglobulins that can be distinguished antigenically yet are found in all normal humans. For example, IgG and IgM are different isotypes; the constant region of their

---

*Only IgA and IgM have J chains. Only these immunoglobulins exist as multimers (dimers and pentamers, respectively). The J chain is covalently bound to the Fc portion of the immunoglobulin and serves to hold the monomer H2L2 units together.

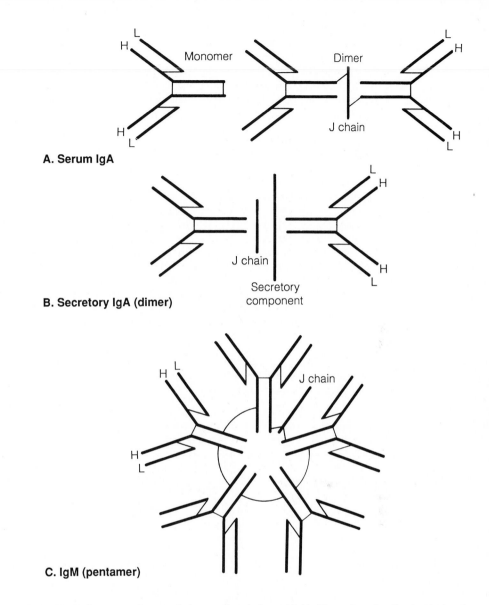

Figure 59–3. Structure of serum IgA, secretory IgA, and IgM. (Reproduced, with permission, from Stites DP, Stobo JD, Wells JV [editors]: *Basic & Clinical Immunology,* 6th ed. Appleton & Lange, 1987.)

H chains (γ and μ) is different antigenically (the 5 immunoglobulin classes—IgG, IgM, IgA, IgD, and IgE—are different isotypes; their heavy chains are antigenically different). Similarly, IgA1 and IgA2 are different isotypes (the antigenicity of the constant region of their H chains is different), and κ and λ chains are different isotypes (their constant regions also differ antigenically).

(2) Allotypes, on the other hand, are additional antigenic features of immunoglobulins that vary among individuals. They vary because the genes that code for the L and H chains are polymorphic, and individuals can have different alleles. For example, the γ H chain contains an allotype called Gm, which is due to a one- or 2-amino-acid difference that provides a different antigenicity to the molecule. Each individual inherits different allelic genes that code for one or another amino acid at the Gm site.*

---

*Allotypes related to γ H chains are called Gm (an abbreviation of gamma); allotypes related to κ L chains are called Inv (an abbreviation of a patient's name).

(3) Idiotypes are the antigenic determinants of the hypervariable region.* Each idiotype is unique for the V domain of the immunoglobulin produced by a specific clone of antibody-producing cells. Anti-idiotype antibody reacts only with the V domain of the specific immunoglobulin molecule that induced it. The network theory of immune regulation employs anti-idiotype antibody as both a positive and a negative regulator. Because the antibody could interact with the antigen-binding site, it could mimic antigen and induce B cell differentiation. Alternatively, it could suppress it.

IMMUNOGLOBULIN GENES To produce the very large number of different immunoglobulin molecules (10^6–10^9) without requiring excessive numbers of genes, special genetic mechanisms, eg, **DNA rearrangement** and **RNA splicing**, are used.

Each immunoglobulin chain consists of a distinct variable (V) and constant (C) region. For each type of immunoglobulin chain, ie, kappa light chain (κL), lambda light chain (λL), and the 5 heavy chains (γH, αH, μH, ϵH, and δH), there is a separate pool of gene segments located on different chromosomes.[†] Each pool contains a set of different V gene segments widely separated from the D (diversity, seen only in H chains), J (joining), and C gene segments (Fig 59–4). In the synthesis of an H chain, for example, a particular V region is translocated to lie close to a D segment, several J segments, and a C region. These genes are transcribed into mRNA, and all but one of the J segments are removed by splicing the RNA. During B cell differentiation the first translocation brings a VH gene near a Cμ gene, leading to the formation of IgM as the first antibody produced in a primary response.

---

*Any one of these antigen determinants is called an idiotope.

[†]The genes for κL, λL, and the 5 heavy chains are on chromosomes 2, 22, and 14, respectively.

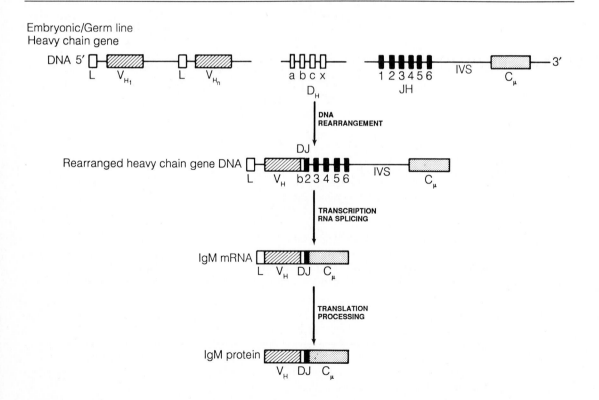

Figure 59–4. Gene rearrangement to produce a μH chain. V, variable regions; L, leader sequence; D, diversity segments; J, joining segments; C, constant region; IVS, intervening sequence. (Reproduced, with permission, from Stites DP, Stobo JD, Wells JV [editors]: *Basic & Clinical Immunology,* 6th ed. Appleton & Lange, 1987.)

The V region of each L chain is encoded by 2 gene segments (V + J). The V region of each H chain is encoded by 3 gene segments (V + D + J). These various segments are united into one functional V gene by DNA rearrangement. Each of these assembled V genes is then transcribed with the appropriate C genes and spliced to produce an mRNA that codes for the complete peptide chain. L and H chains are synthesized separately on polysomes and then assembled in the cytoplasm by means of disulfide bonds to form H2L2 units. Finally, the carbohydrate moiety is added and the immunoglobulin molecule is released from the cell.

The gene organization mechanism outlined above permits the assembly of a very large number of different molecules. Antibody **diversity** depends on (1) multiple gene segments, (2) their rearrangement into different sequences, (3) the combining of different L and H chains in the assembly of immunoglobulin molecules, and (4) mutations.

IMMUNOGLOBULIN CLASS SWITCHING (ISOTYPE SWITCHING) Initially, all B cells carry IgM specific for an antigen and produce IgM antibody in response to exposure to that antigen. Later, gene rearrangement permits the elaboration of antibodies of the same antigenic specificity but of different immunoglobulin classes (Fig 59–5). In **class switching**, the same assembled VH gene can sequentially associate with different CH genes so that the immunoglobulins produced later (IgG, IgA, or IgE) have the same specificity as the original IgM but have different biologic characteristics. This is illustrated in the "class switch" section of Fig 59–5. A different molecular mechanism is involved in the switching from IgM to IgD. In this case, a single mRNA consisting of VDJ CμCδ is initially transcribed and is then spliced into separate VDJ Cμ and VDJ Cδ mRNAs. Mature B cells can, in this manner, express both IgM and IgD (See Fig 59–5, alternative RNA splicing).

A single B cell expresses only one L-chain and one H-chain allele; ie, either the paternal or maternal set is expressed but not both. This is called **allelic exclusion**. One set is "excluded" and does not code for different immunoglobulin. The mechanism of this exclusion is unknown.

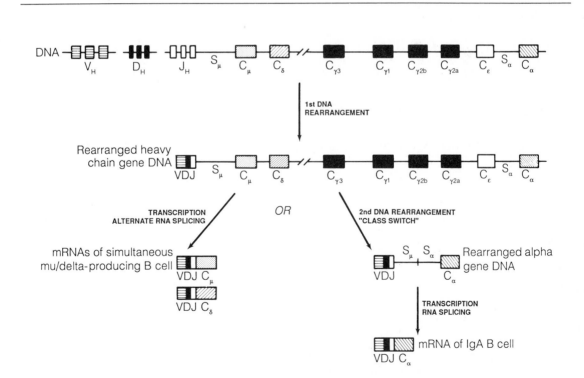

Figure 59–5. Gene rearrangement to produce different immunoglobulin classes. V, variable regions; D, diversity segments; J, joining segments; C, constant regions; S, switch sites. (Reproduced, with permission, from Stites DP, Stobo JD, Wells JV [editors]: *Basic & Clinical Immunology,* 6th ed. Appleton & Lange, 1987.)

Review Questions

1. What are monoclonal antibodies, and what cells make them? Describe how these cells are produced.
2. Contrast the structure of an IgG, IgM, and IgA molecule.
3. What forms the antigen-binding site?
4. To which portion of the immunoglobulin molecule does complement bind?
5. What do the terms constant, variable, and hypervariable refer to?
6. What are domains, and where are they located?
7. Distinguish between the terms isotype, allotype, and idiotype.
8. Which immunoglobulin class (a) makes up more than half the immunoglobulin in adult serum, (b) is present in the highest concentration in newborn serum, (c) has the highest avidity, (d) is secreted on mucosal surfaces, (e) triggers anaphylaxis, (f) is on the mast cell surface, and (g) can cross the placenta?
9. Describe the structure of the immunoglobulin genes and how a large number of antibody specificities are produced from a relatively small number of genes.
10. Which class of immunoglobulin is produced first in response to antigen? Describe the process by which other classes are made.

60

Humoral Immunity

THE PRIMARY RESPONSE   When an antigen is first encountered, a rise of antibody detectable in the serum occurs within days or weeks, depending on the nature and dose of the antigen and the route of administration (eg, parenteral or oral). The serum antibody concentration continues to rise for several weeks, then declines and may drop to very low levels (Fig 60–1). The **first** antibodies to appear are **IgM** followed by IgG or IgA. IgM levels tend to decline earlier than IgG levels.

THE SECONDARY RESPONSE   When there is a second encounter with the same antigen or a closely related (or cross-reacting) one, months or years after the primary response, there is a rapid antibody response to higher levels than the primary response. This is attributed to the persistence of antigen-sensitive ''memory cells'' after the first contact.

Figure 60–1. Antibody synthesis in the primary and secondary responses. (Reproduced, with permission, from Jawetz E et al: *Review of Medical Microbiology*, 18th ed. Appleton & Lange, 1989.)

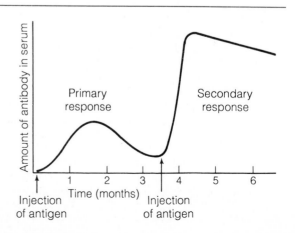

During the secondary response, the amount of IgM produced is similar to that after the first contact with antigen. However, a much **larger** amount of IgG antibody is produced and the levels tend to persist much **longer** than in the primary response. Also, such antibodies tend to bind antigen more firmly (ie, have **higher avidity**) and thus dissociate less easily.

RESPONSE TO MULTIPLE ANTIGENS ADMINISTERED SIMULTANEOUSLY When 2 or more antigens are administered at the same time, the host reacts by producing antibodies to all of them. Competition of antigens for antibody-producing mechanisms occurs experimentally but appears to be of little significance in medicine. Combined immunization is widely used, eg, the diphtheria, pertussis, tetanus (DPT) vaccine or the measles, mumps, rubella (MMR) vaccine.

FUNCTION OF ANTIBODIES The primary function of antibodies is to protect against infectious agents or their products (see Table 59–2). Antibodies provide resistance because they can (1) **neutralize** toxins and viruses and (2) **opsonize** microorganisms. Opsonization is the process by which antibodies make microorganisms more easily ingested by phagocytic cells. This occurs by either of 2 reactions. (1) The Fc portion of the immunoglobulin interacts with its receptors on the phagocyte surface to facilitate ingestion; or (2) IgG or IgM activate complement to yield C3b, which interacts with its receptors on the surface of the phagocyte.

Antibodies can be induced **actively** in the host or acquired **passively** and thus be immediately available for defense. In medicine, passive immunity is used in the neutralization of the toxins of diphtheria, tetanus, and botulism by antitoxins and in the inhibition of such viruses as rabies and hepatitis A and B early in the incubation period.

Review Questions

1. Compare the primary and secondary responses from the following points of view: (a) time for antibody to appear, (b) quantity of antibody produced, (c) class of antibody produced, and (d) duration of antibody production.
2. Two important functions of antibodies are neutralization and opsonization. Describe these processes.

Cell-Mediated Immunity 61

Antibody-mediated immunity is directed primarily against (1) toxin-induced diseases, (2) infections in which virulence is related to polysaccharide capsules (eg, pneumococcus, meningococcus, *Haemophilus influenzae),* and (3) certain viral infections. However, in many microbial infections, especially intracellular ones such as tuberculosis, cell-mediated immunity imparts resistance and aids in recovery. Furthermore, cell-mediated immunity is essential in defense against parasites, tumors, and transplanted grafts. The strongest evidence for the importance of cell-mediated immunity comes from clinical situations in which its suppression (by immunosuppressive drugs or disease, eg, AIDS) results in overwhelming infections or tumors.

The constituents of the cell-mediated immune system include several cell types: (1) **macrophages**, which present the antigen to T cells; (2) **T cells**, which participate in antigen recognition and in regulation (helper and suppressor) functions (see Chapter 58); (3) **natural killer** (NK) cells, which can inactivate pathogens; and (4) **K (killer)** and

cytotoxic T cells, which can kill with or without antibody. Macrophages and T cells produce lymphokines, which activate other T-cells (eg, cytotoxic T cells) and macrophage effector activities that involve killing the pathogen or tumor cell.

Although the complexity of cell and lymphokine interactions is enormous, the result is relatively simple: In the person with competent cellular immunity, many opportunistic pathogens rarely or never cause disease, and the spread of other agents—for example, certain viruses (eg, herpesviruses) or tumors (eg, Kaposi's sarcoma)—is limited. The assessment of the competence of cell-mediated immunity is therefore important.

TESTS FOR EVALUATION OF CELL-MEDIATED IMMUNITY

Evaluation of the immunocompetence of persons depends either on the demonstration of delayed-type hypersensitivity to universally present antigens (equating the ability to respond with the competence of cell-mediated immunity) or on laboratory assessments of T cells.

Skin Tests for the Presence of Delayed-Type Hypersensitivity

Most normal persons respond with delayed-type reactions to skin test antigens of *Candida,* streptokinase-streptodornase, or mumps because of past exposure to these antigens. Absence of reactions to several of these skin tests suggests impairment of cell-mediated immunity.

Skin Tests for the Ability to Develop Delayed-Type Hypersensitivity

Most normal persons with competent cell-mediated reactions can readily develop reactivity to simple chemicals (eg, dinitrochlorobenzene; DNCB) applied to their skin in lipid solvents. When the same chemical is applied to the same area 7–14 days later, they respond with a delayed-type skin reaction. Immunocompromised persons with incompetent cell-mediated immunity fail to develop such delayed-type hypersensitivity.

In Vitro Tests for Lymphoid Cell Competence

A. Lymphocyte Blast Transformation: When sensitized T lymphocytes are exposed to the specific antigen, they transform into large blast cells with greatly increased DNA synthesis, as measured by incorporation of tritiated thymidine. This *specific* effect involves relatively few cells. A larger number of T cells undergo *nonspecific* blast transformation when exposed to certain mitogens. The mitogens phytohemagglutinin and concanavalin A are plant extracts that stimulate T cells specifically. (Bacterial endotoxin, a lipopolysaccharide, stimulates B cells specifically.)

B. Macrophage Migration Inhibitory Factor: Macrophage migration inhibitory factor is elaborated by cultured T cells when exposed to the antigen to which they are sensitized. Its effect can be measured by observing the reduced migration of macrophages in the presence of the factor compared with controls.

C. Enumeration of T Cells, B Cells, and Subpopulations: B cells can be counted by using fluorescence-labeled antibody against all immunoglobulin classes. Specific monoclonal antibodies directed against T cell markers permit the enumeration of T cells, CD4 helper cells, CD8 suppressor cells, and others. The normal ratio of CD4 to CD8 cells is 1.5 or greater, whereas in some immunodeficiencies (eg, AIDS) it is 1 or less.

ROLE OF ADJUVANTS & LIPIDS IN ESTABLISHING CELL-MEDIATED REACTIVITY

Weak antigens or simple chemicals tend not to elicit cell-mediated hypersensitivity when administered alone, but they do so when given as a mixture with an adjuvant. The role of the **adjuvant** is presumably to enhance the uptake of the antigen by antigen-presenting cells, eg, macrophages. A common experimental adjuvant is a mixture of mineral oil, lanolin, and killed mycobacteria (Freund's adjuvant), which stimulates the formation of local granulomas. It is prohibited for human use. Cell wall lipids (wax D) of mycobacteria serve as adjuvants for tuberculoprotein to establish cell-mediated reactivity. Skin lipids may aid the catechols of poison oak or poison ivy in sensitizing the skin.

Review Questions

1. Contrast the role of cell-mediated immunity in defense against infection with the role of humoral (antibody) immunity.
2. Describe the cells involved in cell-mediated immunity and their functions.
3. How can you evaluate the competency of a patient's cell-mediated immune system?
4. What role do adjuvants play in cell-mediated immunity?

Major Histocompatibility Complex & Transplantation

62

The success of tissue and organ transplants depends on the donor's and recipient's **human leukocyte antigens** (HLA) encoded by the HLA genes.[*] These proteins are alloantigens, ie, they differ among members of the same species. If the HLA proteins on the donor's cells differ from those on the recipient's cells, an immune response occurs in the recipient. The genes for the HLA proteins are clustered in the major histocompatibility complex (MHC), located on the short arm of chromosome 6.[†] Three of these genes (HLA-A, HLA-B, and HLA-C) code for the class I MHC antigens. Several HLA-D loci determine the class II MHC antigens, ie, DP, DQ, and DR (Fig 62–1). Each person has 2 **haplotypes,** ie, 2 sets of these genes, one on the paternal and the other on the maternal chromosome 6. These genes are very diverse (**polymorphic**), but any individual inherits only a single allele at each locus from each parent and thus can make no more than 2 different forms of each class I and class II glycoprotein. Expression of these genes is codominant; ie, the proteins encoded by both the paternal and maternal genes are produced.

---

[*]Certain HLA antigens are associated with specific diseases (eg, HLA-B27 with ankylosing spondylitis).

[†]In addition to these major antigens, there are ''weak'' minor antigens coded for by genes located at sites other than the MHC.

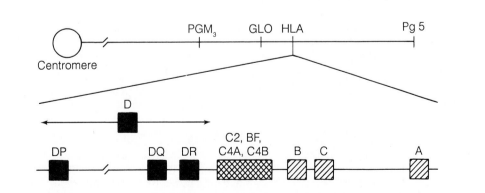

Figure 62–1. The human leukocyte antigen (HLA) gene complex. A, B, and C are the class I loci. DP, DQ, and DR are class II loci. C2, BF, and C4A and C4B are complement loci. PGM$_3$, GLO, and Pg 5 are adjacent, unrelated genes. (Reproduced, with permission, from Stites DP, Stobo JD, Wells JV [editors]: *Basic & Clinical Immunology,* 6th ed. Appleton & Lange, 1987.)

MHC ANTIGENS

Class I MHC Antigens These are glycoproteins found on the surfaces of **virtually all nucleated cells**. There are approximately 20 different proteins encoded by the allelic genes at the A locus, 40 at the B locus, and 8 at the C locus. The complete class I antigen is composed of a 45,000-molecular-weight heavy chain noncovalently bound to a beta-2 microglobulin. The heavy chain is highly polymorphic and is similar to an immunoglobulin molecule; it has hypervariable regions in its N-terminal region. The **polymorphism** of these molecules is important in the **recognition of self and nonself**. Stated another way, if these molecules were very similar, our ability to reject foreign grafts would be correspondingly lower.

Class I antigens are detected in the laboratory by reacting lymphocytes (as antigen) with a battery of specific antibodies plus complement.* If lymphocyte and antibody match, the cell is lysed. This test, along with the test for class II antigens (see below), is used to identify the haplotypes of donors being considered for transplant surgery.

Class II MHC Antigens These occur on the **surfaces of certain cells**, including macrophages, B cells, dendritic cells of the spleen, and Langerhans cells of the skin. They are highly polymorphic glycoproteins composed of 2 polypeptides (MW 33,000 and 28,000) that are noncovalently bound. Like class I antigens, they have hypervariable regions that provide much of the polymorphism.

Class II antigens were first demonstrated by the "**mixed-leukocyte reaction**." In this test, "stimulator" lymphocytes from a potential donor are first killed by irradiation and then mixed with live "responder" lymphocytes from the recipient; the mixture is incubated in cell culture to permit DNA synthesis, which is measured by incorporation of tritiated thymidine. The greater the amount of DNA synthesis in the responder cells, the more foreign are the MHC class II antigens of the donor cells. A large amount of DNA synthesis indicates an unsatisfactory "match"; ie, donor and recipient MHC class II (HLA-D) antigens are *not* similar, and the graft is likely to be rejected. Currently, clinical laboratories can determine the important class II antigens (DR loci) by using serologic tests analogous to those used for the class I antigens.

BIOLOGIC IMPORTANCE OF MHC The ability of T cells to recognize antigen is dependent on association of the antigen with either class I or class II proteins. For example, cytotoxic T cells respond to antigen in association with MHC class I glycoproteins. Thus, a cytotoxic T cell that kills a virus-infected cell will not kill a cell infected with the same virus if the cell does not also express the same class I proteins. Helper T cells recognize class II antigens. Helper-cell activity depends in general on *both* the recognition of the antigen on antigen-presenting cells *and* the presence on these cells of "self" MHC class II antigens. This requirement to recognize the "self" MHC protein is called **MHC restriction**. Note that T cells recognize antigens bound to the surface of cells, whereas B cells can recognize soluble antigens that interact with immunoglobulin receptors.

TRANSPLANTATION An **autograft** (transfer of an individual's own tissue) is regularly accepted. A **syngeneic graft**[†] is a transfer of tissue between genetically identical individuals, ie, identical twins, and usually "takes" permanently. A **xenograft,**[†] transfer of tissue between different species, is always rejected by an immunocompetent recipient.

An **allograft**[†] is a graft between genetically different members of the same species, eg, from one human to another. Unless specific measures are taken, it is rejected by the "allograft reaction." Initially, vascularization of the graft is normal but in 11–14 days, marked reduction in circulation and mononuclear cell infiltration occurs, with eventual necrosis.[††] A T cell-mediated reaction is the main cause of rejection of many types of grafts, eg, skin, but

---

*The antibodies are obtained primarily from multiparous women who have been exposed to the father's antigens on fetal lymphocytes that cross the placenta during pregnancy. Some monoclonal antibodies are available also.

[†]Previously used synonyms for these terms include isograft (syngeneic graft), heterograft (xenograft), and homograft (allograft).

[††]Two other types of graft rejection also can occur: (1) "hyperacute," in which the graft is rejected very rapidly as a result of the presence of large amounts of preformed antibodies, eg, anti-ABO antibodies; and (2) chronic rejection, which can take months or years and is probably due to incompatibility of the weak (minor) histocompatibility antigens.

antibodies make an important contribution to the rejection of certain transplants, especially bone marrow. In experimental animals, rejection of most types of grafts can be transferred by cells, not serum. Also, T cell-deficient animals do not reject grafts but B cell-deficient animals do. The role of cytotoxic T cells in allograft rejection is described on page 258.

If a second allograft from the same donor is applied to a sensitized recipient, it is rejected in 5–6 days. This **accelerated** ("second-set") rejection is caused primarily by presensitized cytotoxic T cells.

The acceptance or rejection of a transplant is determined, in large part, by the class I and class II MHC proteins, with **class II** playing the **major** role. The proteins encoded by the DR locus are especially important. Prior to transplantation surgery, laboratory tests are performed to determine the closest match of MHC antigens in the donor and recipient. Class I antigens and certain class II antigens, especially DR, are detected by using a panel of known antibodies plus complement to lyse donor lymphocytes. Additional information regarding the compatibility of the class II antigens is determined by the mixed leukocyte reaction with cultured cells. In addition to the tests used for matching, preformed cytotoxic antibodies in the recipient's serum reactive against the graft are detected by observing the lysis of donor lymphocytes by the recipient's serum plus complement. This is called "**crossmatching**" and is done to prevent hyperacute rejections from occurring. (ABO blood group tests are also done on the donor and recipient.)

Among siblings in a single family, there is a 25% chance for both haplotypes to be shared and a 50% chance for one haplotype to be shared. For example, if the father is haplotype AB, the mother is CD, and the recipient child is AC, there is a 25% chance for a sibling to be AC, ie, a 2-haplotype match, and a 50% chance for a sibling to be either BC or AD, ie, a one-haplotype match.

Results of Organ Transplants If donor and recipient are well matched by mixed lymphocyte culture and histocompatibility antigen typing, the long-term survival of a transplanted organ or tissue is greatly enhanced. In 1986, the 5-year survival rate of 2-haplotype-matched kidney transplants from related donors was near 95%, that of one-haplotype-matched kidney transplants was near 80%, and that of transplant of kidneys from cadaver donors was near 60%. The survival rate of the last category was higher if the graft recipient had had several previous blood transfusions. The reason for this is unknown (but may be associated with tolerance). The heart transplant survival rate for 5 years is near 50–60%; the liver transplant rate is lower. Corneas are easily grafted, because they are avascular and the lymphatic supply of the eye prevents many antigens from triggering an immune response; consequently, the proportion of "takes" is very high.

Graft-Versus-Host Reaction Well-matched transplants of bone marrow may establish themselves initially in 85% of recipients, but subsequently a **graft-versus-host (GVH)** reaction develops in about two-thirds of them.* This reaction occurs because grafted immunocompetent T cells proliferate in the irradiated, immunocompromised host and "reject" cells with class II antigens, resulting in severe organ dysfunction especially in the skin, liver, and gastrointestinal tract. The GVH reaction can be reduced by administering antithymocyte globulin or monoclonal antibodies before grafting; this eliminates mature T cells from the donor marrow. Immunotoxins, eg, ricin linked to monoclonal anti-T-cell antibody, can also be used to reduce this reaction.

EFFECT OF IMMUNOSUPPRESSION ON GRAFT REJECTION To reduce the chance of rejection of transplanted tissue, immunosuppressive measures, eg, corticosteroids, azathioprine, cyclosporine, and radiation, are used. Unfortunately, immunosuppression enhances the recipient's susceptibility to opportunistic infections and neoplasms. Immunosuppressive drugs, eg, cyclosporine, also reduce graft-versus-host reactions.

Review Questions

1. Describe the genes that constitute the major histocompatibility complex.
2. Each person has 2 haplotypes with codominant genes. Explain this sentence.

---

*GVH reactions can also occur in immunodeficient children given a blood transfusion.

3. Compare class I and class II MHC antigens from the following points of view: (a) type of cells on which they are located, (b) laboratory test used to detect them, and (c) role in antigen recognition by CD4 and CD8 T cells.
4. Distinguish between an autograft, a syngeneic graft, an allograft, and a xenograft.
5. Describe the allograft reaction.
6. Describe how a prospective kidney donor is tested for compatibility with the recipient prior to transplant surgery.
7. What are the circumstances under which a graft-versus-host reaction occurs? Describe the reaction.

63

Complement

The complement system consists of approximately 20 proteins that are present in normal human (and other animal) serum. The term ''complement'' refers to the ability of these proteins to complement, ie, augment, the effects of other components of the immune system, eg, antibody. There are 3 main effects of complement: (1) **lysis** of cells such as bacteria, allografts, and tumor cells; (2) **generation of mediators** that participate in inflammation and attract phagocytes; and (3) **opsonization**, ie, enhancement of phagocytosis. Complement proteins are synthesized mainly by the liver. Complement is heat-labile; ie, it is inactivated by heating serum at 56 °C for 30 minutes. Immunoglobulins are not inactivated at this temperature.

ACTIVATION Several complement components are proenzymes, which must be cleaved to form active enzymes. Activation of the complement system can be initiated either by antigen-antibody complexes or by a variety of nonimmunologic molecules.

Sequential activation of complement components (Fig 63–1) occurs via one of 2 pathways.

(1) In the **classic** pathway, antigen-antibody complexes* activate C1† to form an esterase, which cleaves C2 and C4 to form a C4b2a complex. The latter is C3 convertase, which cleaves C3 molecules into 2 fragments, C3a and C3b. C3a, an **anaphylatoxin**, is discussed below. C3b forms a complex with C4b2a, producing a new enzyme, C5 convertase (C4b2a3b), which cleaves C5 to form C5a and C5b. C5a is an anaphylatoxin and a chemotactic factor (see below). C5b binds to C6 and C7 to form a complex that interacts with C8 and C9 to produce the ''**membrane attack**'' unit (C5b6789), which causes cytolysis.

(2) In the **alternative** pathway, many unrelated substances from complex chemicals, eg, endotoxin, to infectious agents, eg, parasites, activate a different C3 convertase (C3bBb), which generates more C3b. The additional C3b binds to form C3bBbC3b, a C5 convertase that generates C5b, leading to the production of the ''membrane attack'' unit described above.

REGULATION OF THE COMPLEMENT SYSTEM Several serum proteins regulate the complement system at different stages. (1) C1 inhibitor binds to and inactivates the esterase. Complement activation proceeds past this point by generating sufficient C1 to overwhelm the inhibitor. (2) Factor I cleaves C3b, thereby reducing the amount of C5 convertase available. (3) Factor

---

*Only IgM and IgG fix complement. C1 is bound to a site located in the Fc region. Of the IgGs, only IgG1, IgG2, and IgG3 subclasses fix complement; IgG4 does not.

†C1 is composed of 3 proteins, C1q, C1r, and C1s. C1q is an aggregate of 18 polypeptides that binds to the Fc portion of IgG and IgM. It is multivalent and can cross-link several immunoglobulin molecules. C1s is a proenzyme that becomes the esterase. Calcium is required for the activation of C1.

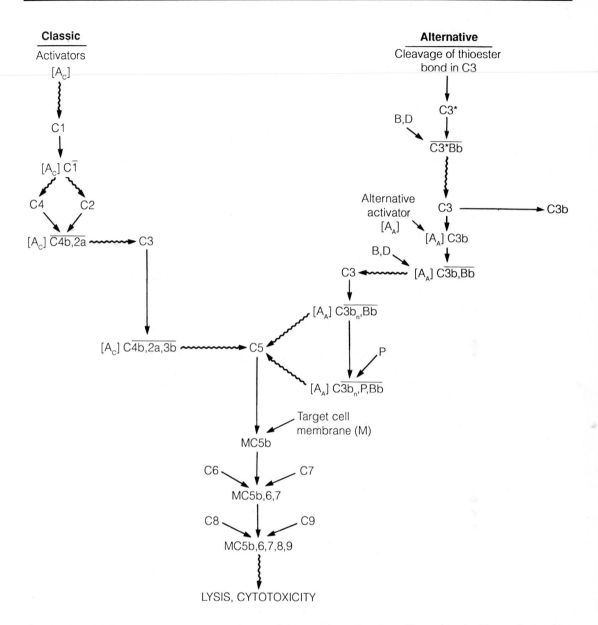

Figure 63–1. The classic and alternative pathways of the complement system. (Reproduced, with permission, from Stites DP, Stobo JD, Wells JV [editors]: *Basic & Clinical Immunology,* 6th ed. Appleton & Lange, 1987.) Note: C2a in the classic pathway was recently renamed C2b.

H enhances the effect of factor I on C3b. C3b deposited on certain membranes or activators is protected from factors H and I. (4) Factor P (properdin) protects C3b and stabilizes the convertases of the alternative pathway. (5) Factors B and D interact with C3b to form C3bBb (C3 convertase) in the alternative pathway.

BIOLOGIC EFFECTS

Opsonization Cells, antigen-antibody complexes, and other particles are phagocytized much better in the presence of C3b. This is due to the presence of C3b receptors on the surface of many phagocytes.

Chemotaxis   C5a and the C567 complex attract leukocytes. They migrate especially well toward C5a.

Anaphylatoxin   C3a, C4a, and C5a can produce degranulation of mast cells with release of mediators, eg, histamine, leading to increased vascular permeability and smooth-muscle contraction.

Cytolysis   Insertion of the C5b6789 complex into the cell membrane leads to killing or lysis of many types of cells including erythrocytes, bacteria, and tumor cells. Cytolysis is not an enzymatic process; rather, it appears that insertion of the complex results in disruption of the membrane and the entry of water and electrolytes into the cell.

CLINICAL ASPECTS

(1) Inherited (or acquired) deficiency of some complement components, especially C5–C8, greatly enhances susceptibility to *Neisseria* **bacteremia** and other infections.

(2) Inherited deficiency of C1 esterase inhibitor results in **angioedema**. When the inhibitor is reduced, an overproduction of esterase occurs. This leads to an increase in anaphylatoxins, which cause capillary permeability and edema.

(3) Immune complexes bind complement, and thus complement levels are low in immune complex diseases, eg, acute glomerulonephritis. Binding (activating) complement attracts polymorphonuclear leukocytes, which release enzymes that damage tissue.

Review Questions

1. What are the 3 major biologic effects of complement?
2. Compare the classic and the alternative pathways of complement activation. What is the nature of the substances that activate? What is the molecule that serves as the common entry point for both pathways to the rest of the sequence?
3. What is a convertase, and what role does it play?
4. Which components of complement facilitate (a) opsonization, (b) chemotaxis, (c) anaphylaxis, and (d) cytolysis?
5. What is the "membrane attack" unit, and what is its biologic effect?

64

Antigen-Antibody Reactions in the Laboratory

Reactions of antigens and antibodies are highly specific. An antigen will react only with antibodies elicited by itself or by a closely related antigen, ie, one expressing the same epitopes. Because of the great specificity, reactions between antigens and antibodies are suitable for identifying one by using the other. This is the basis of serologic reactions. Cross-reactions between related antigens can occur, and these can limit the specificity of the test.

Antigen-antibody reactions are applied to the identification of specific components in mixtures of either one. Microorganisms and other cells possess a variety of antigens and thus may react with many different antibodies. Monoclonal antibodies excel in identification of antigens because cross-reacting antibodies are absent; ie, monoclonal antibodies are highly specific.

DIAGNOSTIC ANTIGEN-ANTIBODY REACTIONS   Different types of antigen-antibody reactions take advantage of different physical or biologic features most suitable for diagnostic reactions.

Agglutination   In this reaction, the antigen is **particulate** (eg, bacteria and red blood cells)* or is an inert particle (latex beads) coated with an antigen. Antibody, because it is divalent or multivalent, cross-links the antigenically multivalent particles and forms a latticework, and clumping (agglutination) can be seen. This reaction can be done in a small cup or tube or with a drop on a slide.

Precipitation   In this reaction, the antigen is **in solution.** The antibody cross-links antigen molecules in variable proportions, and aggregates (precipitates) form. In the **zone of equivalence,** optimal proportions of antigen and antibody combine; the maximal amount of precipitates forms, and the supernatant contains neither an excess of antibody nor an excess of antigen (Fig 64–1). In the **zone of antibody excess,** there is too much antibody for efficient lattice formation, and precipitation is less than maximal.[†] In the **zone of antigen excess,** all antibody has combined but precipitation is reduced because many antigen-antibody complexes are too small to precipitate; ie, they are "soluble."

Precipitin reactions can be done in solution or in semisolid medium (agar).

A. Precipitation in Solution: This reaction can be made quantitative; ie, antigen or antibody can be measured in terms of micrograms of nitrogen present. It is used primarily in research.

B. Precipitation in Agar: This is done as either single or double diffusion. It can be done in the presence of an electric field also.

(1) Single diffusion   In single diffusion, antibody is incorporated into agar and antigen is measured into a well. As the antigen diffuses with time, precipitation rings form depending on the antigen concentration. By calibrating the method, such **radial immunodiffusion** is used to

---

*When red cells are used, it is called hemagglutination.

[†]The term "prozone" refers to the failure of a precipitate or flocculate to form because too much antibody is present. For example, a false-negative serologic test for syphilis (VDRL) is occasionally reported because the antibody titer is too high. Dilution of the serum yields a positive result.

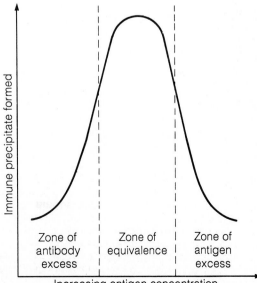

Figure 64–1. Precipitin curve. In the presence of a constant amount of antibody, the amount of immune precipitate formed is plotted as a function of increasing amounts of antigen. (Reproduced, with permission, from Stites DP, Stobo JD, Wells JV [editors]: *Basic & Clinical Immunology,* 6th ed. Appleton & Lange, 1987.)

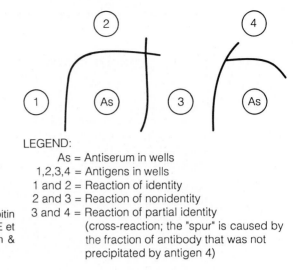

LEGEND:
As = Antiserum in wells
1,2,3,4 = Antigens in wells
1 and 2 = Reaction of identity
2 and 3 = Reaction of nonidentity
3 and 4 = Reaction of partial identity
(cross-reaction; the "spur" is caused by the fraction of antibody that was not precipitated by antigen 4)

Figure 64–2. Double-diffusion (Ouchterlony) precipitin reactions. (Reproduced, with permission, from Jawetz E et al: *Review of Medical Microbiology,* 18th ed. Appleton & Lange, 1989.)

measure IgG, IgM, complement components, and other substances in serum. (IgE cannot be measured because its concentration is too low.)

(2) Double diffusion   In double diffusion, antigen and antibody are placed in different wells in agar and allowed to diffuse and form concentration gradients. Where optimal proportions (see zone of equivalence, above) occur, lines of precipitate form. This method (Ouchterlony) indicates whether antigens are identical, related but not identical, or not related (Fig 64–2).

C. Precipitation in Agar With an Electric Field:

(1) Immunoelectrophoresis   A serum sample is placed in a well in agar on a glass slide (Fig 64–3). A current is passed through the agar, and the proteins move in the electric field according to their charge and size. Then a trough is cut into the agar and filled with antibody. As the antigen and antibody diffuse toward each other, they form a series of arcs of precipitate.

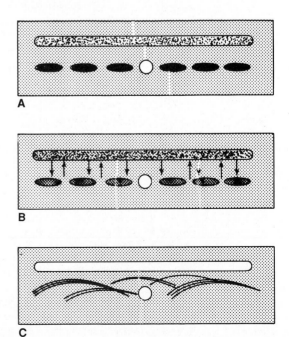

Figure 64–3. Immunoelectrophoresis. *A:* Human serum placed in the central well is electrophoresed, and the proteins migrate to different regions (dark ellipses). Antiserum to human serum is then placed in the elongated trough (speckled area). *B:* Human serum proteins and antibodies diffuse into agar. *C:* Precipitate arcs form in the agar. (Reproduced, with permission, from Stites DP, Stobo JD, Wells JV [editors]: *Basic & Clinical Immunology,* 6th ed. Appleton & Lange, 1987.)

This permits the serum proteins to be characterized in terms of their presence, absence, or unusual pattern (eg, human myeloma protein).

(2) Counter-immunoelectrophoresis This method relies on movement of antigen toward the cathode and of antibody toward the anode during the passage of electric current through agar. The meeting of the antigen and antibody is greatly accelerated and made visible in 30-60 minutes. This has been applied to the detection of bacterial polysaccharide antigens in cerebrospinal fluid.

Radioimmunoassay (RIA) This method is used for the quantitation of antigens or haptens that can be radioactively labeled. It is based on the competition for specific antibody between the labeled (known) and the unlabeled (unknown) concentration of material. The complexes that form between the antigen and antibody can then be separated and the amount of radioactivity measured. The more unlabeled antigen present, the less radioactivity there is in the complex. The concentration of the unknown (unlabeled) antigen or hapten is determined by comparison with the effect of standards. RIA is a highly sensitive method and is commonly used to assay hormones or drugs in serum. The radioallergosorbent test (RAST) is a specialized RIA that is used to measure the amount of serum IgE antibody that reacts with a known allergen (antigen).

Enzyme Immunoassay (ELISA) There are many variations of this method that depend on the conjugation of an enzyme to either an antigen or an antibody. The enzyme is detected by assaying for enzyme activity with its substrate. The method is nearly as sensitive as RIA yet requires no special equipment or radioactive labels.

For measurement of antibody, known antigens are fixed to a solid phase (eg, plastic microplate), incubated with test serum dilutions, washed, and then reincubated with an anti-immunoglobulin labeled with an enzyme, eg, horseradish peroxidase. Enzyme activity is measured by adding the substrate for the enzyme and estimating the color reaction in a spectrophotometer. The amount of antibody bound is proportionate to the enzyme activity.

Immunofluorescence Fluorescent dyes, eg, fluorescein and auramine, can be covalently attached to antibody molecules and made visible by ultraviolet (UV) light in the fluorescence microscope. Such "labeled" antibody can be used to identify antigens, eg, on the surface of bacteria (such as streptococci and treponemes), in cells in histologic section, or in other specimens. The immunofluorescence reaction is called **direct** when known labeled antibody interacts directly with unknown antigen and **indirect** when a 2-stage process is used (eg, known antigen is attached to a slide, unknown serum is added, and the preparation is washed; if the unknown serum antibody matches the antigen, it will remain fixed to it on the slide and can be detected on addition of a fluorescent dye-labeled antiglobulin antibody and examination by UV microscopy). The indirect test is often more sensitive than direct immunofluorescence, because more labeled antibody adheres per antigenic site. Furthermore, the labeled antiglobulin becomes a "universal reagent"; ie, independent of the nature of the antigen used, the antiglobulin is reactive with all IgG of that species.

Complement Fixation The complement system consists of 20 or more plasma proteins that interact with one another and with cell membranes. Each protein component must be activated sequentially under appropriate conditions for the reaction to progress. Antigen-antibody complexes are among the activators, and the complement fixation test can be used to identify one of them if the other is known.

The reaction consists of the following 2 steps (Fig 64–4): (1) Antigen and antibody (one known and the other unknown) are mixed, and a measured amount of complement (usually from guinea pig) is added. If antigen and antibody match, they will combine and take up ("fix") the complement. (2) An indicator system, consisting of "sensitized" red blood cells (ie, red blood cells plus anti-red blood cell antibody), is added. If the antibody matched the antigen in the first step, complement was fixed and less is available to attach to the sensitized red blood cells. The red blood cells remain **unhemolyzed;** ie, the test is **positive.** If the antibody did *not* match the antigen in the first step, complement is free to attach to the sensitized red blood cells and they are **lysed;** ie, the test is **negative.**

Complement must be carefully standardized, and the patient's serum must be heated to 56°C for 30 minutes to inactivate any human complement activity. The antigen must be quantitated. The result is expressed as the highest dilution of serum that gives positive results.

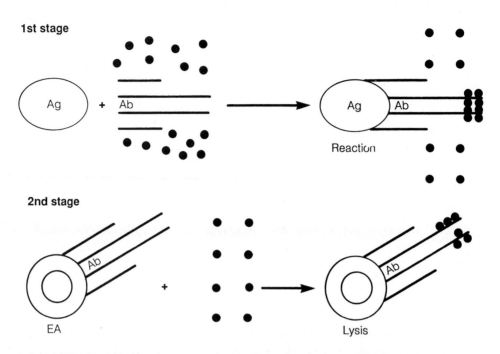

1st stage

Ag + Ab ⟶ Ag Ab

Reaction

2nd stage

EA + ⟶ Lysis

Figure 64–4. Complement fixation. In the first stage, if antigen and antibody are homologous, complement (black circles) is fixed. In the second stage, sensitized red cells (EA) are added. If complement was fixed in the first stage, less complement remains free. Therefore, lysis of EA is reduced. (Reproduced, with permission, from Stites, DP, Stobo JD, Wells JV [editors]: *Basic & Clinical Immunology*, 6th ed. Appleton & Lange, 1987.)

Controls to determine whether antigen or antibody alone fixes complement are needed to make the test results valid. If antigen or antibody alone fixes complement, it is said to be anticomplementary.

Neutralization Tests These use the ability of antibodies to block the effect of toxins or the infectivity of viruses. They can be used in cell culture (eg, inhibition of cytopathic effect and plaque-reduction assays) or in host animals (eg, mouse protection tests).

Immune Complexes Immune complexes in tissue can be stained with fluorescent complement. Immune complexes in serum can be detected by binding to C1q or by attachment to certain (eg, Raji lymphoblastoid) cells in culture.

Hemagglutination Tests Many viruses clump red blood cells from one species or another (active hemagglutination). This can be inhibited by antibody specifically directed against the virus (hemagglutination inhibition) and can be used to measure the presence and concentration of such antibody. Red blood cells also can absorb many antigens and, when mixed with matching antibodies, will clump (this is known as **passive hemagglutination**).*

Antiglobulin (Coombs) Test In many hemolytic anemias, eg, hemolytic disease of the newborn (Rh incompatibility) and drug-related hemolytic anemias, antibodies are bound to the red cell surface. These immunoglobulins can be detected by the direct antiglobulin (Coombs) test, in which antiserum against human immunoglobulin is used to agglutinate the patient's red cells. In some cases, the amount of antibody bound is too small to detect in the direct Coombs test, and the indirect antiglobulin test for antibodies in the patient's serum should be performed. In this test, the patient's serum is mixed with normal red cells, and antiserum to human immunoglobulins is added. If antibodies are present in the patient's serum, agglutination occurs.

*The red cells are passive carriers of the antigen.

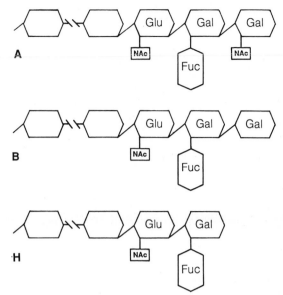

Figure 64–5. ABO blood groups. Structures of the terminal sugars that determine ABO blood groups are shown. (Reproduced, with permission, from Stites DP, Stobo JD, Wells JV [editors]: *Basic & Clinical Immunology,* 6th ed. Appleton & Lange, 1987.)

ANTIGEN-ANTIBODY REACTIONS INVOLVING RED BLOOD CELL ANTIGENS Many different blood group systems exist in humans. Each system consists of a gene locus specifying antigens on the erythrocyte surface. The 2 most important blood groupings, ABO and Rh, are described below.

The ABO Blood Groups & Transfusion Reactions All human erythrocytes contain alloantigens (ie, antigens that vary among individual members of a species) of the ABO group. This is an important system that serves as the basis for blood typing and transfusions.

The A and B antigens are carbohydrates that differ by a single sugar. Despite this small difference, A and B antigens do not cross-react. Erythrocytes have 3 sugar-terminal sugars in common on their surface: N-acetylglucosamine, galactose, and fucose. These 3 sugars form the H antigen (Fig 64–5). Type A cells have an additional N-acetylgalactosamine, whereas type B cells have an additional galactose. The A and B genes code for transferases that add the respective sugars.

There are 4 combinations of the 2 antigens present on erythrocytes (Table 64–1). The plasma contains antibody against the absent antigens, so that antigen and corresponding antibody do not coexist in the same person's blood. Transfusion reactions result when incompatible donor red blood cells are transfused; eg, if group A blood were transfused into a group B person (because anti-A antibody is present). (Transfused donor antibody is rapidly diluted and therefore becomes inactive against the recipient cells.)

To avoid antigen-antibody reactions that would result in transfusion reactions, all blood for transfusions must be carefully "**matched**"; ie, erythrocytes are typed for their surface antigens by specific sera. As shown in Table 64–1, persons with group O blood have no A or B antigens on their red cells and so are "universal donors"; ie, they can give blood to people in all 4 groups. Persons with group AB blood have neither A nor B antibody and thus are "universal recipients."

In addition to red blood cells, the A and B antigens appear on the cells of many tissues. Furthermore, these antigens can be secreted in saliva and other body fluids. Secretion is controlled by a secretor gene. Approximately 85% of people carry the dominant form of the gene, which allows secretion to occur.

Table 64–1. ABO blood groups.

Group	Antigen on Red Cell	Antibody in Plasma
A	A	Anti-B
B	B	Anti-A
AB	A and B	No anti-A or anti-B
O	No A or B	Anti-A and anti-B

Rh Blood Type & Hemolytic Disease of the Newborn   About 85% of humans have erythrocytes that express the Rh(D) antigen, ie, are Rh(D)$^+$. When an Rh(D)$^-$ person is transfused with Rh(D)$^+$ blood or when an Rh(D)$^-$ woman has an Rh(D)$^+$ fetus (the D gene being inherited from the father), the Rh(D) antigen will stimulate the development of antibodies. This occurs most often when the Rh(D)$^+$ erythrocytes of the fetus leak into the maternal circulation during delivery of the first Rh(D)$^+$ child. Subsequent Rh(D)$^+$ pregnancies are likely to be affected by the mother's anti-D antibody, and hemolytic disease of the newborn (**erythroblastosis fetalis**) may result. This disease results from the passage of maternal IgG anti-Rh(D) antibodies through the placenta to the fetus, with subsequent lysis of the fetal erythrocytes. The direct antiglobulin (Coombs) test is typically positive (see above for description of the Coombs test). The problem can be prevented by administration of high-titer Rh(D) immune globulins to an Rh(D)$^-$ mother immediately upon the delivery of an Rh(D)$^+$ child. These antibodies promptly attach to Rh(D)$^+$ erythrocytes and prevent their acting as sensitizing antigen. This prophylaxis is widely practiced and effective.

Review Questions

1. Contrast agglutination and precipitation reactions.
2. In the precipitin reaction, what happens in (a) the zone of antibody excess, (b) the zone of antigen excess, and (c) the zone of equivalence?
3. What is the principle of (a) the RIA and (6) the ELISA?
4. What is the difference between the direct and indirect fluorescent-antibody assays?
5. Describe the procedure used in the complement-fixation test. If the red cells lyse, is that a positive or a negative test? Why?
6. Contrast the direct and indirect Coombs tests. What are these tests used for?
7. What determines the ABO blood groups?
8. If group A blood is transfused into a group B person, what will happen and why?
9. If group O blood is transfused into a group B person, what will happen and why?
10. If group A blood is transfused into a group AB person, what will happen and why?
11. What blood group is present in universal donors? Why? In universal recipients? Why?
12. Will there be problems in children whose father is Rh(D)$^+$ and whose mother is Rh(D)$^-$? Explain.
13. How can the induction of Rh antibodies in the mother be mitigated?

65

Hypersensitivity (Allergy)

When an immune response results in exaggerated or inappropriate reactions harmful to the host, the term **hypersensitivity** or **allergy** is used. These reactions are typical in a given individual upon a second contact with a specific antigen. The first contact sensitizes.

Hypersensitivity reactions can be subdivided into 4 main types. Types I, II, and III are antibody-mediated, whereas type IV is cell-mediated (Table 65–1).

TYPE I: IMMEDIATE (ANAPHYLACTIC) HYPERSENSITIVITY   An antigen induces the formation of **IgE antibody**, which binds firmly by its Fc portion to basophils and mast cells. After a period of weeks, reexposure to the same antigen results in its fixation to the cell-bound IgE,

Table 65–1. Hypersensitivity reactions.

Mediator	Type	Reaction
Antibody	I (immediate, anaphylactic)	IgE antibody is induced by allergen and binds via its Fc receptor to mast cells and basophils. After encountering the antigen again, the fixed IgE becomes cross-linked, inducing degranulation and release of mediators, eg, histamine.
Antibody	II (cytotoxic)	Antigens on a cell surface combine with antibody; this leads to complement-mediated lysis, eg, transfusion or Rh reactions, or other cytotoxic membrane damage, eg, autoimmune hemolytic anemia.
Antibody	III (immune complex)	Antigen-antibody immune complexes are deposited in tissues, complement is activated, and polymorphonuclear cells are attracted to the site, causing tissue damage.
Cell	IV (delayed)	T lymphocytes sensitized by an antigen release lymphokines upon second contact with the same antigen. The lymphokines induce inflammation and activate macrophages, which, in turn, release various mediators.

cross-linking of the IgE, and release of pharmacologically active mediators within minutes (''immediate reaction''). Cyclic nucleotides and calcium play essential roles in release of the mediators.* The reactivity can be **transmitted by serum** but not by cells. No single mediator accounts for the effects of anaphylaxis. Some important mediators and their effects are as follows:

(1) **Histamine** occurs in platelets and in granules of tissue mast cells and basophils in a preformed state. Its release causes vasodilatation, increased capillary permeability, and smooth-muscle contraction. Clinically, disorders such as allergic rhinitis (hay fever), urticaria, and angioedema can occur. The bronchospasm so prominent in acute anaphylaxis is due to histamine release. Antihistamine drugs can block histamine receptor sites and can be relatively effective in allergic rhinitis but not in asthma (see below).

(2) **Slow-reacting substance of anaphylaxis (SRS-A)** consists of several leukotrienes, which do not exist in a preformed state but are produced during anaphylactic reactions. This accounts for the slow onset of the effect of SRS-A. Leukotrienes are formed from arachidonic acid by the lipoxygenase pathway and cause increased vascular permeability and smooth-muscle contraction. They are the principal mediators in the bronchoconstriction of asthma and are not influenced by antihistamines.

(3) **Eosinophil chemotactic factor of anaphylaxis (ECF-A)** is a tetrapeptide that exists preformed in mast cell granules. When released during anaphylaxis, it attracts eosinophils that are prominent in immediate allergic reactions.

(4) **Serotonin** (hydroxytryptamine) is preformed in mast cells and blood platelets. When released during anaphylaxis, it causes capillary dilation, increased vascular permeability, and smooth-muscle contraction but is of minor importance in human anaphylaxis.

(5) **Prostaglandins and thromboxanes** are related to leukotrienes. They are derived from arachidonic acid via the cyclooxygenase pathway. Prostaglandins cause dilatation and increased permeability of capillaries and bronchoconstriction. Thromboxanes aggregate platelets.

The above-mentioned mediators are active only for some minutes after release; they are enzymatically inactivated and resynthesized slowly. Manifestations of anaphylaxis vary among species, because mediators are released at different rates in different amounts and tissues vary in their sensitivity to them. For example, the respiratory tract (bronchospasm, laryngeal edema) is a principal shock organ in humans but the liver (hepatic veins) plays that role in dogs.

---

*An increase in cyclic GMP within these cells increases mediator release, whereas an increase in cyclic AMP decreases release. Therefore, drugs that increase intracellular cyclic AMP, such as epinephrine, can be used to treat type I hypersensitivities.

Atopy Atopic disorders are immediate-hypersensitivity reactions that exhibit a strong **familial predisposition** and are associated with elevated IgE levels. The predisposition to atopy is genetic, and symptoms are induced by exposure to the specific allergens. These antigens are typically found in the environment (eg, pollens and house dust) or in foods (eg, shellfish and nuts). Exposure of nonatopic individuals to these substances does not elicit an allergic reaction. Common clinical manifestations include hay fever, asthma, eczema, and urticaria. Many sufferers give immediate-type reactions to skin tests (injection, patch, or scratch) containing the offending antigen.

Atopic hypersensitivity is transferable by serum, not by lymphoid cells. In the past, this observation was used for diagnosis in the passive cutaneous anaphylaxis (Prausnitz-Küstner) reaction, which consists of taking serum from the patient and injecting it into the skin of a normal person. Some hours later the test antigen, injected into the "sensitized" site, will yield an immediate wheal-and-flare reaction. This test is now impractical because of the danger of transmitting certain viral infections. Radioallergosorbent tests (RAST) permit the identification of specific IgE against potentially offending allergens if suitable specific antigens for in vitro tests are available.

The cause of atopy is speculative. Reduced number of suppressor T cells and abnormal "mediator feedback" have been proposed, as well as a predisposition to an abnormally high IgE response.

Drug Hypersensitivity Drugs, particularly antimicrobial agents, are now among the most common causes of hypersensitivity reactions. Usually it is not the intact drug that induces antibody formation. Rather, a metabolic product of the drug, which acts as a hapten and binds to a body protein, does so. The resulting antibody can react with the hapten, the intact drug, or the carrier protein to form complexes that are cell-bound and give rise to type I hypersensitivity.* When reexposed to the drug, the person may exhibit rashes, fevers, or local or systemic anaphylaxis of varying severity. Reactions to very small amounts of the drug can occur, eg, in a skin test with the hapten. A clinically useful example is the skin test using penicilloyl-polylysine to reveal an allergy to penicillin.

Desensitization Major manifestations of anaphylaxis occur when large amounts of mediators are suddenly released as a result of a massive dose of antigen abruptly combining with IgE on many mast cells. This is systemic anaphylaxis, which is potentially fatal. Desensitization can prevent systemic anaphylaxis.

Acute desensitization involves the administration of very small amounts of antigen at 15-minute intervals, with small-scale formation of complexes and not enough mediator release to produce a major reaction. This permits the administration of a drug or foreign protein to a hypersensitive person, but hypersensitivity is restored days or weeks later.

Chronic desensitization involves the long-term administration at weekly intervals of the antigen to which the person is hypersensitive. This stimulates the production of IgG-blocking antibodies in the serum, which can prevent subsequent antigen from reaching IgE on mast cells, thus preventing a reaction.

Treatment & Prevention of Anaphylactic Reactions Treatment aims to counteract the action of mediators by maintaining an airway and supporting ventilation and cardiac function. Also, epinephrine, antihistamines, corticosteroids, or cromolyn sodium, either singly or in combination, should be given. Cromolyn sodium prevents release of mediators, eg, histamine, from mast cell granules. Prevention relies on identification of the allergen by a skin test and avoidance of that allergen.

TYPE II: CYTOTOXIC HYPERSENSITIVITY Antibody directed at antigens of the **cell membrane** activates complement (or other effectors) and damages those cells. The antibody (IgG or IgM) attaches to the antigen via the Fab region and acts as a bridge to complement via the Fc region. As a result, there may be complement-mediated lysis as in hemolytic anemias, ABO transfusion reactions, or Rh hemolytic disease. In addition to causing lysis, complement activation can attract phagocytes to the site, with consequent release of enzymes that damage cell membranes.

---

*Some drugs are involved in cytotoxic hypersensitivity reactions (type II) and in serum sickness (type III).

Drugs, eg, penicillins, phenacetin, quinidine, can attach to surface proteins on red blood cells and initiate antibody formation. Such autoimmune antibodies (IgG) then may combine with the cell surface and result in hemolysis. The direct antiglobulin (Coombs) test is typically positive (see Chapter 64). Other drugs, eg, quinine, may attach as haptens to platelets and then lyse them to produce thrombocytopenia with bleeding tendency. Others, eg, hydralazine, may modify host tissue and favor the production of autoantibodies directed at cell DNA, with results resembling those of systemic lupus erythematosus. Certain infections, eg, *Mycoplasma pneumoniae* infection, can induce antibodies that cross-react with red cell antigens, resulting in hemolytic anemia. In rheumatic fever, antibodies against the group A streptococci cross-react with cardiac tissue. In Goodpasture's syndrome, antibody to basement membranes of kidney and lung form, resulting in severe damage to the membranes through activity of complement-attracted leukocytes.

TYPE III: IMMUNE-COMPLEX HYPERSENSITIVITY   When antibody and antigen coexist, immune complexes are formed. Normally, they are promptly removed by the reticuloendothelial system but occasionally they persist and are **deposited in tissues**, resulting in several disorders. In persistent microbial or viral infections, immune complexes may be deposited in organs, eg, the kidneys, resulting in dysfunction. In autoimmune disorders, "self" antigens may elicit antibodies that bind to organ antigens or deposit in organs as complexes, especially in joints (arthritis), kidneys (nephritis), or blood vessels (vasculitis).

Wherever immune complexes are deposited, they activate the complement system. Polymorphonuclear cells are attracted to the site, and inflammation and tissue injury occur. Two typical type III hypersensitivity reactions are the Arthus reaction and serum sickness.

Arthus Reaction   If animals are given an antigen repeatedly until they have high levels of precipitating IgG antibody[†] and that antigen is then injected subcutaneously or intradermally, intense edema and hemorrhage develop, reaching a peak in 3–6 hours. Antigen, antibody, and complement are deposited in vessel walls; polymorphonuclear cell infiltration and intravascular clumping of platelets then occur. These reactions can lead to vascular occlusion and necrosis. A likely clinical counterpart of the Arthus reaction is hypersensitivity pneumonitis (allergic alveolitis) associated with the inhalation of thermophilic actinomycetes ("farmer's lung").

Serum Sickness   Following the injection of foreign serum (or certain drugs), the antigen is excreted slowly. During this time, antibody production starts. The simultaneous presence of antigen and antibody leads to the production of immune complexes, which may circulate or be deposited at various sites. Typical serum sickness results in fever, urticaria, arthralgia, lymphadenopathy, and splenomegaly a few days to 2 weeks after injection of the foreign serum. Although it takes several days for symptoms to appear, serum sickness is classed as an immediate reaction because symptoms occur promptly after immune complexes form. Symptoms improve as the immune elimination of the antigen continues and subside when it is complete. Nowadays, serum sickness follows the injection of foreign sera less frequently than it follows the administration of drugs, eg, penicillin.

Immune Complex Diseases   Many clinical disorders associated with immune complexes have been described, although the antigen is often in doubt. Several representative examples are described below.

A. Glomerulonephritis: Acute poststreptococcal glomerulonephritis is a well-accepted immune complex disease. Its onset follows several weeks after a group A beta-hemolytic streptococcal infection, particularly of the skin, and often with nephritogenic serotypes of *Streptococcus pyogenes*. Typically, the complement level is low, suggesting an antigen-antibody reaction. Lumpy deposits of immunoglobulin and C3 are seen along glomerular basement membranes by immunofluorescence, suggesting the presence of antigen-antibody complexes, although streptococcal antigens have rarely been demonstrated. It is assumed that streptococcal antigen-antibody complexes, after being filtered out by glomeruli, fix complement, attract polymorphs, and start the inflammatory process.

[†]Much more antibody is typically needed to elicit an Arthus reaction than anaphylactic reaction.

Similar lesions with "lumpy" deposits containing immunoglobulin and C3 occur in infective endocarditis, serum sickness, and certain viral infections, eg, hepatitis B, infectious mononucleosis, and dengue hemorrhagic fever. Lesions containing immune complexes also occur in the nephritis of systemic lupus erythematosus, where the "lumpy" deposits contain DNA as the antigen.

B. Arthritis: Rheumatoid arthritis is a chronic inflammatory joint disease, especially of young women. Serum and synovial fluid of patients contain "rheumatoid factors," ie, IgM and IgG antibodies that bind to the Fc fragment of normal human IgG. It is assumed that there are deposits of immune complexes (containing IgG and rheumatoid factor) on synovial membranes and in blood vessels that activate complement and attract polymorphonuclear cells, causing inflammation. Patients have high titers of rheumatoid factor and low titers of complement in serum during active rheumatoid disease.

C. Autoimmune disease: In many autoimmune diseases, antigen-antibody complexes related to the organ site of activity (eg, thyroid hormone receptors and acetylcholine receptors) have been demonstrated. Autoimmune diseases are discussed in Chapter 66.

TYPE IV: DELAYED (CELL-MEDIATED) HYPERSENSITIVITY

Delayed hypersensitivity is a function of **T lymphocytes, not antibody**. It can be transferred by immunologically committed (sensitized) T cells, not by serum.* The response is "delayed"; ie, it starts hours (or days) after contact with the antigen and often lasts for days. It consists mainly of mononuclear cell infiltration and tissue induration, as typified by the tuberculin skin test.

Clinically Important Delayed Hypersensitivity Reactions

A. Contact Hypersensitivity: This manifestation of cell-mediated hypersensitivity occurs after sensitization with simple chemicals (eg, nickel and formaldehyde), plant materials (eg, poison ivy and poison oak), topically applied drugs (eg, sulfonamides and neomycin), some cosmetics, soaps, and other substances. In all cases, the small molecules enter the skin and then, acting as haptens, attach to body proteins to serve as complete antigen. Cell-mediated hypersensitivity is induced, particularly in the skin. Upon a later skin contact with the offending agent, the sensitized person develops erythema, itching, vesication, eczema, or necrosis of skin within 12–48 hours. Patch testing on a small area of skin can sometimes identify the offending antigen. Subsequent avoidance of the material will prevent recurrences.

B. Tuberculin-Type Hypersensitivity: Delayed-type hypersensitivity to antigens of microorganisms occurs in many infectious diseases and has been used as an aid in diagnosis. It is typified by the tuberculin reaction. When a patient previously exposed to *Mycobacterium tuberculosis* is injected with a small amount of tuberculin in the epidermis, there is little reaction in the first few hours. Gradually, however, induration and redness develop and reach a peak in 48–72 hours. A positive skin test indicates that the person has been infected with the agent, but it has no implication as to the presence of current disease. However, if the skin test converts from negative to positive, it suggests recent infection and possible current activity. Infected persons do not always have a positive skin test, because overwhelming infection, disorders that suppress skin reactivity (eg, uremia, measles, sarcoidosis, lymphoma, and AIDS), or the administration of immunosuppressive drugs (eg, corticosteroids and antineoplastics) may cause anergy.

A positive skin test response assists in diagnosis and provides support for chemoprophylaxis or chemotherapy. In leprosy, a positive lepromin test indicates the presence of tuberculoid leprosy with competent cell-mediated immunity, whereas a negative lepromin test suggests the presence of lepromatous leprosy with impaired cell-mediated immunity. In systemic mycotic infections (eg, coccidioidomycosis, histoplasmosis, and blastomycosis), a positive delayed-type skin test with the specific antigen indicates exposure to the organism. Cell-mediated hypersensitivity develops in many viral infections, eg, herpes simplex and mumps. However, serologic tests are more specific both for diagnosis and for assessment of immunity. In protozoan and helminthic infections, skin tests may be positive but they are generally not as useful as specific serologic tests.

---

*It can also be transferred by "transfer factor" (see Chapter 58).

Review Questions

1. What is the evidence that anaphylaxis is antibody-mediated rather than cell-mediated?
2. Describe the pathogenesis of anaphylaxis, including (a) the antibody, (b) cells, and (c) mediators.
3. What are some common atopic disorders and their allergens? What is the role of IgE in atopy?
4. What is the rationale behind desensitization to mitigate type I hypersensitivity reactions?
5. What are the similarities and differences between type II (cytotoxic) and type I (anaphylactic) hypersensitivity?
6. What is the pathogenesis of serum sickness? Nowadays, serum is not the main cause. What is?
7. What is the pathogenesis of poststreptococcal glomerulonephritis?
8. Why is cell-mediated hypersensitivity called "delayed"?
9. What is the pathogenesis of poison oak and poison ivy hypersensitivity?
10. Describe the immunologic process involved in a positive tuberculin skin test.

Tolerance & Autoimmune Disease **66**

TOLERANCE Tolerance is specific immunologic **unresponsiveness**; ie, an immune response to a certain antigen (or epitope) does not occur, although the immune system is otherwise functioning normally. In general, antigens that are present during embryonic life are considered "self" and do not stimulate an immunologic response. On the other hand, antigens that are not present during the process of maturation, ie, that are encountered first when the body is immunologically mature, are considered "nonself" and usually elicit an immunologic response.

Whether an antigen will induce tolerance rather than an immunologic response is largely determined by the following:

(1) The immunologic **maturity** of the host is important; eg, neonatal animals are immunologically immature and will accept allografts that would be rejected by mature animals.

(2) The **structure and dose** of the antigen are factors; eg, a very simple molecule induces tolerance more readily than a complex one, and very high or very low doses of antigen may result in tolerance instead of an immune response. Purified polysaccharides or amino acid copolymers injected in very large doses result in "immune paralysis"—a lack of response.

(3) T cells become tolerant more readily and remain tolerant longer than B cells.

(4) Administration of a cross-reacting antigen tends to terminate tolerance.

(5) Administration of immunosuppressive drugs enhances tolerance, eg, in transplants.

(6) Tolerance is maintained best if the antigen continues to be present.

Hypotheses on the induction of tolerance include the following:

(1) The macrophages fail to effectively present the antigen to T lymphocytes;

(2) suppressor T cells might inhibit the reactivity of lymphocytic clones; and

(3) very high ("high zone") or very low ("low zone") doses of antigen may delete potentially reactive B cell clones or helper T cell clones (clonal deletion theory).

AUTOIMMUNE DISEASES The adult host usually exhibits tolerance to tissue antigens present during fetal life that are recognized as "self." However, in certain circumstances tolerance may be lost and immune reactions may develop to host antigens, resulting in autoimmune diseases. Either humoral or cell-mediated reactions can be involved. Many autoimmune diseases exhibit a marked familial incidence, which suggests a **genetic predisposition** to these disorders. There is a strong association of some diseases with certain human leukocyte antigen (HLA) specificities, especially the class II genes. For example, rheumatoid arthritis occurs predominantly in individuals carrying the HLA-DR4 gene.

Mechanisms The following mechanisms for autoimmunity have been proposed.

A. Release of Sequestered Antigens: Certain tissues, eg, sperm, central nervous system, and the lens and uveal tract of the eye, are sequestered so that their antigens have no access to the immune system. When such antigens enter the circulation accidentally, eg, after damage, they elicit both humoral and cellular responses, producing aspermatogenesis, encephalitis, or endophthalmitis, respectively.

B. Escape of Tolerance at the T Cell Level: Unresponsiveness to a "self" antigen may be maintained by tolerance at the T cell level. Such tolerance may be terminated by cross-reactions, ie, when the host responds to antigens that cross-react with tolerated "self" antigens. For example, in rheumatic fever, antibodies against streptococcal antigens cross-react with heart tissue antigens.

C. Diminished Suppressor T Cell Function: In normal immune regulation, suppressor T cells may limit an immune response to "self" antigens. If suppressor T cell functions decrease, antibodies to "self" antigens may be formed, eg, an antibody to normal IgG. Such antibody (IgM or IgG) occurs in rheumatoid arthritis, in which antigen-antibody complexes form in joints.

Diseases Some examples of diseases that involve autoimmune reactions are described below.

A. Allergic Encephalitis: This is due to a cell-mediated response to the basic protein of brain myelin. For example, when animal brain substance, mixed with adjuvant, is injected into an animal of the same species, a demyelinating encephalitis develops. It resembles postvaccinal encephalitis seen in persons injected with older rabies vaccines made in rabbit brains. Rarely, it occurs following certain viral infections, eg, measles or influenza, or following immunizations against these viral infections.

B. Chronic Thyroiditis: When animals are injected with thyroid gland material, they develop humoral and cell-mediated immunity against thyroid antigens and a chronic thyroiditis. Humans with Hashimoto's chronic thyroiditis have antibodies to thyroglobulin, suggesting that these antibodies may provoke an inflammatory process that leads to fibrosis of the gland.

C. Rheumatic Fever: Group A streptococcal infections regularly precede the development of rheumatic fever. Cross-reactions occur between cell membrane antigens of streptococci and human heart muscle sarcolemma, which may play a causative role in disease.

D. Hemolytic Anemias, Thrombocytopenias, and Granulocytopenias: Various forms of these disorders have been attributed to the attachment of autoantibodies to cell surfaces and subsequent cell destruction. Pernicious anemia may represent an autoimmune reaction to intrinsic factor, a protein secreted by parietal cells of the stomach that facilitates the absorption of vitamin B_{12}. Idiopathic thrombocytopenic purpura is due to antibody directed against platelets.

E. Diabetes, Myasthenia Gravis, and Hyperthyroidism (Graves' Disease): In these diseases, antibodies to receptors occur and may have a pathogenic role. In extreme insulin resistance in diabetes, antibodies to insulin receptors have been demonstrated that interfere with insulin binding. In myasthenia gravis (a nervous system disease), antibodies to acetylcholine receptors of neuromuscular junctions occur in the serum. Some patients with

Graves' disease have circulating antibodies to thyrotropin receptors, which, when they bind to the receptors, resemble thyrotropin in activity and stimulate the thyroid to produce more thyroxine.

F. Systemic Lupus Erythematosus (SLE), Rheumatoid Arthritis, and Other Collagen Vascular Diseases: These disorders feature vasculitis and collagen degeneration plus a variety of focal inflammatory lesions and the presence of autoantibodies against many different "self" antigens. For example, antibodies to DNA are found in SLE and antibodies to IgG (rheumatoid factor) occur in rheumatoid arthritis. Complement levels are low, and the nephritis associated with these disorders appears to be an immune complex disease. Although the causes of these disorders are unknown, typical cases have followed sensitization by drugs, foreign proteins, and other immune stimuli.

Review Questions

1. What are the criteria that determine tolerance?
2. What are the hypotheses that may explain tolerance?
3. What are the suggested mechanisms for autoimmune diseases?

Tumor Immunity

67

TUMOR-ASSOCIATED ANTIGENS   Animals carrying a chemically or virally induced malignant tumor can develop resistance to that tumor and cause its **regression**. In the course of neoplastic transformation, **new antigens**, called tumor-associated antigens (TAA), develop at the cell surface and the host recognizes such cells as "nonself." In chemically induced tumors in experimental animals, TAAs are highly specific; ie, cells of one tumor will have TAAs different from cells of another tumor even when they arise within the same animal. In contrast, virally induced tumors possess TAAs that cross-react with one another if induced by the same virus. TAAs on tumor cells induced by different viruses do not cross-react.

MECHANISM OF TUMOR IMMUNITY   Cell-mediated reactions attack these "nonself" tumor cells and limit their proliferation. Such immune responses probably act as a **surveillance** system to detect and eliminate newly arising clones of neoplastic cells. In general, the immune response against tumor cells is weak and can be overcome experimentally by a large dose of tumor cells. Some tumor cells can escape surveillance by "modulation," ie, internalizing the surface antigen so that it no longer presents a target for immune attack.

The cell-mediated immune responses that affect tumor cells in vitro include natural killer (NK) cells, which act without antibody; killer (K) cells, which mediate antibody-dependent cytolysis (antibody-dependent cell-mediated cytotoxicity); cytotoxic T cells; and activated macrophages. Whether these immune responses function to prevent or control tumors in vivo is unknown.

Tumor antigens can stimulate the development of specific antibodies as well. Some of these antibodies are cytotoxic, but others enhance tumor growth, perhaps by blocking recognition of tumor antigens by the host. Spontaneously arising human tumors may have new cell surface antigens against which the host develops both cytotoxic antibodies and cell-mediated immune responses. Enhancement of these responses at times permits containment of some tumors. For example, the administration of BCG vaccine (bacillus Calmette-Guérin, a bovine myco-bacterium) into surface melanomas can lead to their partial regression. Immunomodulators, like interleukins and interferons, are also being tested in such settings. One interleukin, tumor necrosis factor (cachectin), is experimentally effective against a variety of solid tumors. In addition, lymphocytes activated by interleukin-2 (lymphokine-activated killer or LAK cells) may be useful in cancer immunotherapy.

CARCINOEMBRYONIC ANTIGEN & ALPHA-FETOPROTEIN Some human tumors contain antigens that normally occur in fetal but not in adult human cells.

(a) carcinoembryonic antigen circulates at elevated levels in the serum of many patients with carcinoma of the colon, pancreas, breast, or liver. It is found in fetal gut, liver, and pancreas and in very small amounts in normal sera. Detection of this antigen (by radioimmunoassay) is not helpful in diagnosis but may be helpful in management of such tumors. If the level declines after surgery, it suggests that the tumor is not spreading. Conversely, a rise in the level of carcinoembryonic antigen in patients with resected carcinoma of the colon suggests recurrence or spread of the tumor.

(b) alpha-fetoprotein has elevated levels in the sera of hepatoma patients and is used as a marker for this disease. It is produced by fetal liver and is found in small amounts in some normal sera. It is, however, nonspecific; it occurs in several other malignant and nonmalignant diseases.

Monoclonal antibodies directed against new surface antigens on malignant cells (eg, B cell lymphomas) can be useful in diagnosis. Perhaps, someday, such antibodies might carry toxic chemicals specifically to such cells and be useful for therapy.

Review Questions

1. Describe immune surveillance against tumor cells from the point of view of (a) antigens and (b) host response.
2. Distinguish between carcinoembryonic antigen and alpha-fetoprotein.

68

Immunodeficiency

Immunodeficiency can occur in any of the 4 major components of the immune system: (1) B cells (antibody), (2) T cells, (3) complement, and (4) phagocytes. The deficiencies can be either congenital or acquired. Clinically, recurrent or opportunistic infections are commonly seen. Recurrent infections with pyogenic bacteria, eg, staphylococci, indicate a B cell deficiency, whereas recurrent infections with certain fungi, viruses, or protozoa indicate a T cell deficiency.

CONGENITAL IMMUNODEFICIENCIES

1. B Cell Deficiencies

A. X-Linked Hypogammaglobulinemia (Bruton's Agammaglobulinemia): Very low levels of all immunoglobulins (IgG, IgA, IgM, IgD, and IgE) and a virtual **absence of B cells** are found. This may be due to a failure of maturation of pre-B cells. Clinically, recurrent pyogenic infections occur in infants about 6 months of age when maternal antibody is no longer protective. Treatment with pooled gamma globulin reduces the number of infections.

B. Selective Immunoglobulin Deficiencies: IgA deficiency is the **most common** of these; IgG and IgM deficiencies are rarer. Patients with a deficiency of IgA typically have recurrent sinus and lung infections. (However, some individuals with IgA deficiency do not have frequent infections, possibly because their IgG and IgM levels confer protection.) The cause of IgA deficiency may be a failure of heavy-chain gene switching; the total number of cells is normal, as are IgM and IgG synthesis. Patients with a deficiency of IgA should not be treated with gamma globulin preparations, because they may react against foreign IgA and, by cross-reaction, deplete their already low level of IgA.

2. T Cell Deficiencies

A. Thymic Aplasia (DiGeorge's Syndrome): Severe viral, fungal, or protozoal infections occur in affected infants early in life as a result of a profound **deficit of T cells**. Both the thymus and the parathyroids fail to develop properly owing to a defect in the third and fourth pharyngeal pouches. The most common presenting symptom is tetany due to hypocalcemia. Other congenital abnormalities commonly occur. Antibody production is either normal or decreased. A transplant of fetal thymus may reconstitute T cell immunity. A thymus from a child older than 14 weeks should not be used, because a graft-versus-host reaction may occur.

B. Chronic Mucocutaneous Candidiasis: In this disease, the skin and mucous membranes of children are infected with *Candida albicans*, which, in immunocompetent individuals, is a nonpathogenic member of the normal flora. These children have a T cell deficiency **specifically** for this organism; other T cell and B cell functions are normal. Treatment consists primarily of antifungal drugs. Thymic transplant may be helpful.

3. Combined B Cell & T Cell Deficiencies

A. Severe Combined Immunodeficiency Disease (SCID): Recurrent infections caused by bacteria, viruses, fungi, and protozoa occur early in life, because **both B and T cells are absent**. This inherited disease is probably due to a defect in the differentiation of an early stem cell. There are 2 types: X-linked and autosomal. One form of the disease is due to the absence of class II MHC proteins caused by a failure to transcribe the HLA-DR genes. Because immunity is so profoundly depressed, these children must be protected from exposure to microorganisms, usually by being enclosed in a plastic "bubble." Live, attenuated viral vaccines should not be given. Bone marrow transplant may restore immunity.

B. Adenosine Deaminase and Nucleoside Phosphorylase Deficiency: Patients with a hereditary absence of these enzymes can have a severe deficiency of B and T cells, although some have only mild dysfunction. The absence of these enzymes results in an accumulation of dATP, an inhibitor of ribonucleotide reductase, and a consequent decrease in the deoxynucleoside triphosphate precursors of DNA. This severely affects bone marrow differentiation. Bone marrow transplantation can be helpful.

C. Wiskott-Aldrich Syndrome: Recurrent pyogenic infections, eczema, and bleeding due to thrombocytopenia during the first year of life characterize this syndrome. The most important defect is the inability to mount an IgM response to the capsular polysaccharides of bacteria, such as pneumococci. IgG levels are normal, and T cell immunity is variable. Bone marrow transplantation may be helpful.

D. Ataxia-Telangiectasia: In this disease, ataxia (staggering), telangiectasia (enlarged small blood vessels of the conjunctivas and skin), and recurrent infections occur prominently. It is an autosomal recessive disease that appears by 2 years of age. Lymphopenia and IgA deficiency commonly occur. Treatment designed to correct the immunodeficiency has not been successful.

4. Complement Deficiencies

A. Hereditary Angioedema: This is an uncommon autosomal dominant disease due to a deficiency of C1 esterase inhibitor. In the absence of inhibitor, C1 esterase continues to act on C4 to generate vasoactive kinins. This leads to capillary permeability and edema in several organs. Laryngeal edema can be fatal. Steroid drugs, such as oxymetholone and danazol, can be useful in increasing the concentration of C1 inhibitor.

B. Recurrent Infections: Patients with deficiencies in C1, C3, or C5 or the later components C6, C7, or C8 have an increased susceptibility to bacterial infections. Those with reduced levels of C6, C7, or C8 are especially prone to bacteremia with *Neisseria meningitidis* or *Neisseria gonorrhoeae*.

C. Autoimmune Diseases: Patients with C2 and C4 deficiencies have diseases resembling systemic lupus erythematosus or other autoimmune diseases. C2 deficiency is the most common complement defect and is frequently asymptomatic.

5. Phagocyte Deficiencies

A. Chronic Granulomatous Disease (CGD): Patients with this disease have a marked susceptibility to opportunistic infections with certain bacteria and fungi, eg, *Staphylococcus epidermidis* and *Aspergillus fumigatus*. Viral and protozoal infections are not a major concern. In most cases, this is an X-linked disease that appears by the age of 2 years. (In some patients, the disease is autosomal.) It is due to a defect in the intracellular microbicidal activity of neutrophils as a result of a **lack of NADPH oxidase** activity (or similar enzymes). These enzymes are required for the generation of peroxides and superoxides that kill the organisms. B cell and T cell functions are usually normal. In the laboratory, diagnosis can be confirmed by the nitroblue tetrazolium dye reduction test. Treatment is based on antimicrobial drugs. White blood cell infusions may be helpful.

B. Chédiak-Higashi Syndrome: In this autosomal recessive disease, recurrent pyogenic infections, caused primarily by staphylococci and streptococci, occur. This is due to the failure of the **lysosomes** of neutrophils to empty their contents. Large granular inclusions composed of abnormal lysosomes are seen. Peroxide and superoxide formation is normal, as are B cell and T cell functions. Treatment involves antimicrobial drugs. There is no useful therapy for the phagocyte defect.

C. Job's Syndrome: Patients with this syndrome have recurrent "cold"* staphylococcal abscesses, eczema, and high levels of IgE. The neutrophils are defective in chemotaxis; their ingestive and oxidative processes are intact. Treatment consists of antimicrobial drugs.

ACQUIRED IMMUNODEFICIENCIES

1. B Cell Deficiencies: Common Variable Hypogammaglobulinemia

Patients present with recurrent infections caused by pyogenic bacteria. The infections usually occur in persons between the ages of 15 and 35 years. The number of B cells is normal, but the ability to synthesize IgG (and other immunoglobulins) is greatly reduced. T cell function is usually normal. The cause of the failure to produce IgG is unknown.

2. T Cell Deficiencies

A. AIDS: Patients with AIDS present with opportunistic infections caused by certain bacteria, viruses, fungi, and protozoa (eg, *Mycobacterium avium-intracellulare*, herpesviruses,

---

*"Cold" refers to the lack of inflammation with its associated redness and warmth.

C albicans, and *Pneumocystis carinii*). This is due to greatly reduced helper T cell number caused by infection with the retrovirus, human immunodeficiency virus (HIV; see Chapter 45). This virus specifically infects cells with the CD4 surface receptor. Markedly reduced helper to suppressor T cell ratios occur, but elevated immunoglobulin levels are found. The response to specific immunizations is poor; this is attributed to the loss of helper T cell activity. AIDS patients also have a high incidence of tumors such as Kaposi's sarcoma and lymphomas, which may be due to a failure of immune surveillance. Treatment involves antimicrobial drugs for the opportunistic infections and azidothymidine to limit the replication of HIV.

B. Measles: Patients with measles have a transient suppression of delayed hypersensitivity as manifested by a loss of PPD skin test reactivity. Quiescent tuberculosis can become active. In these patients, T cell function is altered but immunoglobulins are normal.

Review Questions

1. X-linked hypogammaglobulinemia and selective IgA deficiency probably have different causes. What are they?
2. Contrast the types of infections that occur in children with X-linked hypogammaglobulinemia and thymic aplasia. Why are they different?
3. What is the most common clinical problem seen in patients with severe combined immunodeficiency disease? Why does this problem occur?
4. What diseases are individuals with a deficiency of the late-acting complement components, ie, C6, C7, and C8, likely to have?
5. What is the pathogenesis of chronic granulomatous disease? To what organisms are patients with this disease especially susceptible?
6. What is the immunodeficiency in AIDS? What are the consequences of this immunodeficiency?

Part VIII: Brief Summaries of Medically Important Organisms

Summaries of Medically Important Bacteria

GRAM-POSITIVE COCCI

Staphylococcus aureus

A. Diseases: Abscesses of many organs, endocarditis, gastroenteritis (food poisoning), toxic shock syndrome.

B. Characteristics: Gram-positive cocci in clusters. Coagulase-positive. Catalase-positive.

C. Habitat and Transmission: Habitat is the human skin and nose. Transmission is via the hands.

D. Pathogenesis: A variety of enzymes and toxins are made (see p 64). The 2 most important are coagulase and enterotoxin(s). Coagulase is the best correlate of pathogenicity. Enterotoxins cause food poisoning (one of these, TSST-1, causes toxic shock syndrome). Predisposing factors are breaks in the skin, foreign bodies such as sutures, neutrophil levels below 500/μL, intravenous drug abuse, and, for toxic shock syndrome, tampon use.

E. Laboratory Diagnosis: Gram-stained smear and culture. Yellow or gold colonies on blood agar. *Staphylococcus aureus* is coagulase-positive; *Staphylococcus epidermidis* is coagulase-negative. Serologic tests not useful.

F. Treatment: Penicillin G for sensitive isolates; β-lactamase-resistant penicillins such as nafcillin for resistant isolates; vancomycin for isolates resistant to nafcillin. About 85% are resistant to penicillin G. Plasmid-encoded β-lactamase mediates most resistance. Resistance to nafcillin may be due to changes in binding proteins. Some are tolerant to penicillin.

G. Prevention: No vaccine or drug is available.

Streptococcus pyogenes (Group A)

A. Diseases: Suppurative diseases, eg, pharyngitis and cellulitis; nonsuppurative diseases, eg, rheumatic fever and acute glomerulonephritis.

B. Characteristics: Gram-positive cocci in chains. Beta-hemolytic. Catalase-negative.

C. Habitat and Transmission: Habitat is the human throat and skin. Transmission is via respiratory droplets.

D. Pathogenesis: For suppurative infections, hyaluronidase ("spreading factor") mediates subcutaneous spread seen in cellulitis; erythrogenic toxin causes the rash of scarlet fever; M protein impedes phagocytosis. For nonsuppurative infections, rheumatic fever is caused by immunologic cross-reaction between bacterial antigen and human heart tissue, and acute glomerulonephritis is caused by immune complexes bound to glomeruli.

E. Laboratory Diagnosis: Gram-stained smear and culture. Beta-hemolytic colonies on blood agar. (Hemolysis due to streptolysins O and S.) If isolate is sensitive to bacitracin, it is presumptively identified as *Streptococcus pyogenes*. Group determined by antiserum against cell wall C polysaccharide in precipitin test. Assay for antibody in patient's serum not done for suppurative infections. Patient's antistreptolysin O (ASO) antibody titer is tested to determine prior exposure to *S pyogenes* if rheumatic fever is suspected.

F. Treatment: Penicillin G.

G. Prevention: Penicillin used in rheumatic fever patients to prevent recurrent *S pyogenes* pharyngitis.

Streptococcus agalactiae (Group B)

A. Diseases: Neonatal meningitis and sepsis.

B. Characteristics: Gram-positive cocci in chains. Beta-hemolytic. Catalase-negative.

C. Habitat and Transmission: Habitat is the human vagina. Transmission occurs during birth.

D. Pathogenesis: No toxins or virulence factors identified.

E. Laboratory Diagnosis: Gram-stained smear and culture. Beta-hemolytic colonies on blood agar. Organisms hydrolyze hippurate and are CAMP test-positive. Group determined by antiserum against cell wall polysaccharide in precipitin test.

F. Treatment: Penicillin G.

G. Prevention: No vaccine. Ampicillin prior to delivery may be useful if mother is culture-positive.

Streptococcus faecalis (Enterococcus; Group D)

A. Diseases: Urinary and biliary tract infections are most frequent.

B. Characteristics: Gram-positive cocci in chains. Catalase-negative.

C. Habitat and Transmission: Habitat is the human colon; urethra and female genital tract can be colonized. May enter bloodstream during gastrointestinal or genitourinary tract manipulations. May infect other sites, eg, endocarditis.

D. Pathogenesis: No toxins or virulence factors identified.

E. Laboratory Diagnosis: Gram-stained smear and culture. Alpha-, beta-, or nonhemolytic colonies on blood agar. Grows in 6.5% NaCl and hydrolyzes esculin in the presence of 40% bile. Serologic tests not useful.

F. Treatment: Penicillin plus an aminoglycoside such as gentamicin is synergistic. Organism is resistant to either drug given individually. Aminoglycoside resistance is due to an inability to penetrate. The penicillin weakens the cell wall, allowing the aminoglycoside to penetrate.

G. Prevention: Penicillin and gentamicin should be given to patients with damaged heart valves prior to intestinal or urinary tract procedures. No vaccine is available.

Streptococcus pneumoniae (Pneumococcus)

A. Diseases: The most common diseases are pneumonia and meningitis in adults and otitis media and sinusitis in children.

B. Characteristics: Gram-positive "lancet-shaped" cocci in pairs (diplococci) or short chains. Alpha-hemolytic. Catalase-negative.

C. Habitat and Transmission: Habitat is the human upper respiratory tract. Transmission is via respiratory droplets.

D. Pathogenesis: Induces inflammatory response. No known exotoxins. Polysaccharide capsule retards phagocytosis. Antipolysaccharide antibody opsonizes the organism and provides type-specific immunity. Viral respiratory infection predisposes to pneumococcal pneumonia by damaging mucociliary elevator; splenectomy predisposes sepsis.

E. Laboratory Diagnosis: Gram-stained smear and culture. Alpha-hemolytic colonies on blood agar. Growth inhibited by bile and optochin. Quellung reaction occurs (see swelling of capsule with type-specific antiserum). Serologic tests not useful. Latex agglutination test for capsular antigen in spinal fluid can be diagnostic.

F. Treatment: Penicillin G. Low-level resistance due to altered penicillin-binding proteins is not of clinical concern; high-level resistance is rare.

G. Prevention: Vaccine contains capsular polysaccharide of the 23 serotypes that cause bacteremia most frequently. No drug prophylaxis is available.

Streptococci (Viridans Group, eg, *S sanguis, S mutans*)

A. Diseases: Endocarditis is the most important.

B. Characteristics: Gram-positive cocci in chains. Alpha-hemolytic. Catalase-negative.

C. Habitat and Transmission: Habitat is the human oropharynx. Organism enters bloodstream during dental procedures.

D. Pathogenesis: Bacteremia from dental procedures spreads organism to damaged heart valves. Organism is protected from host defenses within vegetations. No known toxins. Dextrans enhance adherence.

E. Laboratory Diagnosis: Gram-stained smear and culture. Alpha-hemolytic colonies on blood agar. Growth not inhibited by bile or optochin, in contrast to pneumococci. Many species are classified as viridans group streptococci. Serologic tests not useful.

F. Treatment: Penicillin G with or without an aminoglycoside.

G. Prevention: Penicillin for patients with damaged or prosthetic heart valves who undergo dental procedures.

GRAM-NEGATIVE COCCI

Neisseria meningitidis (Meningococcus)

A. Diseases: Meningitis and meningococcemia.

B. Characteristics: Gram-negative "kidney-bean" diplococci. Oxidase-positive. Large polysaccharide capsule.

C. Habitat and Transmission: Habitat is the human upper respiratory tract; transmission is via respiratory droplets.

D. Pathogenesis: After colonizing the upper respiratory tract, the organism reaches the meninges via the bloodstream. Endotoxin in cell wall causes symptoms of septic shock seen in meningococcemia. No known exotoxins; IgA protease produced. Capsule is antiphagocytic. Deficiency in late complement components predisposes to bacteremia.

E. Laboratory Diagnosis: Gram-stained smear and culture. Oxidase-positive colonies on chocolate agar. Ferments maltose in contrast to gonococci. Serologic tests not useful.

F. Treatment: Penicillin G (no significant resistance). Many isolates are resistant to sulfonamides owing to plasmid-encoded enzymes that actively export the drug.

G. Prevention: Vaccine contains capsular polysaccharide of strains A, C, Y, and W-135. Rifampin given to close contacts to decrease oropharyngeal carriage.

Neisseria gonorrhoeae (Gonococcus)

A. Disease: Gonorrhea.

B. Characteristics: Gram-negative "kidney-bean" diplococci. Oxidase-positive. Insignificant capsule.

C. Habitat and Transmission: Habitat is the human genital tract. Transmission is by sexual contact.

D. Pathogenesis: Organism invades mucous membranes and causes inflammation. Endotoxin present. No extoxins identified. IgA protease and pili are virulence factors.

E. Laboratory Diagnosis: Gram-stained smear and culture. Organism visible intracellularly within neutrophils in urethral exudate. Oxidase-positive colonies on Thayer-Martin medium. Gonococci do not ferment maltose, whereas meningococci do. Serologic tests not useful.

F. Treatment: Oral penicillin (amoxicillin) for uncomplicated cases. If resistant, spectinomycin or cephalosporin is used. Tetracycline added for urethritis due to *Chlamydia trachomatis*. High-level resistance to penicillin is caused by plasmid-encoded penicillinase especially prevalent in Southeast Asian strains. Low-level resistance to penicillin is caused by reduced permeability.

G. Prevention: No drug or vaccine. Condoms offer protection. Trace contacts and treat to interrupt transmission. Treat eyes of newborns with erythromycin ointment or silver nitrate to prevent conjunctivitis.

GRAM-POSITIVE RODS

Bacillus anthracis

A. Disease: Anthrax.

B. Characteristics: Large, gram-positive, spore-forming rods. Capsule composed of poly-D-glutamate.

C. Habitat and Transmission: Habitat is soil. Transmission is by contact with infected animals or inhalation of spores from animal hair and wool.

D. Pathogenesis: Anthrax toxin consists of 3 proteins: edema factor, which is an adenylate cyclase; protective antigen, which mediates the entry of the other 2 components into the cell; and lethal factor, whose mechanism of action is unknown. Capsule consisting of polyglutamic acid is an important virulence factor.

E. Laboratory Diagnosis: Gram-stained smear plus aerobic culture on blood agar. *Bacillus anthracis* is nonmotile, in contrast to other *Bacillus* species. Rise in antibody titer in indirect hemagglutination test is diagnostic.

F. Treatment: Penicillin (no significant resistance).

G. Prevention: Vaccine consisting of protective antigen is given to individuals in high-risk occupations.

Clostridium tetani

A. Disease: Tetanus.

B. Characteristics: Anaerobic, gram-positive, spore-forming rods.

C. Habitat and Transmission: Habitat is the soil. Organism enters through traumatic breaks in the skin.

D. Pathogenesis: Spores germinate under anaerobic conditions in the wound. Organism produces polypeptide exotoxin, which blocks release of inhibitory neurotransmitters (glycine and GABA). Excitatory neurons are unopposed, and extreme muscle spasm results.

E. Laboratory Diagnosis: Primarily a clinical diagnosis. Organism is rarely isolated. Serologic tests not useful.

F. Treatment: Hyperimmune human globulin to neutralize toxin. Also penicillin G and spasmolytic drugs. No significant resistance to penicillin.

G. Prevention: Toxoid vaccine (toxoid is formaldehyde-treated toxin). Usually given to children in combination with diphtheria toxoid and pertussis vaccine (DPT). If patient is injured and has not been immunized, give hyperimmune globulin plus toxoid. Debride wound.

Clostridium botulinum

A. Disease: Botulism.

B. Characteristics: Anaerobic, gram-positive, spore-forming rods.

C. Habitat and Transmission: Habitat is the soil. Organism and toxin transmitted in improperly preserved food.

D. Pathogenesis: Polypeptide exotoxin inhibits the release of acetylcholine at the myoneural junction, causing flaccid paralysis. Failure to sterilize food during preservation allows spores to survive. Spores germinate in anaerobic environment and produce toxin. The toxin is heat-labile; therefore, foods eaten without proper cooking are usually involved.

E. Laboratory Diagnosis: Presence of toxin in patient's serum or stool or in food. Detection involves either known antitoxin in serologic tests or production of the disease in mice. Serologic tests for antibody in the patient are not useful.

F. Treatment: Antitoxin to types A, B, and E made in horses. Use penicillin for infant and wound botulism; organism is growing in patient. No significant resistance to penicillin. Respiratory support may be required.

G. Prevention: Observing proper food preservation techniques, cooking all home-canned food, and discarding bulging cans.

Clostridium perfringens

A. Diseases: Gas gangrene (myonecrosis) and food poisoning.

B. Characteristics: Anaerobic, gram-positive, spore-forming rods.

C. Habitat and Transmission: Habitat is soil and human colon. Myonecrosis results from contamination of wound with soil or feces. Food poisoning is transmitted by ingestion of contaminated food.

D. Pathogenesis: Gas gangrene in wounds is caused by germination of spores under anaerobic conditions and the production of several cytotoxic factors, especially alpha toxin, a lecithinase that disrupts cell membranes. Food poisoning is caused by production of enterotoxin within the gut.

E. Laboratory Diagnosis: Gram-stained smear plus anaerobic culture. Spores not usually seen in clinical specimens; the organism is growing, and nutrients are not restricted. Produces "stormy fermentation" in milk media. Production of lecithinase is detected on egg yolk agar and identified by enzyme inhibition with specific antiserum. Serologic tests not useful.

F. Treatment: Penicillin G plus debridement of the wound in gas gangrene (no significant resistance to penicillin). Only symptomatic treatment needed in food poisoning.

G. Prevention: Extensive debridement of the wound plus administration of penicillin decreases probability of gas gangrene.

Corynebacterium diphtheriae

A. Disease: Diphtheria.

B. Characteristics: Club-shaped gram-positive rods arranged in V or L shape. Granules stain metachromatically. Aerobic, nonspore-forming organism.

C. Habitat and Transmission: Habitat is the human throat. Transmission is via respiratory droplets.

D. Pathogenesis: Organism secretes an exotoxin that inhibits protein synthesis by adding ADP-ribose to EF-2. Toxin has 2 components: subunit A, which has the ADP ribosylating activity, and subunit B, which binds the toxin to cell surface receptors.

E. Laboratory Diagnosis: Gram-stained smear and culture. Black colonies on tellurite plate. Document toxin production with precipitin test or by disease produced in laboratory animals. Serologic tests not useful. The Schick test, a skin test that determines whether a person has antitoxin and is therefore immune, is rarely used.

F. Treatment: Antitoxin made in horses neutralizes the toxin. Penicillin G kills the organism. No significant resistance to penicillin.

G. Prevention: Toxoid vaccine (toxoid is formaldehyde-treated toxin), usually given to children in combination with tetanus toxoid and pertussis vaccine (DPT).

Listeria monocytogenes

A. Diseases: Meningitis and sepsis in newborns and immunocompromised adults.

B. Characteristics: Small gram-positive rods. Aerobic, nonspore-forming organism.

C. Habitat and Transmission: Organism colonizes the gastrointestinal and female genital tracts; in nature it is widespread in animals, plants, and soil. Transmission is across the placenta or by contact during delivery. Outbreaks of disease are related to unpasteurized milk products, eg, cheese.

D. Pathogenesis: No toxins identified. Immunosuppression and immunologic immaturity predispose to infection.

E. Laboratory Diagnosis: Gram-stained smear and culture. Small, beta-hemolytic colonies on blood agar. Tumbling motility. Serologic tests not useful.

F. Treatment: Penicillin (no significant resistance).

G. Prevention: No vaccine or drug is available.

GRAM-NEGATIVE RODS ASSOCIATED PRIMARILY WITH THE ENTERIC TRACT

Escherichia coli

A. Diseases: Urinary tract infection (UTI), sepsis, neonatal meningitis, and "traveler's diarrhea" are the most common.

B. Characteristics: Facultative gram-negative rods; ferment lactose.

C. Habitat and Transmission: Habitat is the human colon; it colonizes the vagina and urethra. From the urethra, it ascends and causes UTI. Acquired during birth in neonatal meningitis and by the fecal-oral route in diarrhea.

D. Pathogenesis: Endotoxin in cell wall causes septic shock. Two enterotoxins are produced. The heat-labile toxin (LT) stimulates adenylate cyclase by ADP ribosylation. Increased cAMP causes outflow of chloride ions and water, resulting in diarrhea. The heat-stabile toxin (ST) causes diarrhea, perhaps by stimulating guanylate cyclase. Virulence factors include pili for attachment to mucosal surfaces and a capsule that impedes phagocytosis.

Predisposing factors to UTI in women include the proximity of the anus to the vagina and urethra, as well as a short urethra. This leads to colonization of the urethra and vagina by fecal flora. Abnormalities, eg, strictures, valves, and stones, predispose as well. Indwelling urinary catheters and intravenous lines predispose to UTI and sepsis, respectively. Colonization of the vagina leads to neonatal meningitis acquired during birth.

E. Laboratory Diagnosis: Gram-stained smear and culture. Lactose-fermenting colonies on EMB and MacConkey's agar. Green sheen on EMB agar. TSI agar shows acid slant and acid butt with gas. Differentiate from other lactose-positive organisms by biochemical reactions. For epidemiologic studies, type organism by O and H antigens by using known antisera. Serologic tests for antibodies in patient's serum not useful.

F. Treatment: Ampicillin or sulfonamides for urinary tract infections. Cephalosporins for meningitis and sepsis. Rehydration is effective in traveler's diarrhea; trimethoprim-sulfamethoxazole may shorten duration of symptoms. Antibiotic resistance mediated by plasmid-encoded enzymes, eg, β-lactamase and aminoglycoside-modifying enzymes.

G. Prevention: Prevention of UTI involves limiting the frequency and duration of urinary catheterization. Prevention of sepsis involves promptly removing or switching sites of intravenous lines. Prevention of traveler's diarrhea is related to eating cooked food and drinking boiled water in certain countries. Prophylactic doxycycline or Pepto-Bismol may prevent traveler's diarrhea.

Salmonella typhi

A. Disease: Typhoid fever.

B. Characteristics: Facultative gram-negative rods. Non-lactose-fermenting. Produces H_2S. Motile, in contrast to *Shigella*.

C. Habitat and Transmission: Habitat is the human colon only, in contrast to other salmonellae, which are found in the colons of animals as well. Transmission is by the fecal-oral route.

D. Pathogenesis: Invades the reticuloendothelial system. Endotoxin in cell wall causes fever. Capsule (Vi antigen) is a virulence factor. No exotoxins known. Decreased stomach acid resulting from ingestion of antacids or gastrectomy predisposes to *Salmonella* infections.

E. Laboratory Diagnosis: Gram-stained smear and culture. Non-lactose-fermenting colonies on EMB and MacConkey's agar. TSI agar shows alkaline slant and acid butt, with no gas and a small amount of H_2S. Biochemical and serologic reactions used to identify species. Identity can be determined by using known antisera against O, H, and Vi antigens in agglutination test. Widal test detects agglutinating antibodies to O and H antigens in patient's serum, but its use is limited.

F. Treatment: Most effective drug is chloramphenicol. Ampicillin and trimethoprim-sulfamethoxazole can be used in patients who are not severely ill. Resistance to chloramphenicol and ampicillin is mediated by plasmid-encoded acetylating enzymes and β-lactamase, respectively.

G. Prevention: Public health measures, eg, sewage disposal, chlorination of the water supply, stool cultures for food handlers, and hand washing prior to food handling. There is a killed vaccine against *Salmonella typhi,* but it is not very effective.

Salmonella enteritidis

A. Diseases: Enterocolitis. Sepsis with abscesses occasionally.

B. Characteristics: Facultative gram-negative rods. Non-lactose-fermenting. Produces H_2S. Motile, in contrast to *Shigella*. More than 1500 serotypes.

C. Habitat and Transmission: Habitat is the enteric tracts of humans and animals, eg, chickens and domestic livestock. Transmission is by the fecal-oral route.

D. Pathogenesis: Invades the mucosa of the small and large intestines. Can enter blood, causing sepsis. Infectious dose is at least 10^5 organisms, much greater than the dose required for *Shigella*. Endotoxin in cell wall; no exotoxin. Predisposing factors include lowered stomach acidity from either antacids or gastrectomy. Sickle cell disease predisposes to osteomyelitis.

E. Laboratory Diagnosis: Gram-stained smear and culture. Non-lactose-fermenting colonies on EMB and MacConkey's agar. TSI agar shows alkaline slant and acid butt, with gas and H_2S. Biochemical and serologic reactions used to identify species. Can identify the organism by using known antisera in agglutination assay. Widal test detects antibodies in patient's serum to the O and H antigens of the organism but is not widely used.

F. Treatment: Antibiotics usually not recommended for uncomplicated enterocolitis. Ampicillin, chloramphenicol, or trimethoprim-sulfamethoxazole used for sepsis depending on sensitivity tests. Resistance to ampicillin and chloramphenicol is mediated by plasmid-encoded β-lactamases and acetylating enzymes, respectively.

G. Prevention: Public health measures, eg, sewage disposal, chlorination of the water supply, stool cultures for food handlers, and hand washing prior to food handling. No vaccine is available.

Shigella species (eg, *S dysenteriae, S sonnei*)

A. Disease: Enterocolitis (dysentery).

B. Characteristics: Facultative gram-negative rods. Non-lactose-fermenting. Nonmotile, in contrast to *Salmonella*.

C. Habitat and Transmission: Habitat is the human colon only; unlike *Salmonella,* there are no animal carriers for *Shigella*. Transmission is by the fecal-oral route.

D. Pathogenesis: Invades the mucosa of the ileum and colon but does not penetrate farther, so sepsis is rare. Endotoxin in cell wall. Infectious dose is much lower (1–10 organisms) than for *Salmonella*. Children in mental institutions and day-care centers experience outbreaks of shigellosis.

E. Laboratory Diagnosis: Gram-stained smear and culture. Non-lactose-fermenting colonies on EMB and MacConkey's agar. TSI agar shows an alkaline slant with an acid butt and no gas or H_2S. Identified by biochemical reactions or by serology with anti-O antibody in agglutination test. Serologic tests for antibodies in the patient's serum are not done.

F. Treatment: In most cases, fluid and electrolyte replacement only. In severe cases, ampicillin or trimethoprim-sulfamethoxazole. Resistance is mediated by plasmid-encoded enzymes, eg, β-lactamase, that degrade ampicillin and a mutant pteroate synthetase that reduces sensitivity to sulfonamides.

G. Prevention: Public health measures, eg, sewage disposal, chlorination of the water supply, stool cultures for food handlers, and hand washing prior to food handling. Prophylactic drugs not used. No vaccine is available.

Vibrio cholerae

A. Disease: Cholera.

B. Characteristics: Gram-negative, comma-shaped rods. Oxidase-positive, which distinguishes them from Enterobacteriaceae.

C. Habitat and Transmission: Habitat is the human colon. Transmission is by the fecal-oral route.

D. Pathogenesis: Watery diarrhea caused by enterotoxin that activates adenylate cyclase by adding ADP-ribose to the regulatory protein. Increase in cAMP causes outflow of chloride ions and water. Toxin has 2 components: subunit A, which has the ADP-ribosylating activity; and subunit B, which binds the toxin to cell surface receptors. Organism produces mucinase, which enhances attachment to the intestinal mucosa. Role of endotoxin is unclear. Infectious dose is high ($>10^7$ organisms). Carrier state rare.

E. Laboratory Diagnosis: Gram-stained smear and culture. (During epidemics, cultures not necessary.) Agglutination with known antisera confirms the identification.

F. Treatment: Treatment of choice is fluid and electrolyte replacement. Tetracycline is not necessary but shortens duration and reduces carriage.

G. Prevention: Public health measures, eg, sewage disposal, chlorination of the water supply, stool cultures for food handlers, and hand washing prior to food handling. Vaccine containing killed cells has limited effectiveness. Tetracycline used for close contacts.

Campylobacter jejuni

A. Disease: Enterocolitis.

B. Characteristics: Curved (comma- or S-shaped) gram-negative rods. Microaerophilic. Grows well at 42 °C.

C. Habitat and Transmission: Habitat is human and animal feces. Transmission is by the fecal-oral route.

D. Pathogenesis: Invades mucosa of the colon but does not penetrate; therefore, sepsis rarely occurs. No enterotoxin known.

E. Laboratory Diagnosis: Gram-stained smear plus culture on special agar, eg, Skirrow's agar, at 42 °C in high CO_2, low O_2 atmosphere. Serologic tests not useful.

F. Treatment: Symptomatic relief usually; erythromycin for severe disease.

G. Prevention: Public health measures, eg, sewage disposal, chlorination of the water supply, stool cultures for food handlers, and hand washing prior to food handling. No preventive vaccine or drug is available.

Klebsiella pneumoniae

A. Disease: Pneumonia, urinary tract infection, and sepsis.

B. Characteristics: Facultative gram-negative rods with large polysaccharide capsule.

C. Habitat and Transmission: Habitat is the human upper respiratory and enteric tracts. Organism is transmitted to the lungs by aspiration from upper respiratory tract and by inhalation of respiratory droplets. It is transmitted to the urinary tract by ascending spread of fecal flora.

D. Pathogenesis: Endotoxin causes fever and shock associated with sepsis. No exotoxin known. Organism has large capsule, which impedes phagocytosis. Chronic pulmonary disease predisposes to pneumonia; catheterization predisposed to UTI.

E. Laboratory Diagnosis: Gram-stained smear and culture. Characteristic mucoid colonies are a consequence of the organism's abundant polysaccharide capsule. Lactose-fermenting colonies on MacConkey's agar. Differentiated from *Enterobacter* and *Serratia* by biochemical reactions.

F. Treatment: Cephalosporins alone or with aminoglycosides, but antibiotic sensitivity testing must be done. Resistance is mediated by plasmid-encoded enzymes that inactivate aminoglycosides.

G. Prevention: No vaccine or drug is available. Urinary and intravenous catheters should be removed promptly.

Proteus species (eg, *P vulgaris, P mirabilis*)

A. Diseases: UTI and sepsis.

B. Characteristics: Facultative gram-negative rods. Non-lactose-fermenting. Highly motile. Produce urease. Antigens of OX strains of *P vulgaris* cross-react with many rickettsiae.

C. Habitat and Transmission: Habitat is the human colon and the environment (soil and water). Transmission to urinary tract is by ascending spread of fecal flora.

D. Pathogenesis: Endotoxin causes fever and shock associated with sepsis. No exotoxins known. Urease is a virulence factor because it degrades urea to produce ammonia, which raises the pH. This leads to stones, damage to epithelium, and infection. Organism is highly motile, which may facilitate entry into the bladder. Predisposing factors are colonization of the vagina, urinary catheters, and abnormalities of the urinary tract such as strictures, valves, and stones.

E. Laboratory Diagnosis: Gram-stained smear and culture. "Swarming" (spreading) effect over blood agar plate as a consequence of the organism's active motility. Non-lactose-fermenting colonies on EMB or MacConkey's agar. TSI agar shows an alkaline slant and acid butt with H_2S. Organism produces urease, whereas *Salmonella,* which can appear similar on TSI agar, does not. Serologic tests not useful.

F. Treatment: Ampicillin frequently used, but antibiotic sensitivities should be done. Resistance is mediated by plasmid-encoded β-lactamase.

G. Prevention: No vaccine or drug is available. Prompt removal of urinary catheters helps prevent urinary tract infections.

Pseudomonas aeruginosa

A. Diseases: Wound infection, UTI, pneumonia, and sepsis. One of the most important causes of nosocomial infections especially in burn patients and those with cystic fibrosis.

B. Characteristics: Aerobic gram-negative rods. Non-lactose-fermenting. Pyocyanin (blue-green) pigment produced.

C. Habitat and Transmission: Habitat is environmental water sources, eg, in hospital respirators and humidifiers. Also inhabits the skin, upper respiratory tracts, and colons of about 10% of people. Transmission is via water aerosols, aspiration, and fecal contamination.

D. Pathogenesis: Endotoxin is responsible for fever and shock associated with sepsis. Produces exotoxin A, which acts like diphtheria toxin (inactivates EF-2), but its role in pathogenesis is unclear. Pili and capsule are virulence factors that mediate attachment and inhibit phagocytosis, respectively.

E. Laboratory Diagnosis: Gram-stained smear and culture. Non-lactose-fermenting colonies on EMB or MacConkey's agar. TSI agar shows an alkaline slant and an alkaline butt, because the sugars are not fermented. Oxidase-positive. Serologic tests not useful.

F. Treatment: Antibiotics must be chosen on the basis of antibiotic sensitivities, because resistance is common. Resistance is mediated by a variety of plasmid-encoded enzymes, eg, β-lactamases and acetylating enzymes.

G. Prevention: Disinfection of water-related equipment in the hospital, hand washing, and prompt removal of urinary and intravenous catheters.

Bacteroides fragilis

A. Disease: Sepsis, peritonitis, and abdominal abscess.

B. Characteristics: Anaerobic, gram-negative rods.

C. Habitat and Transmission: Habitat is the human colon, where it is the predominant anaerobe. Transmission occurs by spread from the colon to the blood or peritoneum.

D. Pathogenesis: Lipopolysaccharide in cell wall is chemically different from typical endotoxin. No exotoxins known. Capsule is antiphagocytic. Predisposing factors to infection include surgery, trauma, and chronic disease, eg, cancer.

E. Laboratory Diagnosis: Gram-stained smear plus anaerobic culture. Identification based on biochemical reactions and gas chromatography. Serologic tests not useful.

F. Treatment: Metronidazole, clindamycin, and cefoxitin are all effective. Abscesses should be surgically drained. Resistance to penicillin G, some cephalosporins, and aminoglycosides is common. Plasmid-encoded β-lactamase mediates resistance to penicillin.

G. Prevention: In bowel surgery, perioperative cefoxitin can reduce the frequency of postoperative infections. No vaccine is available.

GRAM-NEGATIVE RODS ASSOCIATED PRIMARILY WITH THE RESPIRATORY TRACT

Haemophilus influenzae

A. Diseases: Meningitis, otitis media, and pneumonia are common.

B. Characteristics: Small gram-negative (coccobacillary) rods. Type b capsule is polyribitol phosphate. Requires factors X (hemin) and V (NAD) for growth.

C. Habitat and Transmission: Habitat is the upper respiratory tract. Transmission is via respiratory droplets.

D. Pathogenesis: Polysaccharide capsule is the most important determinant of virulence; 95% of invasive disease is caused by capsular type b. IgA protease is produced. Most cases of meningitis occur in children under 2 years of age, because maternal antibody has waned and the immune response of the child can be inadequate. No toxins identified.

E. Laboratory Diagnosis: Gram-stained smear plus culture on chocolate agar with both factors X and V. Determine serotype by using antiserum in various tests, eg, Quellung, immunoelectrophoresis, or latex agglutination. Capsular antigen present in serum or cerebrospinal fluid. Serologic test not useful.

F. Treatment: Ampicillin and chloramphenicol for empirical therapy of meningitis. (Empirical therapy begins with both, because approximately 15% of isolates are resistant to ampicillin owing to a plasmid-encoded β-lactamase.) Can also use cephalosporins, eg, ceftriaxone or cefuroxime.

G. Prevention: Rifampin can prevent meningitis in close contacts. Vaccine containing the type b capsular polysaccharide is effective in persons over 2 years of age.

Legionella pneumophila

A. Disease: Legionnaires' disease ("atypical" pneumonia).

B. Characteristics: Gram-negative rods, but stain poorly with standard Gram's stain. Require increased iron and cysteine for growth in culture.

C. Habitat and Transmission: Habitat is environmental water sources. Transmission is via aerosol. Person-to-person transmission does not occur.

D. Pathogenesis: Aside from endotoxin, no toxins, enzymes, or virulence factors are known. Predisposing factors include being male, being over age 55 years, smoking, and having a high alcohol intake. Immunosuppressed patients, eg, renal transplant recipients, are highly susceptible.

E. Laboratory Diagnosis: Microscopy with silver impregnation stain or fluorescent antibody. Culture on charcoal yeast extract agar containing increased amounts of iron and cysteine. Diagnosis usually made serologically.

F. Treatment: Erythromycin.

G. Prevention: No vaccine or prophylactic drug is available.

Bordetella pertussis

A. Disease: Whooping cough (pertussis).

B. Characteristics: Small gram-negative rods.

C. Habitat and Transmission: Habitat is the human respiratory tract. Transmission is via respiratory droplets.

D. Pathogenesis: Two toxins are produced. Pertussis toxin stimulates adenylate cyclase by adding ADP ribose onto the inhibitory coupling protein. Toxin has 2 components: subunit A, which has the ADP-ribosylating activity, and subunit B, which binds the toxin to cell surface receptors. In addition, extracellular adenylate cyclase is produced, which can inhibit killing by phagocytes. Hemagglutinating proteins on the fimbriae mediate attachment to the ciliated epithelium of the respiratory tract.

E. Laboratory Diagnosis: Gram-stained smear plus culture on Bordet-Gengou agar. Identified by biochemical reactions and slide agglutination with known antisera. Serologic tests not useful.

F. Treatment: Erythromycin.

G. Prevention: Vaccine contains killed organisms. Side effects, eg, brain damage, may limit use. Usually given to children in combination with diphtheria and tetanus toxoids (DPT).

GRAM-NEGATIVE RODS CAUSING ZOONOSES

Brucella species (eg, B abortus, B suis, B melitensis)

A. Disease: Brucellosis (undulant fever).

B. Characteristics: Small gram-negative rods.

C. Habitat and Transmission: Habitat is domestic livestock. Transmission is via milk, milk products, or direct contact with the animal.

D. Pathogenesis: Organisms localize in reticuloendothelial cells. Virulence associated with intracellular survival. Endotoxin necessary for pathogenesis. No exotoxin or capsule identified. Predisposing factors are drinking unpasteurized milk or working in an abattoir.

E. Laboratory Diagnosis: Gram-stained smear plus culture on blood agar plate. Identified by biochemical reactions and by agglutination with known antiserum. Diagnosis may be made serologically also.

F. Treatment: Tetracycline.

G. Prevention: Pasteurize milk; vaccinate cattle. No human vaccine is available.

Francisella tularensis

A. Disease: Tularemia.

B. Characteristics: Small gram-negative rods.

C. Habitat and Transmission: Habitat is many species of wild animals, especially rabbits, deer, and rodents. Transmission is by ticks (eg, *Dermacentor),* aerosols, contact, and ingestion.

D. Pathogenesis: Organisms localize in reticuloendothelial cells. Role of endotoxin is uncertain. No exotoxins known.

E. Laboratory Diagnosis: Culture is rarely done, because special media are required and there is a high risk of infection of laboratory personnel. Diagnosis is usually made by serologic tests.

F. Treatment: Streptomycin.

G. Prevention: Live, attenuated vaccine for persons in high-risk occupations. Protect against tick bites.

Pasteurella multocida

A. Disease: Wound infection, eg, cellulitis.

B. Characteristics: Small gram-negative rods.

C. Habitat and Transmission: Habitat is the mouths of many animals, especially cats and dogs. Transmission is by animal bites.

D. Pathogenesis: Spreads rapidly within skin. No exotoxins known.

E. Laboratory Diagnosis: Gram-stained smear and culture.

F. Treatment: Penicillin.

G. Prevention: Ampicillin should be given to individuals with cat bites.

Yersinia pestis

A. Disease: Plague.

B. Characteristics: Small gram-negative rods with bipolar staining.

C. Habitat and Transmission: Habitat is wild rodents, eg, prairie dogs and squirrels. Transmission is by flea bite.

D. Pathogenesis: Dependent on several factors including endotoxin, an exotoxin, 2 antigens (V and W), and an envelope antigen that protects against phagocytosis.

E. Laboratory Diagnosis: Gram-stained smear. Other stains, eg, Wayson's, show typical "safety-pin" appearance more clearly. Cultures are hazardous and should be done only in specially equipped laboratories. Organism is identified by immunofluorescence. Diagnosis can be made by serologic tests.

F. Treatment: Streptomycin either alone or in combination with tetracycline. Strict quarantine for 72 hours.

G. Prevention: Control rodent population and avoid contact with dead rodents. Killed vaccine is available for persons in high-risk occupations.

MYCOBACTERIA & ACTINOMYCETES

Mycobacterium tuberculosis

A. Disease: Tuberculosis.

B. Characteristics: Aerobic, acid-fast rods. High lipid content of cell wall. Lipids include mycolic acids, wax D, and phosphatides. Grows very slowly.

C. Habitat and Transmission: Habitat is the human lungs. Transmission is via droplets produced by coughing.

D. Pathogenesis: Granulomas and caseation mediated by cellular immunity. Cord factor (trehalose mycolate) correlates with virulence. No exotoxins or endotoxin. Major predisposing factor is poverty. Immunosuppression increases risk of reactivation.

E. Laboratory Diagnosis: Acid-fast rods with Ziehl-Neelsen (or Kinyoun) stain; can use auramine O for screen. Slow-growing (3–6 weeks) colony on Löwenstein-Jensen medium. Organisms produce niacin and are catalase-negative. No serologic tests. PPD skin test is positive if induration measuring 10 mm or more appears 48 hours after inoculation (delayed hypersensitivity). Positive skin test indicates exposure but not necessarily disease.

F. Treatment: Long-term therapy (6–9 months) with 2 drugs, eg, isoniazid plus either rifampin or ethambutol for uncomplicated pulmonary tuberculosis. Triple-drug therapy is used in severe cases, eg, meningitis, and where the chance of isoniazid-resistant organisms is high, as in Southeast Asians.

G. Prevention: Isoniazid taken for 1 year can prevent tuberculosis in infected persons. BCG vaccine containing live, attenuated organisms may prevent disease. Used rarely in the USA but widely in parts of Europe.

Mycobacterium leprae

A. Disease: Leprosy.

B. Characteristics: Aerobic, acid-fast rods. Cannot be cultured in vitro. Optimal growth at less than body temperature.

C. Habitat and Transmission: Habitat is the human skin and nerves. Transmission is by prolonged contact.

D. Pathogenesis: Lesions are usually situated in the cooler parts of the body, eg, skin and peripheral nerves. In tuberculoid leprosy, destructive lesions are due to the cell-mediated response to the organism. Damage to fingers is due to burns and other trauma, because nerve damage causes loss of sensation. In lepromatous leprosy, the cell-mediated response is lost and large numbers of organisms appear in the lesions and blood. No toxins or virulence factors are known.

E. Laboratory Diagnosis: Acid-fast rods are abundant in lepromatous leprosy, but few are found in the tuberculoid form. Cultures and serologic tests not done. Lepromin skin test is positive in the tuberculoid but not in the lepromatous form.

F. Treatment: Dapsone. For dapsone-resistant strains, multiple-drug therapy with dapsone and rifampin, with or without clofazimine.

G. Prevention: Dapsone for close family contacts. No vaccine is available.

Actinomyces israelii

A. Disease: Actinomycosis (abscesses with draining sinus tracts).

B. Characteristics: Anaerobic, gram-positive branching rods.

C. Habitat and Transmission: Habitat is anaerobic crevices around the teeth. Transmission into tissues occurs during dental disease or trauma. Organism also aspirated into lungs.

D. Pathogenesis: No toxins or virulence factors known.

E. Laboratory Diagnosis: Gram-stained smear plus anaerobic culture on blood agar plate. "Sulfur granules" visible in the pus. No serologic tests.

F. Treatment: Penicillin G and surgical drainage.

G. Prevention: No vaccine or drug is available.

Nocardia asteroides

A. Disease: Nocardiosis (especially lung and brain abscesses).

B. Characteristics: Aerobic, gram-positive branching rods. Partially acid-fast.

C. Habitat and Transmission: Habitat is the soil. Transmission is probably via airborne particles.

D. Pathogenesis: No toxins or virulence factors known. Immunosuppression and cancer predispose to infection.

E. Laboratory Diagnosis: Gram-stained smear and modified Ziehl-Neelsen stain. Aerobic culture on blood agar plate. No serologic tests.

F. Treatment: Sulfonamides.

G. Prevention: No vaccine or drug is available.

MYCOPLASMAS

Mycoplasma pneumoniae

A. Disease: "Atypical" pneumonia.

B. Characteristics: Smallest free-living organisms. Not seen on Gram-stained smear, because they have no cell wall. The only bacteria with cholesterol in cell membrane. Can be cultured in vitro.

C. Habitat and Transmission: Habitat is the human respiratory tract. Transmission is via respiratory droplets.

D. Pathogenesis: No toxins known. Hydrogen peroxide and cytolytic enzymes may damage the respiratory tract.

E. Laboratory Diagnosis: Microscopy not useful. Can be cultured on special bacteriologic media but takes at least 10 days to grow, which is too long to be clinically useful. Positive cold-agglutinin test is presumptive evidence. Complement fixation test for antibodies to *Mycoplasma pneumoniae* is more specific.

F. Treatment: Erythromycin.

G. Prevention: No vaccine or drug is available.

SPIROCHETES

Treponema pallidum

A. Disease: Syphilis.

B. Characteristics: Spirochetes. Not seen on Gram-stained smear. Not cultured in vitro.

C. Habitat and Transmission: Habitat is the human genital tract. Transmission is by sexual contact and from mother to fetus across the placenta.

D. Pathogenesis: Organism multiplies at site of inoculation and then spreads widely via the bloodstream. Many features of syphilis are attributed to blood vessel involvement. Primary and secondary lesions heal spontaneously. Tertiary lesions consist of gummas, aortitis, or central nervous system inflammation. No toxins or virulence factors known.

E. Laboratory Diagnosis: Seen by dark-field microscopy or immunofluorescence. Serologic tests important: VDRL (or RPR) is nontreponemal test used for screening; FTA-ABS is the most widely used specific test for *Treponema pallidum.*

F. Treatment: Benzathine penicillin (long-acting form) for primary and secondary syphilis (no resistance to penicillin).

G. Prevention: Benzathine penicillin given to contacts. No vaccine is available.

Borrelia burgdorferi

A. Disease: Lyme disease.

B. Characteristics: Spirochetes. Not seen on Gram-stained smear. Can be cultured in vitro.

C. Habitat and Transmission: Found in ixodid ticks, especially in 3 areas in the USA: Northeast (eg, Connecticut), Midwest (eg, Wisconsin), and West Coast (eg, California). Transmitted by tick bite primarily from 2 reservoirs, mice and deer.

D. Pathogenesis: Organism invades skin and spreads via the bloodstream to involve primarily the heart, joints, and central nervous system. Arthritis is caused by immune complexes. No toxins or virulence factors identified.

E. Laboratory Diagnosis: Diagnosis usually made serologically, ie, by detecting IgM antibody.

F. Treatment: Penicillin or tetracycline.

G. Prevention: Avoid tick bite.

Leptospira interrogans

A. Disease: Leptospirosis.

B. Characteristics: Spirochetes that can be seen on dark-field microscopy but not light microscopy. Can be cultured in vitro.

C. Habitat and Transmission: Habitat is wild and domestic animals. Transmission is via animal urine (in the USA, transmission is chiefly via dog, livestock, and rat urine).

D. Pathogenesis: Two phases: an initial bacteremic phase and a subsequent immuno-pathologic phase with meningitis. No toxins or virulence factors known.

E. Laboratory Diagnosis: Dark-field microscopy and culture in vitro are available but not usually done. Diagnosis usually made by serologic testing.

F. Treatment: Penicillin G or tetracycline.

G. Prevention: Doxycycline effective for short-term exposure. Vaccination of domestic livestock and pets. Rat control.

CHLAMYDIAE

Chlamydia trachomatis

A. Disease: Nongonococcal urethritis, cervicitis, inclusion conjunctivitis, lymphogranuloma venereum, and trachoma. Also pneumonia in infants.

B. Characteristics: Obligate intracellular parasites. Not seen on Gram-stained smear. Exists as inactive elementary body extracellularly and as metabolically active, dividing reticulate body intracellularly.

C. Habitat and Transmission: Habitat is the human genital tract and eyes. Transmission is by sexual contact and at birth. Transmission in trachoma is chiefly by hand-to-eye contact.

D. Pathogenesis: No toxins or virulence factors known.

E. Laboratory Diagnosis: Cytoplasmic inclusions seen on Giemsa- or fluorescent-antibody-stained smear. Glycogen-filled cytoplasmic inclusions can be visualized with iodine. Organism grows in cell culture and embryonated eggs. Diagnosis can be made by serologic tests, eg, complement fixation or microimmunofluorescence test.

F. Treatment: Tetracycline or erythromycin.

G. Prevention: Erythromycin effective in infected mother to prevent neonatal disease. No vaccine is available.

Chlamydia psittaci

A. Disease: Psittacosis.

B. Characteristics: Obligate intracellular parasites. Not seen on Gram-stained smear. Exists as inactive elementary body extracellularly and as metabolically active, dividing reticulate body intracellularly.

C. Habitat and Transmission: Habitat is birds, both psittacine and others. Transmission is via aerosol of bird secretions and feces.

D. Pathogenesis: No toxins or virulence factors known.

E. Laboratory Diagnosis: Cytoplasmic inclusion seen by Giemsa or fluorescent-antibody staining. Organism can be isolated from sputum, but this is rarely done. Diagnosis usually made serologically, eg, by complement fixation test.

F. Treatment: Tetracycline.

G. Prevention: No vaccine or drug is available.

RICKETTSIAE

Rickettsia rickettsii

A. Disease: Rocky Mountain spotted fever.

B. Characteristics: Obligate intracellular parasites. Not seen well on Gram-stained smear. Antigens cross-react with OX strains of *P vulgaris* (Weil-Felix reaction).

C. Habitat and Transmission: *Dermacentor* ticks are the natural reservoir. Transmission is via tick bite.

D. Pathogenesis: Organism invades endothelial lining of capillaries, causing vasculitis. No toxins or virulence factors identified.

E. Laboratory Diagnosis: Stain and culture rarely done. Diagnosis usually made by complement fixation or Weil-Felix test.

F. Treatment: Tetracycline.

G. Prevention: Protective clothing and prompt removal of ticks. Tetracycline effective in exposed persons. No vaccine is available.

Coxiella burnetii

A. Disease: Q fever.

B. Characteristics: Obligate intracellular parasites. Not seen well on Gram-stained smear.

C. Habitat and Transmission: Habitat is domestic livestock. Transmission is by inhalation of aerosols of urine, feces, amniotic fluid, or placental tissue. The only rickettsia not transmitted to humans by an arthropod.

D. Pathogenesis: No toxins or virulence factors known.

E. Laboratory Diagnosis: Stain and culture rarely done. Diagnosis usually made by serologic tests. Weil-Felix test is negative.

F. Treatment: Tetracycline.

G. Prevention: Vaccine for high-risk occupations. No drug is available.

SUMMARIES OF MEDICALLY IMPORTANT VIRUSES

DNA ENVELOPED VIRUSES

Herpes Simplex Virus Type 1

A. Diseases: Herpes labialis (fever blisters or cold sores), keratitis, encephalitis.

B. Characteristics: Enveloped virus with icosahedral nucleocapsid and linear double-stranded DNA. No virion polymerase. One serotype; cross-reaction with HSV-2 occurs. No herpes group-specific antigen.

C. Transmission: By saliva or direct contact with virus from the vesicle.

D. Pathogenesis: Initial vesicular lesions occur in the mouth or on the face. The virus then travels up the axon and becomes latent in sensory (trigeminal) ganglia. Recurrences occur in skin innervated by affected sensory nerve and are stimulated by fever, sunlight, stress, etc. Dissemination occurs in patients with depressed cell-mediated immunity.

E. Laboratory Diagnosis: Virus causes CPE in cell culture. It is identified by antibody neutralization or fluorescent-antibody test. Tzanck smear reveals multinucleated giant cells. This implicates a herpesvirus but is not specific for HSV-1. A rise in antibody titer can be used to diagnose a primary infection but not recurrences.

F. Treatment: Acyclovir for encephalitis and disseminated disease. Trifluorothymidine for keratitis. Primary infections and localized recurrences are self-limited. A variety of over-the-counter drying agents can be used to promote healing.

G. Prevention: Recurrences can be prevented by avoiding the specific inciting agent such as intense sunlight. No vaccine or chemoprophylaxis is available.

Herpes Simplex Virus Type 2

A. Diseases: Herpes genitalis, aseptic meningitis, and neonatal infection.

B. Characteristics: Enveloped virus with icosahedral nucleocapsid and linear double-stranded DNA. No virion polymerase. One serotype; cross-reaction with HSV-1 occurs. No herpes group-specific antigen.

C. Transmission: Sexual contact in adults and during passage through the birth canal in neonates.

D. Pathogenesis: Initial vesicular lesions occur on genitals. The virus then travels up the axon and becomes latent in sensory (lumbar or sacral) ganglion cells. Recurrences may be induced by stress.

E. Laboratory Diagnosis: virus causes CPE in cell culture. Identify by antibody neutralization or fluorescent-antibody test. Tzanck smear reveals multinucleated giant cells but is not specific for HSV-2. A rise in antibody titer can be used to diagnose a primary infection but not recurrences.

F. Treatment: Acyclovir is useful in the treatment of both primary and recurrent disease. It has no effect on the latent state.

G. Prevention: Primary disease can be prevented by protection from exposure to vesicular lesions. Recurrences can be reduced by the long-term use of oral acyclovir.

Varicella-Zoster Virus

A. Diseases: Varicella (chickenpox) in children and zoster (shingles) in adults.

B. Characteristics: Enveloped virus with icosahedral nucleocapsid and linear double-stranded DNA. No virion polymerase. One serotype.

C. Transmission: Respiratory droplets and contact with vesicular fluid.

D. Pathogenesis: Initial infection is in the respiratory tract. It spreads via the blood to the internal organs such as the liver and then to the skin. After the acute episode of varicella, the virus remains latent in the sensory ganglia and can reactivate to cause zoster years later, especially in older and immunocompromised individuals.

E. Laboratory Diagnosis: Virus causes CPE in cell culture and can be identified by fluorescent-antibody test. Multinucleated giant cells seen in smears from the base of the vesicle. A 4-fold rise in antibody titer in convalescent-phase serum is diagnostic.

F. Treatment: No antiviral therapy is indicated for varicella or zoster in the immunocompetent patient. In the immunocompromised patient, acyclovir can prevent dissemination.

G. Prevention: None in immunocompetent individuals. Immunocompromised patients exposed to the virus should receive passive immunization with varicella-zoster immune globulin (VZIG) and acyclovir to prevent disseminated disease.

Cytomegalovirus

A. Diseases: Cytomegalic inclusion body disease in infants. Mononucleosis in transfusion recipients. Pneumonia and hepatitis in immunocompromised patients.

B. Characteristics: Enveloped virus with icosahedral nucleocapsid and linear double-stranded DNA. No virion polymerase. One serotype.

C. Transmission: Virus is found in many human body fluids including blood, saliva, semen, cervical mucus, breast milk, and urine. It is transmitted via these fluids, across the placenta, or by organ transplantation.

D. Pathogenesis: Initial infection usually in the oropharynx. The virus spreads to many organs, eg, central nervous system and kidneys in fetuses. In adults, lymphocytes are frequently involved. A latent state occurs in leukocytes. Disseminated infection in immunocompromised patients can result from either a primary infection or reactivation of a latent infection.

E. Laboratory Diagnosis: The virus causes CPE in cell culture and can be identified by fluorescent-antibody test. "Owl's eye" nuclear inclusions are seen. A 4-fold rise in antibody titer in convalescent-phase serum is diagnostic.

F. Treatment: No drug is available. In clinical trials, ganciclovir is beneficial in treating pneumonia and retinitis. Acyclovir and adenine arabinoside are ineffective.

G. Prevention: No vaccine is available. Do not transfuse CMV antibody-positive blood into newborns or antibody-negative immunocompromised patients.

Epstein-Barr Virus

A. Diseases: Infectious mononucleosis; associated with Burkitt's lymphoma in east African children.

B. Characteristics: Enveloped virus with icosahedral nucleocapsid and linear double-stranded DNA. No virion polymerase. One serotype.

C. Transmission: Virus found in human epithelial cells and lymphocytes. It is transmitted primarily by saliva.

D. Pathogenesis: Infection begins in the pharyngeal epithelium, spreads to the cervical lymph nodes, then travels via the blood to the liver and spleen.

E. Laboratory Diagnosis: The virus is rarely isolated. Lymphocytosis, including atypical lymphocytes, occurs. Heterophil antibody is typically positive (Monospot test). A significant rise in EBV-specific antibody to viral capsid antigen is diagnostic.

F. Treatment: No effective drug is available.

G. Prevention: None.

Hepatitis B Virus

A. Diseases: Hepatitis B; associated with hepatocellular carcinoma.

B. Characteristics: Enveloped virus with incomplete circular double-stranded DNA; ie, one strand has about one-third missing and the other strand is "nicked" (not covalently bonded). DNA polymerase in virion. There are 3 important antigens: the surface antigen, the core antigen, and the e antigen, which is located in the core. In patients' serum, long rods and spherical forms composed solely of HBsAg predominate.

C. Transmission: Transmitted by blood, during birth, and by sexual intercourse.

D. Pathogenesis: Hepatocellular injury due to viral replication; immune complex formation leading to arthritis, rash, and glomerulonephritis. Chronic hepatitis and cirrhosis can occur. Hepatocellular carcinoma may be related to the integration of the viral DNA into hepatocyte DNA.

E. Laboratory Diagnosis: HBV has not been grown in cell culture. Three serologic tests are commonly used: surface antigen (HBsAg), surface antibody (HBsAb), and core antibody (HBcAb). See Chapter 41 for a discussion of the results of these tests.

F. Treatment: No specific treatment.

G. Prevention: There are 3 main approaches: (1) vaccine that contains HBsAg as the immunogen; (2) hyperimmune serum globulins obtained from donors with high titers of HBsAb; and (3) education of chronic carriers regarding precautions.

Smallpox Virus

A. Disease: Smallpox (eradicated in 1977).

B. Characteristics: Poxviruses are the largest viruses. Enveloped virus with linear double-stranded DNA. DNA-dependent RNA polymerase in virion. One serologic type.

C. Transmission: By respiratory droplets or direct contact with the virus from skin lesions.

D. Pathogenesis: The virus infects the mucosal cells of the upper respiratory tract, then spreads to the local lymph nodes and by viremia to the liver and spleen and later the skin. Skin lesions progress in the following order: macule, papule, vesicle, pustule, crust.

E. Laboratory Diagnosis: Virus identified by CPE in cell culture or "pocks" on chorioallantoic membrane. Electron microscopy reveals typical particles; cytoplasmic inclusions seen in light microscopy. Viral antigens in the vesicle fluid can be detected by precipitin tests. A 4-fold or greater rise in antibody titer in the convalescent-phase serum is diagnostic.

F. Treatment: None.

G. Prevention: Vaccine contains live attenuated vaccinia virus. Vaccine is no longer used except by the military, because the disease has been eradicated.

DNA NONENVELOPED VIRUS

Adenovirus

A. Diseases: Upper and lower tract respiratory disease, especially pharyngitis and pneumonia. Some strains cause sarcomas in certain animals but not humans.

B. Characteristics: Nonenveloped virus with icosahedral nucleocapsid and linear double-stranded DNA. No virion polymerase. There are 34 serotypes, some associated with specific diseases.

C. Transmission: Respiratory droplet and feces primarily; iatrogenic transmission in eye disease.

D. Pathogenesis: Virus preferentially infects epithelium of respiratory tract and eyes. After acute infection, persistent, low-grade virus production without symptoms can occur.

E. Laboratory Diagnosis: Virus causes CPE in cell culture and can be identified by fluorescent-antibody or complement fixation test. Antibody titer rise in convalescent-phase serum is diagnostic.

F. Treatment: None.

G. Prevention: Live vaccine against types 3, 4, and 7 is used in the military.

RNA ENVELOPED VIRUSES

Influenza Virus

A. Disease: Influenza.

B. Characteristics: Enveloped virus with a helical nucleocapsid and segmented, single-stranded RNA of negative polarity. RNA polymerase in virion. The 2 major antigens are the hemagglutinin and the neuraminidase on separate surface spikes. Antigenic shifts in these proteins as a result of reassortment of RNA segments accounts for the epidemics of influenza. Antigenic drift due to mutations also contributes. The antigenicity of the internal capsid protein determines whether the virus is an A, B, or C influenza virus.

C. Transmission: Respiratory droplets.

D. Pathogenesis: Infection is limited primarily to the epithelium of the respiratory tract.

E. Laboratory Diagnosis: Virus grows in cell culture and embryonated eggs and can be detected by hemadsorption or hemagglutination. It is identified by hemagglutination inhibition or complement fixation. Antibody titer rise in convalescent-phase serum is diagnostic.

F. Treatment: Amantadine is available but infrequently used.

G. Prevention: Vaccine contains inactivated strains of A and B virus currently causing disease. The vaccine is not a good immunogen and must be given annually. Recommended for people over age 65 years and for those with chronic diseases especially of the heart and lungs. Amantadine provides good prophylaxis in unvaccinated people who have been exposed.

Measles Virus

A. Disease: Measles. Subacute sclerosing panencephalitis is a rare late complication.

B. Characteristics: Enveloped virus with a helical nucleocapsid and one piece of single-stranded, negative-polarity RNA. RNA polymerase in virion. It has a single serotype.

C. Transmission: Respiratory droplets.

D. Pathogenesis: Initial site of infection is the upper respiratory tract. Virus spreads to local lymph nodes and then via the blood to other organs including the skin. The maculopapular rash is due to both viral replication and immunologic injury. The virus can suppress T cell function, and delayed hypersensitivity against tuberculin can be lost temporarily.

E. Laboratory Diagnosis: The virus is rarely isolated. Serologic tests are used if necessary.

F. Treatment: No antiviral therapy is available.

G. Prevention: Vaccine containing live attenuated virus. Usually given in combination with mumps and rubella vaccines.

Mumps Virus

A. Disease: Mumps. Sterility due to bilateral orchitis is a rare complication.

B. Characteristics: Enveloped virus with a helical nucleocapsid and one piece of single-stranded, negative-polarity RNA. RNA polymerase in virion. It has a single serotype.

C. Transmission: Respiratory droplets.

D. Pathogenesis: The initial site of infection is the upper respiratory tract. The virus spreads to local lymph nodes and then via the bloodstream to other organs, especially the parotid glands, testes, ovaries, meninges, and pancreas.

E. Laboratory Diagnosis: The virus can be isolated in cell culture and detected by hemadsorption. Diagnosis can also be made serologically.

F. Treatment: No antiviral therapy is available.

G. Prevention: Vaccine containing live attenuated virus. Usually given in combination with measles and rubella vaccines.

Rubella Virus

A. Disease: Rubella. Congenital rubella syndrome is characterized by developmental abnormalities, especially cardiovascular and neurologic, and by prolonged virus excretion.

B. Characteristics: Enveloped virus with an icosahedral nucleocapsid and a single strand of positive-polarity RNA. No polymerase in virion. It has a single serotype.

C. Transmission: Respiratory droplets.

D. Pathogenesis: The initial site of infection is the nasopharynx, from which it spreads to local lymph nodes. It then disseminates to the skin via the bloodstream. The rash is attributed to both viral replication and immune injury. During maternal infection, the virus replicates in the placenta and then spreads to fetal tissue. If infection occurs during the first trimester, a high frequency of congenital abnormalities occurs.

E. Laboratory Diagnosis: Virus growth in cell culture is detected by interference with plaque formation by coxsackievirus; rubella virus does not cause CPE. To determine whether an adult woman is immune, a single serum specimen to detect IgG antibody in the hemagglutination inhibition test is used. To detect whether recent infection has occurred, either a single serum specimen for IgM antibody or a set of acute-and convalescent-phase sera for IgA antibody can be used.

F. Treatment: No antiviral therapy is available.

G. Prevention: Vaccine containing live attenuated virus. Usually given in combination with measles and mumps vaccine.

Parainfluenza Virus

A. Diseases: Croup in young children, bronchiolitis in infants, and the common cold in adults.

B. Characteristics: Enveloped virus with helical nucleocapsid and one piece of single-stranded, negative-polarity RNA. RNA polymerase in virion. Unlike the case with influenza viruses, the antigenicity of its hemagglutinin and neuraminidase is stable.

C. Transmission: Respiratory droplets.

D. Pathogenesis: Infection and death of respiratory epithelium without systemic spread of the virus. Multinucleated giant cells caused by the viral fusion protein are a hallmark.

E. Laboratory Diagnosis: Isolation of the virus in cell culture is detected by hemadsorption. Immunofluorescence is used for identification. A 4-fold or greater rise in antibody titer is diagnostic in primary infections, but the heterotypic response limits its usefulness in repeated infections.

F. Treatment: None.

G. Prevention: No vaccine or drug is available.

Respiratory Syncytial Virus

A. Diseases: Bronchiolitis and pneumonia in infants.

B. Characteristics: Enveloped virus with a helical nucleocapsid and one piece of single-stranded, negative-polarity RNA. RNA polymerase in virion. Unlike other paramyxoviruses, it has only a fusion protein in its surface spikes. It has no hemagglutinin.

C. Transmission: Respiratory droplets.

D. Pathogenesis: Infection involves primarily the lower respiratory tract in infants without systemic spread. There may be an immunopathologic component; immunization has resulted in more severe disease.

E. Laboratory Diagnosis: Isolation in cell culture. Multinucleated giant cells visible. Immunofluorescence is used for identification. Serology is not useful for diagnosis in infants.

F. Treatment: Aerosolized ribavirin for sick infants.

G. Prevention: No vaccine or prophylactic drug is available.

Rabies Virus

A. Disease: Rabies.

B. Characteristics: Bullet-shaped enveloped virus with a helical nucleocapsid and one piece of single-stranded, negative polarity RNA. RNA polymerase in virion. The virus has a single serotype.

C. Transmission: Animal bite, usually by wild animals such as skunks, raccoons, and bats. In the USA, dogs are infrequently involved. Transmitted rarely by inhalation of bat guano.

D. Pathogenesis: Replication of virus at the site of the bite, followed by ascension up the nerve to the central nervous system. After replicating in the brain, the virus migrates peripherally to the salivary glands where it enters the saliva. When the animal is in the agitated state as a result of encephalitis, virus in the saliva can be transmitted via a bite.

E. Laboratory Diagnosis: Tissue can be stained with fluorescent antibody or with various dyes to detect inclusions called Negri bodies. The virus can be isolated in newborn mice, but because this takes 1 or 2 weeks, it cannot be used to determine whether a person should receive the vaccine. Serology is useful only to make the diagnosis in the clinically ill patient; it does not help the person who has been bitten. It is also used to evaluate the antibody response to the vaccine given before exposure to those in high-risk occupations.

F. Treatment: No antiviral therapy is available.

G. Prevention: Preexposure prevention of rabies consists of the vaccine only. Postexposure prevention consists of (1) washing the wound; (2) giving immune serum, half in the wound and half intramuscularly; and (3) giving the inactivated vaccine made in human cell culture. The decision to give the immune serum and the vaccine depends on the circumstances. Prevention of rabies in dogs and cats by using a live attenuated vaccine has reduced human rabies significantly.

Human Immunodeficiency Virus

A. Disease: Acquired immune deficiency syndrome (AIDS).

B. Characteristics: Enveloped virus with a single-stranded diploid RNA genome and reverse transcriptase. The *tat* gene encodes a transacting protein that activates transcription. It is a type D retrovirus (lentivirus). There are several antigenic types.

C. Transmission: Transfer of body fluids, eg, blood and semen. Also transplacental.

D. Pathogenesis: Infects and kills helper T cells, which predisposes to opportunistic infections. Other cells, eg, astrocytes, are infected also.

E. Laboratory Diagnosis: Virus is isolated from blood or semen only at certain laboratories. Antibody detection, which indicates prior infection but not necessarily active disease, is widely available.

F. Treatment: Azidothymidine (AZT) inhibits HIV replication. Clinical improvement occurs, but the virus persists. Treatment of the opportunistic infection depends on the organism.

G. Prevention: Screening of blood prior to transfusion for the presence of antibody. ''Safe sex,'' including the use of condoms.

RNA NONENVELOPED VIRUSES

Poliovirus

A. Diseases: Paralytic poliomyelitis and aseptic meningitis.

B. Characteristics: Naked nucleocapsid with single-stranded, positive polarity RNA. No virion polymerase. There are 3 serotypes.

C. Transmission: Fecal-oral route.

D. Pathogenesis: The virus replicates in the pharynx and the gastrointestinal tract. It can spread to the local lymph nodes and then through the bloodstream to the central nervous system. Most infections are asymptomatic or very mild. Aseptic meningitis is more frequent than paralytic polio, in which the motor neurons are killed.

E. Laboratory Diagnosis: Recovery of the virus from spinal fluid indicates infection of the central nervous system. Isolation of the virus from stools indicates infection but not necessarily disease. It can be found in the gastrointestinal tracts of asymptomatic carriers. The virus can be detected in cell culture by CPE and identified by neutralization with type-specific antiserum. A significant rise in antibody titer in convalescent-phase serum is also diagnostic.

F. Treatment: No antiviral therapy is available.

G. Prevention: Disease can be prevented by both the inactivated (Salk) vaccine and the attenuated (Sabin) vaccine; both induce humoral antibody that neutralizes the virus in the bloodstream. The oral Sabine vaccine is used for routine childhood immunizations, because it (1) induces IgA immunity in the gut, thereby interfering with transmission; (2) induces immunity of longer duration; and (3) is administered orally. Immune globulins are available but rarely used.

Coxsackieviruses

A. Diseases: Aseptic meningitis, herpangina, pleurodynia, myocarditis, and pericarditis are the most important diseases.

B. Characteristics: Naked nucleocapsid with single-stranded, positive-polarity RNA. No virion polymerase. Group A and B viruses are defined by their different pathogenicity in mice. There are multiple serotypes in each group.

C. Transmission: Fecal-oral route.

D. Pathogenesis: The initial site of infection is the oropharynx, but the main site is the gastrointestinal tract. The virus spreads through the bloodstream to various organs.

E. Laboratory Diagnosis: The virus can be detected by CPE in cell culture and identified by neutralization. A significant rise in antibody titer in convalescent-phase serum is diagnostic.

F. Treatment: No antiviral therapy is available.

G. Prevention: No vaccine is available.

Hepatitis A Virus

A. Disease: Hepatitis A.

B. Characteristics: Naked nucleocapsid virus with a single-stranded, positive-polarity RNA. No virion polymerase. Virus has a single serotype.

C. Transmission: Fecal-oral route.

D. Pathogenesis: The virus replicates in the gastrointestinal tract and then spreads to the liver during a brief viremic period. The virus is cytopathic for the hepatocyte.

E. Laboratory Diagnosis: The most useful test is IgM antibody. Isolation of the virus from clinical specimens is not done.

F. Treatment: No antiviral drug is available.

G. Prevention: Administration of immune globulins during the incubation period can mitigate the disease. No vaccine is available.

Reoviruses (Especially Rotavirus)

A. Disease: The most important reovirus is rotavirus, which causes gastroenteritis especially in young children.

B. Characteristics: Naked double-layered capsid with 10 or 11 segments of double-standard RNA. RNA polymerase in virion. Rotavirus is resistant to stomach acid and hence can reach the gastrointestinal tract.

C. Transmission: Reoviruses are transmitted either by respiratory droplet or by the fecal-oral route. Human rotaviruses are found only in humans and are transmitted by the fecal-oral route.

D. Pathogenesis: Rotavirus infection is limited to the gastrointestinal tract.

E. Laboratory Diagnosis: Detection of rotavirus in the stool by ELISA. A significant rise in antibody titer in convalescent-phase serum is useful. Isolation of the virus is not done from clinical specimens.

F. Treatment: No antiviral drug is available.

G. Prevention: No vaccine is available.

Rhinoviruses

A. Disease: Common cold.

B. Characteristics: Naked nucleocapsid viruses with single-stranded, positive-polarity RNA. No virion polymerase. There are more than 100 serotypes. Rhinoviruses are destroyed by stomach acid and do not replicate in the gastrointestinal tract, in contrast to poliovirus, coxsackievirus, and echovirus, which are resistant to stomach acid.

C. Transmission: Aerosol droplets and hand-to-nose contact.

D. Pathogenesis: Infection is limited to the mucosa of the upper respiratory tract and conjunctivas. The virus replicates best at the low temperatures of the nose and less well at 37 °C, accounting for its failure to infect the lower respiratory tract.

E. Laboratory Diagnosis: Laboratory tests are rarely used clinically. The virus can be recovered from nose or throat washings by growth in cell culture. Serologic tests are not useful.

F. Treatment: No antiviral therapy is available.

G. Prevention: No vaccine is available because there are too many serotypes.

SUMMARIES OF MEDICALLY IMPORTANT FUNGI

FUNGI CAUSING CUTANEOUS & SUBCUTANEOUS INFECTIONS

Dermatophytes (eg, *Trichophyton, Microsporum, Epidermophyton* species)

A. Diseases: Dermatophytoses, eg, tinea capitis, tinea cruris, and tinea pedis.

B. Characteristics: These fungi are molds that use keratin as a nutritional source. Not dimorphic. Habitat of most dermatophytes that cause human disease is human skin, with the exception of *Microsporum canis*, which inhabits the skin of dogs and cats.

C. Transmission: Skin scales.

D. Pathogenesis: Grow only in the superficial, cornified layers of skin, ie, the keratin layer. They do not invade underlying tissue. The lesions are due to the inflammatory response to the fungi. Frequency of infection is enhanced by moisture and warmth. An important host defense is provided by the fatty acids produced by sebaceous glands. The "id" reaction is a hypersensitivity response in one skin location, eg, fingers, to the presence of the organism in another, eg, feet.

E. Laboratory Diagnosis: Skin scales should be examined microscopically in a KOH preparation for the presence of hyphae. The organism is identified by the appearance of its mycelium and its asexual spores on Sabouraud's agar. Serologic tests are not useful.

F. Skin test: Trichophytin antigen can be used to determine the competence of a patient's cell-mediated immunity. Not used for diagnosis of tinea.

G. Treatment: Topical agents such as miconazole, clotrimazole and tolnaftate are used. Undecylenic acid is effective against tinea pedis. Griseofulvin is the treatment of choice for tinea unguium and tinea capitis.

H. Prevention: Skin should be kept dry and cool.

Sporothrix schenckii

A. Disease: Sporotrichosis.

B. Characteristics: Thermally dimorphic. Habitat is soil or vegetation.

C. Transmission: Traumatic penetration of skin.

D. Pathogenesis: Local abscess or ulcer with nodules in draining lymphatics.

E. Laboratory Diagnosis: Cigar-shaped budding cells visible in pus. Culture on Sabouraud's agar shows typical morphology.

F. Skin Test: None.

G. Treatment: Potassium iodide, ketoconazole.

H. Prevention: Skin should be protected when gardening.

FUNGI CAUSING SYSTEMIC INFECTIONS

Histoplasma capsulatum

A. Disease: Histoplasmosis.

B. Characteristics: Thermally dimorphic. The mold form produces tuberculate chlamydospores (asexual spores). The mold grows preferentially in soil enriched with bird droppings. Endemic in Ohio and Mississippi River valley areas.

C. Transmission: Inhalation of airborne asexual spores (microconidia).

D. Pathogenesis: Microconidia enter the lung and differentiate into yeast cells. The yeast cells are ingested by alveolar macrophages and multiply within them. An immune response is mounted, and granulomas form. Most infections are contained at this level, but suppression of cell-mediated immunity can lead to disseminated disease.

E. Laboratory Diagnosis: Sputum or tissue can be examined microscopically and cultured on Sabouraud's agar. The presence of tuberculate chlamydospores is diagnostic. A rise in antibody titer is useful for diagnosis, but cross-reaction with other fungi *(Coccidioides)* occurs. Immunodiffusion test is more specific than complement fixation test.

F. Skin Test: Histoplasmin, a mycelial extract, is the antigen. Useful for epidemiologic purposes to determine the incidence of infection. A positive result indicates only that infection has occurred; it cannot be used to diagnose disease. Skin testing can induce antibodies, so serologic tests must be done first.

G. Treatment; Amphotericin B for disseminated disease; ketoconazole for pulmonary disease. No treatment is indicated for primary histoplasmosis.

H. Prevention: Endemic areas should be avoided. No vaccine or prophylactic drug is available.

Coccidioides immitis

A. Disease: Coccidioidomycosis.

B. Characteristics: Thermally dimorphic. At 37°C in the body, it forms spherules containing endospores. At 25°C, it grows as a mold. The cells at the tip of the hyphae differentiate into asexual spores (arthrospores). Natural habitat is the soil of the lower Sonoran life zone.

C. Transmission: Inhalation of airborne arthrospores.

D. Pathogenesis: Arthrospores differentiate into spherules in the lungs. Spherules rupture, releasing endospores that form new spherules, thereby disseminating the infection within the body. A cell-mediated immune response contains the infection in most people, but those who are immunocompromised are at high risk for disseminated disease.

E. Laboratory Diagnosis: Sputum or tissue should be examined microscopically for spherules and cultured on Sabouraud's agar. A rise in IgM precipitin antibodies indicates recent infection. A rising titer of complement-fixing IgG antibodies indicates dissemination; a decreasing titer indicates a response to therapy.

F. Skin Test: Either coccidioidin, a mycelial extract, or spherulin, an extract of spherules, is the antigen. Useful in determining whether the patient has been infected. A positive test indicates prior infection but not necessarily active disease.

G. Treatment: Amphotericin B for disseminated disease; ketoconazole for limited pulmonary disease. No treatment is indicated for primary coccidioidomycosis.

H. Prevention: Endemic areas should be avoided. No vaccine or prophylactic drug is available.

Blastomyces dermatitidis

A. Disease: Blastomycosis.

B. Characteristics: Thermally dimorphic. The yeast form has a single, broad-based bud and a thick, refractile wall. Natural habitat is rich soil (eg, near beaver dams).

C. Transmission: Inhalation of airborne asexual spores.

D. Pathogenesis: Inhaled conidia differentiate into yeasts, which initially cause an abscess followed by formation of granulomas. Dissemination is rare but when it occurs, skin and bone are most commonly involved.

E. Laboratory Diagnosis: Sputum or skin lesions examined microscopically for yeast with a broad-based bud. Culture on Sabouraud's agar also. Serologic tests are not useful.

F. Skin Test: Little value.

G. Treatment: Ketoconazole is the drug of choice.

H. Prevention: No vaccine or prophylactic drug is available.

Paracoccidioides brasiliensis

A. Disease: Paracoccidioidomycosis.

B. Characteristics: Thermally dimorphic. The yeast form has multiple buds (resembles the steering wheel of a ship).

C. Transmission: Inhalation of airborne conidia.

D. Pathogenesis: Inhaled conidia differentiate to the yeast form in lungs. Can disseminate to many organs.

E. Laboratory Diagnosis: Yeasts with multiple buds visible in pus or tissues. Culture on Sabouraud's agar shows typical morphology.

F. Skin Test: Not useful.

G. Treatment: Ketoconazole or sulfonamides.

H. Prevention; No vaccine or prophylactic drug is available.

FUNGI CAUSING OPPORTUNISTIC INFECTIONS

Aspergillus fumigatus

A. Diseases: Invasive aspergillosis is the major disease. Allergic bronchopulmonary aspergillosis is important also.

B. Characteristics: Mold with septate hyphae that branch at a V-shaped angle. Not dimorphic. Habitat is the soil.

C. Transmission: Inhalation of airborne condidia.

D. Pathogenesis: Opportunistic pathogen. In immunocompromised patients, invasive disease occurs. The organism invades blood vessels, causing thrombosis and infarction. In a person with a lung cavity, a "fungus ball" (aspergilloma) can develop. An allergic person can develop allergic bronchopulmonary aspergillosis.

E. Laboratory Diagnosis: Septate hyphae invading tissue are visible microscopically. Invasion distinguishes disease from colonization. Culture on Sabouraud's agar. Serologic tests detect IgG precipitins in patients with aspergillomas and IgE antibodies in patients with allergic bronchopulmonary aspergillosis.

F. Skin Test: None available.

G. Treatment: Amphotericin B for invasive aspergillosis. Some lesions can be surgically removed. Steroid therapy is recommended for allergic bronchopulmonary aspergillosis.

H. Prevention: No vaccine or prophylactic drug is available.

Candida albicans

A. Disease: Thrush, disseminated candidiasis, and chronic mucocutaneous candidiasis.

B. Characteristics: Candida albicans is a yeast when part of the normal flora of mucous membranes but forms pseudohyphae and hyphae when it invades tissue. The yeast form produces germ tubes when incubated in serum at 37°C. Not thermally dimorphic.

C. Transmission: Part of the normal flora of skin, mucous membranes, and gastrointestinal tract. No person-to-person transmission.

D. Pathogenesis: Opportunistic pathogen. Predisposing factors include depressed immune system, altered skin and mucous membrane, suppression of normal flora, and presence of foreign bodies. Thrush is most common in infants, immunosuppressed patients, and persons on antibiotic therapy. Skin lesions occur frequently on moisture-damaged skin. Disseminated infection occurs in immunosuppressed patients and intravenous drug abusers. Chronic mucocutaneous candidiasis occurs in children with a T cell defect in immunity to Candida.

E. Laboratory Diagnosis: Microscopic examination of tissue reveals yeasts and pseudohyphae. If only yeasts are found, colonization is suggested. The yeast is gram-positive. Germ tube formation and production of chlamydospores distinguish C albicans from virtually all other species of Candida. Serologic tests not useful.

F. Skin Test: Used to determine competency of cell-mediated immunity rather than to diagnose candidal disease.

G. Treatment: Skin and mucous membrane disease can be treated with oral or topical antifungal agents such as nystatin or miconazole. Disseminated disease requires amphotericin B and flucytosine, but resistance to flucytosine limits its effectiveness. Chronic mucocutaneous candidiasis is treatable with ketoconazole.

H. Prevention: Predisposing factors should be reduced or eliminated.

Cryptococcus neoformans

A. Disease: Cryptococcosis, especially cryptococcal meningitis.

B. Characteristics: Heavily encapsulated yeast. Not dimorphic. Habitat is soil, especially where enriched by pigeon droppings.

C. Transmission: Inhalation of airborne yeast cells.

D. Pathogenesis: Organisms cause influenzalike syndrome or pneumonia. They spread via the bloodstream to the meninges. Reduced cell-mediated immunity predisposes to severe disease, but some cases of cryptococcal meningitis occur in immunocompetent people.

E. Laboratory Diagnosis: Visualization of the encapsulated yeast in India ink preparations of spinal fluid. Culture of sputum or spinal fluid on Sabouraud's agar. Latex agglutination test detects polysaccharide capsular antigen in spinal fluid.

F. Skin Test: Not available.

G. Treatment: Amphotericin B plus flucytosine.

H. Prevention: No vaccine or prophylactic drug is available.

Mucor & Rhizopus species

A. Disease: Mucormycosis.

B. Characteristics: Molds with nonseptate, ribbonlike hyphae. Not dimorphic. Habitat is the soil.

C. Transmission: Inhalation of airborne sporangiospores.

D. Pathogenesis: Opportunistic pathogens. They cause disease primarily in ketoacidotic diabetic and leukemic patients. The nose and sinuses are typically involved. Hyphae invade the mucosa and progress into underlying tissue and vessels, leading to necrosis and infarction.

E. Laboratory Diagnosis: Microscopic examination for the presence of invasive hyphae. Culture on Sabouraud's agar. Serologic tests are not available.

F. Skin Test: None.

G. Treatment: Amphotericin B and surgical debridement.

H. Prevention: No vaccine or prophylactic drug is available. Control of underlying disease, eg, diabetes, tends to prevent mucormycosis.

SUMMARIES OF MEDICALLY IMPORTANT PARASITES

PROTOZOA

1. Intestinal & Urogenital Infections

Entamoeba histolytica

A. Diseases: Amebic dysentery and liver abscess.

B. Characteristics: Intestinal protozoan. Motile ameba (trophozoite); forms cysts with 4 nuclei. Life cycle: Humans ingest cysts, which form trophozoites in small intestine. Trophozoites pass to the colon and multiply. Cysts form in the colon.

C. Transmission and Epidemiology: Fecal-oral transmission of cysts. Human reservoir. Occurs worldwide, especially in tropics.

D. Pathogenesis: Trophozoites invade colon epithelium and produce "teardrop" ulcer. Can spread to liver and cause abscess.

E. Laboratory Diagnosis: Trophozoites or cysts visible in stool. Serology (indirect hemagglutination test) positive with invasive disease.

F. Treatment: Metronidazole plus iodoquinol.

G. Prevention: Proper disposal of human waste. Water purification. Hand washing.

Giardia lamblia

A. Disease: Giardiasis.

B. Characteristics: Intestinal protozoan. Pear-shaped, flagellated trophozoite, forms cyst with 4 nuclei. Life cycle: Humans ingest cysts, which form trophozoites in duodenum. Trophozoites encyst and are passed in feces.

C. Transmission and Epidemiology: Fecal-oral transmission of cysts. Human and animal reservoir. Occurs worldwide.

D. Pathogenesis: Trophozoites attach to wall but do not invade. They interfere with absorption of fat and protein.

E. Laboratory Diagnosis: Trophozoites or cysts visible in stool. String test used if necessary.

F. Treatment: Metronidazole.

G. Prevention: Water purification. Hand washing.

Cryptosporidium species

A. Disease: Cryptosporidiosis, especially diarrhea.

B. Characteristics: Intestinal protozoan. Life cycle: Oocysts release sporozoites; they form trophozoites. After schizonts and merozoites form, microgametes and macrogametes are produced; they unite to form a zygote and then an oocyst.

C. Transmission and Epidemiology: Fecal-oral transmission of cysts. Human and animal reservoir. Occurs worldwide.

D. Pathogenesis: Trophozoites attach to wall of small intestine but do not invade.

E. Laboratory Diagnosis: Oocysts visible in stool with acid-fast stain.

F. Treatment: None.

G. Prevention: None.

Trichomonas vaginalis

A. Disease: Trichomoniasis.

B. Characteristics: Urogenital protozoan. Pear-shaped, flagellated trophozoites. No cysts or other forms.

C. Transmission and Epidemiology: Transmitted sexually. Human reservoir. Occurs worldwide.

D. Pathogenesis: Attach to wall of vagina and cause inflammmation and discharge.

E. Laboratory Diagnosis: Trophozoites visible in secretions.

F. Treatment: Metronidazole for both sexual partners.

G. Prevention: Condoms limit transmission.

2. Blood & Tissue Infections

Plasmodium (P vivax, P ovale, P malariae, & P falciparum)

A. Disease: Malaria.

B. Characteristics: Blood and tissue protozoan. Life cycle: Sexual cycle consists of gametogony in humans and sporogony in mosquitoes; asexual cycle (schizogony) occurs in humans. Sporozoites in saliva of female *Anopheles* mosquito enter blood and rapidly invade hepatocytes (exoerythrocytic phase). There they multiply and form merozoites (*Plasmodium* *vivax* and *Plasmodium ovale* also from hypnozoites, a latent form). Merozoites leave the hepatocytes and infect red cells (erythrocytic phase). There they form schizonts that release more merozoites, which infect other red cells in a synchronous pattern (3 days for *Plasmodium malariae;* 2 days for the others). Some merozoites become male and female gametocytes, which, when ingested by female *Anopheles,* release male and female gametes. These unite to produce a zygote, which forms an oocyst containing many sporozoites.These are released and migrate to salivary glands.

C. Transmission and Epidemiology: Transmitted by female *Anopheles* mosquitoes. Occurs primarily in the tropical areas of Asia, Africa, and Latin America.

D. Pathogenesis: Merozoites destroy red cells. Cyclic fever pattern is due to periodic release of merozoites. *Plasmodium falciparum* can infect red cells of all ages and cause aggregates of red cells to occlude capillaries. This can cause severe kidney damage (blackwater fever). Hypnozoites can cause relapses.

E. Laboratory Diagnosis: Organisms visible in blood smear.

F. Treatment: Chloroquine if sensitive. For chloroquine resistant *P falciparum,* quinine, sulfadoxine, and pyrimethamine are effective. Primaquine for hypnozoites of *P vivax* and *P ovale.*

G. Prevention: Chloroquine. Primaquine to prevent relapses. For those in areas with a high risk of chloroquine resistance, chloroquine plus Fansidar. Protection from bites. Drainage of swamps. Mosquito control.

Pneumocystis carinii

A. Disease: Pneumonia.

B. Characteristics: Respiratory pathogen (? protozoan). Reclassified in 1988 as a yeast. Life cycle: uncertain.

C. Transmission and Epidemiology: Transmitted by inhalation. Humans are reservoir. Occurs worldwide. Most infections asymptomatic.

D. Pathogenesis: Organisms in alveoli cause inflammation. Immunosuppression predisposes to disease.

E. Laboratory Diagnosis: Organisms visible in silver stain of lung tissue.

F. Treatment: Trimethoprim-sulfamethoxazole; pentamidine.

G. Prevention: Trimethoprim-sulfamethoxazole in immunosuppressed individuals.

Toxoplasma gondii

A. Disease: Toxoplasmosis.

B. Characteristics: Tissue protozoan. Life cycle: Cysts in cat feces or in meat are ingested by humans and differentiate in the gut into forms that invade the gut wall. They infect macrophages and form trophozoites (tachyzoites) that multiply rapidly, kill cells, and infect others. Cysts containing bradyzoites form later. Cat ingests cysts in raw meat, and bradyzoites excyst, multiply, and form male and female gametocytes. These fuse to form oocysts in cat gut, which are excreted in cat feces.

C. Transmission and Epidemiology: Transmitted by ingestion of cysts and transplacentally from mother to fetus. Cat is definitive host; humans and other mammals are intermediate hosts. Occurs worldwide.

D. Pathogenesis: Trophozoites infect many organs, especially brain, eyes, and liver. Cysts persist in tissue.

E. Laboratory Diagnosis: Serologic tests for IgM and IgG antibodies are usually used. Trophozoites or cysts visible in tissue.

F. Treatment: Sulfonamide and pyrimethamine for congenital or disseminated disease.

G. Prevention: Meat should be cooked. Pregnant women should not handle cats, litter boxes, or raw meat.

Trypanosoma cruzi

A. Disease: Chagas' disease.

B. Characteristics: Blood and tissue protozoan. Life cycle: Trypomastigotes in blood of reservoir host are ingested by reduviid bug and form epimastigotes and then trypomastigotes in the gut. When the bug bites, it defecates and feces containing trypomastigotes contaminate the wound. Organisms enter the blood and form amastigotes within cells; these then become trypomastigotes.

C. Transmission and Epidemiology: Transmitted by reduviid bugs. Humans and many animals are reservoirs. Occurs in rural Latin America.

D. Pathogenesis: Amastigotes kill cells, especially cardiac muscle.

E. Laboratory Diagnosis: Trypomastigotes visible in blood, but bone marrow biopsy, culture in vitro, xenodiagnosis, or serologic tests may be required.

F. Treatment: Nifurtimox for acute disease. No effective drug for chronic disease.

G. Prevention: Protection from bite. Insect control.

Trypanosoma gambiense & Trypanosoma rhodesiense

A. Disease: Sleeping sickness (African trypanosomiasis).

B. Characteristics: Blood and tissue protozoan. Life cycle: Trypomastigotes in blood of human or animal reservoir are ingested by tsetse fly. They differentiate in the gut to form epimastigotes and then metacyclic trypomastigotes in salivary glands. When fly bites, trypomastigotes enter the blood. Repeated variation of surface antigen occurs, which allow the organism to evade the immune response.

C. Transmission and Epidemiology: Transmitted by tsetse flies. *Trypanosoma gambiense* has a human reservoir and occurs primarily in west Africa. *Trypanosoma rhodesiense* has an animal reservoir (especially wild antelope) and occurs primarily in east Africa.

D. Pathogenesis: Trypomastigotes infect brain, causing encephalitis.

E. Laboratory Diagnosis: Trypomastigotes visible in blood in early stages and in cerebrospinal fluid in late stages. Serologic tests useful.

F. Treatment: Suramin in early disease. Suramin plus melarsoprol if central nervous system symptoms exist.

G. Prevention: Protection from bite. Insect control.

Leishmania donovani

A. Disease: Kala-azar (visceral leishmaniasis).

B. Characteristics: Blood and tissue protozoan. Life cycle: Human macrophages containing amastigotes are ingested by sandfly. Amastigotes differentiate in fly gut to promastigotes, which migrate to pharynx. When fly bites, promastigotes enter blood macrophages and form amastigotes. These can infect other reticuloendothelial cells, especially in spleen and liver.

C. Transmission and Epidemiology: Transmitted by sandflies (Phlebotomus or Lutzomyia). Animal reservoir (chiefly dogs, small carnivores, and rodents) in Africa, Middle East, and parts of China. Human reservoir in India.

D. Pathogenesis: Amastigotes kill reticuloendothelial cells, especially in liver, spleen, and bone marrow.

E. Laboratory Diagnosis: Amastigotes visible in bone marrow smear. Serologic tests useful. Skin test indicates prior infection.

F. Treatment: Sodium stibogluconate.

G. Prevention: Protection from bite. Insect control.

CESTODES

Diphyllobothrium latum

A. Disease: Diphyllobothriasis.

B. Characteristics: Cestode (fish tapeworm). Scolex has 2 elongated sucking grooves; no circular suckers or hooks. Gravid uterus forms a rosette. Oval eggs have an operculum at one end. Life cycle: Humans ingest undercooked fish containing sparganum larvae. Larvae attach to gut wall and become adults containing gravid proglottids. Eggs are passed in feces. In fresh water, eggs hatch and the embryos are eaten by copepods. When these are eaten by freshwater fish, larvae form in the fish muscle.

C. Transmission and Epidemiology: Transmitted by eating raw or undercooked freshwater fish. Humans are definitive hosts; copepods are the first and fish the second intermediate hosts, respectively. Occurs worldwide but endemic in Scandinavia, Japan, and north-central USA.

D. Pathogenesis: Tapeworm in gut causes little damage.

E. Laboratory Diagnosis: Eggs visible in stool.

F. Treatment: Niclosamide or praziquantel.

G. Prevention: Adequate cooking of fish. Proper disposal of human waste.

Echinococcus granulosus

A. Disease: Hydatid cyst disease.

B. Characteristics: Cestode (dog tapeworm). Scolex has 4 suckers and a double circle of hooks. Adult worm has only 3 proglottids. Life cycle: Dogs are infected when they ingest the entrails of sheep, eg, liver, containing hydatid cysts. The adult worms develop in the gut, and eggs are passed in the feces. Eggs are ingested by sheep (and humans) and hatch hexacanth larvae in the gut that migrate in the blood to various organs, especially the liver and brain. Larvae form large, unilocular hydatid cysts containing many protoscoleces and daughter cysts.

C. Transmission and Epidemiology: Transmitted by ingestion of eggs in food contaminated with dog feces. Dogs are main definitive hosts; sheep are intermediate hosts; humans are dead-end hosts. Endemic in sheep-raising areas, eg, Mediterranean, Middle East, some western states of the USA.

D. Pathogenesis: Hydatid cyst is a space-occupying lesion. Also, if cyst ruptures antigens in fluid can cause anaphylaxis.

E. Laboratory Diagnosis: Serologic tests, eg, indirect hemagglutination. Pathologic examination of excised cyst.

F. Treatment: Surgical removal of cyst.

G. Prevention: Sheep entrails should not be fed to dogs.

Taenia saginata

A. Disease: Taeniasis.

B. Characteristics: Cestode (beef tapeworm). Scolex has 4 suckers but no hooks. Gravid proglottids have 15–20 uterine branches. Life cycle: Humans ingest undercooked beef containing cysticerci. Larvae attach to gut wall and become adult worms with gravid proglottids. Terminal proglottids detach, pass in feces, and are eaten by cattle. In the gut, oncosphere embryos hatch, burrow into blood vessels, and migrate to skeletal muscles where they develop into cysticerci.

C. Transmission and Epidemiology: Transmitted by eating raw or undercooked beef. Humans are definitive hosts; cattle are intermediate hosts. Occurs worldwide but endemic in areas of Asia, Latin America, and eastern Europe.

D. Pathogenesis: Tapeworm in gut causes little damage. In contrast to the case with *Taenia solium,* cysticercosis does not occur.

E. Laboratory Diagnosis: Gravid proglottids visible in stool. Eggs seen less frequently.

F. Treatment: Praziquantel.

G. Prevention: Adequate cooking of beef. Proper disposal of human waste.

Taenia solium

A. Diseases: Taeniasis and cysticercosis.

B. Characteristics: Cestode (pork tapeworm). Scolex has 4 suckers and a circle of hooks. Gravid proglottids have 5–10 uterine branches. Life cycle: Humans ingest undercooked pork containing cysticerci. Larvae attach to gut wall and develop into adult worms with gravid proglottids. Terminal proglottids detach, pass in feces, and are eaten by pigs. In gut, oncosphere (hexacanth) embryos burrow into blood vessels and migrate to skeletal muscle, where they develop into cysticerci. If humans eat *T solium* eggs in food contaminated with human feces, the oncospheres burrow into blood vessels and disseminate to organs (eg, brain, eyes) where they encyst to form cysticerci.

C. Transmission and Epidemiology: Taeniasis acquired by eating raw or undercooked pork. Cysticercosis acquired only by ingesting eggs in fecally contaminated food or water. Humans are definitive hosts; pigs or humans are intermediate hosts. Occurs worldwide but endemic in areas of Asia, Latin America, and southern Europe.

D. Pathogenesis: Tapeworm in gut causes little damage. Cysticerci can expand and cause symptoms of mass lesions, especially in brain.

E. Laboratory Diagnosis: Gravid proglottids visible in stool. Eggs seen less frequently.

F. Treatment: Praziquantel for intestinal worms and cerebral cysticercosis.

G. Prevention: Adequate cooking of pork. Proper disposal of human waste.

TREMATODES

Clonorchis sinensis

A. Disease: Clonorchiasis.

B. Characteristics: Trematode (liver fluke). Life cycle: Humans ingest undercooked fish containing encysted larvae (metacercariae). In duodenum, immature flukes enter biliary duct, become adults, and release eggs that are passed in feces. Eggs are eaten by snails; the eggs hatch and form miracidia. These multiply through generations (rediae) and then produce many free-swimming cercariae, which encyst under scales of fish and are eaten by humans.

C. Transmission and Epidemiology: Transmitted by eating raw or undercooked freshwater fish. Humans are definitive hosts; snails and fish are first and second intermediate hosts, respectively. Endemic in the Orient.

D. Pathogenesis: Inflammation of biliary tract.

E. Laboratory Diagnosis: Eggs visible in feces.

F. Treatment: Praziquantel.

G. Prevention: Adequate cooking of fish. Proper disposal of human waste.

Paragonimus westermani

A. Disease: Paragonimiasis.

B. Characteristics: Trematode (lung fluke). Life cycle: Humans ingest undercooked freshwater crab containing encysted larvae (metacercariae). In gut, immature flukes enter peritoneal cavity, burrow through diaphragm into lung parenchyma, and become adults. Eggs enter bronchioles and are coughed up or swallowed. In fresh water, eggs hatch, releasing miracidia that enter snails, multiply through generations (rediae), and then form many cercariae that infect and encyst in crabs.

C. Transmission and Epidemiology: Transmitted by eating raw or undercooked crab meat. Humans are definitive hosts; snails and crabs are first and second intermediate hosts, respectively. Endemic in the Orient and India.

D. Pathogenesis: Inflammation and secondary bacterial infection of lung.

E. Laboratory Diagnosis: Eggs visible in sputum or feces.

F. Treatment: Praziquantel.

G. Prevention: Adequate cooking of crabs. Proper disposal of human waste.

Schistosoma (S mansoni, S japonicum, & S hematobium)

A. Disease: Schistosomiasis.

B. Characteristics: Trematode (blood fluke). Adults exist as 2 sexes but are attached to each other. Eggs are distinguished by spines: *Schistosoma mansoni* has large lateral spine; *Schistosoma japonicum* has small lateral spine; *Schistosoma hematobium* has terminal spine. Life cycle: Humans are infected by cercariae penetrating skin. Cercariae form larvae that penetrate blood vessels and are carried to the liver, where they become adults. The flukes migrate retrograde in the portal vein to reach the mesenteric venules (*S mansoni* and *S japonicum)* or urinary bladder venules *(S hematobium)*. Eggs penetrate the gut or bladder wall, are excreted, and hatch in fresh water. The ciliated larvae (miracidia) penetrate snails and multiply through generations to produce many free-swimming cercariae.

C. Transmission and Epidemiology: Transmitted by penetration of skin by cercariae. Humans are definitive hosts; snails are intermediate hosts. Endemic in tropical areas: *S mansoni* in Africa and Latin America, *S hematobium* in Africa and Middle East, *S japonicum* in the Orient.

D. Pathogenesis: Eggs in tissue induce inflammation, granulomas, fibrosis, and obstruction, especially in liver and spleen. *S mansoni* damages the colon (inferior mesenteric venules), *S japonicum* damages the small intestine (superior mesenteric venules), and *S hematobium* damages the bladder. Bladder damage predisposes to carcinoma.

E. Laboratory Diagnosis: Eggs visible in feces or urine.

F. Treatment: Praziquantel.

G. Prevention: Proper disposal of human waste. Swimming in endemic areas should be avoided.

NEMATODES

1. Intestinal Infection

Ancylostoma duodenale & Necator americanus

A. Disease: Hookworm.

B. Characteristics: Intestinal nematode. Life cycle: Larvae penetrate skin, enter the blood, and migrate to the lungs. They enter alveoli, pass up the trachea, then are swallowed. They become adults in small intestine and attach to walls with teeth *(Ancylostoma)* or cutting plates *(Necator)*. Eggs are passed in feces and form noninfectious rhabditiform larvae and then infectious filariform larvae.

C. Transmission and Epidemiology: Larvae in soil penetrate skin of feet. Humans are the only hosts. Endemic in the tropics.

D. Pathogenesis: Anemia due to blood loss form gastrointestinal tract.

E. Laboratory Diagnosis: Eggs visible in feces.

F. Treatment: Mebendazole.

G. Prevention: Use of footwear. Proper disposal of human waste.

Ascaris lumbricoides

A. Disease: Ascariasis.

B. Characteristics: Intestinal nematode. Life cycle: Humans ingest eggs, which form larvae in gut. Larvae migrate through the blood to the lungs, where they enter the alveoli, pass up the trachea, and are swallowed. In the gut, they become adults and lay eggs that are passed in the feces. They embryonate, ie, become infective in soil.

C. Transmission and Epidemiology: Transmitted by food contaminated by soil containing eggs. Humans are the only hosts. Endemic in the tropics.

D. Pathogenesis: Larvae in lung can cause pneumonia. Heavy worm burden can cause intestinal obstruction or malnutrition.

E. Laboratory Diagnosis: Eggs visible in feces.

F. Treatment: Mebendazole.

G. Prevention: Proper disposal of human waste.

Enterobius vermicularis

A. Disease: Pinworm infection

B. Characteristics: Intestinal nematode. Life cycle: Humans ingest eggs, which develop into adults in gut. At night, females migrate from the anus and lay many eggs on skin and in environment. Embryo within egg becomes an infective larva within 4-6 hours. Reinfection is common.

C. Transmisson and Epidemiology: Transmitted by ingesting eggs. Humans are the only hosts. Occurs worldwide.

D. Pathogenesis: Worms and eggs cause perianal pruritus.

E. Laboratory Diagnosis: Eggs visible by "Scotch tape" technique. Adult worms found in diapers.

F. Treatment: Mebendazole or pyrantel pamoate.

G. Prevention: None.

Strongyloides stercoralis

A. Disease: Strongyloidiasis.

B. Characteristics: Intestinal nematode. Life cycle: Larvae penetrate skin, enter the blood, and migrate to the lungs. They move into alveoli and up the trachea and are swallowed. They become adults and enter the mucosa, where females produce eggs that hatch in the colon into noninfectious, rhabditiform larvae that are usually passed in feces. Occasionally, rhabditiform larvae molt in the gut to form infectious, filariform larvae that can enter the blood and migrate to the lung (autoinfection). The noninfectious larvae passed in feces form infectious filariform larvae in the soil. These larvae can either penetrate the skin or form adults. Adults in soil can undergo several entire life cycles there. This free-living cycle can be interrupted when filariform larvae contact the skin.

C. Transmission and Epidemiology: Filariform larvae in soil penetrate skin. Endemic in the tropics.

D. Pathogenesis: Little effect in immunocompetent persons. In immunocompromised persons, massive superinfection can occur accompanied by secondary bacterial infections.

E. Laboratory Diagnosis: Larvae visible in stool.

F. Treatment: Thiabendazole.

G. Prevention: Proper disposal of human waste.

Trichinella spiralis

A. Disease: Trichinosis.

B. Characteristics: Intestinal nematode that encysts in tissue. Life cycle: Humans ingest undercooked meat containing encysted larvae, which mature into adults in small intestine. Female releases larvae that enter blood and migrate to skeletal muscle or brain, where they encyst.

C. Transmission and Epidemiology: Transmitted by ingestion of raw or undercooked meat, usually pork. Reservoir hosts are primarily pigs and rats. Humans are dead-end hosts. Occurs worldwide but endemic in eastern Europe and west Africa.

D. Pathogenesis: Inflammation of muscle.

E. Laboratory Diagnosis: Encysted larvae visible in muscle biopsy. Serologic tests positive.

F. Treatment: Thiabendazole effective early against adults. None for established disease.

G. Prevention: Adequate cooking of pork.

Trichuris trichiura

A. Disease: Whipworm infection.

B. Characteristics: Intestinal nematode. Life cycle: Humans ingest eggs, which develop into adults in gut. Eggs are passed in feces into soil, where they embryonate, ie, become infectious.

C. Transmission and Epidemiology: Transmitted by food or water contaminated with soil containing eggs. Humans are the only hosts. Occurs worldwide, especially in the tropics.

D. Pathogenesis: Worm in gut usually causes little damage.

E. Laboratory Diagnosis: Eggs visible in feces.

F. Treatment: Mebendazole

G. Prevention: Proper disposal of human waste.

---

2. Tissue Infection

Dracunculus medinensis

A. Disease: Dracunculiasis.

B. Characteristics: Tissue nematode. Life cycle: Humans ingest copepods containing infective larvae in drinking water. Larvae are released in gut, migrate to body cavity, mature, and mate. Fertilized female migrates to subcutaneous tissue and forms a papule, which ulcerates. Motile larvae are released into water, where they are eaten by copepods and form infective larvae.

C. Transmission and Epidemiology: Transmitted by copepods in drinking water. Humans are major definitive hosts. Many domestic animals are reservoir hosts. Endemic in tropical Africa, Middle East, and India.

D. Pathogenesis: Adult worms in skin cause inflammation and ulceration.

E. Laboratory Diagnosis: Not useful.

F. Treatment: Niridazole. Extraction of worm from skin ulcer.

G. Prevention: Purification of drinking water.

Loa loa

A. Disease: Loiasis.

B. Characteristics: Tissue nematode. Life cycle: Bite of deer fly (mango fly) deposits infective larvae, which crawl into the skin and develop into adults that migrate subcutaneously. Females produce microfilariae, which enter the blood. These are ingested by deer flies, in which the infective larvae are formed.

C. Transmission and Epidemiology: Transmitted by deer flies. Humans are the only definitive hosts. No animal reservoir. Endemic in central and west Africa.

D. Pathogenesis: Hypersensitivity to adult worms causes ''swelling'' in skin. Adult worm seen crawling across conjunctivas.

E. Laboratory Diagnosis: Microfilariae visible on blood smear.

F. Treatment: Diethylcarbamazine.

G. Prevention: Deer fly control.

Onchocerca volvulus

A. Disease: Onchocerciasis (river blindness).

B. Characteristics: Tissue nematodes. Life cycle: Bite of female blackfly deposits infective larvae, which mature in body cavity. Worms enter subcutaneous tissue, where they mature within skin nodules. Female produce microfilariae, which migrate in interstitial fluids and are ingested by blackflies, in which the infective larvae are formed.

C. Transmission and Epidemiology: Transmitted by female blackflies. Humans are the only definitive hosts. No animal reservoir. Endemic along rivers of tropical Africa and Central America.

D. Pathogenesis: Microfilariae in eye ultimately can cause blindness. Adults induce inflammatory nodules in skin.

E. Laboratory Diagnosis: Microfilariae visible in skin biopsy, not in blood.

F. Treatment: Ivermectin affects microfilariae, not adult worms. Suramin for adult worms.

G. Prevention: Blackfly control and ivermectin.

Toxocara canis

A. Disease: Visceral larva migrans.

B. Characteristics: Nematode larvae cause disease. Life cycle in humans: *Toxocara* eggs are passed in dog feces and ingested by humans. They hatch into larvae in small intestine; larvae enter the blood and migrate to organs, especially liver, brain, and eyes, where they are trapped and die.

C. Transmission and Epidemiology: Transmitted by ingestion of eggs in food or water contaminated with dog feces. Dogs are definitive hosts. Humans are dead-end hosts.

D. Pathogenesis: Granulomas form around dead larvae. Granulomas in the retina can cause blindness.

E. Laboratory Diagnosis: Larvae visible in tissue. Serologic tests useful.

    F. Treatment: None.

    G. Prevention: Dogs should be dewormed.

Wuchereria bancrofti

    A. Disease: Filariasis.

    B. Characteristics: Tissue nematodes. Life cycle: Bite of female mosquito deposits infective larvae that penetrate bite wound, form adults, and produce microfilariae. These circulate in the blood, chiefly at night, and are ingested by mosquitoes, in which the infective larvae are formed.

    C. Transmission and Epidemiology: Transmitted by female mosquitoes of several genera, especially *Anopheles* and *Culex,* depending on geography. Humans are the only definitive hosts. Endemic in many tropical areas.

    D. Pathogenesis: Adult worms cause inflammation that blocks lymphatic vessels (elephantiasis). Chronic, repeated infection required for symptoms to occur.

    E. Laboratory Diagnosis: Microfilariae visible on blood smear.

    F. Treatment: Diethylcarbamazine affects microfilariae. No treatment for adult worms.

    G. Prevention: Mosquito control.

Part IX: Clinical Cases

CASE 1   **Chief Complaint**   A 21-year-old male in shock with a temperature of 41° C.

History   The patient was well until 3 days ago, when mild frontal headaches began. On the morning of admission, he felt very hot and had a shaking chill. That afternoon he became confused and fainted, at which time he was brought to the hospital.

Physical Exam   T 41° C, BP 70/30, P 140, R 24. The patient was intermittently alert. Pertinent findings include:
Skin: Several ecchymoses on the trunk and bleeding from the nose and mouth.
Neck: Supple. No signs of meningeal irritation.
Lungs: Clear.
Heart: No murmur.
Abdomen: Negative except for surgical scar in left upper quadrant, indicating a splenectomy.
Neurologic: No localizing signs.

Laboratory
Blood: Hematocrit 22%; WBC 2800; differential 15% bands, 60% polys, 22% lymphs, 3% eos; platelets 20,000.
Urine: 2+ protein, occasional WBC and RBC.
Chest x-ray: Lungs and heart normal.

Course   Four hours after admission, the patient became obtunded and his blood pressure continued to fall despite antibiotics, transfusions, and blood pressure support with dopamine. Cardiac arrest occurred 2 hours later, cardiopulmonary resuscitation efforts failed, and the patient died. No autopsy was performed.

Comment   This is a case of septic shock, a medical emergency. It is typified by the abrupt onset of fever and hypotension. The shaking chill suggests bacteremia. The rapid downhill course is compatible with bacterial infection, especially by "encapsulated pyogens" (see below) or enteric gram-negative rods.

Questions
1. What is the most important specimen to obtain to make a microbiologic diagnosis?
2. What are the 3 organisms most likely to cause sepsis in this patient?
3. How would you distinguish among these 3 in the laboratory?
4. What is the main predisposing factor to infection in this patient?

Laboratory Results   Gram-positive, lancet-shaped diplococci were seen in the blood culture. Subculture to blood agar plate revealed small, translucent, alpha-hemolytic colonies that were bile-soluble and inhibited by optochin. A quellung test with Omni-serum, which contains antibodies against 83 types of pneumococci, was positive.

Diagnosis   Sepsis due to *Streptococcus pneumoniae*.

Questions
5. What is the source of the patient's bacteremia?
6. Why was the patient bleeding into the skin (ecchymoses) and from the nose and mouth?
7. How could this infection have been prevented?
8. What drugs would you have given this patient shortly after his arrival at the hospital?
9. Is drug resistance a problem with S pneumoniae?
10. What is the mode of action of the drugs you would use?
11. What are the serious side effects of these drugs?

Answers to Questions

1. Blood culture. One should be obtained before empirical therapy is started. Three blood cultures are recommended to ensure a 95% probability of isolating the organism.

2. The 3 major encapsulated pyogens cause 75% of septic shock cases in asplenic patients, ie, pneumococci (50%), meningococci (15%), and *Haemophilus influenzae* (10%). (*H influenzae* sepsis occurs primarily in children.) Other important agents include *Escherichia coli* and *Staphylococcus aureus*.

3. **(a)** Gram stain: Pneumococci are gram-positive, lancet-shaped diplococci; meningococci are gram-negative, kidney bean-shaped diplococci, and *H influenzae* are small, coccobacillary gram-negative rods.
   (b) Culture: *H influenzae* requires X and V factors; meningococci are oxidase-positive while pneumococci are inhibited by bile and optochin.
   (c) Quellung reaction: Antibody causes the capsules of pneumococci and meningococci to swell. The organism can be identified with specific antibody, and the serotype can be determined.

4. Splenectomy increases the risk of septic shock 100-fold. The spleen is an important filter for bacteria in the blood as well as a source of antibody. The patient's spleen was removed 10 years before as treatment for his hereditary spherocytosis.

5. Pneumococci are commonly part of the normal flora of the nasopharynx. From there they can enter the bloodstream. Pneumonia can be a source of pneumococcal bacteremia, but this patient's lungs were clear and the chest x-ray was normal. Pneumococci are acquired by respiratory aerosol, and they colonize the nasopharynx.

6. Disseminated intravascular coagulation (DIC) can accompany septic shock. DIC consumes clotting factors, and bleeding results. DIC is usually associated with endotoxin, ie, with gram-negative organisms. Teichoic acids of gram-positive organisms also may activate complement, leading to platelet aggregation and leaky capillaries.

7. Pneumococcal vaccine should be given to all patients who have had a splenectomy. It contains the capsular polysaccharide of the 23 types that most commonly cause bacteremia. Meningococcal vaccine, which contains the capsular polysaccharides of 4 common types, can also be given. A vaccine against *H influenzae* type B is available as well. In splenectomized children, daily peroral penicillin is used to prevent pneumococcal infection.

8. In view of the severity of the patient's illness, bactericidal drugs given intravenously were indicated. The choice of drugs was governed by the organisms most likely to be involved. He was treated with ampicillin, gentamicin, chloramphenicol, and nafcillin. Pneumococci and meningococci are susceptible to penicillins. Many enteric gram-negative rods are susceptible to aminoglycosides, and enterococci are killed by a combination of penicillin and aminoglycosides. Chloramphenicol affects many organisms, including ampicillin-resistant *H influenzae*. Nafcillin was added to cover *S aureus*. (*Note*: Other regimens are also useful. A combination of penicillin, cefuroxime, and gentamicin is another common choice.)

9. Almost all pneumococci are susceptible to penicillins. There is low-level resistance in some strains, but these are easily treatable with high doses of penicillin. Highly resistant strains are quite rare. Meningococci are also susceptible to penicillin. About 25% of *H influenzae* isolates are resistant to ampicillin due to a plasmid-mediated β-lactamase. Almost all of these isolates are susceptible to chloramphenicol.

10. Penicillins prevent cell wall synthesis by inhibiting transpeptidation. Aminoglycosides inhibit protein synthesis by binding to the 30S ribosomal subunit and preventing the formation of polysomes, ie, monosomes accumulate. Chloramphenicol blocks protein synthesis by inhibiting peptidyltransferase.

11. Penicillins cause anaphylaxis and serum sickness. Aminoglycosides affect the kidneys. Chloramphenicol depresses the bone marrow count and, rarely, causes aplastic anemia.

CASE 2 **Chief Complaint** A 4-year-old boy with diarrhea for 2 days.

History His mother said he was well until 2 days ago, when he stopped eating and felt feverish. He then developed abdominal pain and nonbloody diarrhea, which became progressively more severe. No vomiting or shaking chills occurred. There was no history of recent antibiotic use or travel outside San Francisco. No one else in the family was ill.

Physical Exam   T 38° C, BP 120/70, P 100, R 16. The patient was an acutely ill child appearing flushed and dehydrated. The only abnormal finding was diffuse abdominal tenderness without rebound.

Laboratory
  Blood: Hematocrit 38%; WBC 10,000 with normal differential.
  Urine: Normal.

Comment   Diarrhea typically is due either to enterotoxins or to bacterial invasion of the bowel wall. It is important to determine which mechanism is occurring, because that information is helpful in determining the diagnosis and treatment.

Questions
  1. What test should be done on the stool immediately that can provide evidence of whether the diarrhea is toxigenic or invasive (inflammatory)?
  2. What are the possible organisms that can cause diarrhea in this patient?
  3. If this had occurred in a developing country rather than in the USA, what other important bacterium should be considered?
  4. Do the organisms you thought of in answer to questions 2 and 3 cause toxigenic or inflammatory diarrhea?
  5. What is the most important specimen to obtain to make a microbiologic diagnosis?

Course   A stain for fecal leukocytes revealed many polymorphonuclear leukocytes (PMNs). The stool was positive for occult blood.

Question
  6. In view of these findings, which 3 organisms are most likely to be the cause of this child's diarrhea?

Course   At this point, a clinical assessment should be made to determine the empirical treatment, ie, what to do until the results of the cultures are known. The mainstay of treatment is fluid replacement, eg, with a solution containing sodium, potassium, and glucose. Antimotility agents are best avoided, because they reduce the natural purgative effect and tend to prolong the excretion of organisms.

  A rectal swab was taken for culture; the patient's mother was given advice regarding oral hydration, and the patient was sent home.

  Culture of the stool revealed lactose-negative colonies on eosin-methylene blue (EMB) agar. Triple-sugar-iron agar showed an alkaline slant, acid butt, and no H_2S. The urease test was negative.

Question
  7. On the basis of these findings, what genus of organisms has been isolated?

Course   An agglutination test with antiserum to the O antigen of *Shigella* and *Salmonella* was performed to identify the organism. Agglutination was observed with *Shigella* group B antiserum, indicating that the organism was *Shigella flexneri*. The identification was confirmed by using an API strip, which contains 20 biochemical reactions.

  The patient's mother was contacted, and the results of the culture were discussed with her. She reported that her child had recovered and was well.

Questions
  8. What is the natural habitat of the organism?
  9. As the family was well, where was the organism likely to have come from?
  10. If treatment were indicated, what drugs would you give?
  11. Is there a prolonged carrier state associated with this infection?
  12. Could this infection have been prevented?

Answers to Questions
  1. Stain for fecal leukocytes. Test for occult blood also.
  2. Bacteria: Likely organisms: *Escherichia coli, Clostridium perfringens, Bacillus cereus, Staphylococcus aureus* (but less likely; no vomiting occurred), *Shigella, Salmonella,*

Campylobacter. Less likely: *Yersinia enterocolitica, Vibrio parahaemolyticus.* Viruses: rotavirus, Norwalk virus. Parasites: *Entamoeba histolytica, Giardia lamblia.*

3. *Vibrio cholerae.*

4. Known toxin producers: *V cholerae, S aureus, B cereus, C perfringens,* strains of *E coli.* Known inflammatory agents: *Shigella, Salmonella, Campylobacter,* strains of *E coli, Y enterocolitica.* Uncertain: *E histolytica, G lamblia, V parahaemolyticus.*

5. Stool culture. A blood culture would not be done, because there were no signs of sepsis, eg, no shaking chill, normal blood pressure. An examination for ova and parasites would not be done at this stage unless there were a specific indication, eg, family exposure or travel.

6. *Shigella, Salmonella, and Campylobacter.*

7. *Shigella.*

8. Human gastrointestinal tract. There is no animal reservoir for shigellae, in contrast to many *Salmonella* species.

9. His playmates, perhaps at the day-care center.

10. Either trimethoprim-sulfamethoxazole or ampicillin can be given. Because strains can be resistant, sensitivity test should be done.

11. Shigellosis is typically a self-limited disease with few or no sequelae. There is no prolonged carrier state, unlike that for some *Salmonella* infections, eg, *Salmonella typhi* infections.

12. Shigellosis is quite common in young children; their personal cleanliness and bowel habits are less than perfect. There is no vaccine. Prophylactic antibiotics are not used.

CASE 3

Chief Complaint A 10-year-old girl with leukemia who has had a fever for 2 days.

History The patient was well until 1 year ago when the diagnosis of acute leukemia was made. She was treated with chemotherapy, and remission occurred. One month prior to admission, increasing fatigue and weight loss were noted and a bone marrow revealed 50% blast forms. Chemotherapy, including steroids, was instituted. Two days ago her temperature rose to 39° C without specific localizing symptoms.

Physical Exam T 39°C, BP 100/60, P 100, R 20. The patient appears thin and chronically ill.
Pertinent findings include:
Skin: Pale with several ecchymoses. No petechiae or jaundice.
Head and neck: Normal
Lungs: Clear
Heart: No murmurs.
Abdomen: No tenderness, masses, or organomegaly.
Lymph nodes: Not enlarged.
Neurologic: Normal.

Laboratory
Blood: Hematocrit 20%; WBC 600; differential 10% bands, 30% polys, 55% lymphs, 5% monos; platelets 26,000.
Urine: Normal.
Chest x-ray: Normal.

Comment Fever in an immunocompromised (neutropenic) host is commonly caused by infection. Because infection is the leading cause of death in these patients, it is important that treatment be instituted immediately, before the culture results are ready. Immunocompromised patients with infections frequently have muted signs and symptoms because they are less capable of mounting an inflammatory response.

Questions
1. What are the common bacteria, viruses, and fungi to cause infection in a neutropenic patient?
2. What empirical therapy would you start prior to receipt of the culture results?
3. What specimens would you obtain for culture?

Course   The patient was treated with ticarcillin, nafcillin, and tobramycin intravenously. She remained febrile during the next 48 hours, and all cultures showed no growth. The following day, the patient complained of pain in her left eye and blurred vision. Funduscopy revealed a white, cottony lesion in the perimacular region. She also complained of a sore throat, and inspection revealed several whitish, adherent plaques on the posterior pharynx.

Question

4. In view of these findings, what is the likely genus of the pathogen?

Course   Amphotericin B was started. On day 4, the blood cultures revealed oval, gram-positive organisms without capsules. They were 2–3 times larger than staphylococci. Some of the cells were budding.

Questions

5. What genus of organism was recovered from the blood culture?
6. How would you distinguish among various species of organisms in this genus?
7. What is the natural habitat of this organism?
8. What is the mode of action of amphotericin B?
9. What is the major site of toxicity with amphotericin B?
10. Could this infection have been prevented?

Course   Two days later, the patient developed a right hemiparesis; she died the following day. Autopsy revealed a massive cerebral infarct and invasive *Candida* esophagitis. The esophageal site was thought to be the origin of the fungemia.

Answers to Questions

1. The opportunistic pathogens commonly seen in neutropenic patients are as follows:
   (a) Bacteria: Staphylococci, eg, *Staphylococcus aureus* and *Staphylococcus epidermidis;* gram-negative rods, eg, *Escherichia coli, Klebsiella pneumonia,* and *Pseudomonas aeruginosa.*
   (b) Viruses: Herpesviruses, eg, herpes simplex virus type 1, cytomegalovirus, and varicella-zoster virus.
   (c) Fungi: *Candida albicans, Aspergillus fumigatus,* and *Mucor* and *Rhizopus* species.
2. Combination therapy of bactericidal drugs is commonly used, eg, ticarcillin and tobramycin, which are effective against many of the common bacterial pathogens. Nafcillin can be added for the β-lactamase-producing *S aureus*. Trimethoprim-sulfamethoxazole is also used to cover several types of bacteria and *Pneumocystis*.
3. Blood, urine, and stool plus specific sites of symptoms, if any. Cultures should be taken before antibiotics are started.
4. *Candida* species, such as *C albicans* and *C tropicalis,* since (a) there was no response to antibiotics, (b) no bacteria grew on culture, (c) cottony exudates in the retina are typical of *Candida,* and (d) the throat lesions resemble thrush.
5. The description best fits a species of *Candida*.
6. *C albicans* produces germ tubes, whereas almost all other *Candida* species do not. Biochemical tests, eg, sugar assimilation tests, can also be used.
7. *C albicans* is part of the normal human flora on the skin and in the mouth, gastrointestinal tract, and vagina.
8. It disrupts fungal cell membranes. Its selective toxicity is based on its binding to ergosterol in the fungal membranes but not to the cholesterol in human cell membranes.
9. The kidneys. Serum creatinine levels should be monitored.
10. No preventive measures for candidal infections have been shown to be effective. Trimethoprim-sulfamethoxazole is given to patients with defective cell-mediated immunity to prevent *Pneumocystis* pneumonia.

CASE 4   **Chief Complaint**   A 26-year-old woman with lower abdominal pain for 3 days.

History   The patient was well until 3 days ago when malaise, anorexia, and mild, crampy, left-lower-quadrant pain began. The symptoms intensified during the last 24 hours. She now feels feverish and has vomited twice, and her pain is moderately severe. No shaking chill, diarrhea, dysuria, or hematuria has occurred. She has noticed an increased amount of yellowish vaginal discharge. The discharge is nonbloody and has no odor. Her last menstrual period ended 3 days ago.

Physical Exam T 39°C, BP 120/80, P 96, R 14.
Pertinent physical findings include:
Abdomen: Left-lower-quadrant tenderness without rebound. No masses or organomegaly. Bowel sounds normal. No costovertebral-angle tenderness.
Pelvis: Introitus and vagina: Normal.
Cervix: Inflamed with a small amount of purulent discharge at os; motion tenderness elicited.
Uterus: Normal size; no tenderness or masses.
Adnexae: Very tender on left. No masses felt.

Laboratory
Blood: Hematocrit 40%; WBC 17,400; differential 12% bands, 65% polys, 20% lymphs, 3% monos.
Urine: Normal.
Abdominal film: No distended bowel loops.

Comment This is a case of pelvic inflammatory disease (acute salpingitis and cervicitis). Because infertility can result, prompt and appropriate treatment is important. A clinical judgment must be made whether to hospitalize patients with pelvic inflammatory disease; this depends on, eg, the severity of the illness and the reliability of the patient to follow an outpatient regimen. This patient was hospitalized.

Questions
1. Which organisms are most likely to cause this infection?
2. What specimen(s) would you obtain for culture?
3. Knowing the organisms that might be involved, what empirical antibiotic therapy would you suggest? (There are several alternatives.)

Course Culdocentesis yielded 20 mL of bloody, foul-smelling purulent fluid, which was sent for aerobic and anaerobic culture. (A rubber stopper was placed on the needle tip to maintain anaerobic conditions within the syringe.) Gram stain of the fluid revealed gram-negative diplococci and gram-negative rods.
The patient was started on cefoxitin and doxycycline intravenously. Within 24 hours, her pain was significantly diminished and her temperature dropped to 37.5°C.
Aerobic cultures revealed oxidase-positive colonies on Thayer-Martin medium that were gram-negative diplococci microscopically. Anaerobic cultures grew numerous, similar-appearing colonies consisting of gram-negative rods.

Questions
4. What is the most likely organism isolated in the aerobic cultures?
5. What genus of anaerobic organisms seems likely?

Course Subsequent laboratory tests confirmed the presence of 2 organisms, *Neisseria gonorrhoeae* and *Bacteroides fragilis*. The patient's signs and symptoms resolved by 48 hours, and both antibiotics were continued for an additional 48 hours. She was discharged to continue taking doxycycline orally for the next 10 days.

Questions
6. Since syphilis can be acquired at the same time as gonorrhea, how would you test for this disease?
7. How would you prevent gonorrhea from spreading to others?
8. What is the mode of action of cefoxitin and doxycycline?
9. Is antibiotic resistance a clinical concern with *N gonorrhoeae* and *B fragilis?*

Answers to Questions
1. *N gonorrhoeae* is the most common cause. Mixed infections, with or without gonococci, are frequent. Other organisms isolated include *Escherichia coli,* enterococci, and various

anaerobes, eg, peptostreptococci and *B fragilis*. *Chlamydia trachomatis* can also be involved.

2. Culture of pus from the cervix should be done. In addition, culdocentesis (aspiration of fluid from the "cul-de-sac" behind the cervix) is an important diagnostic procedure. If fluid is obtained, it should be cultured.

3. One suggested regimen for hospitalized patients includes cefoxitin (a cephalosporin effective against gonococci, including penicillinase-producing strains, and against anaerobes) and doxycycline (a tetracycline effective against *C trachomatis* and various enteric gram-negative rods, eg, *E coli*). For other regimens, see the *Morbidity and Mortality Report* published by the Centers for Disease Control or an infectious-disease text.

4. *N gonorrhoeae.*

5. *Bacteroides* species, eg, *B fragilis* or *Fusobacterium* species.

6. VDRL. If positive, confirm with fluorescent treponemal antibody-absorption (FTA-ABS) test. If VDRL is negative, consider repeating in 2 weeks.

7. Sexual contacts should be traced and treated. Also, cultures from the patient should be performed, either upon discharge from the hospital or a few days thereafter.

8. Cefoxitin, a cephalosporin, inhibits peptidoglycan synthesis by blocking transpeptidation. Doxycycline, a tetracycline, inhibits protein synthesis at the level of the 30S ribosomal subunit.

9. Some strains of gonococci produce penicillinase, which renders many penicillins ineffective. These strains (PPNG) have caused outbreaks in the USA but have not become endemic here. Some strains of *B fragilis* produce penicillinase also. Antibiotic susceptibility testing should be performed with both organisms.

CASE 5

Chief Complaint   A 52-year-old man with a cough for the past 3 days.

History   The patient was in his usual state of health until 3 days ago, when fever and a cough began abruptly, accompanied by anorexia and a severe frontal headache. The cough is productive of a small amount of whitish, nonbloody sputum. No chest pain or myalgias occurred. A shaking chill accompanied by sweating occurred yesterday. Mild, nonbloody diarrhea without nausea or vomiting began yesterday also.

The patient is a clerk at a supermarket. His medical history is significant for a kidney transplant 2 years ago. To prevent rejection, he takes azathioprine and prednisone. His smoking and drinking habits include 2 packs of cigarettes and a 6-pack of beer per day—more on weekends. His wife and children are well. He has no pets and no history of recent travel.

Physical Exam   T 40°C, BP 130/70, P 96, R 24. The patient was an acutely ill man, appearing flushed and short of breath.
Pertinent findings include:
Eyes, ears, and throat: Normal. No sinus tenderness.
Neck: Supple.
Lungs: Inspiratory rales heard over left posterior lung. No dullness to percussion.
Heart: Normal
Abdomen: Normal
Neurologic: Normal

Laboratory
Blood: Hematocrit 46%; WBC 18,000; differential 9% bands, 77% polys, 12% lymph, 2% eos.
Urine: No sugar, 1+ protein, 10 RBC/HPF,* 2 WBC/HPF.
Chest x-ray: Segmental infiltrate in left lower lobe.

Questions
1. What are the 2 important specimens to obtain to make a microbiologic diagnosis?
2. What procedure can you do with one of the specimens that might provide information regarding the cause of this disease?

*HPF = high-power field.

Course A sputum specimen was obtained for Gram stain and culture. The Gram stain revealed many polys but no predominant organism. Few gram-positive and gram-negative cocci were seen. A blood culture was taken.

Comment The clinical presentation suggests atypical pneumonia; there is scant, nonpurulent sputum, and a Gram stain shows polys but no organisms.

Questions
3. What are some of the causes of atypical pneumonia?
4. Patients who take azathioprine and prednisone have reduced immunity. What organisms typically cause pneumonia in immunocompromised adults?

Comment The following findings are in accord with a diagnosis of *Legionella* pneumonia: (1) a middle-aged man who smokes and drinks; (2) an immunocompromised patient; (3) multisystem involvement as indicated by headache, diarrhea, and microscopic hematuria; and (4) no predominant organism on Gram stain.

Course In view of the suggestive findings described above, examination of the sputum with fluorescent antibody to *Legionella pneumophila* was performed and was positive.

Questions
5. What is the treatment of choice for Legionella *pneumonia?*
6. What is the mechanism of action of this drug?
7. What is the natural habitat of this organism?
8. Can the organism be cultured in the laboratory?
9. In addition to fluorescent-antibody analysis of sputum, what is another serologic method for making the diagnosis of Legionella *pneumonia?*
10. Why was the organism not seen in the Gram-stained smear?

Course The patient was treated with erythromycin intravenously for 7 days and then with oral erythromycin for an additional 2 weeks. He rapidly defervesced within 24 hours, and his cough resolved gradually during the following week.

Answers to Questions
1. Sputum and blood.
2. Light microscopy of a Gram-stained smear of sputum.
3. *Mycoplasma pneumoniae* is the most common cause. However, *L pneumophila, Chlamydia psittaci* (psittacosis), and viruses, eg, influenza virus, also cause this clinical picture.
4. (a) Bacteria: Most are gram-negative rods, eg, *Klebsiella, Pseudomonas,* and *Legionella. Staphylococcus aureus* is important also.
   (b) Viruses: Cytomegalovirus, herpes simplex virus type 1, varicella-zoster virus.
   (c) Fungi: *Candida, Aspergillus.*
   (d) Parasites: *Pneumocystis, Strongyloides.*
5. Erythromycin.
6. It inhibits bacterial protein synthesis at the level of the 50S ribosomal subunit.
7. Environmental water sources, eg, air-conditioning units, hospital water taps, and bodies of water such as lakes.
8. Yes, on special agar high in iron and cysteine, but cultures are not commonly done.
9. A greater than 4-fold rise in antibody titer to *Legionella* in the acute- and convalescent-phase sera detected by indirect immunofluorescence.
10. Although it has a gram-negative cell wall, it stains poorly by the standard Gram stain procedure. The reason for this is unknown.

CASE 6   **Chief Complaint** A 30-year-old woman with nausea and vomiting for 3 days.

History The patient was well until 1 week ago, when she noted some stiffness and swelling in the fingers of both hands; this lasted a few days. Four days ago, malaise, fatigue, and anorexia began, followed the next day by nausea and vomiting, which have continued to the present. No hematemesis or diarrhea has occurred. Upper abdominal aching began yesterday. The smell of food induces nausea. She noticed that her urine was darker than usual today.

She is a waitress who smokes 2 packs of cigarettes and drinks a 6-pack of beer per day. She has had 5 sex partners in the last 3 months. No recent travel, transfusions, or intravenous drug abuse. No one else she knows has similar symptoms.

Physical Exam   T 37 °C, BP 130/80, P 80, R 12.
Pertinent findings include:
Skin: No jaundice, petechiae, or spider angiomas.
Eyes: Sclerae were icteric.
Abdomen: Punch tenderness elicited in right upper quadrant. Tender liver edge palpable 4 cm below costal margin. Spleen not palpable. No masses. Abdomen not distended. Bowel sounds normal.
Pelvic: Within normal limits.
Rectal: Stool light color. Occult blood negative.

Laboratory
Blood: Hematocrit 40%; WBC 8200; differential 50% polys, 45% lymphs, 5% monos.
Urine: Normal, except that bilirubin test was positive.
Chemistry: Total bilirubin 4 mg (direct 3 mg; indirect 1 mg); alanine aminotransferase 600 mg%; alkaline phosphatase 100 mg%; electrolytes within normal limits.
X-ray: Abdominal film within normal limits.

Comment   This case is typical of viral hepatitis. Many viruses can infect the liver. It is important to determine the specific cause, because there are both personal and public health implications with some agents, eg, hepatitis B virus.

Questions
1. What viruses should be considered possible causes of this patient's disease?
2. What tests would you order to determine which virus caused this disease?

Course   The results of the serologic tests were as follows: IgM HAV antibody, negative; HBV surface antigen, positive; IgM HBV core antibody, negative; HBV surface antibody, negative.

Questions
3. In view of these results, what disease does the patient have?
4. If a different jaundiced patient's test results were IgM HAV antibody negative, HBV surface antigen negative, IgM HBV core antibody positive, HBV surface antibody negative, what would your interpretation be?
5. If a different jaundiced patient's test results were IgM HAV antibody negative, HBV surface antigen negative, IgM HBV core antibody negative, HBV surface antibody positive, what would your interpretation be?
6. What is your explanation for the arthralgias described at the beginning of the history?
7. What specific antiviral therapy, if any, is available for hepatitis B?
8. How did she acquire this disease?

Course   The patient's symptoms intensified during the next 3 days and then gradually resolved over the next 2 weeks; the serum bilirubin declined to normal. However, the patient's HBV surface antigen remained positive at 3, 6, and 12 months after discharge and no HBV surface antibody was detectable.

Questions
9. What is your interpretation of these HBV surface antigen results?
10. What is the best laboratory test to determine whether she is likely to transmit HBV to others?
11. What would you advise this patient regarding (a) donating blood, (b) dental surgery and other operations, (c) protecting her newborn child if she becomes pregnant, (d) sharing a toothbrush, (e) sexual activity, (f) problems with chronic liver disease, (g) possibility of carcinoma of the liver, (h) effect of infection with hepatitis Delta virus?

Answers to Questions

1. Hepatitis A and B; non A, non B (NANB); and Delta viruses. Also Epstein-Barr virus and cytomegalovirus. Yellow fever virus can infect the liver, but this patient had not traveled to an endemic area.
2. Four serologic tests are typically ordered: (a) IgM antibody to HAV, (b) IgM antibody to HBV core antigen, (c) HBV surface antigen, and (d) HBV surface antibody.
3. Acute hepatitis B.
4. Acute hepatitis B. During the "window" phase, the surface antigen and surface antibody are negative; only the core antibody is positive. The positive IgM result indicates recent infection.
5. The patient had hepatitis B in the past and is now immune. The patient is not a chronic carrier; surface antigen is negative. Because neither hepatitis A nor hepatitis B was demonstrated by the serologic tests, it is likely that the patient has NANB hepatitis (or some other viral hepatitis).
6. Arthralgias are typical during the prodromal period of hepatitis B. They are probably due to HBV-antibody immune complexes deposited in the joints.
7. There are no antiviral drugs for hepatitis B. Only supportive therapy is available. Immune globulins are not used for treatment, only for prevention.
8. Because she has no history of either blood transfusions or intravenous drug abuse, it is probable that the virus was acquired sexually.
9. The patient is a chronic carrier of HBV.
10. Serologic test for e antigen. This is the best indicator of the presence of infectious HBV in the blood. No direct assay for infectious virus is presently available.
11. (a) Do not donate blood.
    (b) Advise your dentist and all medical personnel that you are HBV surface antigen-positive.
    (c) The newborn should be actively immunized with the hepatitis B vaccine and passively immunized with hepatitis B immune globulins.
    (d) Do not share toothbrushes or other personal articles that may contact blood, eg, razors.
    (e) Sex partners should be immunized with hepatitis B vaccine.
    (f) Chronic active hepatitis may result.
    (g) A higher incidence of carcinoma of the liver occurs in chronic carriers.
    (h) Patients infected with HBV who are superinfected with hepatitis Delta virus can experience a severe form of hepatitis.

CASE 7

Chief Complaint   A 20-year-old male with a cough of several weeks' duration.

History   The patient is a recent immigrant from Southeast Asia who noted the gradual onset of tiredness and loss of appetite about 1 month ago. A week or so later, he felt feverish and the cough began. At first the cough was nonproductive, but for the past week he has brought up several tablespoons per day of greenish sputum that is streaked with blood. He has lost 10 lb during the past month. He is a nonsmoker and has had no exposure to industrial respiratory pollutants.

Physical Exam   T 38 °C, BP 124/70, P 80, R 16. Patient does not appear acutely ill.
Pertinent findings include:
Lungs: Rales heard in right upper lobe. No dullness to percussion.
Heart: Normal.
Abdomen: Normal.
Lymph nodes: Not enlarged.

Laboratory
Blood: Hematocrit 38; WBC 11,000; Differential 3% bands, 63% polys, 30% lymphs, 4% monos.
Urine: Normal.
Chest x-ray: Infiltrate in posterior segment of right upper lobe with suggestion of a cavity.

Question
1. Which 2 procedures should you do with the sputum that could provide immediate information regarding the organism causing the illness?

Course Gram stain of the sputum revealed mixed flora with no predominant organism. The acid-fast stain showed numerous long, slender, pink rods. A sputum specimen was sent for culture.

Questions

2. In view of these results, what is the most likely diagnosis?
3. What is the treatment of choice for this disease?
4. Is antibiotic resistance a problem?
5. Approximately how long after the start of treatment is the patient considered to be infectious for others?
6. How is the organism transmitted?
7. What is the natural habitat of the organism?
8. Why is the organism acid-fast?
9. Can the organism be cultured in the laboratory?
10. What is the role of serologic tests in making the diagnosis of tuberculosis?
11. What should be done for the members of his family?
12. What is the immunologic basis for a positive skin test?
13. Can atypical mycobacteria, eg, *Mycobacterium kansasii* and *Mycobacterium intracellulare* cause a similar clinical picture?

Course The patient was hospitalized because there was doubt about whether he would reliably take the antitubercular drugs. He was treated with isoniazid (INH), rifampin, and ethambutol, and his symptoms abated. Routine sputum cultures were negative. After 2 weeks, he was discharged to return to the clinic for follow-up cultures and chest x-rays 1 month late. Four weeks after they were taken, his cultures were reported positive for *Mycobacterium tuberculosis*. Drug susceptibility tests subsequently reported the isolate to be sensitive to INH, and the third drug, ethambutol, was discontinued. Follow-up cultures were negative, and chest x-rays showed resolution of the lesions.

Answers to Questions

1. Gram stain and acid-fast stain.
2. Tuberculosis.
3. Multiple drug therapy for 6–9 months is the accepted mode of treatment. Isoniazid (INH) is bactericidal and is the mainstay of treatment. It is frequently combined with rifampin or ethambutol or both.
4. Southeast Asians have a high rate of infection with INH-resistant strains of *M tuberculosis*. Triple-drug therapy should be used in case the organism is INH-resistant.
5. Approximately 2–3 weeks, but treatment must continue for at least 9 months to avoid recurrences.
6. Transmitted by inhalation of aerosolized organisms from expectorated sputum.
7. Human lungs.
8. The high concentration of lipid makes mycobacteria acid-fast. These lipids prevent the dyes used in the Gram stain from penetrating; hence, they are not seen on a gram-stained smear.
9. Yes, on special media, eg, Löwenstein-Jensen medium. It is very slow-growing, so cultures should be held for at least 6 weeks. It will not grow on blood agar.
10. There are no serologic tests for tuberculosis.
11. If they are asymptomatic, they should be skin-tested with PPD. If positive, they should be given INH. If they are symptomatic, they should be investigated for tuberculosis with sputum cultures.
12. Cell-mediated immune response to the *M tuberculosis* proteins in PPD. This response forms an indurated area at least 10 mm in diameter in the skin.
13. Yes. The clinical picture can be indistinguishable, so cultures must be done. Atypical mycobacteria are frequently more resistant to drugs than is *M tuberculosis*.

CASE 8

Chief Complaint An 18-year-old woman with a sore throat for the last 3 days.

History The patient was well until 3 days ago, when she experienced the gradual onset of malaise, anorexia, and mild sore throat. The symptoms have intensified, and she now feels that her throat is "on fire." At present she is feverish, has a frontal headache, and has completely lost her interest in food and cigarettes. She received DPT vaccine as a child.

Physical Exam   T 39 °C, BP 126/70, P 92, R 18. Patient appears acutely ill.
Pertinent findings include:
Skin: No rash or jaundice.
Throat: Intensely red and swollen; yellowish exudate on left tonsil. No adherent membrane
    on pharynx.
Neck: Several tender, enlarged lymph nodes. No signs of meningeal irritation.
Chest: Clear.
Heart: Normal.
Abdomen: Not distended. No tenderness. Tender liver edge felt 2 cm below costal margin.
    Spleen tip palpable. Bowel sounds normal.
Neurologic: Normal.

Laboratory

Blood: Hematocrit 39%; WBC 14,000; Differential: 52% polys, 45% lymphs, 3% monos;
    platelets: 100,000.
Urine: Normal.
Chest x-ray: Normal.

Questions

1. What is your differential diagnosis?
2. What laboratory tests would you order to make a microbiologic diagnosis?

Course   She was admitted to the college infirmary. The following day, a throat culture
revealed alpha-hemolytic streptococci. A Monospot test was negative. Transaminases were
elevated to twice normal levels. Bilirubin and alkaline phosphatase were normal. WBC
16,000. Differential: 48% polys, 50% lymphs (3% are atypical), 2% monos.

Questions

3. In view of these laboratory findings, what is your diagnostic impression?
4. In view of your diagnostic impression, what treatment would you prescribe?

Course   Aspirin and warm, salt-water gargles were given. However, during the next 2 days
the throat remained sore, swallowing was difficult, and only liquids were taken. The throat
remained inflamed, and the liver and spleen were still palpable. The following day the
temperature, which had reached 40 °C, dropped to 38 °C and the patient began to feel
somewhat better. A repeat blood count showed WBC 15,000 with 45% polys, 53% lymphs
(15% are atypical), and 2% monos. The Monospot test was positive.

Comment   This is a typical case of infectious mononucleosis with the cardinal findings of
fever, pharyngitis, and cervical lymphadenopathy. Hepatosplenomegaly is commonly found.
Laboratory findings include a lymphocytosis with atypical cells and a positive heterophil
antibody test. Both the atypical cells and heterophil antibody can appear several days after the
patient presents.

Questions

5. How is this infection transmitted?
6. Is EBV infection common in the USA?
7. In what age group is infectious mononucleosis common and why?
8. What are heterophil antibodies?
9. Should you try to make the diagnosis of infectious mononucleosis by recovering EBV in
   cell culture?
10. Can infectious mononucleosis be contracted more than once?
11. Is there a vaccine or drug for the prevention of infectious mononucleosis?

Answers to Questions

1. This clinical picture is typical of infectious mononucleosis caused by Epstein-Barr virus
   (EBV). However, other viruses, such as herpes simplex virus, coxsackieviruses, and
   adenoviruses, also cause pharyngitis, as do certain bacteria, eg, *Streptococcus pyogenes*
   and *Neisseria gonorrhoeae*. Cytomegalovirus and *Toxoplasma gondii* can cause a
   mononucleosislike picture but typically without a prominent pharyngitis. Viral hepatitis
   also can manifest with many of this patient's features but is not associated with pharyngitis.

Diphtheria is highly unlikely, because the patient was immunized and it is rare in the USA.

2. Throat culture for *S pyogenes* and a heterophil antibody test (Monospot test).

3. Streptococcal pharyngitis can be ruled out; only alpha-hemolytic colonies were found on throat culture. The heterophil test can be negative early in infectious mononucleosis. The liver function tests and the finding of several atypical lymphs support the diagnosis of infectious mononucleosis.

4. The treatment for infectious mononucleosis is supportive. There is no antiviral therapy. Acyclovir, which is effective against certain other herpesviruses, namely herpes simplex virus types 1 and 2 and varicella-zoster virus, is not effective against EBV.

5. EBV is present in saliva. Transmission between young adults is primarily by kissing. EBV infects oropharyngeal cells, causing the pharyngitis.

6. Yes. Over 90% of adults in the USA have antibodies to EBV.

7. Infectious mononucleosis occurs primarily in young adults. EBV infection in children either is asymptomatic or results in an undifferentiated viral pharyngitis without the other concomitant symptoms of infectious mononucleosis.

8. Heterophil antibodies are agglutinins for sheep or horse red blood cells formed during EBV infection. These antibodies are not directed against any EBV antigens; they may be formed against some cellular component modified by EBV infection. Because heterophil antibodies are nonspecific, EBV infections should be confirmed by IgM antibody to viral capsid antigen in difficult-to-diagnose cases.

9. Isolation of EBV in cell culture is not used for clinical diagnosis. EBV can be cultured in the laboratory, but it is not routinely available.

10. EBV-induced infectious mononucleosis can be contracted only once. Lifelong immunity is not due to heterophil agglutinins; those usually disappear within a few years. Antibody to viral capsid antigen persists for life, but it is unclear whether this antibody, other antibodies, or the cell-mediated response provides this immunity. Recurrences of "mononucleosis" may be due to other causes, eg, cytomegalovirus or *Toxoplasma*.

11. No vaccine or drug is available that prevents infectious mononucleosis.

CASE 9

Chief Complaint   A 1-year-old child who had a seizure about 20 minutes ago.

History   The child was well except for an upper respiratory tract infection during the past 2 days. Last night, she felt feverish and became very sleepy. She was difficult to arouse this morning and then had a generalized convulsion. Her mother brought her to the emergency room immediately. Immunizations: oral polio and DPT vaccines given at 2, 4, and 6 months.

Physical Exam   T 40 °C, BP 100/70, P 120, R 16. A somnolent child who was irritable when examined.
   Pertinent findings include:
   Skin: No petechiae or ecchymoses.
   Eyes: Pupils regular and equal. No papilledema.
   Ears: Normal.
   Throat: Mild inflammation. No exudate.
   Neck: Marked rigidity.
   Lungs: Clear.
   Heart: Normal.
   Abdomen: Normal.
   Neurologic: Deep-tendon reflexes normal. Remainder of the exam deferred because the patient was unable to cooperate.

Laboratory
   Blood: Hematocrit 40%; WBC 21,000; differential 16% bands, 80% polys, 4% monos.
   Urine: Normal.
   Chest x-ray: Normal.

Questions
   1. What are the 2 most important specimens to obtain to make a microbiologic diagnosis?
   2. What laboratory test should be done immediately on one of the specimens that may provide information regarding the cause of this infection?

3. What is the most likely organism to cause this infection? What are 2 other possibilities?
4. How would you distinguish among these 3 organisms on Gram's stain?

Comment   This case is typical of acute bacterial meningitis, a life-threatening emergency. It demands immediate empirical therapy, which is guided by the physician's impression of what is likely to be the causative organism. The main criteria used to formulate this impression are the age of the patient; preexisting medical conditions, eg, immunocompromised state; and analysis of the spinal fluid including a Gram-stained smear, the number of white cells, and whether they are polys or lymphocytes. Spinal fluid protein and glucose are also important, but those values may take time to obtain and therapy should be initiated as soon as possible.

Course   A lumbar puncture was performed. The spinal fluid appeared cloudy, and the opening pressure was 300 mm of water. There were 2800 cells/mm³, of which 88% were polys. The Gram stain revealed very short gram-negative rods. Specimens of spinal fluid were sent for glucose, protein, and culture. A blood culture was done, and at the same time an intravenous infusion was started and antibiotic therapy begun.

Questions
5. What antibiotics would you begin as your empirical therapy?
6. What immunologic test can be done on the spinal fluid that might identify the organism?

Course   Treatment with ampicillin and chloramphenicol was begun, and the patient was admitted to the hospital. The latex agglutination test on the spinal fluid was positive for *Haemophilus influenzae*. The spinal fluid protein and glucose values were 300 mg% and 15 mg%, respectively. The following day, her temperature dropped to 38.5 °C and she was more responsive.

The microbiology laboratory reported growth of a small gram-negative rod resembling *H influenzae* in the blood culture. Spinal fluid cultures on chocolate agar (with IsoVitaleX) grew many colonies of a small gram-negative rod. There was no growth on the blood agar plate.

Questions
7. What are the growth requirements of *H influenzae* that can be used to identify the organism in the clinical laboratory?
8. Most (90%) *H influenzae* isolates causing invasive disease, eg, bacteremia and meningitis, are type B. What determines the type?

Course   The isolate from both the blood and spinal fluid cultures was identified as *H influenzae*. The disk test for β-lactamase production by the isolate was negative, and susceptibility tests showed that the organism was sensitive to ampicillin. Chloramphenicol was discontinued.

The patient continued to improve and was afebrile by 48 hours. Ampicillin was continued for 14 days. A lumbar puncture performed prior to discharge revealed almost normal values.

Questions
9. What is the natural habitat of this organism, and how is it acquired?
10. What is the role of the organism's capsular polysaccharide in causing disease?
11. Do exotoxins play a role in pathogenesis by *H influenzae*? Does the organism contain endotoxin?
12. How can *H influenzae* meningitis be prevented?

Answers to Questions
1. Blood culture and spinal fluid.
2. Gram's stain of the spinal fluid.
3. *H influenzae* is by far the most frequent cause of meningitis in children between the ages of 6 months and 6 years. *Streptococcus pneumoniae* and *Neisseria meningitidis* are less frequent causes at this age.
4. *H influenzae* is a short "coccobacillary" gram-negative rod. *S pneumoniae* is a gram-positive coccus in doublets or short chains. *N meningitidis* is a kidney bean-shaped gram-negative coccus.

5. Combination therapy of ampicillin and chloramphenicol is commonly used. Ampicillin is the treatment of choice for *H influenzae* meningitis, but approximately 25% of isolates are ampicillin-resistant as a result of β-lactamase. Chloramphenicol is added to cover these resistant organisms. When the results of susceptibility tests are known, one drug is discontinued. Certain cephalosporins, eg, ceftriaxone or cefuroxime, can also be used.

6. Latex agglutination test for capsular polysaccharide of *H influenzae, S pneumoniae, N meningitidis,* and other encapsulated bacteria is rapid, accurate, and inexpensive. Counterimmunoelectrophoresis for capsular polysaccharide in the spinal fluid can also be done, but it takes longer and may not be readily available.

7. *H influenzae* requires both X (heme) and V (NAD) factors.

8. The antigenicity of the capsular polysaccharide.

9. It colonizes the human nasopharynx and is transmitted by respiratory tract secretions.

10. It retards phagocytosis of the organism.

11. Exotoxins are not known to be involved. Like all gram-negative organisms, *H influenzae* contains endotoxin.

12. (a) The vaccine containing the capsular polysaccharide of type B *H influenzae* should be given to all children at 2 years of age. Note that many cases of *H influenzae* meningitis occur in children younger than 2 years. Unfortunately, the vaccine is relatively ineffective in these children because they do not form antibodies well in response to polysaccharide vaccines, such as this one and the pneumococcal vaccine.

   (b) Rifampin should be given to close household contacts of the patient and to the patient to eradicate nasopharyngeal carriage. If the patient attends a day-care center, contacts there should be given rifampin.

CASE 10

Chief Complaint A 32-year-old male with diarrhea for the past 3 weeks.

History The patient was well until 6 months ago, when fever, shortness of breath, and cough began. Chest X-ray followed by bronchoscopy resulted in the diagnosis of *Pneumocystis* pneumonia. He was treated with trimethoprim-sulfamethoxazole and recovered. Studies of his peripheral lymphocytes showed a CD4-to-CD8 ratio of 0.1.

For the past 3 weeks he has had frequent loose, watery bowel movements. There were no bloody or tarry stools. Stools were not fatty or foul-smelling. Crampy lower abdominal pain was associated with each movement. No nausea, vomiting, or fever has occurred. He has lost about 7 lb. There was no recent antibiotic use. The diarrhea has not responded to over-the-counter antidiarrheal drugs.

Physical Exam T 37 °C, BP 130/70, P 84, R 12. Patient was in no acute distress.
Pertinent findings include:
Skin: Moderately dehydrated. No jaundice.
Lungs: Normal.
Heart: Normal.
Abdomen: Not distended. Mild diffuse tenderness without rebound. No masses or hepatosplenomegaly. Bowel sounds moderately hyperactive.

Laboratory
Blood: Hematocrit 40%; WBC 9200; differential 56% polys, 41% lymphs, 3% eos.
Urine: Normal.
Chest x-ray: Normal.

Question
1. What test should be done on the stool immediately that can provide evidence as to whether the diarrhea is invasive (inflammatory) in origin?

Course Stain for fecal leukocytes revealed no PMNs. The stool was negative for occult blood. Specimen was sent for culture.

Question
2. What are the organisms likely to cause diarrhea in this patient?

Course Stool culture was negative for *Shigella, Salmonella,* and *Campylobacter.* Routine examination for ova and parasites revealed no evidence of *Giardia, Entamoeba,* or helminths, eg, *Strongyloides,* but a modified acid-fast stain of the stool revealed many *Cryptosporidium* oocysts, which stain red with this technique.

Question
3. What would you prescribe for this patient?

Course There are no effective drugs for cryptosporidia. A trial of metronidazole, which is effective against other protozoa, eg, *Entamoeba* and *Giardia,* was instituted but did not relieve the symptoms. A few weeks later, the diarrhea became significantly worse, ie, as many as 15–20 explosive, watery bowel movements per day. Intravenous fluids and parenteral hyperalimentation were required to maintain nutrition and fluid balance. The patient's condition steadily deteriorated, and he died approximately 5 weeks later.

Questions
4. What is the natural habitat of this organism, and how is it transmitted?
5. Does *Cryptosporidium* cause diarrhea in immunocompetent individuals also, or is it exclusively an opportunistic pathogen?
6. What is the pathogenesis of *Cryptosporidium*-induced diarrhea?
7. Could this infection have been prevented?

Answers to Questions
1. A stain for fecal leukocytes and a test for occult blood should be performed.
2. In view of the absence of fecal leukocytes, *Shigella, Salmonella,* and *Campylobacter* seem unlikely. In view of the prolonged time the diarrhea has lasted, toxigenic bacteria, eg, *Escherichia coli* and *Clostridium perfringens,* also seem unlikely. Similarly, most viral diarrheas are usually self-limited. Because no antibiotics were taken recently, *Clostridium difficile* is unlikely. However, since this patient has acquired immunodeficiency syndrome (AIDS), the infections that normally are self-limited may become chronic and severe. Prominent among these are 2 protozoan causes of diarrhea, *Cryptosporidium* and *Giardia,* and the helminth *Strongyloides.*
3. No specific antiparasitic drug is effective against cryptosporidia. Maintenance of adequate hydration is important.
4. It is a well-recognized cause of diarrhea in both domestic and wild animals. Outbreaks of diarrhea in families and at day-care centers occur also. Fecal-oral transmission from animal to human and from human to human occurs.
5. Cryptosporidia are increasingly recognized as a significant cause of self-limited, noninvasive diarrhea in immunocompetent individuals. When looked for, they were found in up to 4% of diarrheal stools (that contained no other known pathogen) obtained from otherwise healthy patients.
6. The organisms adhere to the lining of the small intestine but do not invade. No enterotoxin has been demonstrated. The precise mechanism by which the organisms cause diarrhea is unknown.
7. There are no means of prevention.

Part X: National Board Practice Questions

BASIC BACTERIOLOGY

Directions (Questions 1–26):   Select the ONE lettered answer that is BEST for each question.

1. Each of the following statements concerning the surface structures of bacteria is correct EXCEPT
   (A) The interaction of bacteria with the mucosal epithelium can be mediated by pili.
   (B) Polysaccharide capsules are able to retard phagocytosis.
   (C) Both gram-negative rods and cocci have lipopolysaccharide (endotoxin) in their cell walls.
   (D) Bacterial flagella are nonantigenic in humans; they closely resemble human flagella in structure and chemical composition.

2. Each of the following statements concerning peptidoglycan is correct EXCEPT
   (A) It has a backbone composed of alternating units of muramic acid and acetyl-glucosamine.
   (B) Cross-links between the tetrapeptides involve D-alanine.
   (C) It is thinner in gram-positive than in gram-negative cells.
   (D) It can be degraded by lysozyme.

3. Each of the following statements concerning bacterial spores is correct EXCEPT
   (A) Their survival ability is based on their enhanced metabolic activity.
   (B) They are formed by gram-positive rods.
   (C) They can be killed by being heated to 121° C for 15 minutes.
   (D) They contain much less water than do bacterial cells.

4. Which one of these statements is the MOST accurate comparison of human, bacterial, and fungal cells?
   (A) Human cells undergo mitosis, whereas neither bacteria nor fungi do.
   (B) Human and fungal cells have similar cell walls, in contrast to bacterial cells, which contain peptidoglycan.
   (C) Human and bacterial cells have plasmids, whereas fungal cells do not.
   (D) Human and fungal cells have similar ribosomes, whereas bacterial ribosomes are different.

5. Which statement is the MOST accurate regarding the drug depicted in the diagram?
   (A) It inhibits DNA synthesis.
   (B) It is bacteriostatic.
   (C) It binds to 30S ribosomes.
   (D) It prevents formation of folic acid.

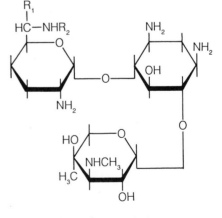

6. Each of the following statements regarding the selective action of antibiotics on bacteria is correct EXCEPT
   (A) Chloramphenicol affects the large subunit of the bacterial ribosome, which is different from the large subunit of the human ribosome.

(B) Isoniazid affects the DNA polymerase of bacteria but not that of human cells.

(C) Both sulfonamides and trimethoprim affect folic acid synthesis in bacteria, a pathway that does not occur in human cells.

(D) Penicillins affect bacteria rather than human cells because bacteria have a cell wall, whereas human cells do not.

7. Each of the following statements concerning endotoxins is correct EXCEPT

(A) They are less potent (ie, less active on a weight basis) than exotoxins.

(B) They are more stable when heated than exotoxins.

(C) They bind to specific cell receptors, whereas exotoxins do not.

(D) They are part of the bacterial cell wall, whereas exotoxins are not.

8. The MAIN host defense against bacterial exotoxins is provided by

(A) activated macrophages secreting proteases

(B) IgG and IgM antibodies

(C) helper T cells

(D) modulation of host cell receptors in response to the toxin

9. Each of the following events involves genetic recombination EXCEPT

(A) transduction of a chromosomal gene

(B) transposition of a mobile genetic element

(C) integration of a temperate bacteriophage

(D) conjugation, eg, transfer of an R (resistance) factor

10. Each of the following statements concerning the normal flora is correct EXCEPT

(A) The most common organism found on the skin is *Staphylococcus epidermidis.*

(B) *Escherichia coli* is a prominent member of the normal flora of the throat.

(C) The major site where *Bacteroides fragilis,* an anaerobe, is found is the colon.

(D) One of the most important sites where *Staphylococcus aureus* is found is the nose.

11. Each of the following statements concerning the mechanism of action of antimicrobial drugs is correct EXCEPT

(A) Vancomycin acts by inhibiting peptidoglycan synthesis.

(B) Chloramphenicol binds to the 50S ribosomal subunit and inhibits peptidyltransferase.

(C) Erythromycin is a bactericidal drug that disrupts cell membranes by a detergentlike action.

(D) Aminoglycosides such as streptomycin are bactericidal drugs that inhibit protein synthesis.

12. Each of the following statements concerning the resistance of bacteria to antimicrobial drugs is correct EXCEPT

(A) Resistance to chloramphenicol is known to be mediated by an enzyme that acetylates the drug.

(B) Resistance to penicillin is known to be due to reduced affinity of transpeptidases.

(C) Resistance to penicillin is known to be due to cleavage by β-lactamase.

(D) Resistance to tetracycline is known to be due to an enzyme that hydrolyzes the ester linkage.

13. Of the following choices, the MOST important function of antibody in host defenses against bacteria is

(A) activation of lysozyme that degrades the cell wall

(B) acceleration of proteolysis of exotoxins

(C) facilitation of phagocytosis

(D) inhibition of bacterial protein synthesis

14. Which of the following events is MOST likely to be due to bacterial conjugation?

(A) A strain of *Corynebacterium* produces a toxin encoded by a prophage.

(B) A strain of *Neisseria gonorrhoeae* produces β-lactamase encoded by a plasmid similar to a plasmid of another gram-negative organism.

(C) An encapsulated strain of *Streptococcus pneumoniae* has acquired the gene for capsule formation from the extract of another encapsulated strain.

(D) A gene encoding resistance to gentamicin in the *E coli* chromosome appears in the genome of a virulent bacteriophage that has infected *E coli.*

15. Each of the following statements about bacteria that grow anaerobically is correct EXCEPT

(A) A low oxidation-reduction potential (E_h), such as -300 mV, is often present where anaerobes grow.

(B) Anaerobes are bacteria that require reduced oxygen tension and will not grow on the surface of agar medium in air.

(C) Many anaerobes lack superoxide dismutase and catalase.

(D) Facultative anaerobes can grow only in the presence of less than 10% oxygen.

16. The identification of bacteria by serologic tests is based on the presence of specific antigens. Which one of the following components of the cell is LEAST likely to contain useful antigens?

(A) capsule

(B) flagella

(C) cell wall

(D) ribosomes

17. Each of the following statements concerning bacterial spores is correct EXCEPT

(A) Spores are formed under adverse environmental conditions such as the absence of a carbon source.

(B) Spores are resistant to boiling.

(C) Spores are metabolically inactive and contain dipicolinic acid, a calcium chelator.

(D) Spores are formed primarily by organisms of the genus *Neisseria*.

18. Each of the following statements concerning the mechanism of action of antimicrobial drugs is correct EXCEPT

(A) Amphotericin B inhibits fungi rather than bacteria because fungal cell membranes contain ergosterol but bacterial cell membranes do not.

(B) Gentamicin inhibits bacteria rather than fungi because it binds to 70S ribosomes rather than 80S ribosomes.

(C) Erythromycin inhibits anaerobes rather than aerobes because it acts as an electron sink.

(D) Cephalosporins inhibit the cross-linking of bacterial peptidoglycan and have no inhibitory effect on fungi.

19. Each of the following statements concerning the mechanism of action of antibacterial drugs is correct EXCEPT

(A) Penicillins are bactericidal drugs that inhibit the transpeptidase reaction and activate autolytic enzymes.

(B) Tetracyclines are bacteriostatic drugs that inhibit protein synthesis by blocking tRNA binding.

(C) Aminoglycosides are bacteriostatic drugs that inhibit protein synthesis by activating ribonuclease, which degrades mRNA.

(D) Rifampin inhibits bacterial RNA polymerase.

20. Each of the following is a typical property of obligate anaerobes EXCEPT

(A) They generate energy by using the cytochrome system.

(B) They grow best at a low oxidation-reduction (E_h) potential.

(C) They lack superoxide dismutase.

(D) They lack catalase.

21. Which one of the following antimicrobial drugs acts primarily by inhibiting formation of the cell wall?

(A) vancomycin

(B) isoniazid

(C) rifampin

(D) metronidazole

22. Each of the following statements concerning the growth of bacteria is correct EXCEPT

(A) Some bacteria grow in both the presence and the absence of oxygen.

(B) Some bacteria uses gaseous CO_2 as a carbon source, whereas others require carbon in the form of organic molecules.

(C) Some bacteria grow in an exponential, logarithmic manner, whereas others undergo meiosis.

(D) Some bacteria have a doubling time as short as 30 minutes, whereas others have a doubling time of 10 hours or more.

23. Each of the following statements concerning the killing of bacteria is correct EXCEPT

(A) Lysozyme in tears can hydrolyze bacterial cell walls.

(B) Silver nitrate can inactivate bacterial enzymes.

(C) Detergents can disrupt bacterial cell membranes.

(D) Ultraviolet light can degrade bacterial capsules.

24. In the Gram stain, the decolorization of gram-negative bacteria by alcohol is related to

(A) proteins encoded by F plasmids

(B) lipids in the cell wall

    (C) 70S ribosomes

    (D) branched polysaccharides in the capsule

25. Chemical modification of benzylpenicillin (penicillin G) has resulted in several beneficial changes in the clinical use of this drug. Which one of the following is NOT one of those beneficial changes?

    (A) lowered frequency of anaphylaxis

    (B) increased activity against gram-negative rods

    (C) increased resistance to stomach acid

    (D) reduced cleavage by penicillinase

26. Each of the following statements concerning resistance to antibiotics is correct EXCEPT

    (A) Resistance to aminoglycosides can be due to phosphorylating enzymes encoded by R plasmids.

    (B) Resistance to sulfonamides is primarily due to enzymes that hydrolyze the 5-membered ring structure.

    (C) Resistance to penicillin can be due to alterations in binding proteins in the cell membrane.

    (D) Resistance to tetracycline is primarily due to failure to achieve adequate concentrations of the drug within the bacteria.

Answers (Questions 1–26):

1 (D)	6 (B)	11 (C)	16 (D)	21 (A)	26 (B)
2 (C)	7 (C)	12 (D)	17 (D)	22 (C)	
3 (A)	8 (B)	13 (C)	18 (C)	23 (D)	
4 (D)	9 (D)	14 (B)	19 (C)	24 (B)	
5 (C)	10 (B)	15 (D)	20 (A)	25 (A)	

Directions (Questions 27–33):   Select the ONE lettered heading that is MOST closely associated with the numbered phrases or statements.

Questions 27–30

    (A) Penicillins

    (B) Aminoglycosides

    (C) Chloramphenicol

    (D) Rifampin

    (E) Sulfonamides

27. Inhibit(s) bacterial RNA polymerase
28. Inhibit(s) cross-linking of peptidoglycan
29. Inhibit(s) protein synthesis by binding to the 30S ribosomal subunit
30. Inhibit(s) folic acid synthesis

Questions 31–33

    (A) Transduction

    (B) Conjugation

    (C) DNA transformation

    (D) Transposition

31. During an outbreak of gastrointestinal disease caused by an *Escherichia coli* strain sensitive to ampicillin, tetracycline, and chloramphenicol, a stool sample from one patient yielded *E coli* with the same serotype resistant to the 3 antibiotics.

32. A mutant cell line lacking a functional thymidine kinase gene was exposed to a preparation of DNA from normal cells; under appropriate growth conditions a colony of cells was isolated that produced thymidine kinase.

33. A retrovirus without an oncogene did not induce leukemia in mice; after repeated passages through mice, viruses recovered from a tumor were highly oncogenic and contained a new gene.

Answers (Questions 27–33):

27 (D)   32 (C)
28 (A)   33 (A)
29 (B)
30 (E)
31 (B)

Directions (Questions 34–39):   For each numbered item, select
  (A) A if the item is associated with (A) only
  (B) B if the item is associated with (B) only
  (C) C if the item is associated with both (A) and (B)
  (D) D if the item is associated with neither (A) nor (B)

34. Functions of the bacterial capsule include
  (A) Retardation of phagocytosis
  (B) Antigenicity
  (C) Both
  (D) Neither

35. Properties of bacterial pili include
  (A) Are primarily lipopolysaccharides
  (B) Show considerable antigenic diversity
  (C) Both
  (D) Neither

36. Mechanisms that mediate resistance to penicillins include
  (A) Cleavage of the β-lactam ring
  (B) Alteration in binding proteins
  (C) Both
  (D) Neither

37. Known mechanisms of action for some bacterial toxins include
  (A) ADP ribosylation
  (B) Degradation of mRNA
  (C) Both
  (D) Neither

38. Antimicrobial drugs that inhibit bacterial protein synthesis include
  (A) Erythromycin
  (B) Tetracycline
  (C) Both
  (D) Neither

39. The physiologic effects of endotoxin include
  (A) Activation of adenylate cyclase
  (B) Release of endogenous pyrogen
  (C) Both
  (D) Neither

Answers (Question 34–39):

34 (C)   37 (A)
35 (B)   38 (C)
36 (C)   39 (B)

Directions (Questions 40–65):   For each question, ONE or MORE of the numbered options is correct.
  Select
  A if only 1, 2, and 3 are correct
  B if only 1 and 3 are correct
  C if only 2 and 4 are correct
  D if only 4 is correct
  E if all are correct

40. Mechanisms of resistance to benzylpenicillin (penicillin G) by *Staphylococcus aureus* include
    (1) production of enzymes that degrade the β-lactam ring of penicillin
    (2) acetylation of the benzyl group
    (3) changes in binding proteins located in the cell membrane and cell wall
    (4) activation of adenylate cyclase by transposon A
41. Members of the normal flora
    (1) are usually nonpathogens but can cause disease in immunocompromised patients
    (2) prevent some pathogens from colonizing mucous membranes
    (3) are present in larger numbers in the colon than in other parts of the body
    (4) are important in keeping the pH of the urine low
42. The effects of endotoxin include
    (1) opsonization
    (2) fever
    (3) degradation of IgA
    (4) hypotension
43. Bacterial surface structures that show antigenic diversity include
    (1) pili
    (2) capsules
    (3) flagella
    (4) peptidoglycan
44. The effects of antibody on bacteria include
    (1) lysis of gram-negative bacteria in conjunction with complement
    (2) augmentation of phagocytosis
    (3) inhibition of adherence of bacteria to mucosal surfaces
    (4) increase in frequency of lysogeny
45. Some exotoxins
    (1) lose their toxicity when treated chemically and can then be used as immunogens in vaccines
    (2) are capable of causing disease in their purified form, free of any bacteria
    (3) act in the gastrointestinal tract to cause diarrhea
    (4) are lipopolysaccharides
46. Correct statements concerning bacterial and human cells include the following:
    (1) Bacteria are prokaryotic, ie, they have one molecule of DNA, are haploid, and have no nuclear membrane; whereas human cells are eukaryotic, ie, they have multiple chromosomes, are diploid, and have a nuclear membrane.
    (2) Bacterial and human ribosomes differ in size and chemical composition.
    (3) Bacterial cells possess peptidoglycan, whereas human cells do not.
    (4) Bacteria derive their energy by oxidative phosphorylation within mitochondria in a manner similar to that of human cells.
47. Correct statements concerning bacteria and fungi include the following:
    (1) Bacteria have sterols in their plasma membranes, whereas fungi do not.
    (2) Yeasts reproduce by budding, whereas bacteria reproduce by binary fission.
    (3) Bacterial spores are less heat-resistant than fungal spores.
    (4) Some fungi undergo dimorphic changes when they grow in tissue, whereas bacteria do not.
48. Correct statements concerning the mechanism of action of penicillin include the following:
    (1) The β-lactam ring of penicillin is required for its activity.
    (2) The structure of penicillin resembles that of a dipeptide of alanine, which is a component of peptidoglycan.
    (3) Penicillin inhibits transpeptidases, which are required for cross-linking peptidoglycan.
    (4) Penicillin is a bacteriostatic drug, because autolytic enzymes are not activated.
49. Correct statements concerning the selective toxicity of antimicrobial drugs include the following:
    (1) Amphotericin B is selective because fungal cells contain ergosterol in their membranes, whereas human cells contain cholesterol.
    (2) Cephalosporins are selective because bacteria contain peptidoglycan, whereas human cells do not.
    (3) Sulfonamide is selective because bacteria must synthesize folic acid, whereas human cells do not.

        (4) Tetracycline is selective because bacterial RNA polymerase is different from human RNA polymerase.

50. Correct statements concerning the mechanisms of resistance to antimicrobial drugs include the following:
- **(1)** R factors are plasmids that carry the genes for enzymes that modify one or more drugs.
- **(2)** Resistance to some drugs is due to a chromosomal mutation that alters the receptor for the drug.
- **(3)** Resistance to some drugs is due to transposon genes that encode for enzymes that inactivate the drugs.
- **(4)** Resistance genes can be transferred by conjugation.

51. Correct statements concerning endotoxins include the following:
- **(1)** The toxicity of endotoxins is due to the lipid portion of the molecule.
- **(2)** The antigenicity of somatic (O) antigen is due to repeating oligosaccharides.
- **(3)** Endotoxins are located in the cell wall.
- **(4)** Endotoxins are found in most gram-positive bacteria.

52. Correct statements concerning exotoxins include the following:
- **(1)** Exotoxins are polypeptides.
- **(2)** Exotoxins are more easily inactivated by heat than are endotoxins.
- **(3)** Exotoxins are more toxic than endotoxins when equal amounts are compared.
- **(4)** Exotoxins can be converted to toxoids.

53. Correct statements concerning the cell walls of microorganisms include the following:
- **(1)** Both bacteria and fungi possess a cell wall.
- **(2)** Endotoxin is located in the cell walls of gram-negative bacteria.
- **(3)** Both gram-negative rods and mycobacteria have cell walls that contain more lipid than the cell walls of gram-positive rods.
- **(4)** Resistance plasmids (R factors) are located in the periplasmic space.

54. Correct statements concerning the killing of bacteria include the following:
- **(1)** Seventy percent ethanol kills more effectively than absolute (100%) ethanol.
- **(2)** An autoclave uses steam under pressure to reach the killing temperature of 121° C.
- **(3)** The pasteurization of milk kills pathogens but allows many organisms and spores to survive.
- **(4)** Iodine kills by causing the formation of thymine dimers in bacterial DNA.

55. Correct statements concerning the death of microorganisms include the following:
- **(1)** Disinfection of drinking water results in the death of all microorganisms, including spores.
- **(2)** Application of an antiseptic to the skin prior to venipuncture results in the death of all microorganisms, including spores.
- **(3)** Surgical scrubbing of the hands with an iodophor prior to an operation results in the death of all microorganisms, including spores.
- **(4)** Sterilization of surgical instruments results in the death of all microorganisms, including spores.

56. Sulfonamides and trimethoprim are frequently used together. Correct statements concerning their combined use include the following:
- **(1)** Sulfonamides and trimethoprim act on the same enzyme, dihydropteroate synthetase.
- **(2)** The synthesis of bacterial DNA is effectively inhibited.
- **(3)** Sulfonamides and trimethoprim interact to form a new compound with a wider spectrum of antibacterial activity.
- **(4)** The combination reduces the emergence of resistant mutants.

57. Correct statements concerning the drug depicted in the diagram include the following:
- **(1)** The drug inhibits cell wall synthesis.
- **(2)** The drug is made by a fungus.
- **(3)** The portion of the molecule required for activity is labeled B.
- **(4)** The drug is bacteriostatic.

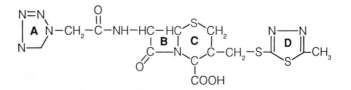

58. Correct statements concerning the normal flora include the following:
  (1) The normal flora of the colon consists predominantly of anaerobic bacteria.
  (2) The presence of the normal flora prevents certain pathogens from colonizing the upper respiratory tract.
  (3) Normal flora organisms are permanent residents of the body surfaces.
  (4) Fungi, eg, yeasts, are not members of the normal flora.

59. Correct statements concerning exotoxins and endotoxins include the following:
  (1) The LD_{50} for exotoxins is higher than that for endotoxins.
  (2) A lipid contributes to the toxic effect of endotoxins but not to that of exotoxins.
  (3) Endotoxins are used for immunization in the form of toxoids, but exotoxins are not.
  (4) Exotoxins are polypeptides, whereas endotoxins are not.

60. Correct statements concerning the structure and chemical composition of bacteria include the following:
  (1) Some gram-positive cocci contain a layer of teichoic acid external to the peptidoglycan.
  (2) Some gram-positive rods contain dipicolinic acid in their spores.
  (3) Some gram-negative rods contain lipid A in their cell wall.
  (4) Some mycoplasmas contain pentaglycine in their peptidoglycan.

61. Correct statements concerning the mode of action of antibiotics include the following:
  (1) Vancomycin inhibits peptidoglycan synthesis.
  (2) The ability of penicillin to selectively inhibit the growth of bacterial but not of human cells is based on the presence of peptidoglycan in the bacterial cell wall.
  (3) Cephalosporins inhibit the transpeptidation reaction.
  (4) Amphotericin B inhibits the growth of bacteria by blocking an early step in peptidoglycan synthesis.

62. A variety of features distinguish bacteria from viruses. Correct statements concerning these features include the following:
  (1) Bacteria are capable of synthesizing proteins, whereas viruses must utilize the cellular ribosomes of the host.
  (2) Bacteria generate ATP, whereas viruses derive their energy from the host cell.
  (3) Bacteria reproduce by binary fission, whereas viral reproduction results in many progeny from one parental virus.
  (4) Bacteria contain double-stranded circular DNA as genetic material, whereas no viruses have double-stranded circular DNA.

63. Correct statements concerning the normal flora include the following:
  (1) *Staphylococcus epidermidis* is the major organism on the skin.
  (2) *Bacteroides* species are found in larger numbers than *Escherichia coli* in the colon.
  (3) The yeast *Candida albicans* is part of the normal flora of both men and women.
  (4) The predominant organisms in the alveoli are viridans streptococci.

64. Correct statements concerning exotoxins include the following:
  (1) Exotoxins are usually lipopolysaccharides.
  (2) Exotoxins produce fever and leukopenia in the host.
  (3) Exotoxins determine the invasiveness of bacteria.
  (4) Exotoxins can be chemically modified to provide an immunizing preparation.

65. Correct statements concerning cholera toxin include the following:
  (1) Binding of cholera toxin to the mucosal epithelium occurs via interaction of the B subunit of the toxin with a ganglioside in the cell membrane.
  (2) Cholera toxin promotes active secretion of Cl^- and HCO_3^- into the lumen of the gut.
  (3) Cholera toxin activates the enzyme adenylate cyclase in the mucosal epithelium.
  (4) Cholera toxin inhibits elongation factor 2 in the gut mucosa.

Answers (Questions 40–65):

40 (B)	44 (A)	48 (A)	52 (E)	56 (C)	60 (A)	64 (D)
41 (A)	45 (A)	49 (A)	53 (A)	57 (A)	61 (A)	65 (A)
42 (C)	46 (A)	50 (E)	54 (A)	58 (A)	62 (A)	
43 (A)	47 (C)	51 (A)	55 (D)	59 (C)	63 (A)	

CLINICAL BACTERIOLOGY

Directions (Questions 66–131): Select the ONE lettered answer that is BEST in each question.

66. An outbreak of sepsis caused by *Staphylococcus aureus* has occurred in the newborn nursery. You are called upon to investigate. According to your knowledge of normal floras, what is the MOST likely source of the organism?
    (A) colon
    (B) nose
    (C) throat
    (D) vagina

67. Each of the statements about the classification of streptococci is correct EXCEPT
    (A) Pneumococci *(Streptococcus pneumoniae)* are α-hemolytic and can be serotyped on the basis of their polysaccharide capsules.
    (B) Enterococci are group D streptococci and can be classified by their ability to grow in 6.5% sodium chloride.
    (C) Although pneumococci *(S pneumoniae)* and the viridans streptococci are α-hemolytic, they can be differentiated by the bile solubility test and their susceptibility to optochin.
    (D) Viridans streptococci are identified by Lancefield grouping, which is based on the C carbohydrate in the cell wall.

68. Each of the following agents is a recognized cause of diarrhea EXCEPT
    (A) *Clostridium perfringens*
    (B) *Streptococcus faecalis*
    (C) rotavirus
    (D) *Vibrio cholerae*

69. Each of the following organisms is an important cause of urinary tract infections EXCEPT
    (A) *Escherichia coli*
    (B) *Proteus mirabilis*
    (C) *Klebsiella pneumoniae*
    (D) *Bacteroides fragilis*

70. Your patient is a 30-year-old woman with nonbloody diarrhea for the past 14 hours. Each of the following organisms could be responsible EXCEPT
    (A) *Clostridium difficile*
    (B) *Streptococcus pyogenes*
    (C) *Shigella dysenteriae*
    (D) *Salmonella enteritidis*

71. Each of the statements concerning *Mycobacterium tuberculosis* is correct EXCEPT
    (A) After being stained with carbolfuchsin, *M tuberculosis* resists decolorization with acid alcohol.
    (B) *M tuberculosis* has a large amount of mycolic acid in its cell wall.
    (C) *M tuberculosis* appears as a red rod in the Gram reaction.
    (D) *M tuberculosis* appears as a red rod in the acid-fast reaction.

72. A 50-year-old homeless alcoholic has a fever and is coughing up 1 cup of green, foul smelling sputum per day. You suspect he may have a lung abscess. Which one of the following pairs of organisms is MOST likely to be the cause.
    (A) *Listeria monocytogenes* and *Legionella pneumophila*
    (B) *Nocardia asteroides* and *Mycoplasma pneumoniae*
    (C) *Fusobacterium nucleatum* and *Peptostreptococcus intermedius*
    (D) *Clostridium perfringens* and *Chlamydia psittaci*

73. Which one of the following diseases is BEST diagnosed by serologic means?
    (A) Q fever
    (B) pulmonary tuberculosis
    (C) gonorrhea
    (D) nongonococcal urethritis

74. Your patient has subacute bacterial endocarditis caused by a member of the viridans group

of streptococci. Which one of the following areas is MOST likely to be the source of the organism?

(A) skin
(B) colon
(C) oropharynx
(D) urethra

75. A culture of skin lesions from a patient with pyoderma (impetigo) shows numerous colonies surrounded by a zone of beta-hemolysis on a blood agar plate. A Gram-stained smear shows gram-positive cocci. If you found the catalase test to be negative, what would you have determined?

(A) The bacteria are streptococci.
(B) The bacteria are staphylococci.
(C) The bacteria are neither streptococci nor staphylococci.
(D) The bacteria are pneumococci.

76. The coagulase test, in which the bacteria cause plasma to clot, is used to distinguish

(A) *Streptococcus pyogenes* from *Streptococcus faecalis*
(B) *S pyogenes* from *Staphylococcus aureus*
(C) *S aureus* from *Staphylococcus epidermidis*
(D) *S epidermidis* from *Neisseria meningitidis*

77. Which one of the following is considered a virulence factor for *S aureus*?

(A) a heat-labile toxin that inhibits glycine release at the internuncial neuron
(B) an oxygen-labile hemolysin
(C) resistance to novobiocin
(D) protein A that binds to the Fc portion of IgG

78. Which one of the following statements BEST differentiates *Streptococcus pneumoniae* from the viridans group of streptococci?

(A) *S pneumoniae* is a gram-positive coccus that forms long chains, whereas viridans streptococci are short-chain, gram-positive cocci.
(B) *S pneumoniae* is inhibited by bile and optochin, whereas viridans streptococci are not.
(C) Viridans streptococci grow in 6.5% NaCl, whereas *S pneumoniae* does not.
(D) *S pneumoniae* is alpha-hemolytic, whereas the viridans streptococci are beta-hemolytic.

79. Which one of the following host defense mechanisms is the MOST important for preventing dysentery caused by *Shigella?*

(A) gastric acid
(B) salivary enzymes
(C) normal flora of the mouth
(D) esophageal mucosa

80. The MOST important protective function of the antibody stimulated by tetanus immunization is

(A) to opsonize the pathogen *(Clostridium tetani)*
(B) to prevent growth of the pathogen
(C) to prevent adherence of the pathogen
(D) to neutralize the toxin of the pathogen

81. Five hours after eating fried rice at a restaurant, a 24-year-old woman and her husband both developed nausea, vomiting, and diarrhea. Which of the following organisms is the MOST likely to be involved?

(A) *Clostridium perfringens*
(B) enterotoxigenic *E coli*
(C) *Bacillus cereus*
(D) *Salmonella typhi*

82. Which one of the following agents has the LOWEST 50% infective dose (ID_{50})?

(A) *Shigella sonnei*
(B) *Vibro cholerae*
(C) *Salmonella typhi*
(D) *Campylobacter jejuni*

83. For which of the following enteric illnesses is a chronic carrier state MOST likely to develop?

(A) *Campylobacter* enterocolitis
(B) *Shigella* enterocolitis
(C) cholera
(D) typhoid fever

84. Which one of the following zoonotic illnesses has NO arthropod vector?
   (A) plague
   (B) Lyme disease
   (C) brucellosis
   (D) epidemic typhus

85. Which one of the following organisms infects principally vascular endothelial cells?
   (A) *Salmonella typhi*
   (B) *Rickettsia typhi*
   (C) *Haemophilus influenzae*
   (D) *Coxiella burnetii*

86. Which one of the following statements MOST accurately depicts the ability of the organism to be cultured in the laboratory?
   (A) *Treponema pallidum* from a chancre can be grown on a special artificial medium supplemented with cholesterol.
   (B) *Mycobacterium leprae* can be grown in the armadillo and the mouse footpad but not on any artificial media.
   (C) *Mycobacterium tuberculosis* can be grown on enriched artificial media and produces visible colonies in 48–96 hours.
   (D) Atypical mycobacteria are found widely in soil and water but cannot be cultured on artificial media in the laboratory.

87. Chlamydiae
   (A) are strict intracellular parasites, eg, they cannot grow outside cells
   (B) possess either RNA or DNA but not both
   (C) are inhibited by aminoglycosides but not tetracyclines
   (D) are typically transmitted by arthropods

88. For which one of the following bacterial vaccines are toxic side effects an important concern?
   (A) the vaccine containing pneumococcal polysaccharide
   (B) the vaccine containing killed *Bordetella pertussis* cells
   (C) the vaccine containing tetanus toxoid
   (D) the vaccine containing diphtheria toxoid

89. Each of the following statements concerning *Staphylococcus aureus* is correct EXCEPT
   (A) Gram-positive cocci in grapelike clusters are seen on Gram-stained smear.
   (B) The coagulase test is positive.
   (C) Treatment should include a β-lactamase-resistant penicillin.
   (D) Endotoxin is an important pathogenetic factor.

90. Your patient is a 70-year-old-man who underwent bowel surgery for colon cancer 3 days ago. He now has a fever and abdominal pain. You are concerned that he may have peritonitis. Which one of the following pairs of organisms is MOST likely to be the cause?
   (A) *Bacteroides fragilis* and *Klebsiella pneumoniae*
   (B) *Bordetella pertussis* and *Salmonella enteritidis*
   (C) *Actinomyces israelii* and *Campylobacter jejuni*
   (D) *Clostridium botulinum* and *Shigella dysenteriae*

91. A 65-year-old man develops dysuria and hematuria. A Gram stain of a urine sample shows gram-negative rods. Culture of the urine on EMB agar reveals lactose-negative colonies without evidence of swarming motility. Which one of the following organisms is MOST likely to be the cause of this urinary tract infection?
   (A) *Streptococcus faecalis*
   (B) *Pseudomonas aeruginosa*
   (C) *Proteus vulgaris*
   (D) *Escherichia coli*

92. A 25-year-old man complains of a urethral discharge. You perform a Gram stain on a specimen of the discharge and see polymorphonuclear leukocytes but no bacteria. Of the organisms listed, the one MOST likely to cause the discharge is
   (A) *Treponema pallidum*
   (B) *Chlamydia trachomatis*
   (C) *Candida albicans*
   (D) *Coxsiella burnetii*

93. Six hours after a delicious Thanksgiving dinner of barley soup, roast turkey, stuffing, sweet potato, green beans, cranberry sauce, and pumpkin pie topped with whipped cream, the Smith family of 4 develops vomiting and diarrhea. Which one of the following

organisms is MOST likely to be the cause of the symptoms?

(A) *Shigella flexneri*

(B) *Campylobacter jejuni*

(C) *Staphylococcus aureus*

(D) *Serratia marcescens*

94. Your patient has a brain abscess that was detected 1 month after a dental extraction. Which one of the following organisms is MOST likely to be involved?

(A) anaerobic streptococci

(B) *Mycobacterium smegmatis*

(C) *Lactobacillus acidophilus*

(D) *Mycoplasma pneumoniae*

95. The MOST important contribution of the capsule of *S pneumoniae* to virulence is

(A) to prevent dehydration of the organisms on mucosal surfaces.

(B) to retard phagocytosis by polymorphonuclear leukocytes

(C) to inhibit polymorphonuclear leukocyte chemotaxis

(D) collagenaselike activity to accelerate tissue invasion

96. The MOST important way the host circumvents the function of the pneumococcal polysaccharide capsule is via

(A) T lymphocytes sensitized to polysaccharide antigens

(B) polysaccharide-degrading enzymes

(C) anticapsular antibody

(D) activated macrophages

97. The pathogenesis of which of the following organisms is MOST related to invasion of the intestinal mucosa?

(A) *Vibrio cholerae*

(B) *Shigella sonnei*

(C) enterotoxigenic *E coli*

(D) *Clostridium botulinum*

98. Which one of the following organisms that infect the gastrointestinal tract causes bacteremia MOST frequently?

(A) *Shigella flexneri*

(B) *Campylobacter jejuni*

(C) *Vibrio cholerae*

(D) *Salmonella typhi*

99. A 30-year-old woman with systemic lupus erythematosus is found to have a positive serologic test for syphilis (VDRL test). She denies having had sexual contact with a partner who had symptoms of a venereal disease. The next BEST step would be to

(A) reassure her that the test is a false-positive reaction related to her autoimmune disorder

(B) trace her sexual contacts for serologic testing

(C) treat her with penicillin

(D) perform a fluorescent treponemal antibody-absorption (FTA-ABS) test on a specimen of her serum

100. Each of the following statements concerning *Treponema* is correct EXCEPT

(A) *T pallidum* produces an exotoxin that stimulates adenylate cyclase.

(B) *T pallidum* cannot be grown on conventional laboratory media.

(C) Trepomenes are members of the normal flora of the human oropharynx.

(D) Patients infected with *T pallidum* produce antibodies that can inhibit its motility.

101. Each of the following statements concerning clostridia is correct EXCEPT

(A) Pathogenic clostridia are found both in the soil and in the normal flora of the colon.

(B) Antibiotic-associated (pseudomembranous) colitis is due to a toxin produced by *Clostridium difficile.*

(C) Anaerobic conditions at the wound site are not required to cause tetanus, because spores will form in the presence of oxygen.

(D) Botulism, which is caused by ingesting preformed toxin, can be prevented by boiling food prior to eating.

102. Each of the following statements concerning *Bacteroides fragilis* is correct EXCEPT

(A) *B fragilis* is a gram-negative rod that is part of the normal flora of the colon.

(B) *B fragilis* forms endospores, which allow it to survive in soil.

(C) The capsule is an important virulence factor.

(D) *B fragilis* infections are characterized by foul-smelling pus.

103. Each of the following statements concerning staphylococci is correct EXCEPT
  - **(A)** *S aureus* is differentiated from *S epidermidis* by the production of coagulase.
  - **(B)** *S aureus* infections are often associated with abscess formation.
  - **(C)** The majority of clinical isolates of *S aureus* elaborate penicillinase; therefore, presumptive antibiotic therapy for staphylococcal infections should not include penicillin G.
  - **(D)** Scalded-skin syndrome caused by *S aureus* is due to catalase that enzymatically degrades epidermal desmosomes.

104. Acute glomerulonephritis is a nonsuppurative complication that follows infection by which one of the following organisms?
  - **(A)** *Streptococcus faecalis*
  - **(B)** *Streptococcus pyogenes*
  - **(C)** *Streptococcus pneumoniae*
  - **(D)** *Streptococcus agalactiae*

105. Each of the following statements concerning gram-negative rods is correct EXCEPT
  - **(A)** *E coli* is part of the normal flora in the colon; therefore, it does not cause diarrhea.
  - **(B)** *E coli* ferments lactose, whereas the enteric pathogens *Shigella* and *Salmonella* do not.
  - **(C)** *Klebsiella pneumoniae,* although a cause of pneumonia, is part of the normal flora in the colon.
  - **(D)** *Proteus* species are highly motile organisms that are found in the human colon and cause urinary tract infections

106. A 70-year-old man is found to have a hard mass in his prostate, which is suspected to be a carcinoma. Twenty-four hours after surgical removal of the mass, he develops fever to 39.°C and has several shaking chills. Of the organisms listed, which one is LEAST likely to be involved?
  - **(A)** *Escherichia coli*
  - **(B)** *Streptococcus faecalis*
  - **(C)** *Klebsiella pneumoniae*
  - **(D)** *Legionella pneumophila*

107. Five days ago a 65-year-old woman with a lower urinary tract infection began taking ampicillin. She now has a fever and severe diarrhea. Of the organisms listed, which one is MOST likely to be the cause of the diarrhea?
  - **(A)** *Clostridium difficile*
  - **(B)** *Bacteroides fragilis*
  - **(C)** *Proteus mirabilis*
  - **(D)** *Bordetella pertussis*

108. The pathogenesis of which one of the following diseases is LEAST likely to involve an exotoxin?
  - **(A)** scarlet fever
  - **(B)** typhoid fever
  - **(C)** toxic shock syndrome
  - **(D)** botulism

109. Which one of the following attributes do cold agglutinins, reagin antibody, and heterophile antibody have in common?
  - **(A)** They are detected in the laboratory by complement fixation.
  - **(B)** They are induced by different bacterial antigens.
  - **(C)** They are detected in the laboratory by reactions with antigens that did not induce them.
  - **(D)** They persist for life.

110. Regarding the effect of benzylpenicillin (penicillin G) on bacteria, which one of the following organisms is LEAST likely to be resistant?
  - **(A)** *Staphylococcus aureus*
  - **(B)** *Streptococcus faecalis*
  - **(C)** *Streptococcus pyogenes*
  - **(D)** *Neisseria gonorrhoeae*

111. Which one of the following organisms is MOST likely to be the cause of pneumonia in an immuncompetent patient?
  - **(A)** *Nocardia asteroides*
  - **(B)** *Serratia marcescens*

    (**C**) *Mycoplasma pneumoniae*
    (**D**) varicella-zoster virus

112. Which one of the following statements about chlamydiae is MOST accurate?
    (**A**) Each *Chlamydia* species has only one serologic type.
    (**B**) Chlamydiae possess cell walls.
    (**C**) Chlamydiae can divide extracellularly by binary fission.
    (**D**) The growth of chlamydiae is inhibited more readily by cephalosporins than by tetracyclines.

113. Each of the following statements concerning chlamydial genital tract infections is correct EXCEPT
    (**A**) Infection can be diagnosed by finding antichlamydial antibody in a serum specimen.
    (**B**) Infection can persist after administration of penicillin.
    (**C**) Symptomatic infections can be associated with urethral or cervical discharge containing many polymorphonuclear leukocytes.
    (**D**) Infection can be asymptomatic more often than symptomatic.

114. Which one of the following illnesses is NOT a zoonosis?
    (**A**) typhoid fever
    (**B**) Q fever
    (**C**) tularemia
    (**D**) Rocky Mountain spotted fever

115. Endotoxin-mediated symptoms are typically associated with infection by which one of the following organisms?
    (**A**) *Staphylococcus aureus*
    (**B**) *Neisseria meningitidis*
    (**C**) *Streptococcus pyogenes*
    (**D**) *Mycoplasma pneumoniae*

116. Which one of the following is NOT a characteristic of the staphylococci associated with toxic shock syndrome?
    (**A**) elaboration of enterotoxin F
    (**B**) coagulase production
    (**C**) appearance of the organism in grapelike clusters on Gram-stained smear
    (**D**) catalase-negative reaction

117. Which one of the following is NOT relevant to the classification or pathogenesis of *Neisseria gonorrhoeae* or *N meningitidis?*
    (**A**) polysaccharide capsule
    (**B**) immunoglobulin A protease
    (**C**) M protein
    (**D**) pili

118. Which one of the following is NOT relevant to the classification, pathogenesis, or immunology of Lancefield group A beta-hemolytic streptococcal (*Streptococcus pyogenes*) infections?
    (**A**) protein A
    (**B**) M protein
    (**C**) lipoteichoic acid
    (**D**) the polysaccharide group-specific substance

119. Which one of the following is NOT related to Lancefield group B streptococci (*S agalactiae*)?
    (**A**) pyoderma (impetigo)
    (**B**) vaginal carriage in 5–25% of normal women of childbearing age
    (**C**) neonatal sepsis and meningitis
    (**D**) beta-hemolysis

120. Three organisms, *S pneumoniae, N meningitidis,* and *H influenzae,* cause the vast majority of cases of bacterial meningitis. What is the MOST important pathogenic feature they share?
    (**A**) protein A
    (**B**) capsule
    (**C**) endotoxin
    (**D**) β-lactamase

121. Diarrhea caused by which one of the following agents is characterized by the presence of fecal leukocytes?
    (**A**) *Campylobacter jejuni*

(B) rotavirus
(C) *Clostridium perfringens*
(D) *enterotoxigenic E coli*

122. Which one of the following organisms that cause enteric infections is MOST often associated with bacteremia?
(A) *Vibrio cholerae*
(B) *Campylobacter jejuni*
(C) *Salmonella enteritidis*
(D) *Shigella flexneri*

123. Each of the following statements concerning *Chlamydia trachomatis* is correct EXCEPT
(A) It is an important cause of nongonococcal urethritis.
(B) It is the cause of lymphogranuloma venereum.
(C) It is an important cause of subacute bacterial endocarditis.
(D) It is an important cause of conjunctivitis.

124. Each of the following statements concerning *Actinomyces* and *Nocardia* is correct EXCEPT
(A) *A israelii* is an anaerobic rod found as part of the normal flora in the mouth.
(B) Both *Actinomyces* and *Nocardia* are branching, filamentous rods.
(C) *N asteroides* causes infections primarily in immunocompromised patients.
(D) Wild rodents are the animal reservoir for both *Actinomyces* and *Nocardia*.

125. Which one of the following types of organisms is NOT an obligate intracellular parasite and therefore can replicate on bacteriologic media?
(A) *Chlamydia*
(B) *Mycoplasma*
(C) adenovirus
(D) *Rickettsia*

126. Tissue-degrading enzymes play an important role in pathogenesis of several bacteria. Which one of the following is NOT involved in tissue or cell damage?
(A) lecithinase of *Clostridium perfringens*
(B) hyaluronidase of *Streptococcus pyogenes*
(C) M protein of *Streptococcus pneumoniae*
(D) leukocidin of *Staphylococcus aureus*

127. Which one of the following enteric pathogens is MOST likely to cause disease following oral ingestion of a small inoculum (100 organisms)?
(A) enterotoxigenic *Escherichia coli*
(B) *Salmonella enteritidis*
(C) *Vibrio cholerae*
(D) *Shigella flexneri*

128. The soil is the natural habitat for certain microorganisms of medical importance. Which one of the following is LEAST likely to reside there?
(A) *Clostridium tetani*
(B) *Mycobacterium intracellulare*
(C) *Bacillus anthracis*
(D) *Chlamydia trachomatis*

129. Animals are the natural habitat for certain microorganisms of medical importance. Which one of the following is LEAST likely to be associated with animals?
(A) *Campylobacter jejuni*
(B) *Yersinia enterocolitica*
(C) *Salmonella choleraesuis*
(D) *Bordetella pertussis*

130. Of the organisms listed below, which one is the MOST frequent bacterial cause of pharyngitis?
(A) *Staphylococcus aureus*
(B) *Streptococcus pneumoniae*
(C) *Streptococcus pyogenes*
(D) *Neisseria meningitidis*

131. Several pathogens are transmitted either during gestation or at birth. Which one of the following is LEAST likely to be transmitted at these times?
(A) *Haemophilus influenzae*
(B) *Treponema pallidum*
(C) *Neisseria gonorrhoeae*
(D) *Chlamydia trachomatis*

Answers (Questions 66–131):

66 (B)	75 (A)	84 (C)	93 (C)	102 (B)	111 (C)	120 (B)	129 (D)
67 (D)	76 (C)	85 (B)	94 (A)	103 (D)	112 (B)	121 (A)	130 (C)
68 (B)	77 (D)	86 (B)	95 (B)	104 (B)	113 (A)	122 (C)	131 (A)
69 (D)	78 (B)	87 (A)	96 (C)	105 (A)	114 (A)	123 (C)	
70 (B)	79 (A)	88 (B)	97 (B)	106 (D)	115 (B)	124 (D)	
71 (C)	80 (D)	89 (D)	98 (D)	107 (A)	116 (D)	125 (B)	
72 (C)	81 (C)	90 (A)	99 (D)	108 (B)	117 (C)	126 (C)	
73 (A)	82 (A)	91 (B)	100 (A)	109 (C)	118 (A)	127 (D)	
74 (C)	83 (D)	92 (B)	101 (C)	110 (C)	119 (A)	128 (D)	

Directions (Questions 132–149): Select the ONE lettered heading that is MOST closely associated with the numbered phrases or statements.

Questions 132–135
(A) *Mycobacterium intracellulare*
(B) *Treponema pallidum*
(C) *Rickettsia prowazekii*
(D) *Mycoplasma pneumoniae*
132. Obligate intracellular parasite
133. Found primarily in the soil
134. Has no cell wall
135. Acid-fast rod

Questions 136–138
(A) Spirochete
(B) Acid-fast rod
(C) Gram-negative diplococcus
(D) Gram-negative rod
136. Cervical lymphadenitis in a 12-year-old girl in Malaysia
137. Purulent rectal discharge in a 30-year-old homosexual man in Los Angeles
138. Migratory skin rash followed by arthritis in a 6-year-old boy in rural Connecticut

Questions 139–142
(A) *Corynebacterium diphtheriae*
(B) *Listeria monocytogenes*
(C) *Bacillus anthracis*
(D) *Lactobacillus species*
139. Causes both skin lesions and a severe pneumonia
140. Member of the normal flora of the mouth, bowel, and vagina
141. Lysogeny with a prophage required for production of a toxin that inhibits protein synthesis
142. Causes meningitis in neonates and the immunosuppressed

Questions 143–145
(A) *Escherichia coli*
(B) *Klebsiella pneumoniae*
(C) *Salmonella enteritidis*
(D) *Proteus vulgaris*
143. Is frequently implicated in nosocomial infections and is an important cause of community-acquired pneumonia in adults
144. Is the leading cause of urinary tract infection, sepsis, and neonatal meningitis in the USA
145. Pathogenicity associated primarily with urinary tract infections (rarely causes sepsis or meningitis)

Questions 146–149

    (A) *Staphylococcus aureus*
    (B) *Streptococcus pyogenes*
    (C) *Streptococcus faecalis*
    (D) *Streptococcus pneumoniae*

146. Grows in 6.5% sodium chloride
147. Is bile-soluble
148. Produce enterotoxin
149. Is associated with rheumatic fever.

Answers (Questions 132–149):

132 (C)	137 (C)	142 (B)	147 (D)
133 (A)	138 (A)	143 (B)	148 (A)
134 (D)	139 (C)	144 (A)	149 (B)
135 (A)	140 (D)	145 (D)	
136 (B)	141 (A)	146 (C)	

Directions (Questions 150–184): For each numbered item, select

    A if the item is associated with (A) only,
    B if the item is associated with (B) only,
    C if the item is associated with both (A) and (B),
    D if the item is associated with neither (A) nor (B).

Questions 150–154

    (A) *Escherichia coli*
    (B) *Salmonella enteritidis*
    (C) Both
    (D) Neither

150. Causes diarrhea by producing an enterotoxin
151. Is a motile, gram-negative rod
152. Forms spores
153. Has multiple serologic types
154. Does not ferment lactose

Questions 155–159

    (A) *Neisseria meningitidis*
    (B) *Neisseria gonorrhoeae*
    (C) Both
    (D) Neither

155. Is an oxidase-positive, gram-negative diplococcus
156. Has a polysaccharide capsule that is antiphagocytic
157. Contains endotoxin in cell wall
158. Resistance to penicillin has clinical significance
159. Produces an exotoxin that stimulates adenylate cyclase

Questions 160–164

    (A) Q fever
    (B) Rocky Mountain spotted fever
    (C) Both
    (D) Neither

160. Caused by a virus
161. Characterized by rash
162. Transmitted by tick bite
163. Characterized by pneumonia
164. Occurs most commonly on the East Coast of the USA

Questions 165–168

    (A) *Bacteroides fragilis*
    (B) *Clostridium perfringens*
    (C) Both
    (D) Neither

165. Is a gram-positive, spore-forming rod
166. Is an obligate anaerobe
167. Is an obligate intracellular parasite
168. Produces gas in tissues

Questions 169–173

    (A) *Mycobacterium tuberculosis*
    (B) *Mycobacterium leprae*
    (C) Both
    (D) Neither

169. Exotoxin important in pathogenesis
170. Can be seen in an acid-fast stain
171. Diagnosis often possible after cultivation on suitable media for 3–6 weeks
172. Prolonged therapy (9 months or longer) required to prevent recurrences
173. Skin tests for hypersensitivity useful diagnostically

Questions 174–177

    (A) Tetanus
    (B) Diphtheria
    (C) Both
    (D) Neither

174. Caused by a gram-positive rod
175. Caused by exotoxin action at synapse of a spinal motor neuron
176. Caused by an anaerobic bacterium
177. Disease prevented by immunization with toxoid

Questions 178–184

    (A) Group A streptococci
    (B) Group B streptococci
    (C) Both
    (D) Neither

178. Beta-hemolytic
179. Contain endotoxin in cell wall
180. Part of normal flora of the female genital tract
181. Bacitracin-sensitive
182. Associated with neonatal sepsis
183. Contain C carbohydrate in cell wall
184. Associated with acute glomerulonephritis

Answers (Questions 150–184):

150 (A)	155 (C)	160 (D)	165 (B)	170 (C)	175 (A)	180 (B)
151 (C)	156 (A)	161 (B)	166 (C)	171 (A)	176 (A)	181 (A)
152 (D)	157 (C)	162 (B)	167 (D)	172 (C)	177 (C)	182 (B)
153 (C)	158 (B)	163 (A)	168 (C)	173 (C)	178 (C)	183 (C)
154 (B)	159 (D)	164 (B)	169 (D)	174 (C)	179 (D)	184 (A)

Directions (Questions 185–240): For each question, ONE or MORE of the numbered options is correct. Select

    A if only 1, 2, and 3 are correct
    B if only 1 and 3 are correct
    C if only 2 and 4 are correct
    D if only 4 is correct
    E if all are correct

185. Correct statements concerning streptococci include the following:

(1) The main reservoir of group B streptococci is the vagina.

(2) Group A beta-hemolytic streptococci *(Streptococcus pyogenes)* have a cell wall carbohydrate that is antigenically distinct from that of group B streptococci.

(3) Streptococci are catalase-negative, gram-positive cocci.

(4) M protein, which degrades complement, is a virulence factor for *Streptococcus pneumoniae.*

186. Correct statements concerning infections caused by clostridia include the following:

(1) Botulism cannot be prevented by cooking food because the toxin is heat-stable (ie, is not inactivated by boiling).

(2) Tetanus is preventable by immunization with tetanus toxoid.

(3) Tetanus toxin increases the release of excitatory transmitters from sensory neurons.

(4) *Clostridium perfringens,* a cause of gas gangrene, produces alpha toxin, a lecithinase that can degrade cell membranes.

187. Correct statements concerning staphylococci include the following:

(1) *Staphylococcus aureus* produces an exotoxin that causes vomiting and diarrhea.

(2) *Staphylococcus epidermidis* is a major cause of boils in the skin.

(3) All staphylococci produce the enzyme catalase.

(4) *S aureus* contains M protein, which cross-reacts with antibody against cardiac muscle proteins.

188. Correct statements concerning staphylococcal pathogenesis and host defenses include the following:

(1) There is a significant animal reservoir of *S aureus* that increases the frequency of human disease.

(2) Because *S aureus* produces hyaluronidase, the skin offers little protection.

(3) T cells form the major host defense against staphylococci.

(4) A staphylococcal toxin causes exfoliation of the skin.

189. Correct statements concerning bacterial pneumonia include the following:

(1) *Streptococcus pneumoniae* is part of the normal flora of the upper respiratory tract yet can cause pneumonia.

(2) *Mycoplasma pneumoniae* can be cultured in vitro, although it has no cell wall.

(3) *Klebsiella pneumoniae* is a gram-negative rod that produces a large polysaccharide capsule.

(4) *Bacillus cereus* is an important cause of pneumonia in homosexual men.

190. Correct statements concerning exotoxins include the following:

(1) Some strains of *Escherichia coli* produce an enterotoxin that causes diarrhea.

(2) Cholera toxin acts by stimulating adenylate cyclase.

(3) Diphtheria is caused by an exotoxin that inhibits protein synthesis by inactivating an elongation factor.

(4) Botulism is caused by a toxin that hydrolyzes lecithin (lecithinase), thereby destroying nerve cells.

191. Correct statements concerning the Venereal Disease Research Laboratory (VDRL) test for syphilis include the following:

(1) The antigen is composed of inactivated *Treponema pallidum* cells.

(2) The test is usually positive in secondary syphilis.

(3) False-positive results are less frequent than with the FTA-ABS test.

(4) The titer of antibody declines with adequate therapy.

192. Correct statements concerning the fluorescent treponemal antibody-absorption (FTA-ABS) test for syphilis include the following:

(1) The test is specific for *T pallidum.*

(2) The patient's serum is absorbed with saprophytic treponemes.

(3) Once positive, the test remains so despite adequate therapy.

(4) The test is rarely positive in primary syphilis.

193. Correct statements concerning *Corynebacterium diphtheriae* include the following:

(1) Toxin production is dependent on the organism's being lysogenized by a bacteriophage.

(2) It is a spore-forming, gram-positive rod.

(3) Antitoxin should be used to treat patients with diphtheria.

(4) Diphtheria toxoid should not be given to children under the age of 3 years, because the incidence of complications is too high.

194. Correct statements concerning persons infected with *Chlamydia trachomatis* include the following:
  (1) They have antibodies to the agent.
  (2) They develop cell-mediated immunity to the agent.
  (3) They improve clinically after taking tetracycline.
  (4) They acquire solid resistance to reinfection by the same agent.

195. Correct statements concerning chlamydiae include the following:
  (1) They are obligate intracellular parasites that form reticulate bodies within the host cell.
  (2) *C trachomatis* is a cause of nongonococcal urethritis.
  (3) *C psittaci* is a cause of pneumonia.
  (4) *C trachomatis* has multiple serotypes, some of which cause lymphogranuloma venereum.

196. Correct statements concerning certain gram-negative rod include the following:
  (1) *Pseudomonas aeruginosa* causes wound infections that are characterized by blue-green pus as a result of pyocyanin production.
  (2) Invasive disease caused by *Haemophilus influenzae* is most often due to strains possessing a type B polysaccharide capsule.
  (3) *Legionella pneumophila* infection is acquired by inhalation of aerosols from environmental water sources.
  (4) The incidence of whooping cough, which is caused by *Bordetella pertussis,* is on the rise because changing antigenicity has made the vaccine relatively ineffective.

197. Correct statements concerning enterotoxins include the following:
  (1) Enterotoxins typically cause bloody diarrhea with leukocytes in the stool.
  (2) *Staphylococcus aureus* produces an enterotoxin that causes vomiting and diarrhea.
  (3) Norwalk agent secretes an enterotoxin that causes diarrhea, particularly in young children.
  (4) *Escherichia coli* enterotoxin activates adenylate cyclase, resulting in diarrhea.

198. Correct statements concerning bacteria and their products include the following:
  (1) *Mycoplasma pneumoniae* is a partially acid-fast rod that produces factors X (hemin) and V (NAD).
  (2) *Klebsiella pneumoniae* is a gram-negative rod that has a large polysaccharide capsule.
  (3) *Bordetella pertussis* is a gram-positive rod that produces a toxin that inhibits acetylcholine release.
  (4) *Clostridium perfringens* is a gram-positive rod that produces alpha toxin, a lecithinase.

199. Correct statements concerning *Mycobacterium tuberculosis* include the following:
  (1) *M tuberculosis* produces beta-hemolysis on blood agar.
  (2) *M tuberculosis* is a photochromogen; eg, it produces pigment only when exposed to light.
  (3) Thayer-Martin medium can be used to detect both *M tuberculosis* and certain atypical organisms.
  (4) Colonies typically require 3–6 weeks to appear.

200. Correct statements concerning plague include the following:
  (1) Plague is caused by a gram-negative rod.
  (2) Plague is transmitted to humans by flea bites.
  (3) The main reservoirs in nature are small rodents.
  (4) Plague is of concern in many developing countries but has not occurred in the USA since 1968.

201. Correct statements concerning the organisms that cause brucellosis include the following:
  (1) Brucellae are transmitted primarily by tick bites.
  (2) The principal reservoirs of brucellae are small rodents.
  (3) Brucellae are obligate intracellular parasites, which are usually identified by growth in human cell culture.
  (4) Brucellae are found in reticuloendothelial cells and often cause granulomatous lesions.

202. Correct statements concerning epidemic typhus and Rocky Mountain spotted fever include the following:
  (1) Both diseases are characterized by a rash.

(2) The Weil-Felix test can aid in diagnosis of both diseases.

(3) In both diseases, antibodies against certain strains of *Proteus* arise.

(4) Both diseases are transmitted by ticks.

203. Correct statements concerning bacterial vaccines include the following:

(1) Both tetanus and diphtheria can be prevented by vaccines containing toxoid as the antigen.

(2) Both the pneumococcal and the meningococcal vaccines contain capsular polysaccharide as the antigen.

(3) The usefulness of pertussis vaccine is limited by its toxic side effects.

(4) The usefulness of *H influenzae* vaccine is limited by its failure to induce protection in children under 18 months of age.

204. Organisms that cause diarrhea by producing an enterotoxin that acts by activating adenylate cyclase include

(1) *Escherichia coli*

(2) *Staphylococcus aureus*

(3) *Vibrio cholerae*

(4) *Salmonella enteritidis*

205. Correct statements concerning Rocky Mountain spotted fever include the following:

(1) Rocky Mountain spotted fever is transmitted by the bite of a mosquito.

(2) Headache, fever, and rash are characteristic features.

(3) Rocky Mountain spotted fever occurs primarily west of the Mississippi.

(4) Rocky Mountain spotted fever is caused by a rickettsia.

206. Correct statements concerning *Clostridium perfringens* include the following:

(1) It is an important cause of gas gangrene.

(2) It is an important cause of food poisoning.

(3) It produces an exotoxin that degrades lecithin and causes necrosis and hemolysis.

(4) It produces a toxin that inhibits the release of acetylcholine at the synapse.

207. Correct statements concerning *Clostridium tetani* include the following:

(1) *C tetani* is an acid-fast rod.

(2) Pathogenesis is due to the production of an exotoxin that blocks inhibitory neurotransmitters.

(3) *C tetani* is a facultative organism; it will grow on a blood agar plate in the presence of room air.

(4) The natural habitat of *C tetani* is primarily the soil.

208. Correct statements concerning spirochetes include the following:

(1) Species of *Treponema* are part of the normal flora of the mouth.

(2) Species of *Borrelia* cause a tick-borne disease called relapsing fever.

(3) Species of *Treponema* cause syphilis and yaws.

(4) The species of *Leptospira* that cause leptospirosis grow primarily in humans and hence are usually transmitted by person-to-person contact.

209. Correct statements concerning the clinical features of syphilis include the following:

(1) Primary syphilis is characterized by a chancre in both men and women.

(2) The latency period occurs after the secondary stage.

(3) The condylomata lata of secondary syphilis are infectious.

(4) Tertiary syphilis is characterized by lesions in the central nervous and cardiovascular systems.

210. Correct statements concerning the serologic tests for syphilis include the following:

(1) The VDRL test is a nonspecific test that uses cardiolipin as the antigen to detect reagin antibodies.

(2) The fluorescent treponemal antibody-absorption (FTA-ABS) test is specific for antibody to *T pallidum;* nonspecific antibodies are absorbed out with nonpathogenic treponemes.

(3) Both the VDRL and FTA-ABS tests give positive results in secondary syphilis.

(4) Results of the VDRL test are positive for life even in patients adequately treated.

211. Correct statements concerning gonorrhea include the following:

(1) Infection in men is more frequently asymptomatic than in women.

(2) A presumptive diagnosis can be made by finding gram-negative kidney bean-shaped diplococci within polymorphonuclear leukocytes in a urethral discharge.

(3) The definitive diagnosis can be made by detecting at least a 4-fold rise in antibody titer to *Neisseria gonorrhoeae.*

(4) Gonococcal conjunctivitis of the newborn rarely occurs in the USA, because silver nitrate or erythromycin is commonly used as a prophylaxis.

212. Correct statements concerning *Chlamydia trachomatis* include the following:
   (1) It has only a single immunotype (serovar).
   (2) It is often acquired by humans through contact with birds.
   (3) It produces intracellular inclusions mainly in polymorphonuclear cells.
   (4) It is an important cause of pneumonia in infants.

213. Correct statements concerning these organisms include the following:
   (1) *Mycoplasma pneumoniae* is a gram-positive rod with a significant animal reservoir.
   (2) *Clostridium difficile* is a gram-negative rod that causes significant epizootic disease among small wild rodents and only accidentally infects humans.
   (3) *Streptococcus pneumoniae* has 3 major serotypes and is classified as a member of the Lancefield group B streptococci.
   (4) *Bacillus anthracis* is a spore-forming, gram-positive rod found in the soil.

214. Correct statements concerning tetanus immunization include the following:
   (1) The vaccine against tetanus contains a toxoid that is prepared by inactivating the toxic effect of tetanus toxin while retaining its antigenicity.
   (2) Persons who have sustained soil-contaminated wounds and whose vaccine status is uncertain should be given passive immunity in the form of tetanus antitoxin.
   (3) The DPT vaccine given as part of childhood immunization provides protection against tetanus.
   (4) The antigen in the vaccine against tetanus is a poor immunogen and therefore is not very effective in preventing disease.

215. In young adults, *Streptococcus pneumoniae* and *Neisseria meningitidis* are the 2 most important causes of meningitis. Correct statements concerning these organisms include the following:
   (1) The capsule is an important virulence factor for one but not the other.
   (2) One is a rod, and the other is a coccus.
   (3) One has DNA as its genetic material, and the other has RNA.
   (4) One is a gram-positive, and the other is gram-negative.

216. Correct statements concerning pneumonia include the following:
   (1) Aspiration of organisms from the nasopharynx is an important step in the pathogenesis of pneumonia.
   (2) *Mycoplasma pneumoniae* is an important cause of lower respiratory tract infection in young adults.
   (3) Gram-negative rods, such as *Klebsiella,* are an important cause of hospital-acquired pneumonia.
   (4) The pathogenesis of *Streptococcus pneumoniae,* the most frequent cause of community-acquired pneumonia, involves both an exotoxin and an endotoxin.

217. Correct statements concerning *Mycobacterium tuberculosis* include the following:
   (1) Some strains isolated from individuals with previously untreated cases of tuberculosis are resistant to isoniazid.
   (2) *M tuberculosis* grows slowly, often requiring 6 weeks before colonies appear.
   (3) *M tuberculosis* contains a large amount of lipid in its cell wall and therefore stains poorly with Gram's stain.
   (4) The antigen in the skin test is a protein extracted from the organism.

218. Correct statements concerning immunization against diseases caused by clostridia include the following:
   (1) Antitoxin against tetanus protects against botulism as well, because the 2 toxins share antigenic sites.
   (2) Vaccines containing alpha toxin (lecithinase) are effective in protecting against gas gangrene.
   (3) The toxoid vaccine against *Clostridium difficile* infection should be administered to immunocompromised patients.
   (4) Tetanus toxoid provides effective protection against tetanus toxin.

219. Correct statements concerning *Staphylococcus aureus* include the following:
   (1) Some people are persistently colonized with this organism in their noses.
   (2) Staphylococci produce exotoxins called enterotoxins, which cause food poisoning.
   (3) Protein A of the *S aureus* cell wall acts as a virulence factor by binding to the Fc fragment of IgG.
   (4) *S aureus* is primarily transmitted via the airborne route.

220. Correct statements concerning bacteria of the genus *Neisseria* include the following:
 (1) They are gram-negative diplococci.
 (2) They produce IgA protease as a virulence factor.
 (3) They are oxidase-positive.
 (4) They grow best under anaerobic conditions.

221. Correct statements concerning gram-negative rods include the following:
 (1) *Haemophilus influenzae,* which requires hemin and NAD for growth, is an important pathogen but produces no exotoxins.
 (2) *Bordetella pertussis* produces an exotoxin that stimulates adenylate cyclase, which causes diarrhea.
 (3) *Pseudomonas aeruginosa,* a major cause of hospital-acquired infections, is found primarily in water sources.
 (4) *Legionella pneumophila* causes pneumonia by producing an exotoxin that inhibits adenylate cyclase.

222. Correct statements concerning *Corynebacterium diphtheriae* include the following:
 (1) *C diphtheriae* is an anaerobic, spore-forming, gram-positive rod.
 (2) *C diphtheriae* produces an exotoxin that inhibits protein synthesis.
 (3) Delayed hypersensitivity and granuloma formation are important host defenses against *C diphtheriae*.
 (4) A toxoid vaccine is effective in preventing diphtheria.

223. Correct statements concerning *Streptococcus faecalis* include the following:
 (1) *S faecalis* contains lipid A, which is known to cause fever.
 (2) An effective vaccine containing capsular polysaccharide is available.
 (3) A 4-fold rise in complement-fixing antibody is an important diagnostic criterion.
 (4) *S faecalis* can grow in media containing an NaCl concentration higher than isotonic.

224. Correct statements concerning *Klebsiella pneumoniae* include the following:
 (1) *K pneumoniae* contains lipid A, which is known to cause fever.
 (2) A skin test is available to detect prior exposure to *K pneumoniae*.
 (3) An important virulence factor is the polysaccharide capsule of *K pneumoniae*.
 (4) *K pneumoniae* is an oxidase-positive, gram-negative coccus.

225. Correct statements concerning *Legionella pneumophila* include the following:
 (1) It is part of the normal flora of the colon.
 (2) It cannot be grown on laboratory media.
 (3) It does not have a cell wall.
 (4) It is an important cause of infection in renal transplant patients.

226. Correct statements concerning wound infections caused by *Clostridium perfringens* include the following:
 (1) An exotoxin plays a role in pathogenesis.
 (2) Gas is frequently found in the damaged tissues.
 (3) Anaerobic culture of the wound site should be performed.
 (4) *C perfringens* grows only in human cell culture.

227. Correct statements concerning infection with *Chlamydia psittaci* include the following:
 (1) *C psittaci* can be isolated from sputum by growth on blood agar.
 (2) The infection is more readily diagnosed by isolating the organism than by performing serologic tests.
 (3) *C psittaci* is often transmitted to humans by the bite of an arthropod.
 (4) The infection is more commonly acquired from a nonhuman source than from another person.

228. Correct statements concerning *Chlamydia trachomatis* include the following:
 (1) It causes chronic eye infections and can lead to serious impairment of vision.
 (2) It causes pneumonia, mainly in small children.
 (3) It is a common cause of sexually transmitted disease.
 (4) It can be transmitted from an infected mother to her newborn child during birth.

229. Ticks are vectors for the transmission of which of the following diseases?
 (1) Rocky Mountain spotted fever
 (2) tularemia
 (3) Lyme disease
 (4) epidemic typhus

230. Which of the following illnesses in NOT transmitted by an insect vector?
 (1) plague
 (2) Q fever

      (3) yellow fever

      (4) brucellosis

231. The Weil-Felix test is helpful in the diagnosis of which of the following conditions?

      (1) Rocky Mountain spotted fever

      (2) Lyme disease

      (3) epidemic typhus

      (4) Q fever

232. Correct statements concerning *Chlamydia psittaci* include the following:

      (1) It is often transmitted from an infected person to contacts.

      (2) It causes eye infections in neonates.

      (3) It is a common cause of sexually transmitted diseases in humans.

      (4) It infects humans most commonly by the respiratory route.

233. Humans are the only reservoir of infection for which of the following pathogens?

      (1) *Salmonella enteritidis*

      (2) *Shigella sonnei*

      (3) *Campylobacter jejuni*

      (4) *Salmonella typhi*

234. Correct statements concerning the VDRL test include the following:

      (1) A positive VDRL test should be followed by a fluorescent treponemal antibody-absorption (FTA-ABS) test.

      (2) A positive test confirms that the patient is or has been infected with *T pallidum*.

      (3) The VDRL test is usually positive in secondary syphilis.

      (4) The treponemal antigen used in the VDRL test is derived from a nonpathogenic strain (Reiter's strain).

235. Correct statements concerning chlamydiae include the following:

      (1) They possess bacterial-sized ribosomes.

      (2) They have a cell wall.

      (3) They contain both DNA and RNA.

      (4) They can synthesize sufficient ATP for cell growth.

236. Correct statements concerning pneumonia caused by *Mycoplasma pneumoniae* include the following:

      (1) The disease is associated with a rise in cold agglutinins.

      (2) The disease is effectively treated with erythromycin.

      (3) The disease is one of the "atypical" pneumonias.

      (4) The organism cannot be cultured in vitro because it has no cell wall.

237. Correct statements concerning rickettsiae include the following:

      (1) Diagnosis depends on growth in cell cultures treated with formaldehyde.

      (2) Because rickettsiae possess a cell wall, penicillin is the drug of choice.

      (3) Rickettsiae are usually transmitted via aerosol from their soil habitat.

      (4) Rickettsiae tend to multiply in endothelial cells of small blood vessels.

238. Correct statements concerning infections transmitted by the bite of an arthropod vector include the following:

      (1) Yellow fever is transmitted by the bite of the female *Aedes* mosquito.

      (2) Rocky Mountain spotted fever is transmitted by the bite of a tick.

      (3) Plague is transmitted by the bite of the rat flea.

      (4) Q fever is transmitted by the bite of a human body louse.

239. Correct statements concerning bacteria in the family Enterobacteriaceae include the following:

      (1) Salmonellae and shigellae are members of the Enterobacteriaceae.

      (2) Members of the Enterobacteriaceae are oxidase-positive but do not ferment glucose.

      (3) Members of the Enterobacteriaceae are the majority of gram-negative rods isolated in hospitals.

      (4) Members of the Enterobacteriaceae are nonlactose fermenters.

240. Members of the family Enterobacteriaceae include

      (1) *Escherichia coli*

      (2) *Vibrio cholerae*

      (3) *Klebsiella pneumoniae*

      (4) *Pseudomonas aeruginosa*

Answers (Questions 185–240):

185 (A)	193 (B)	201 (D)	209 (E)	217 (E)	225 (D)	233 (C)
186 (C)	194 (A)	202 (A)	210 (A)	218 (D)	226 (A)	234 (B)
187 (B)	195 (E)	203 (E)	211 (C)	219 (A)	227 (D)	235 (A)
188 (D)	196 (A)	204 (B)	212 (D)	220 (A)	228 (E)	236 (A)
189 (A)	197 (C)	205 (C)	213 (D)	221 (B)	229 (A)	237 (D)
190 (A)	198 (C)	206 (A)	214 (A)	222 (C)	230 (C)	238 (A)
191 (C)	199 (D)	207 (C)	215 (D)	223 (D)	231 (B)	239 (B)
192 (A)	200 (A)	208 (A)	216 (A)	224 (B)	232 (D)	240 (B)

BASIC VIROLOGY

Directions (Questions 241–258): Select the ONE lettered answer that is BEST in each question.

241. Viruses enter cells by adsorbing to specific sites on the outer membranes of cells. Each of the following statements is correct EXCEPT
(A) The interaction determines the specific target organs for infection.
(B) The interaction determines whether the purified genome of a virus is infectious.
(C) The interaction can be prevented by neutralizing antibody.
(D) If the sites are occupied, interference with virus infection occurs.

242. Many viruses mature by budding through the outer membrane of the host cell. Each of the following statements regarding these viruses is correct EXCEPT
(A) Some of these viruses enhance multinucleated giant cell formation.
(B) Some new viral antigens appear on the surface of the host cell.
(C) Some of these viruses contain host cell lipids.
(D) Some of these viruses do not have an envelope.

243. Biochemical analysis of a virus reveals the genome to be composed of 4 unequally sized pieces of single-stranded RNA, each of which is complementary to viral mRNA in infected cells. Which one of the following statements is UNLIKELY to be correct?
(A) Different proteins are encoded by each segment of the viral genome.
(B) The virus particle contains a virus-encoded enzyme that can copy the genome into its complement.
(C) Purified RNA extracted from the virus particle is infectious.
(D) The virus can undergo high-frequency recombination via reassortment of its RNA segments.

244. Latency is an outcome particularly characteristic of which one of the following virus groups?
(A) polioviruses
(B) herpesviruses
(C) rhinoviruses
(D) influenza viruses

245. Each of the following statements concerning viral serotypes is correct EXCEPT
(A) In naked nucleocapsid viruses, the serotype is usually determined by the outer capsid proteins.
(B) In enveloped viruses, the serotype is usually determined by the outer envelope proteins, especially the spike proteins.
(C) Some viruses have multiple serotypes.
(D) Some viruses have an RNA polymerase that determines the serotype.

246. The ability of a virus to produce disease can result from a variety of mechanisms. Which one of the following is LEAST likely?
(A) cytopathic effect in infected cells

    (B) malignant transformation of infected cells

    (C) immune response to virus-induced antigens on the surfaces of the infected cells

    (D) production of an exotoxin that activates adenylate cyclase

247. Which one of the following forms of immunity to viruses would be LEAST likely to be lifelong?

    (A) passive immunity

    (B) passive-active immunity

    (C) active immunity

    (D) cell-mediated immunity

248. Which one of the following statements concerning interferons is LEAST accurate?

    (A) Interferons are proteins that influence cell metabolism in many ways, one of which is the induction of an antiviral state.

    (B) Interferons are synthesized only by virus-infected cells.

    (C) Interferons inhibit a broad range of viruses, not just the virus that induced the interferon.

    (D) Synthesis of several host enzymes is induced by interferon in target cells.

249. You have isolated a virus from the stool of a patient with diarrhea and shown that its genome is composed of multiple pieces of double-stranded RNA. Which one of the following is UNLIKELY to be true?

    (A) Each piece of RNA encodes a different protein.

    (B) The virus encodes an RNA-templated RNA polymerase.

    (C) The virion contains an RNA polymerase.

    (D) The genome is integrated into the host chromosome.

250. A temperate bacteriophage has been induced from a new pathogenic strain of *Escherichia coli* that produces a toxin. Which one of the following is the MOST reasonable way to show that the phage encodes the toxin?

    (A) Carry out conjugation of the pathogenic strain with a nonpathogenic strain.

    (B) Infect an experimental animal with the phage.

    (C) Lysogenize a nonpathogenic strain with the phage.

    (D) Look for transposable elements in the phage DNA.

251. Each of the following statements concerning retrovirus is correct EXCEPT

    (A) The virus particle carries an RNA-directed DNA polymerase encoded by the viral genome.

    (B) The viral genome consists of 3 segments of double-stranded RNA.

    (C) The virion is enveloped and enters cells via an interaction with specific receptors on the host cells.

    (D) During infection, the virus synthesizes a DNA copy of its RNA, and this DNA becomes covalently integrated into host cell DNA.

252. A stock of virus particles has been found by electron microscopy to contain 10^8 particles/mL, but a plaque assay reveals only 10^5 plaque-forming units/mL. What is the BEST interpretation of these results?

    (A) A nonpermissive cell line was used for the plaque assay.

    (B) Several kinds of viruses were present in the stock.

    (C) Only one particle in 1000 is infectious.

    (D) The virus is a mutant.

253. Reasonable mechanisms for viral persistence in infected individuals include all of the following EXCEPT

    (A) generation of defective-interfering particles

    (B) virus-mediated inhibition of host DNA synthesis

    (C) integration of a provirus into the genome of the host

    (D) host tolerance to viral antigens

254. Each of the following statements concerning viral surface proteins is correct EXCEPT

    (A) They elicit antibody that neutralizes the infectivity of the virus.

    (B) They determine the species specificity of the virus-cell interaction.

    (C) They participate in active transport of nutrients across the viral envelope membrane.

    (D) They protect the genetic material against nucleases.

255. Each of the following statements concerning viral vaccines is correct EXCEPT

    (A) In live attenuated vaccines, the virus has lost its ability to cause disease but has retained its ability to induce neutralizing antibody.

    (B) In live, attenuated vaccines, the possibility of reversion to virulence is of concern.

    (C) With inactivated vaccines, IgA mucosal immunity is usually induced.

    (D) With inactivated vaccines, protective immunity is due mainly to the production of IgG.
256. The major barrier to the control of viral upper respiratory infections by immunization is
    (A) poor local and systemic immune response to these pathogens
    (B) the number and antigenic diversity of the viruses
    (C) side effects of the vaccine
    (D) inability to grow the virus in cell culture
257. The feature of the influenza virus genome that contributes MOST to the antigenic variation of the virus is
    (A) a high G + C content, which augments binding to nucleoproteins
    (B) inverted repeat regions, which create ''sticky ends''
    (C) segmented nucleic acid
    (D) unique methylated bases
258. What is the BEST explanation for the selective action of acyclovir (acycloguanosine) in herpes simplex virus-infected cells?
    (A) Acyclovir binds specifically to herpesvirus receptors on the infected cell surface.
    (B) Viral phosphokinase phosphorylates acyclovir more effectively than does the host cell phosphokinase.
    (C) Acyclovir inhibits the RNA polymerase in the virus particle.
    (D) Acyclovir blocks the matrix protein of the virus, thereby preventing release by budding.

Answers (Questions 241–258):

241 (B)	246 (D)	251 (B)	256 (B)
242 (D)	247 (A)	252 (C)	257 (C)
243 (C)	248 (B)	253 (B)	258 (B)
244 (B)	249 (D)	254 (C)	
245 (D)	250 (C)	255 (C)	

Directions (Questions 259–272): Select the ONE lettered heading that is MOST closely associated with the numbered phrases or statements.

Questions 259–262

    (A) DNA enveloped virus
    (B) DNA nonenveloped virus
    (C) RNA enveloped virus
    (D) RNA nonenveloped virus
    (E) Viroid
259. Herpes simplex virus
260. Human T cell leukemia virus
261. Human papillomavirus
262. Rotavirus

Questions 263–267

    (A) Attachment and penetration of virion
    (B) Viral mRNA synthesis
    (C) Viral protein synthesis
    (D) Viral genome DNA synthesis
    (E) Assembly and release of progeny virus
263. Main site of action of acyclovir
264. Main site of action of amantadine
265. Function of virion polymerase of influenza virus
266. Main site of action of antiviral antibody
267. Step at which budding occurs

Questions 268–272

(A) Poliovirus
(B) Epstein-Barr virus
(C) Agent of scrapie and kuru
(D) Hepatitis B virus
(E) Respiratory syncytial virus

268. Part of the genome DNA is synthesized by the virion polymerase.
269. Translation product of viral mRNA is a polyprotein that is cleaved to form virion structural proteins.
270. It is remarkably resistant to UV light.
271. It causes latent infection of B cells.
272. It carries a fusion protein on the surface of the virion envelope.

Answers (Questions 259–272):

259 (A)   264 (A)   269 (A)
260 (C)   265 (B)   270 (C)
261 (B)   266 (A)   271 (B)
262 (D)   267 (E)   272 (E)
263 (D)   268 (D)

Directions (Questions 273–296):   For each numbered item, select

A if the item is associated with (A) only
B if the item is associated with (B) only
C if the item is associated with both (A) and (B)
D if the item is associated with neither (A) nor (B)

Questions 273–276

(A) Measles virus
(B) Rubella virus
(C) Both
(D) Neither

273. Enveloped RNA virus
274. Virion contains an RNA polymerase
275. Multiple antigenic types
276. Transmitted by respiratory aerosol

Questions 277–281

(A) Hepatitis A virus
(B) Hepatitis B virus
(C) Both
(D) Neither

277. Enveloped RNA virus
278. Contains virion polymerase
279. Multiple antigenic types that result in multiple episodes of disease
280. Establishes chronic infection
281. Associated with tumors in humans

Questions 282–287

(A) Influenza virus
(B) Rabies virus
(C) Both
(D) Neither

282. Enveloped RNA virus
283. Contains virion polymerase

284. Multiple antigenic types
285. Segmented genome
286. Killed vaccine available
287. Hemagglutinin and neuraminidase are surface proteins

Questions 288–292
    (A) Poliovirus
    (B) Rhinovirus
    (C) Both
    (D) Neither
288. Enveloped RNA virus
289. Multiple antigenic types
290. Contains virion polymerase
291. Replicates in the small intestine
292. Replicates well at lower than body temperature

Questions 293–296
    (A) Cytomegalovirus
    (B) Adenovirus
    (C) Both
    (D) Neither
293. Enveloped DNA virus
294. Contains virion polymerase
295. Segmented genome
296. Transmitted across the placenta

Answers (Questions 273–296):

273 (C)	278 (B)	283 (C)	288 (D)	293 (A)
274 (A)	279 (D)	284 (A)	289 (C)	294 (D)
275 (D)	280 (B)	285 (A)	290 (D)	295 (D)
276 (C)	281 (B)	286 (C)	291 (A)	296 (A)
277 (D)	282 (C)	287 (A)	292 (B)	

Directions (Questions 297–308): For each question, ONE or MORE of the numbered options is correct. Select
A if only 1, 2, and 3 are correct
B if only 1 and 3 are correct
C if only 2 and 4 are correct
D if only 4 is correct
E if all are correct

297. Correct statements concerning interferon include the following:
    (1) Interferon inhibits the growth of many different viruses.
    (2) Interferon can be induced by double-stranded RNA.
    (3) Interferon made by cells of one species acts more effectively in the cells of that species than in the cells of other species.
    (4) Interferon acts by preventing viruses from entering the cell.

298. Correct statements concerning the viruses that infect humans include the following:
    (1) The ratio of physical particles to infectious particles is greater than one.
    (2) The purified nucleic acid of some viruses is infectious but at a lower efficiency than that of the intact virions.
    (3) Some viruses contain lipoprotein envelopes derived from the plasma membrane of the host cell.
    (4) The nucleic acid of some viruses is single-stranded DNA, whereas the nucleic acid of others is double-stranded RNA.

299. Correct statements about virion structure and assembly include the following:
    (1) Most viruses acquire surface glycoproteins by budding through the nuclear membrane.

(2) Helical nucleocapsids are found primarily in DNA viruses.

(3) The symmetry of virus particles prevents inclusion of any nonstructural proteins such as enzymes.

(4) Enveloped viruses use a matrix protein to mediate interactions between viral glycoproteins in the plasma membrane and structural proteins in the nucleocapsid.

300. Correct statements concerning viruses include the following:

(1) Viruses can reproduce only within cells.

(2) The proteins on the surface of the virus mediate the entry of the virus into host cells.

(3) Neutralizing antibody is directed against proteins on the surface of the virus.

(4) Viruses replicate by binary fission.

301. Viruses are obligate intracellular parasites. Correct statements concerning this fact include the following:

(1) Viruses cannot generate energy outside cells.

(2) Viruses cannot synthesize proteins outside cells.

(3) Enveloped viruses require host cell membranes to obtain their envelopes.

(4) Viruses must degrade host cell DNA to obtain nucleotides.

302. Correct statements concerning lysogeny include the following:

(1) Viral genes responsible for lysis are repressed.

(2) Viral DNA is integrated into bacterial DNA.

(3) Replication of a second bacteriophage of the same type does not occur within the lysogenic cell.

(4) Viral genes replicate independently of bacterial genes.

303. Viruses that possess an outer envelope of lipoprotein include

(1) varicella-zoster virus

(2) papillomavirus

(3) influenza virus

(4) poliovirus

304. Viruses that possess a genome of single-strand RNA that is infectious include

(1) influenza virus

(2) rotavirus

(3) measles virus

(4) poliovirus

305. Viruses that possess an RNA polymerase in the virion include

(1) hepatitis A virus

(2) smallpox virus

(3) adenovirus

(4) rotavirus

306. Viruses that possess a DNA polymerase in the virion include

(1) human immunodeficiency virus

(2) Epstein-Barr virus

(3) hepatitis B virus

(4) papillomavirus

307. Viruses that possess a double-stranded nucleic acid as their genome include

(1) herpes simplex virus

(2) rotavirus

(3) adenovirus

(4) parvoviruses

308. Viroids

(1) are defective viruses that are missing the DNA coding for the matrix protein.

(2) consist of RNA without a protein or lipoprotein outer coat.

(3) cause tumors in experimental animals.

(4) can replicate only within cells.

Answers (Questions 297–308):

297 (A)	300 (A)	303 (B)	306 (B)
298 (E)	301 (A)	304 (D)	307 (A)
299 (D)	302 (A)	305 (C)	308 (C)

Directions (Questions 309–350):   Select the ONE lettered answer that is BEST in each question.

309. Which of the following outcomes is MOST common following a primary herpesvirus infection?
(A) complete eradication of virus and virus-infected cells
(B) persistent asymptomatic viremia
(C) establishment of latent infection
(D) persistent cytopathic effect in infected cells

310. Each of the following pathogens is likely to establish chronic or latent infection EXCEPT
(A) cytomegalovirus
(B) hepatitis A virus
(C) hepatitis B virus
(D) herpes simplex virus

311. Each of the following statements regarding poliovirus and its vaccine is correct EXCEPT
(A) Poliovirus is transmitted by the fecal-oral route.
(B) Poliovirus reaches the spinal cord by migrating up motor axons.
(C) The live attenuated vaccine, which contains 3 serotypes, is recommended for use in children.
(D) An unimmunized adult traveling to developing countries should receive the inactivated vaccine.

312. Which one of the following strategies is MOST likely to induce lasting intestinal mucosal immunity to poliovirus?
(A) parenteral (intramuscular) vaccination with inactivated vaccine
(B) oral administration of poliovirus immune globulin
(C) parenteral vaccination with live vaccine
(D) oral vaccination with live vaccine

313. Each of the following clinical syndromes is associated with infection by picornaviruses EXCEPT
(A) myocarditis/pericarditis
(B) hepatitis
(C) mononucleosis
(D) meningitis

314. Which of the following statements concerning rubella vaccine is LEAST accurate?
(A) The vaccine prevents reinfection, thereby limiting the spread of virulent virus.
(B) Because the rash of rubella is so typical, a history of rubella is sufficient to advise the patient that the vaccine is unnecessary.
(C) The vaccine induces antibodies that prevent dissemination of the virus by neutralizing it during the viremic stage.
(D) The incidence of both childhood rubella and congenital rubella syndrome has decreased significantly since the advent of the vaccine.

315. Each of the following statements concerning the rabies vaccine for use in humans is correct EXCEPT
(A) The vaccine contains live attenuated rabies virus.
(B) If your patient is bitten by a wild animal, eg, a skunk, postexposure prophylaxis should be given.
(C) When the vaccine is used for postexposure prophylaxis, rabies immune globulin should also be given.
(D) The virus in the vaccine is grown in human cell cultures, thus decreasing the risk of allergic encephalomyelitis.

316. Each of the following statements concerning influenza is correct EXCEPT
(A) Major epidemics of influenza are caused by influenza A viruses rather than influenza B and C viruses.
(B) Likely sources of new antigens for influenza A viruses are the viruses that cause influenza in animals.

(C) Major antigenic changes (shifts) of viral surface proteins are seen primarily in influenza A viruses rather than in types B and C.

(D) The antigenic changes that occur with antigenic drift are due to the reassortment of the multiple pieces of the influenza genome.

317. Each of the following statements concerning the prevention and treatment of influenza is correct EXCEPT

(A) As with all live vaccines, the influenza vaccine should not be given to pregnant women.

(B) Booster doses of the vaccine are recommended because the duration of immunity is only a few years.

(C) Amantadine is an effective prophylactic drug only against influenza A viruses.

(D) The major antigen in the vaccine is the hemagglutinin.

318. A 6-month-old child develops a persistent cough and a fever. Physical examination and chest x-ray suggest pneumonia. Which one of the following organisms is LEAST likely to cause this infection?

(A) respiratory syncytial virus

(B) adenovirus

(C) parainfluenza virus

(D) rotavirus

319. A 45-year-old male was attacked by a bobcat and bitten repeatedly about the face and neck. The animal was shot by a companion and brought back to the public health authorities. Once you decide to immunize against rabies virus, how would you proceed?

(A) Use hyperimmune serum only.

(B) Use active immunization only.

(C) Use hyperimmune serum and active immunization.

(D) Use hyperimmune serum and follow this with active immunization only if adequate antibody titers are not obtained in the patient's serum.

320. Each statement concerning mumps virus and its disease is correct EXCEPT

(A) Mumps virus is a paramyxovirus and hence has a single-stranded RNA genome.

(B) Meningitis is a recognized complication of mumps.

(C) Mumps orchitis in children prior to puberty presents a significant threat of sterility.

(D) In mumps, the virus is spread through the bloodstream (viremia) to various internal organs.

321. Which of the following statements concerning respiratory syncytial virus is the MOST accurate?

(A) Respiratory syncytial virus has a double-stranded DNA genome.

(B) Respiratory syncytial virus is a nonenveloped virus.

(C) Respiratory syncytial virus causes pneumonia primarily in children.

(D) Respiratory syncytial virus has both a hemagglutinin and a neuraminidase.

322. The principal reservoir for the antigenic shift variants of influenza virus appears to be

(A) people in isolated communities such as the Arctic

(B) Animals, specifically pigs, horses, and fowl

(C) soil, especially in the tropics

(D) sewage

323. The role of an infectious agent in the pathogenesis of kuru was BEST demonstrated by which one of the following observations?

(A) A 16-fold rise in antibody titer to the agent was observed.

(B) The viral genome was isolated from infected neurons.

(C) Electron micrographs of the brains of infected individuals regularly demonstrated intracellular masses of structures resembling paramyxovirus nucleocapsids.

(D) The disease was serially transmitted to experimental animals.

324. A 64-year-old man with chronic lymphatic leukemia develops progressive deterioration of mental and neuromuscular function. At autopsy the brain shows enlarged oligodendrocytes, the nuclei of which contain naked, icosahedral virus particles. The MOST likely diagnosis is

(A) herpes encephalitis

(B) Creutzfeldt-Jakob disease

(C) subacute sclerosing panencephalitis

(D) progressive multifocal leukoencephalopathy

(E) rabies

325. A 20-year-old man, who for many years had received daily injections of growth hormone prepared from human pituitary glands, develops ataxia, slurred speech, and dementia. At autopsy the brain shows widespread neuronal degeneration, a spongy appearance due to many vacuoles between the cells, no inflammation, and no evidence of virus particles. Mice injected with homogenized brain tissue develop a similar disease after 6 months. The MOST likely diagnosis is
(A) herpes encephalitis
(B) Creutzfeldt-Jakob disease
(C) subacute sclerosing panencephalitis
(D) progressive multifocal leukoencephalopathy
(E) rabies

326. A 24-year-old woman has had fever and a sore throat for the past week. Moderately severe pharyngitis and bilateral cervical lymphadenopathy are seen on physical examination. Which one of the following viruses is LEAST likely to cause this picture?
(A) varicella-zoster virus
(B) herpes simplex virus type 1
(C) coxsackievirus
(D) Epstein-Barr virus

327. Scrapie and kuru possess all of the following characteristics EXCEPT
(A) histologic picture of spongiform encephalopathy
(B) transmissibility to animals, with a long incubation period
(C) slowly progressive deterioration of brain function
(D) prominent intranuclear inclusions in oligodendrocytes

328. The following features are characteristic of subacute sclerosing panencephalitis (SSPE) EXCEPT
(A) Immunosuppression is a frequent predisposing factor.
(B) Aggregates of helical nucleocapsids are found in infected cells.
(C) High titers of measles antibody are found in the cerebrospinal fluid.
(D) Slowly progressive deterioration of brain function occurs.

329. The major route of transmission for influenza virus is
(A) inhalation of infectious aerosols
(B) contact with infectious material on hands and environmental surfaces
(C) blood transfusion
(D) sexual transmission

330. Of the following illnesses, which one is the MOST common result of adenovirus infection?
(A) meningitis
(B) croup
(C) urethritis
(D) pharyngitis

331. Which of the following illnesses is MOST often caused by respiratory syncytial virus?
(A) pneumonia in young adults
(B) bronchiolitis and pneumonia in infants
(C) pharyngitis and tonsillitis in all age groups
(D) epiglottitis

332. The slow virus disease that MOST clearly has immunosuppression as an important factor in its pathogenesis is
(A) progressive multifocal leukoencephalopathy
(B) subacute sclerosing panencephalitis
(C) Creutzfeldt-Jakob disease
(D) scrapie

333. A 30-year-old man develops fever and jaundice. He consults a physician, who finds that blood tests for HBs antigen and anti-HBs antibody are negative. Which one of the following additional tests is MOST likely to reveal that the hepatitis was indeed due to hepatitis B virus?
(A) HBe antigen
(B) anti-HBc antibody
(C) anti-HBe antibody
(D) delta antigen

334. Which one of the following is the MOST reasonable explanation for the ability of hepatitis B virus to cause chronic infection?
    (A) Infection does not elicit the production of antibody.
    (B) The liver is an "immunologically sheltered" site.
    (C) Viral DNA may become integrated into the chromosomal DNA of the host cell.
    (D) Many humans are immunologically tolerant to HBs antigen.

335. The routine screening of transfused blood for HBs antigen has not eliminated the problem of posttransfusion hepatitis. Which of the following statements is MOST likely to be the explanation?
    (A) Most posttransfusion hepatitis is caused by hepatitis A virus.
    (B) Most posttransfusion hepatitis is caused by non-A, non-B viruses.
    (C) Many chronic carriers of hepatitis B virus do not have HBs antigen in their blood.
    (D) The present tests for HBs antigen are not sufficiently sensitive to detect many units of contaminated blood.

336. A 35-year-old man addicted to the use of intravenous drugs has been a carrier of HBs antigen for 10 years. He suddenly develops acute fulminant hepatitis and dies within 10 days. Which one of the following laboratory tests would contribute MOST to a diagnosis?
    (A) anti-HBs antibody
    (B) HBe antigen
    (C) anti-HBc antibody
    (D) anti-delta agent antibody

337. Which one of the following is the BEST evidence on which to base a decisive diagnosis of acute mumps disease?
    (A) a positive skin test
    (B) a 4-fold rise in antibody titer to mumps surface antigen
    (C) a history of exposure to a child with mumps
    (D) orchitis in a young adult male

338. Varicella-zoster virus and herpes simplex virus share many characteristics. Which one of the following characteristics is LEAST likely to be shared?
    (A) Inapparent disease, manifested only by virus shedding, is common.
    (B) Latent virus frequently persists after recovery from acute disease.
    (C) The viruses cause a vesicular rash.
    (D) The genome is linear double-stranded DNA.

339. Herpes simplex virus and cytomegalovirus share many features. Which one of the following features is LEAST likely to be shared?
    (A) The virus is an important cause of morbidity and mortality in the newborn.
    (B) The virus frequently crosses the placenta and infects the fetus in utero.
    (C) The virus is an important cause of serious disease in immunosuppressed individuals.
    (D) Infection is often mild or inapparent.

340. Eradication of smallpox was facilitated by several features of the virus. Which one of the following LEAST contributed to eradication?
    (A) The virus has one antigenic type.
    (B) Inapparent infection is rare.
    (C) Administration of live vaccine reliably induces immunity.
    (D) The virus multiplies in the cytoplasm of infected cells.

341. According to present knowledge, which one of these statements concerning infectious mononucleosis is the MOST accurate?
    (A) Epstein-Barr virus capsid antigen induces the heterophil antibody.
    (B) Infected T lymphocytes are abundant in peripheral blood.
    (C) Isolation of the virus is necessary to confirm diagnosis.
    (D) Infectious mononucleosis is transmitted by the virus in saliva.

342. Which one of the following statements about genital herpes is the LEAST accurate?
    (A) Acyclovir reduces the appearance of recurrent disease episodes by eradicating latently infected cells.
    (B) Genital herpes can be transmitted in the absence of apparent lesions.
    (C) Multinucleated giant cells with intranuclear inclusions are found in the lesions.
    (D) Initial disease episodes are generally more severe than recurrent episodes.

343. The influenza vaccine currently in use in the USA is
    (A) an inactivated vaccine consisting of formaldehyde-treated influenza virions, which primarily induce antibody to hemagglutinin

(B) a live attenuated vaccine prepared from a variant of equine influenza virus

(C) a vaccine consisting of highly purified peptide fragments of the hemagglutinin and neuraminidase glycoproteins

(D) a live attenuated vaccine composed of the current influenza A, B, and C isolates

344. Which one of the following is the MOST severe lower respiratory pathogen in infants?

(A) respiratory syncytial virus

(B) adenoviruses

(C) rhinoviruses

(D) coxsackievirus

345. Antigenic drift of influenza virus is MOST probably due to

(A) phenotypic mixing

(B) point mutation

(C) transposition

(D) neuraminidase

346. Which one of the following conditions is LEAST likely to be caused by adenoviruses?

(A) conjunctivitis

(B) pneumonia

(C) pharyngitis

(D) glomerulonephritis

347. Regarding the serologic diagnosis of infectious mononucleosis, which one of the following is correct?

(A) A heterophil antibody is formed that reacts with a capsid protein of Epstein-Barr virus.

(B) A heterophil antibody is formed that agglutinates sheep or horse red blood cells.

(C) A heterophil antigen occurs that cross-reacts with *Proteus* OX19 strains.

(D) A heterophil antigen occurs following infection with cytomegalovirus.

348. Which one of the following statements about the *src* gene of Rous sarcoma virus is INCORRECT?

(A) The *src* protein is found in the nucleus.

(B) The *src* protein catalyzes phosphotransfer from ATP to tyrosine residues in protein.

(C) The *src* protein is required to maintain neoplastic transformation of infected cells.

(D) The viral *src* gene is derived from a cellular gene found in all vertebrate species.

349. Each of the following statements supports the idea that cellular proto-oncogenes participate in human carcinogenesis EXCEPT

(A) The *c-abl* gene is rearranged on the Philadelphia chromosome in myeloid leukemias and encodes a protein with heightened tyrosine kinase activity.

(B) The N-*myc* gene is amplified as much as 100-fold in many advanced cases of neuroblastomas.

(C) The receptor for platelet-derived growth factor (PDGF) is a transmembrane protein that exhibits tyrosine kinase activity.

(D) The c-Ha-*ras* gene is mutated at specific codons in several types of human cancer.

350. Herpes simplex type 1 is distinct from type 2 in several different ways. Which one of the following is the LEAST accurate statement?

(A) Type 1 causes lesions above the umbilicus more frequently than type 2.

(B) Infection by type 1 is not associated with any tumors in humans.

(C) Antiserum to type 1 neutralizes type 1 virus much more effectively than type 2 virus.

(D) Type 1 causes frequent recurrences, whereas type 2 rarely recurs.

Answers (Questions 309–350):

309 (C)	316 (D)	323 (D)	330 (D)	337 (B)	344 (A)
310 (B)	317 (A)	324 (D)	331 (B)	338 (A)	345 (B)
311 (B)	318 (D)	325 (B)	332 (A)	339 (A)	346 (D)
312 (D)	319 (C)	326 (A)	333 (B)	340 (D)	347 (B)
313 (C)	320 (C)	327 (D)	334 (C)	341 (D)	348 (A)
314 (B)	321 (C)	328 (A)	335 (B)	342 (A)	349 (C)
315 (A)	322 (B)	329 (A)	336 (D)	343 (A)	350 (D)

Directions (Questions 351–364): Select the ONE lettered heading that is MOST CLOSELY associated with numbered phrases or statements.

Questions 351–354:
    (A) Yellow fever virus
    (B) Rabies virus
    (C) Rotavirus
    (D) Rubella virus
    (E) Rhinovirus
351. Diarrhea
352. Jaundice
353. Congenital abnormalities
354. Encephalitis

Questions 355–359
    (A) Pneumonia
    (B) Meningitis
    (C) Orchitis
    (D) Shingles
    (E) Subacute sclerosing panencephalitis
355. Adenovirus
356. Measles virus
357. Respiratory syncytial virus
358. Coxsackievirus
359. Varicella-zoster virus

Questions 360–364
    (A) Adenovirus
    (B) Human papillomavirus
    (C) Rhinovirus
    (D) Coxsackievirus
    (E) Epstein-Barr virus
360. Causes myocarditis and pleurodynia
361. Grows better at 33 °C than at 37 °C
362. Causes tumors in laboratory rodents
363. Is implicated in carcinoma of the cervix
364. Causes infectious mononucleosis

Answers (Questions 351–364):

351 (C)	355 (A)	359 (D)	363 (B)
352 (A)	356 (E)	360 (D)	364 (E)
353 (D)	357 (A)	361 (C)	
354 (B)	358 (B)	362 (A)	

Directions (Questions 365–372): For each numbered item, select
    A if the item is associated with (A) ONLY
    B if the item is associated with (B) ONLY
    C if the item is associated with BOTH (A) AND (B)
    D if the item is associated with NEITHER (A) NOR (B)

Questions 365–368
    (A) Cytomegalovirus
    (B) Varicella-zoster (VZ) virus
    (C) Both
    (D) Neither

365. Most infections are mild or inapparent.

366. Immunocompromised individuals are at risk of severe, progressive infection.

367. Acyclovir is effective in disseminated infection.

368. The virus is a common cause of infection of the fetus in utero.

Questions 369–372

   (A) Variola (smallpox) virus
   (B) Cytomegalovirus
   (C) Both
   (D) Neither

369. RNA polymerase is present in the virus particle.

370. The virus persists in a latent state after an acute episode.

371. There is no animal reservoir or vector.

372. Use of the vaccine is currently recommended.

Answers (Questions 365–372)

365 (A)	368 (A)	371 (C)
366 (C)	369 (A)	372 (D)
367 (B)	370 (B)	

Directions (Questions 373–404):   For each question, ONE or MORE of the numbered options is correct. Select

   A if only 1, 2, AND 3 are correct
   B if only 1 AND 3 are correct
   C if only 2 AND 4 are correct
   D if only 4 is correct
   E if ALL are correct

373. Correct statements concerning the AIDS retrovirus, ie, human immunodeficiency virus (HIV), include the following:

   (1) Screening tests for antibodies are useful to prevent transmission of HIV through transfused blood.
   (2) HIV infection involves the CD4 receptor protein on the surface of helper T cells.
   (3) HIV has a special mechanism for control of expression of its genes, eg, the transactivation of transcription *(tat)* gene.
   (4) The presence of circulating antibodies that neutralize HIV is evidence that an individual is protected against HIV-induced disease.

374. Correct statements concerning viral meningitis and viral encephalitis include the following:

   (1) Herpes simplex virus type 2 is the leading cause of viral meningitis.
   (2) The spinal fluid protein is usually decreased in viral meningitis.
   (3) The diagnosis of viral meningitis can be made using the India ink stain on the spinal fluid.
   (4) Herpes simplex virus type 1 is an important cause of viral encephalitis.

375. Many of the oncogenic retroviruses carry oncogenes closely related to normal cellular genes. The latter are called proto-oncogenes. Correct statements concerning proto-oncogenes include the following:

   (1) Several proto-oncogenes have been found in mutant form in human cancers that lack evidence for viral etiology.
   (2) Several viral oncogenes and their progenitor proto-oncogenes encode protein kinases specific for tyrosine residues.
   (3) Some proto-oncogenes have been shown to encode cellular growth factors and receptors for growth factors.
   (4) Proto-oncogenes are closely related to transposable elements found in the chromosomes of plants, bacteria, yeasts, insects, and vertebrates.

376. Correct statements concerning human immunodeficiency virus include the following:
  (1) The CD4 protein on the T cell surface is the receptor for the virus.
  (2) There is appreciable antigenic diversity in the envelope glycoprotein of the virus.
  (3) One of the viral genes codes for a protein that augments the strength of the viral transcriptional promoter.
  (4) A major problem with testing for antibody to the virus is its cross-reactivity with human T-cell leukemia virus type I.

377. Correct statements concerning these viruses include the following:
  (1) Coxsackieviruses are enteroviruses and can replicate in both the respiratory and gastrointestinal tracts.
  (2) Influenza viruses have multiple serotypes based on hemagglutinin and neuraminidase proteins located on the envelope surface.
  (3) Flaviviruses are RNA enveloped viruses that replicate in animals as well as humans.
  (4) Adenoviruses are RNA enveloped viruses with a single serotype.

378. Correct statements concerning the prevention of viral disease include the following:
  (1) Adenovirus vaccine contains purified penton fibers and is usually given to children in conjunction with polio vaccine.
  (2) Coxsackievirus vaccine contains live virus, which induces IgA that prevents reinfection by homologous serotypes.
  (3) Flavivirus immunization consists of hyperimmune serum plus a vaccine consisting of subunits containing surface glycoprotein.
  (4) Influenza virus vaccine contains killed virus that induces neutralizing antibody directed against the hemagglutinin.

379. Correct statements concerning non-A, non-B and delta hepatitis viruses include:
  (1) Non-A, non-B viruses cause most of the posttransfusion hepatitis in the USA.
  (2) Delta agent is a defective virus with an RNA genome and a capsid composed of hepatitis B surface antigen.
  (3) Delta hepatitis causes a carrier state similar to that of hepatitis B.
  (4) Because a serologic test for two of the non-A, non-B viruses is now available, the frequency of hepatitis should decline.

380. Correct statements concerning measles virus and measles include the following:
  (1) Measles virus is an enveloped virus with a double-stranded DNA genome.
  (2) One of the important complications of measles is encephalitis.
  (3) Latent infection by measles virus can be explained by the integration of provirus into the host cell DNA.
  (4) The initial site of replication of measles virus is the upper respiratory tract, from which it spreads via the blood to the skin.

381. Correct statements concerning measles vaccine include the following:
  (1) Measles vaccine contains live attenuated virus.
  (2) Virus in measles vaccine contains the 3 most common serotypes.
  (3) Measles vaccine should not be given to children younger than 15 months of age, because maternal antibodies can prevent an immune response.
  (4) Measles vaccine should not be given in conjunction with other viral vaccines, because interference can occur.

382. Correct statements concerning rubella include the following:
  (1) Congenital abnormalities occur primarily when a pregnant woman is infected during the first trimester.
  (2) Women who say that they have never had rubella can, nevertheless, have neutralizing antibody in their sera.
  (3) In a 6-year-old child, rubella is a mild, self-limited disease with few complications.
  (4) Acyclovir is effective in the treatment of congenital rubella syndrome.

383. Correct statements concerning rabies virus and rabies include the following:
  (1) Rabies virus has a lipoprotein envelope and single-stranded RNA as its genome.
  (2) Rabies virus has a single antigenic type (serotype).
  (3) The incubation period of rabies is usually long (several weeks) rather than short (several days).
  (4) In the USA, dogs are the most common reservoir.

384. Correct statements concerning arboviruses include the following:
  (1) The pathogenesis of dengue hemorrhagic shock syndrome is associated with the heterotypic anamnestic response.

    (2) Wild birds are the reservoir for encephalitis viruses but not for yellow fever virus.

    (3) The extrinsic incubation period is the time during which the virus replicates in the vector.

    (4) There is a live attenuated vaccine that effectively prevents yellow fever.

385. Correct statements concerning rhinoviruses include the following:

    (1) Rhinoviruses are picornaviruses, ie, small, nonenveloped viruses with an RNA genome.

    (2) Rhinoviruses do not infect the gastrointestinal tract because they are sensitive to the low pH in the stomach.

    (3) A good reason why there is no vaccine against rhinoviruses is that there are too many antigenic types.

    (4) Rhinoviruses are an important cause of lower respiratory tract infections, especially in patients with chronic obstructive pulmonary disease.

386. Correct statements concerning these viruses include the following:

    (1) Adenoviruses cause encephalitis, especially in members of the armed forces.

    (2) Respiratory syncytial virus is a cause of lower respiratory tract infections in young children.

    (3) Coronaviruses are a cause of myocarditis and pericarditis in immunocompromised patients.

    (4) Parainfluenza viruses are a cause of croup in infants.

387. Correct statements concerning slow diseases of the central nervous system include the following:

    (1) The causative agents of some of these diseases are unconventional entities that are highly resistant to inactivation by ultraviolet irradiation.

    (2) The sheep disease called scrapie shares clinical and pathologic features with the human disorder called Creutzfeldt-Jakob disease.

    (3) Progressive multifocal leukoencephalopathy is a disorder clearly associated with a virus and occurs primarily in immunocompromised individuals.

    (4) Subacute sclerosing panencephalitis is a disorder clearly associated with measles virus.

388. Correct statements concerning herpes simplex virus type 2 include the following:

    (1) Natural infection with herpes simplex virus type 2 confers only partial immunity against a second primary infection.

    (2) Herpes simplex virus type 2 can cause malignant transformation of cultured cells.

    (3) Herpes simplex virus type 2 can cause virus-specific alterations of the cell membrane, leading to cell fusion and the formation of multinucleated giant cells.

    (4) Recurrent disease episodes due to reactivation of latent herpes simplex virus type 2 are usually more severe than the primary episode.

389. Correct statements concerning Epstein-Barr virus include the following:

    (1) Many infections are mild or inapparent.

    (2) Latently infected lymphocytes regularly persist following an acute episode of infection.

    (3) Infection confers immunity against reinfection.

    (4) The earlier in life primary infection is acquired, the more likely the typical picture of infectious mononucleosis will be manifest.

390. Correct statements regarding rotaviruses include the following:

    (1) A live attenuated vaccine is available.

    (2) Rotaviruses are a leading cause of diarrhea in young children.

    (3) Rotaviruses cause disease by activating adenylate cyclase.

    (4) Rotaviruses belong to the reovirus family, which have a double-stranded, segmented RNA genome.

391. A 65-year-old woman presents with vesicular lesions on her face. Which of the following viruses should be considered LIKELY etiologic agents?

    (1) Epstein-Barr virus

    (2) varicella-zoster virus

    (3) cytomegalovirus

    (4) herpes simplex virus type 1

392. Correct statements concerning the antigenicity of influenza A virus include the following:

    (1) Antigenic shifts, which represent major changes in antigenicity, occur infrequently and are due to the recombination (reassortment) of segments of the viral genome.

    (2) Antigenic shifts can affect both the hemagglutinin and the neuraminidase.

    (3) The worldwide epidemics caused by influenza A virus are due to antigenic shifts.

    (4) The protein involved in antigenic drift is primarily the internal ribonucleoprotein.

393. Correct statements concerning adenoviruses include the following:

    (1) Adenoviruses are composed of a single-stranded DNA genome and a capsid surrounded by an envelope.

    (2) Adenoviruses cause both sore throat and pneumonia.

    (3) There is one serologic type.

    (4) Adenoviruses are implicated as a cause of tumors in animals but not in humans.

394. Correct statements concerning rhinoviruses include the following:

    (1) Rhinoviruses are single-stranded RNA viruses without an envelope.

    (2) Vitamin C is effective in preventing the common cold caused by rhinoviruses.

    (3) Rhinoviruses have at least 80 serotypes.

    (4) Rhinoviruses are an important cause of viral pneumonia.

395. Correct statements concerning the prevention of viral respiratory tract disease include the following:

    (1) To prevent disease by adenoviruses, a live enteric-coated vaccine that causes asymptomatic enteric infection is used in the military.

    (2) To prevent disease caused by influenza A virus, an inactivated vaccine is available for the civilian population.

    (3) No vaccine against respiratory syncytial virus is available.

    (4) To prevent disease caused by rhinoviruses, a vaccine containing purified capsid proteins is used.

396. Correct statements concerning herpesvirus latency include the following:

    (1) Virus can be recovered from latently infected cells by cocultivation with susceptible cells.

    (2) Exogenous stimuli can result in reactivation of latent infection, with induction of symptomatic disease.

    (3) Episodes of herpesvirus reactivation are more frequent and more severe in patients with impaired cell-mediated immunity.

    (4) During latency, antiviral antibody is not demonstrable in the sera of infected individuals.

397. Correct statements concerning rhinoviruses include the following:

    (1) Rhinoviruses are one of the most frequent causes of the common cold.

    (2) Rhinoviruses grow better at 33 °C than at 37 °C and hence have a tendency to cause disease in the upper respiratory tract rather than the lower respiratory tract.

    (3) Rhinoviruses are members of the picornavirus family and hence resemble poliovirus in their structure and replication.

    (4) The immunity provided by the vaccine is excellent, as there is only one serotype.

398. Correct statements concerning Epstein-Barr virus infections include the following:

    (1) The treatment of choice is acyclovir.

    (2) An effective live attenuated vaccine is available.

    (3) The *Culex* mosquito is an important vector.

    (4) Diagnosis can be made by detecting a rise in titer of antibody against the capsid antigen.

399. Correct statements concerning poliovirus infection include the following:

    (1) Congenital infection of the fetus is an important complication.

    (2) A skin test is available to determine prior exposure to the virus.

    (3) Amantadine is an effective preventive agent.

    (4) The virus replicates extensively in the gastrointestinal tract.

400. Correct statements concerning yellow fever include the following:

    (1) Yellow fever virus is transmitted by the *Aedes aegypti* mosquito in the urban form of yellow fever.

    (2) Infection by yellow fever virus causes significant damage to hepatocytes.

    (3) Nonhuman primates in the jungle are a major reservoir of yellow fever virus.

    (4) Acyclovir is an effective treatment.

401. Correct statements concerning subacute sclerosing panencephalitis include the following:

    (1) Vaccination against measles virus has reduced the incidence of subacute sclerosing panencephalitis.

    (2) Patients with subacute sclerosing panencephalitis usually have a history of measles virus infection.

      (3) Measles virus can be recovered from infected neurons by cocultivation with permissive helper cells.

      (4) Maturation of measles virus in infected neurons fails as a result of defective matrix protein.

402. Correct statements concerning Norwalk virus and rotavirus include the following:

      (1) Norwalk virus and rotavirus cause a significant amount of gastroenteritis in the USA.

      (2) Norwalk virus and rotavirus are transmitted primarily by the fecal-oral route.

      (3) Norwalk virus and rotavirus can be seen in the electron microscope.

      (4) Norwalk virus and rotavirus cause a significant amount of pneumonia in neonates.

403. Correct statements concerning respiratory viruses include the following:

      (1) The ability of influenza virus to cause frequent epidemics is related to frequent changes in its antigens.

      (2) The spikes of influenza virus contain 2 proteins, a hemagglutinin and a neuraminidase. Neutralizing antibody against both of these proteins contributes to resistance or immunity against the disease.

      (3) Parainfluenza viruses do not undergo major antigenic changes. Clinically, they are the main cause of acute laryngotracheal bronchitis (croup).

      (4) On average, a person gets only one "common cold" per year because rhinoviruses have very few antigenic types, and therefore antibody to one type offers protection against the others.

404. Correct statements concerning mumps include the following:

      (1) Because there is no vaccine against mumps, passive immunization is the only means of preventing the disease.

      (2) The diagnosis of mumps is made on clinical grounds, because the virus cannot be grown in cell culture and serologic tests are inaccurate.

      (3) Second episodes of mumps can occur because there are 2 serotypes of the virus, and protection is type-specific

      (4) Although the salivary glands are the most obvious sites of infection, the testes, ovaries, and pancreas can be involved as well.

Answers (Questions 373–404):

373 (A)	377 (A)	381 (B)	385 (A)	389 (A)	393 (C)	397 (A)	401 (E)
374 (D)	378 (D)	382 (A)	386 (C)	390 (C)	394 (B)	398 (D)	402 (A)
375 (A)	379 (A)	383 (A)	387 (E)	391 (C)	395 (A)	399 (D)	403 (A)
376 (A)	380 (C)	384 (E)	388 (A)	392 (A)	396 (A)	400 (A)	404 (D)

MYCOLOGY

Directions (Questions 405–417): Select the ONE lettered answer that is BEST in each question.

405. Which of the following fungal agents is MOST LIKELY to be found growing within reticuloendothelial cells?

    (A) *Histoplasma capsulatum*

    (B) *Candida albicans*

    (C) *Cryptococcus neoformans*

    (D) *Sporothrix schenckii*

406. Your patient is a woman with a vaginal discharge. You suspect, on clinical grounds, that it may be due to *Candida albicans*. Which one of the statements is LEAST accurate or appropriate?

    (A) A Gram stain of the discharge should reveal budding yeasts.

    (B) Culture of the discharge on Sabouraud's agar should produce a white mycelium with aerial conidia.

(C) Her urine should be checked for glucose.

(D) You should ask her whether she is taking antibiotics.

407. You have made a clinical diagnosis of meningitis in a 50-year-old immunocompromised woman. A latex agglutination test on the spinal fluid for capsular polysaccharide antigen is positive. The causative organism is MOST likely to be

(A) *Histoplasma capsulatum*

(B) *Cryptococcus neoformans*

(C) *Actinomyces israelii*

(D) *Candida albicans*

408. Fungi often colonize lesions due to other causes. Which of the following is LEAST likely to be present as a colonizer?

(A) *Aspergillus*

(B) *Mucor*

(C) *Sporothrix*

(D) *Candida*

409. Your patient complains of an "itching rash" on her abdomen. On examination, you find that the lesions are red and circular, with a vesiculated border and a healing central area. You suspect tinea corporis. Of the following choices, the MOST appropriate laboratory procedure to make the diagnosis is

(A) potassium hydroxide mount of skin scrapings

(B) Giemsa stain for multinucleated giant cells

(C) fluorescent-antibody stain of the vesicle fluid

(D) observation of 4-fold rise in antibody titer against the organism

410. Each of the following statements concerning *Cryptococcus neoformans* is correct EXCEPT

(A) The organism is frequently found in pigeon feces.

(B) Septate hyphae are found in the lesions.

(C) A latex agglutination test can detect the organism's capsular polysaccharide.

(D) The initial site of infection is usually the lung.

411. A woman who pricked her finger while pruning some rose bushes develops a local pustule that progresses to an ulcer. Several nodules then develop along the local lymphatic drainage. The MOST likely agent is

(A) *Cryptococcus neoformans*

(B) *Candida albicans*

(C) *Sporothrix schenckii*

(D) *Aspergillus fumigatus*

412. Several fungi are associated with disease in immunocompromised patients. Which one of the following is associated LEAST frequently?

(A) *Cryptococcus neoformans*

(B) *Aspergillus fumigatus*

(C) *Malassezia furfur*

(D) *Mucor* species

413. Fungal cells that reproduce by budding are seen in the infected tissues of patients with

(A) candidiasis, cryptococcosis, and sporotrichosis

(B) mycetoma, candidiasis, and mucormycosis

(C) tinea corporis, tinea unguium, and tinea versicolor

(D) sporotrichosis, mycetoma, and aspergillosis

414. Infection by a dermatophyte is MOST often associated with

(A) intravenous drug abuse

(B) inhalation of organism from contaminated bird feces

(C) adherence of organism to perspiration-moist skin

(D) fecal-oral transmission

415. Aspergillosis is recognized in tissue by the presence of

(A) budding cells

(B) septate hyphae

(C) granules

(D) pseudohyphae

416. Which one of the following is NOT a characteristic of histoplasmosis?

(A) person-to-person transmission

(B) specific geographic distribution

(C) yeasts or yeastlike forms in tissue

(D) mycelial phase in soil

417. Each of the following statements concerning mucormycosis is correct EXCEPT
  (A) Mucormycosis can be caused by a number of fungal species.
  (B) Tissue sections from a patient with mucormycosis show large, irregular, nonseptate hyphae.
  (C) Hyphae in tissue show a propensity to grow through blood vessel walls and cause thrombi.
  (D) Mucormycosis is as likely to occur in diabetic patients with good control as in those in a ketoacidotic state.

Answers (Questions 405–417):

405 (A)	410 (B)	415 (B)
406 (B)	411 (C)	416 (A)
407 (B)	412 (C)	417 (D)
408 (C)	413 (A)	
409 (A)	414 (C)	

Directions (Questions 418–427): For each question, ONE or MORE of the numbered options is correct. Select

  A if only 1, 2, and 3 are correct
  B if only 1 and 3 are correct
  C if only 2 and 4 are correct
  D if only 4 is correct
  E is all are correct

418. Correct statements concerning fungi include the following:
  (1) Yeasts are fungi that reproduce by budding.
  (2) Molds are fungi that have elongated filaments called hyphae.
  (3) Thermally dimorphic fungi can exist as yeasts at 37 °C and as molds at 25 °C.
  (4) Both yeasts and molds have a cell wall made of peptidoglycan.

419. Correct statements concerning yeasts include the following:
  (1) Yeasts have chitin in their cell walls and contain ergosterol in their cell membranes.
  (2) Yeasts form ascospores when they invade tissue.
  (3) Yeasts have eukaryotic nuclei and contain mitochondria in their cytoplasm.
  (4) Yeasts have endotoxin but do not synthesize exotoxins.

420. Correct statements concerning fungi and protozoa include the following:
  (1) Both fungi and protozoa are eukaryotic organisms.
  (2) Fungi possess a cell wall, whereas protozoa do not.
  (3) Both fungi and protozoa generate energy in mitochondria.
  (4) Both fungi and protozoa use flagella as their organ of motility.

421. Your patient has been diagnosed as having cryptococcosis. Findings that are useful in establishing the diagnosis include the following:
  (1) A latex agglutination test for the presence of antigen was positive.
  (2) The patient recently traveled in the Mississippi River valley area.
  (3) Encapsulated budding cells were found in the patient's spinal fluid.
  (4) An isolate recovered from the patient's sputum is acid-fast.

422. Correct statements concerning *Candida albicans* include the following:
  (1) *C albicans* is a budding yeast that forms pseudohyphae when it invades tissue.
  (2) *C albicans* causes thrush.
  (3) Impaired cell-mediated immunity is an important predisposing factor to disease.
  (4) *C albicans* is transmitted primarily by respiratory aerosol.

423. Correct statements concerning *Coccidioides immitis* include the following:
  (1) The mycelial phase of the organism grows primarily in the soil, which is its natural habitat.
  (2) In the body, spherules containing endospores are formed.
  (3) A rising titer of complement-fixing antibody indicates disseminated disease.
  (4) Most infections are symptomatic and require treatment with amphotericin B.

424. Correct statements concerning *Histoplasma capsulatum* include the following:
  (1) The natural habitat of *H capsulatum* is the soil, where it grows as a mold.
  (2) *H capsulatum* is transmitted by airborne conidia, and its initial site of infection is the lung.

(3) Within the body, *H capsulatum* grows primarily intracellularly within macrophages.
(4) Infection elicits a cell-mediated immune response, but no skin test is available.

425. Correct statements concerning infection caused by *C immitis* include the following:
(1) Diagnosis is usually made by finding septate hyphae in the sputum.
(2) The organism is acquired by inhalation of arthrospores.
(3) Resistance to amphotericin B is plasmid-mediated.
(4) Infection occurs primarily in the southwestern states and California.

426. Correct statements concerning *Blastomyces dermatitidis* include the following:
(1) *B dermatitidis* is endemic in the Mississippi and Ohio River valleys.
(2) *B dermatitidis* is a dimorphic fungus that forms yeasts cells in tissue.
(3) *B dermatitidis* is commonly diagnosed by serologic tests, because it does not grow in culture.
(4) *B dermatitidis* causes granulomatous skin lesions.

427. *Aspergillus fumigatus* can be involved in a variety of clinical situations, including the following:
(1) tissue invasion in an immunocompromised host
(2) allergy following inhalation of airborne particles of the fungus
(3) colonization of tuberculous cavities in the lungs
(4) thrush

Answers (Questions 418–427):

418 (A) 422 (A) 426 (C)
419 (B) 423 (A) 427 (A)
420 (A) 424 (A)
421 (B) 425 (C)

PARASITOLOGY

Directions (Questions 428–431): Select the ONE lettered answer that is BEST in each question.

428. Children at day-care centers in the USA have a high rate of infections with
(A) *Ascaris lumbricoides*
(B) *Entamoeba histolytica*
(C) *Enterobius vermicularis*
(D) *Necator americanus*

429. The anatomic location of inflammation caused by *Schistosoma mansoni* is primarily
(A) lung alveoli
(B) intestinal venules
(C) renal tubules
(D) bone marrow

430. The form of plasmodia that is transmitted from mosquito to human is
(A) sporozoite
(B) gametocyte
(C) merozoite
(D) hypnozoite

431. The parasite that primarily infects macrophages is
(A) *Plasmodium vivax*
(B) *Leishmania donovani*
(C) *Trypanosoma cruzi*
(D) *Trichomonas vaginalis*

Answers (Questions 428–431):

428 (C)   430 (A)
429 (B)   431 (B)

Directions (Questions 432–439):   Select the ONE lettered heading that is MOST closely associated with the numbered phrases or statements.

Questions 432–439

(A) *Dracunculus medinensis*
(B) *Loa loa*
(C) *Onchocerca volvulus*
(D) *Wuchereria bancrofti*
(E) *Toxocara canis*

432. Causes river blindness
433. Transmitted by mosquito
434. Acquired by drinking contaminated water
435. Treated by extracting worm from skin ulcer
436. Transmitted by deer fly or mango fly
437. Causes visceral larva migrans
438. Causes filariasis
439. Acquired by ingestion of worm eggs

Answers (Questions 432–439):

432 (C)   435 (A)   438 (D)
433 (D)   436 (B)   439 (E)
434 (A)   437 (E)

Directions (Questions 440–471):   For each numbered item, select

A if the item is associated with (A) only,
B if the item is associated with (B) only,
C if the item is associated with both (A) and (B),
D if the item is associated with neither (A) nor (B).

Questions 440–444

(A) *Giardia lamblia*
(B) *Entamoeba histolytica*
(C) Both
(D) Neither

440. Fecal-oral transmission is involved.
441. Infection associated with liver abscess.
442. Bloody diarrhea is a symptom.
443. Cats are the definitive hosts.
444. Flagellated trophozoite is part of the life cycle.

Questions 445–451

(A) *Plasmodium vivax*
(B) *Plasmodium falciparum*
(C) Both
(D) Neither

445. Sporozoites are formed.
446. Hypnozoites are formed.
447. "Banana-shaped" gametocytes are formed.

400 / PART X

448. Microinfarcts occur.

449. Red cells of all ages are infected.

450. A tertian fever cycle, ie, fever that recurs after 48 hours, is characteristic.

451. Chloroquine resistance is a major emerging problem.

Questions 452–458

(A) *Taenia saginata*

(B) *Taenia solium*

(C) Both

(D) Neither

452. Transmission occurs by eating undercooked pork.

453. Transmission occurs by eating cysticerci.

454. Cysticercosis is caused in humans.

455. Egg has a large lateral spine.

456. Scolex has suckers but no hooks.

457. Diagnosis is made by finding gravid proglottids in stools.

458. Praziquantel is an effective treatment.

Questions 459–464

(A) *Clonorchis sinensis*

(B) *Paragonimus westermani*

(C) Both

(D) Neither

459. Transmission occurs by eating liver.

460. Snails are intermediate hosts.

461. The lungs are infected.

462. Crabs are intermediate hosts.

463. Eggs are found in stools.

464. Cercariae are a stage in the life cycle.

Questions 465–471

(A) *Enterobius vermicularis*

(B) *Trichuris trichiura*

(C) Both

(D) Neither

465. The organism is a nematode.

466. Humans are the only hosts.

467. Perianal itching is a symptom.

468. Eggs embryonate in the soil.

469. Diagnosis involves ''Scotch tape'' technique.

470. Transmission occurs by ingestion of eggs.

471. Mebendazole is an effective treatment.

Answers (Questions 440–471):

440 (C)	445 (C)	450 (C)	455 (D)	460 (C)	465 (C)	470 (C)
441 (B)	446 (A)	451 (B)	456 (A)	461 (B)	466 (C)	471 (C)
442 (B)	447 (B)	452 (B)	457 (C)	462 (B)	467 (A)	
443 (D)	448 (B)	453 (C)	458 (C)	463 (C)	468 (B)	
444 (A)	449 (B)	454 (B)	459 (D)	464 (C)	469 (A)	

Directions (Questions 472–493): For each question, ONE or MORE of the numbered options is correct. Select

A if only 1, 2, and 3 are correct

B if only 1 and 3 are correct

C is only 2 and 4 are correct

D if only 4 is correct
E if all are correct

472. Intermediate hosts are part of the life cycle of
    (1) *Trichomonas vaginalis*
    (2) *Taenia solium*
    (3) *Pneumocystis carinii*
    (4) *Toxoplasma gondii*

473. Parasites that pass through the lungs during human infection include
    (1) *Dracunculus medinensis*
    (2) *Necator americanus*
    (3) *Wuchereria bancrofti*
    (4) *Ascaris lumbricoides*

474. Parasites that are transmitted by flies include
    (1) *Onchocerca volvulus*
    (2) *Strongyloides stercoralis*
    (3) *Loa loa*
    (4) *Schistosoma mansoni*

475. Parasites transmitted by mosquitoes include
    (1) *Leishmania donovani*
    (2) *Wuchereria bancrofti*
    (3) *Trypanosoma cruzi*
    (4) *Plasmodium falciparum*

476. Parasites for which pigs are the source of infection for humans include
    (1) *Echinococcus granulosis*
    (2) *Taenia solium*
    (3) *Ascaris lumbricoides*
    (4) *Trichinella spiralis*

477. Laboratory diagnosis of a patient with a suspected liver abscess due to *Entamoeba histolytica* includes
    (1) stool examination
    (2) blood smear
    (3) indirect hemagglutination test
    (4) xenodiagnosis

478. *Toxoplasma gondii* infection
    (1) can be transmitted across the placenta to the fetus
    (2) can be transmitted by cat feces
    (3) can cause encephalitis in immunocompromised patients
    (4) can be diagnosed by finding trophozoites in the stool

479. *Giardia lamblia* infections
    (1) frequently affect children
    (2) cause fat in stools as a result of malabsorption in the small intestine
    (3) can be treated effectively with metronidazole
    (4) can be diagnosed by the string test

480. Correct statements concerning malaria include the following:
    (1) The female *Anopheles* mosquito is the vector.
    (2) Early in infection, sporozoites enter hepatocytes.
    (3) Release of merozoites from red blood cells causes periodic fever and chills.
    (4) Gametocytes are formed in human erythrocytes.

481. Trichomonas infections
    (1) are transmitted sexually
    (2) can be diagnosed by visualizing the cysts
    (3) can be treated effectively with metronidazole
    (4) cause anemia

482. Agents used to prevent malaria include
    (1) mebendazole
    (2) inactivated vaccine
    (3) praziquantel
    (4) chloroquine

483. *Pneumocystis carinii* infections
    (1) are transmitted via the respiratory tract
    (2) can be diagnosed by seeing cysts in tissue

      (3) are symptomatic primarily in immunocompromised patients

      (4) commonly involve the liver, producing abscesses

484. *Trypanosoma cruzi* infections

      (1) are transmitted by the reduviid bug

      (2) occur primarily in tropical Africa

      (3) can be diagnosed by seeing trypomastigotes in a blood smear

      (4) cause lymphedema, leading to elephantiasis

485. Sleeping sickness

      (1) is caused by a trypanosome

      (2) is transmitted by tsetse flies

      (3) occurs primarily in tropical Africa

      (4) can be diagnosed by finding eggs in the stools

486. Kala-azar

      (1) is caused by *Trypanosoma cruzi*

      (2) is transmitted by sandflies

      (3) occurs primarily in rural Latin America

      (4) can be diagnosed by finding amastigotes in the bone marrow

487. *Diphyllobothrium latum*

      (1) is transmitted by undercooked fish

      (2) has operculated eggs

      (3) has crustaceans (copepods) as intermediate hosts

      (4) has scoleces with a circle of hooks

488. Hydatid cyst disease

      (1) is caused by *Echinococcus granulosus*

      (2) is transmitted by eating liver

      (3) is caused by a parasite whose adult form lives in dogs' intestines

      (4) occurs primarily in tropical Africa

489. *Schistosoma hematobium*

      (1) occurs primarily in Latin America

      (2) has snails as intermediate hosts

      (3) has eggs with no spine

      (4) predisposes to bladder carcinoma

490. Hookworm infection

      (1) can cause anemia

      (2) is transmitted by ingestion of eggs

      (3) is caused by *Nectar americanus*

      (4) can be diagnosed by a blood smear

491. *Ascaris lumbricoides*

      (1) is one of the largest nematodes

      (2) is transmitted by ingestion of eggs

      (3) has humans as the only hosts

      (4) can cause pneumonia

492. *Strongyloides stercoralis*

      (1) is acquired by ingestion of eggs

      (2) undergoes a free-living life cycle in soil

      (3) has snails as intermediate hosts

      (4) produces filariform larvae

493. Trichinosis

      (1) is acquired by eating undercooked pork

      (2) occurs primarily in Asia

      (3) can be diagnosed by seeing cysts in muscle biopsy

      (4) is caused by a cestode

Answers (Questions 472–493):

472 (C)	476 (C)	479 (E)	482 (D)	485 (A)	488 (B)	491 (E)
473 (C)	477 (B)	480 (E)	483 (A)	486 (C)	489 (C)	492 (C)
474 (B)	478 (A)	481 (B)	484 (B)	487 (A)	490 (B)	493 (B)
475 (C)						

IMMUNOLOGY

Directions (Questions 494–578): Select the ONE lettered answer that is BEST in each question.

494. Hemolytic disease of the newborn as a result of Rh incompatibility can be classified as a hypersensitivity of the following type:
- **(A)** atopic or anaphylactic
- **(B)** cytotoxic
- **(C)** immune complex
- **(D)** delayed

495. The principal difference between cytotoxic (type II) and immune complex (type III) hypersensitivity is
- **(A)** the class (isotype) of antibody
- **(B)** the distribution of antigen-antibody complexes
- **(C)** the participation of complement
- **(D)** the participation of T cells

496. A child stung by a bee experiences respiratory distress within minutes and lapses into unconsciousness. This reaction is probably mediated by
- **(A)** IgE antibody
- **(B)** IgG antibody
- **(C)** sensitized T cells
- **(D)** complement
- **(E)** IgM antibody

497. A patient with rheumatic fever develops a sore throat. Beta-hemolytic streptococci are cultured from a throat swab. The patient is started on treatment with penicillin, and the sore throat resolves within several days. However, 7 days after initiation of penicillin therapy the patient develops a fever of 38 °C, a generalized rash, and proteinuria. This MOST probably resulted from
- **(A)** recurrence of the rheumatic fever
- **(B)** a different infectious disease
- **(C)** an IgE response to penicillin
- **(D)** an IgG-IgM response to penicillin
- **(E)** a delayed hypersensitivity reaction to penicillin

498. A kidney biopsy taken from a patient with acute glomerulonephritis and stained with fluorescein-conjugated anti-human IgG antibody would probably show
- **(A)** no fluorescence
- **(B)** uniform fluorescence of the glomerular basement membrane
- **(C)** patchy, irregular fluorescence of the glomerular basement membrane
- **(D)** fluorescent B cells
- **(E)** fluorescent macrophages

499. A patient with severe asthma gets no relief from antihistamines. His symptoms are likely to be caused by
- **(A)** histamine
- **(B)** slow-reacting substance A
- **(C)** serotonin
- **(D)** bradykinin
- **(E)** T cell lymphokines

500. Hypersensitivity to penicillin and to poison oak are both
- **(A)** mediated by IgE antibody
- **(B)** mediated by IgG and IgM antibody
- **(C)** initiated by haptens
- **(D)** autoimmune diseases

501. A recipient of a 2-haplotype MHC-matched kidney from a relative still needs immunosuppression to prevent graft rejection because
- **(A)** graft-versus-host disease could be a problem
- **(B)** class II MHC will not be matched properly owing to lack of good reagents

(C) minor histocompatibility antigens will not be matched

(D) immunosuppression decreases the chance of infection at the surgical site

502. Bone marrow transplantation of immunocompromised patients presents which major problem?

(A) potentially lethal graft-versus-host disease

(B) high risk of T cell leukemia

(C) inability to use a live donor

(D) delayed hypersensitivity

503. What role do class II MHC antigens play in graft rejection?

(A) They are usually the recognition element for cytotoxic T cells.

(B) They are a recognition element for helper T cells, which then promote the response of cytotoxic T cells.

(C) They can induce the production of blocking antibodies that protect the graft.

(D) They enhance the function of suppressor T cells.

504. Grafts between genetically identical individuals (such as identical twins)

(A) are rejected slowly as a result of minor histocompatibility antigens

(B) are subject to hyperacute rejection

(C) are not rejected, even without immunosuppression

(D) are not rejected if a kidney is grafted, but skin grafts are rejected

505. A child is born with a congenital viral infection, which fails to clear. This is likely to be a manifestation of

(A) tolerance

(B) AIDS

(C) severe combined immunodeficiency syndrome

(D) chronic granulomatous disease

506. AIDS (acquired immunodeficiency syndrome) is caused by a human retrovirus that kills

(A) B lymphocytes

(B) lymphocyte stem cells

(C) CD4 ($CD4^+$) T lymphocytes

(D) CD8 ($CD8^+$) T lymphocytes

507. Chemically induced tumors have tumor-associated transplantation antigens that

(A) are always the same for a given carcinogen

(B) are different for 2 tumors of different histologic type even if induced by the same carcinogen

(C) are very strong antigens

(D) do not induce an immune response

508. Polyomavirus (a DNA virus) causes tumors in "nude mice" (nude mice do not have a thymus, as a result of a genetic defect) but not in normal mice. Which is the BEST interpretation of this?

(A) Macrophages are required to reject polyomavirus-induced tumors.

(B) Natural killer cells can reject polyomavirus-induced tumors without help from T lymphocytes.

(C) T lymphocytes play an important role in the rejection of polyomavirus-induced tumors.

(D) B lymphocytes play no role in rejection of polyomavirus-induced tumors.

509. C3 is cleaved to form C3b and C3a by C3 convertase. C3b is involved in all of the following EXCEPT

(A) altering vascular permeability

(B) promoting phagocytosis

(C) alternative pathway C3 convertase

(D) C5 convertase

510. During differentiation, a B lymphocyte may switch its

(A) immunoglobulin light-chain isotype

(B) immunoglobulin heavy-chain class

(C) variable region of the immunoglobulin heavy chain

(D) constant region of the immunoglobulin light chain

511. Diversity is an important feature of the immune system. Which of the following statements about it is INCORRECT?

(A) A higher vertebrate can make antibodies with about 10^8 different VH $\times$ VL combinations.

(B) A single cell can synthesize IgM antibody and then switch to IgA antibody.

(C) The hematopoietic stem cell carries the genetic potential to create more than 10^4 immunoglobulin genes.

(D) A single B lymphocyte can produce antibodies of many different specificities, but a plasma cell is monospecific.

512. C3a and C5a can cause
(A) bacterial lysis
(B) smooth-muscle contraction
(C) phagocytosis of IgE-coated bacteria
(D) aggregation of C4 and C2

513. Neutrophils and macrophages are attracted by
(A) IgM
(B) C1
(C) C5a
(D) C8

514. The alternative complement pathway does NOT require
(A) C2
(B) C3b
(C) factor B
(D) factor D

515. Complement fixation refers to
(A) the ingestion of C3b-coated bacteria by macrophages
(B) the destruction of complement in serum by heating it at 56 °C for 30 minutes
(C) the binding of complement components by antigen-antibody complexes
(D) the interaction of C3b with mast cells

516. The classic complement pathway is initiated by interaction of C1 with
(A) antigen
(B) factor B
(C) antigen-IgG complexes
(D) bacterial lipopolysaccharides

517. Patients with severely reduced C3 levels tend to have
(A) increased numbers of severe viral infections
(B) increased numbers of severe bacterial infections
(C) low gamma globulin levels
(D) frequent episodes of hemolytic anemia

518. Individuals with a genetic deficiency of C6 have
(A) decreased resistance to viral infections
(B) increased hypersensitivity reactions
(C) increased frequency of cancer
(D) decreased resistance to *Neisseria* bacteremia

519. Different tumors induced by a given tumor virus usually
(A) have widely differing surface antigens
(B) have only internal antigens
(C) have one or more common surface antigens
(D) contain only viral antigens

520. Natural killer (NK) cells are
(A) B cells
(B) cytotoxic T cells
(C) increased by immunization
(D) able to kill virus-infected cells without prior sensitization

521. A positive tuberculin skin test (a delayed hypersensitivity reaction) indicates that
(A) a humoral immune response has occurred
(B) a cell-mediated immune response has occurred
(C) both the T cell and B cell systems are functional
(D) only the B cell system is functional

522. Reaction to poison ivy or poison oak is
(A) an IgG-mediated response
(B) an IgE-mediated response
(C) a cell-mediated response
(D) an Arthus reaction

523. A child disturbs a wasp nest, is stung repeatedly, and goes into shock within minutes, manifesting respiratory failure and vascular collapse. This is MOST likely to be due to
   (A) systemic anaphylaxis
   (B) a local atopic reaction
   (C) an Arthus reaction
   (D) cytotoxic hypersensitivity

524. "Isotype switching" of immunoglobulin classes by B cells involves
   (A) simultaneous insertion of VL genes adjacent to each CH gene
   (B) successive insertion of a single VH gene adjacent to different CH genes
   (C) activation of homologous genes on chromosome 6
   (D) switching of light-chain types (kappa and lambda)

525. Which of the following pairs of genes is linked on a single chromosome?
   (A) V gene for lambda chain and C gene for kappa chain
   (B) C gene for gamma chain and C gene for kappa chain
   (C) V gene for lambda chain and V gene for heavy chain
   (D) C gene for gamma chain and C gene for alpha chain

526. Idiotypic determinants are located within
   (A) hypervariable regions of heavy and light chains
   (B) constant regions of light chains
   (C) constant regions of heavy chains
   (D) the hinge region

527. A primary immune response in an adult human requires approximately how much time to produce detectable antibody levels in the blood?
   (A) 12 hours
   (B) 2 days
   (C) 1 week
   (D) 2 weeks

528. The membrane IgM and IgD on the surface of an individual B cell
   (A) have identical heavy chains but different light chains
   (B) are identical except for their CH regions
   (C) are identical except for their VH regions
   (D) have different VH and VL regions

529. During the maturation of a B lymphocyte, the first immunoglobulin heavy chain synthesized is the
   (A) mu chain
   (B) gamma chain
   (C) epsilon chain
   (D) alpha chain

530. In the immune response to a hapten-protein conjugate, in order to get antihapten antibodies it is essential that
   (A) the hapten be recognized by helper T cells
   (B) the protein be recognized by helper T cells
   (C) the protein be recognized by B cells
   (D) the hapten be recognized by suppressor T cells

531. In the determination of serum insulin levels by radioimmunoassay, which of the following would NOT be needed?
   (A) isotope-labeled insulin
   (B) goat anti-insulin antibody
   (C) rabbit anti-goat gamma globulin
   (D) isotope-labeled goat anti-insulin antibody

532. Which of the following sequences is appropriate for testing a patient for antibody against the AIDS virus by using the ELISA? (The assay is to be carried out in a plastic plate with incubation and a wash step after each addition except the final one.)
   (A) patient's serum/enzyme substrate/AIDS antigen/enzyme-labeled anti-AIDS antibody
   (B) AIDS antigen/patient's serum/enzyme-labeled antibody versus human gamma globulin/enzyme substrate
   (C) enzyme-labeled antibody versus human gamma globulin/patient's serum/AIDS antigen/enzyme substrate

533. The BEST method to demonstrate IgG on the glomerular basement membrane in a kidney tissue section would be
   (A) precipitin test

(B) complement fixation

(C) agglutination test

(D) indirect fluorescent-antibody test

534. The helper T:suppressor T cell ratio in AIDS is

(A) higher because viral replication stimulates helper T replication

(B) higher because viral replication destroys T suppressors

(C) lower because viral replication stimulates T suppressors

(D) lower because viral replication destroys T helpers

535. A patient with a central nervous system disorder is maintianed on the drug methyldopa. Hemolytic anemia develops, which resolves shortly after the drug is discontinued. This is MOST probably an example of

(A) atopic hypersensitivity

(B) cytotoxic hypersensitivity

(C) immune-complex hypersensitivity

(D) cell-mediated hypersensitivity

536. Which of the following substances is NOT released by activated T cells:

(A) alpha interferon

(B) gamma interferon

(C) interleukin-2

(D) macrophage activation factor

537. A delayed hypersensitivity reaction is characterized by

(A) noncellular edema

(B) a predominantly neutrophil cell infiltrate

(C) a predominantly mononuclear cell infiltrate

(D) a predominantly eosinophilic cell infiltrate

538. Two dissimilar inbred strains of mice, A and B, are crossed to yield an F_1 hybrid strain, AB. If a large dose of spleen cells from an adult A mouse is injected into an adult AB mouse, which of the following is MOST likely to occur?

(A) The spleen cells will be destroyed.

(B) The spleen cells will survive without any effect on the recipient.

(C) The spleen cells will induce a graft-versus-host reaction in the recipient.

(D) The spleen cells will survive and induce tolerance of strain A grafts in the recipient.

539. With the same strains of mice described in the preceding question, if adult AB spleen cells are injected into a newborn B mouse, which of the following is MOST likely to occur?

(A) The spleen cells will be destroyed.

(B) The spleen cells will survive without any effect on the recipient.

(C) The spleen cells will induce a graft-versus-host reaction in the recipient.

(D) The spleen cells will survive and induce tolerance of strain A grafts in the recipient.

540. The minor histocompatibility antigens on cells

(A) are detected by reaction with antibodies and complement

(B) are controlled by several genes in the major histocompatibility complex

(C) are unimportant in human transplantation

(D) induce reactions that can cumulatively lead to a strong rejection response

541. Which of the following is NOT true of class I MHC antigens?

(A) are assayed by a cytotoxic test requiring antibody and complement

(B) can usually be identified in a few hours

(C) are controlled by at least 3 gene loci in the major histocompatibility complex

(D) are found mainly on B cells, macrophages, and activated T cells

542. An antigen found in relatively high concentration in the plasma of normal fetuses and a high proportion of patients with progressive carcinoma of the colon is

(A) viral antigen

(B) carcinoembryonic antigen

(C) alpha-fetoprotein

(D) heterophil antigen

543. An antibody directed against the idiotypic determinants of a human IgG antibody would react with

(A) the Fc part of the IgG

(B) an IgM antibody produced by the same clone that produced the IgG

(C) all human kappa chains

(D) all human gamma chains

544. Which of the following is NOT true of the gene segments that combine to make up a heavy-chain gene?
(A) A large assortment of V region segments is available.
(B) A few J segments are available.
(C) Several H segments are available.
(D) A V and a J segment are preselected by an antigen to make up the variable-region portion of the gene.

545. When immune complexes from the serum are deposited on glomerular basement membrane, damage to the membrane is caused mainly by
(A) lysis by complement
(B) phagocytosis
(C) cytotoxic T cells
(D) enzymes released by polymorphonuclear cells

546. If an individual were genetically unable to make J chain, which immunoglobulins would be affected?
(A) IgG
(B) IgM
(C) IgA
(D) IgG and IgM
(E) IgM and IgA

547. The antibody-binding site is formed primarily by
(A) the variable regions of H and L chains
(B) the hypervariable regions of H and L chains
(C) the hypervariable regions of H chains
(D) the variable regions of H chains
(E) the variable regions of L chains

548. The predominant class of immunoglobulin in the blood of a human newborn is
(A) IgG
(B) IgM
(C) IgA
(D) IgD
(E) IgE

549. Individuals of blood group type AB
(A) are RhD negative
(B) are ''universal recipients'' of transfusions
(C) have circulating anti-A and anti-B antibodies
(D) have the same haplotype

550. Cytotoxic T cells induced by infection with virus A will kill target cells
(A) from the same host infected with any virus
(B) infected by virus A and identical at class I MHC loci of the cytotoxic T cells
(C) infected by virus A and identical at class II MHC loci of the cytotoxic T cells
(D) infected with a different virus and identical at class I MHC loci of the cytotoxic cells
(E) infected with a different virus and identical at class II MHC loci of the cytotoxic cells

551. Antigen-presenting cells that activate helper T cells must express on their surfaces
(A) Ig
(B) Thy-1
(C) class I MHC antigens
(D) class II MHC antigens

552. Which one of the following does NOT contain C3b?
(A) classic-complement-pathway C5 convertase
(B) alternative-pathway C5 convertase
(C) classic-pathway C3 convertase
(D) alternative-pathway C3 convertase

553. Complement factors H and I cause
(A) cell lysis
(B) cleavage of C3 into C3a and C3b
(C) degradation of C3b
(D) chemotaxis

554. Which one of the following is NOT true regarding the complement alternative pathway?
(A) The alternative pathway can be triggered by infectious agents in absence of antibody.
(B) The alternative pathway does not require, C1, C2, or C4.
(C) The alternative pathway cannot be initiated unless C3b fragments are already present.
(D) The alternative pathway has the same terminal sequence of events as the classic pathway.

555. In setting up a complement fixation test for antibody, the reactants should be added in what sequence (Ag = antigen; Ab = antibody; C = complement; EA = antibody-coated indicator erythrocytes)?
(A) Ag + EA + C/wait/ + patient's serum
(B) C + patient's serum + EA/wait/ + Ag
(C) Ag + patient's serum + EA/wait/ + C
(D) Ag + patient's serum + C/wait/ + EA

556. Proteins from 2 samples of animal blood, A and B, were tested by double diffusion in gel against antibovine albumin. Which sample contains horse blood?
(A) sample A
(B) sample B
(C) both samples
(D) neither sample

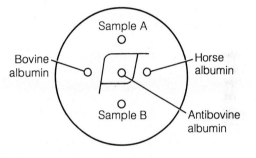

557. In IgG molecules, disulfide bonds connect the following chains EXCEPT
(A) different parts of the same light chain
(B) the 2 light chains to each other
(C) the 2 heavy chains to each other
(D) each light chain to a heavy chain

558. The concentration in serum of IgA is
(A) greater than that of IgG
(B) the same as that of IgG
(C) less than that of IgG
(D) less than that of IgE

559. Complement lyses cells by
(A) enzymatic digestion of the cell membrane
(B) activation of adenylate cyclase
(C) insertion of complement proteins into the cell membrane
(D) inhibition of elongation factor 2

560. Complement activation results in the production of anaphylatoxins, which cause smooth-muscle contraction and histamine release. Anaphylatoxins are derived from
(A) C3 only
(B) C5 only
(C) C3 and C5
(D) C3 and C6

561. Graft and tumor rejection are mediated primarily by
(A) non-complement-fixing antibodies
(B) phagocytic cells
(C) helper T cells
(D) cytotoxic T cells

562. Which of the following properties of antibodies is NOT dependent on the structure of the heavy-chain constant region?
(A) ability to cross the placenta
(B) isotype (class)
(C) ability to fix complement
(D) affinity for antigen

563. In which of the following situations would a graft-versus-host reaction be likely to occur? (Mouse strains A and B are highly inbred; AB is an F1 hybrid between strain A and strain B.)
    (A) newborn strain A spleen cells injected into a strain B adult
    (B) x-irradiated adult strain A spleen cells injected into a strain B adult
    (C) adult strain A spleen cells injected into an x-irradiated strain AB adult
    (D) adult strain AB spleen cells injected into a strain A newborn

564. In a mixed lymphocyte culture, lymphocytes from patient X, who is homozygous for the HLA-Dw7 allele, are irradiated and then cultured with lymphocytes from patient Z. It is found that DNA synthesis is NOT stimulated. The proper conclusion to be drawn is that
    (A) Z is homozygous for HLA-Dw7
    (B) Z is homozygous or heterozygous for HLA-Dw7
    (C) Z is heterozygous for HLA-Dw7
    (D) Z does not carry the HLA-Dw7 allele

565. A patient skin-tested with PPD to determine previous exposure to *Mycobacterium tuberculosis* develops induration at the skin test site 48 hours later. Histologically, the reaction site would MOST probably show
    (A) edema with perhaps a few eosinophils
    (B) a polymorphonuclear cell infiltrate
    (C) a cellular infiltrate consisting mostly of mononuclear cells
    (D) an infiltrate consisting mostly of B lymphocytes

566. Hemolytic disease of the newborn as a result of blood group incompatibility is mediated by
    (A) IgE antibody
    (B) IgG antibody
    (C) IgM antibody
    (D) IgA antibody

567. An Rh-negative woman married to a heterozygous Rh-positive man has 3 children. The probability that all 3 of their children are Rh-positive is
    (A) 1:2
    (B) 1:4
    (C) 1:8
    (D) 1:16

568. Which of the following statements BEST explains the relationship between inflammation of the heart (carditis) and infection with group A beta-hemolytic streptococci?
    (A) Streptococci contain an antigen cross-reactive with heart tissue.
    (B) Streptococci are polyclonal activators of B cells.
    (C) Streptococci are polyclonal activators of T cells.
    (D) Immune complexes of streptococcal antigen and antibody deposit in heart tissue.

569. Your patient became ill 10 days ago with a viral disease. Laboratory examination reveals that the patient's antibodies against this virus have a high ratio of IgM to IgG. What is your conclusion?
    (A) It is unlikely that the patient has encountered this organism previously.
    (B) It is likely that the patient has encountered this organism previously.
    (C) The information given is irrelevant to previous antigen exposure.
    (D) It is likely the patient has an autoimmune disease.

570. If you measure the ability of cytotoxic T cells from an HLA-B27 patient to kill virus X-infected target cells, which one of the following statements is CORRECT?
    (A) Any virus X-infected target cell will be killed.
    (B) Only virus X-infected cells of HLA-B27 type will be killed.
    (C) Any HLA-B27 cell will be killed.
    (D) No HLA-B27 cell will be killed.

571. You have a patient who makes autoantibodies against his own red blood cells. Which of the following cell types is LIKELY to be deficient?
    (A) macrophages
    (B) cytotoxic T cells
    (C) helper T cells
    (D) suppressor T cells

572. You examine a child who has no detectable T or B cells. The primary site of this immunodeficiency MOST probably lies in
    (A) the thymus

(B) the bursal equivalent
(C) T cell-B cell interaction
(D) stem cells originating in the bone marrow

573. The role of the macrophage during an antibody response is to
(A) make antibody
(B) lyse virally infected target cells
(C) suppress cytotoxic T cells
(D) process antigen and "present" it

574. The structural basis of blood group A and B antigen specificity is:
(A) a single terminal sugar residue
(B) a single terminal amino acid
(C) multiple differences is the carbohydrate portion
(D) multiple differences in the protein portion

575. Complement can enhance phagocytosis because of the presence on macrophages and neutrophils of receptors for fragments of
(A) factor D
(B) C3
(C) C6
(D) properdin

576. The main advantage of passive antibody over active immunization is that
(A) it can be administered orally
(B) it provides antibody more rapidly
(C) antibody persists for a longer time
(D) it contains primarily IgM

577. On January 15, a patient developed an illness suggestive of influenza that lasted 1 week. On February 20, she had a similar illness. She had no influenza immunization during this period. Her hemagglutination inhibition titer to influenza A virus was 10 on January 18, 40 on January 30, and 320 on February 20. Which is the MOST appropriate interpretation?
(A) The patient was ill with influenza A on January 15.
(B) The patient was ill with influenza A on February 20.
(C) The patient was not infected with influenza virus.
(D) The patient has an autoimmune disease.

578. An individual who is heterozygous for Gm allotypes contains 2 allelic forms of the protein in serum, but individual lymphocytes produce only one of the 2 forms. This phenomenon, known as "allelic exclusion," is consistent with
(A) a rearrangement of a heavy-chain gene on only one chromosome
(B) rearrangements of heavy-chain genes on both chromosomes
(C) a rearrangement of a light-chain gene on only one chromosome
(D) rearrangements of light-chain genes on both chromosomes

Answers (Questions 494–578):

494 (B)	507 (B)	520 (D)	533 (D)	546 (E)	559 (C)	572 (D)
495 (B)	508 (C)	521 (B)	534 (D)	547 (B)	560 (C)	573 (D)
496 (A)	509 (A)	522 (C)	535 (B)	548 (A)	561 (D)	574 (A)
497 (D)	510 (B)	523 (A)	536 (A)	549 (B)	562 (D)	575 (B)
498 (C)	511 (D)	524 (B)	537 (C)	550 (B)	563 (C)	576 (B)
499 (B)	512 (B)	525 (D)	538 (C)	551 (D)	564 (B)	577 (A)
500 (C)	513 (C)	526 (A)	539 (D)	552 (C)	565 (C)	578 (A)
501 (C)	514 (A)	527 (C)	540 (D)	553 (C)	566 (B)	
502 (A)	515 (C)	528 (B)	541 (D)	554 (C)	567 (C)	
503 (B)	516 (C)	529 (A)	542 (B)	555 (D)	568 (A)	
504 (C)	517 (B)	530 (B)	543 (B)	556 (B)	569 (A)	
505 (A)	518 (D)	531 (D)	544 (D)	557 (B)	570 (B)	
506 (C)	519 (C)	532 (B)	545 (D)	558 (C)	571 (D)	

Directions (Questions 579–621): Select the ONE lettered heading that is MOST closely associated with the numbered words or phrases.

Questions 579–585

    (A) T cells
    (B) B cells
    (C) Macrophages
    (D) T and B cells
    (E) T cells, B cells, and macrophages

579. Major source of interleukin-1
580. Acted on by interleukin-1
581. A source of interleukin-2
582. Acted on by interleukin-2
583. Express class I MHC markers
584. Express class II MHC markers
585. Express surface immunoglobulin

Questions 586–588

    (A) Primary antibody response
    (B) Secondary antibody response

586. Appears more quickly and persists longer
587. Relatively richer in IgG
588. Relatively richer in IgM

Questions 589–592

    (A) Blood group A
    (B) Blood group O
    (C) Blood groups A and O
    (D) Blood group AB

589. People with this type have circulating anti-A antibodies.
590. People with this type have circulating anti-B antibodies.
591. People with this type are called "universal donors."
592. People with this type are called "universal recipients."

Questions 593–598

    (A) Variable region of light chain
    (B) Variable region of heavy chain
    (C) Variable regions of light and heavy chains
    (D) Constant region of heavy chain
    (E) Constant regions of light and heavy chains

593. Determines immunoglobulin class
594. Determines allotypes
595. Determines idiotypes
596. Binding of IgG to macrophages
597. Fixation of complement by IgG
598. Antigen-binding site

Questions 599–602: The following double-immunodiffusion plate contains antibody prepared against whole human serum in the center well. Identify the contents of each peripheral well from the following list (each well to be used once):

599. Whole human serum
600. Human IgG
601. Baboon IgG
602. Human transferrin

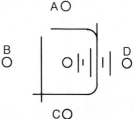

Questions 603–605
    (A) Immediate hypersensitivity
    (B) Cytotoxic hypersensitivity
    (C) Immune complex hypersensitivity
    (D) Delayed-type hypersensitivity
603. Irregular deposition of IgG along glomerular basement membrane
604. Involves mast cells and basophils
605. Mediated by lymphokines

Questions 606–609
    (A) IgM
    (B) IgG
    (C) IgA
    (D) IgE
606. Crosses the placenta
607. Can contain a polypeptide chain not synthesized by a B lymphocyte
608. Found in the milk of lactating females
609. Binds firmly to mast cells and triggers anaphylaxis

Questions 610–613
    (A) Agglutination
    (B) Immunoelectrophoresis
    (C) Immunofluorescence
    (D) ELISA or radioimmunoassay
610. Measure IgG in serum
611. Detect surface IgM on cells in a bone marrow smear
612. Assay growth hormone in serum
613. Determine type A blood group antigen on erythrocytes

Questions 614–617
    (A) IgA
    (B) IgE
    (C) IgG
    (D) IgM
614. Present in highest concentration in serum
615. Present in highest concentration in secretions
616. Present in lowest concentration in serum
617. Contains 10 H and 10 L chains

Questions 618–621: In this double-diffusion (Ouchterlony) assay, the center well contains goat antibody against whole human serum. The peripheral (numbered) wells each contain one of the following proteins:
    (A) Human serum albumin at low concentration
    (B) Human serum albumin at high concentration
    (C) Human serum transferrin
    (D) Sheep serum albumin
618. Which protein is present in well 1?
619. Which protein is present in well 2?
620. Which protein is present in well 3?
621. Which protein is present in well 4?

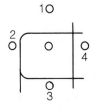

Answers (Questions 579–621):

579 (C)	589 (B)	599 (D)	609 (D)	619 (A)
580 (A)	590 (C)	600 (C)	610 (D)	620 (D)
581 (A)	591 (B)	601 (A)	611 (C)	621 (C)
582 (A)	592 (D)	602 (B)	612 (D)	
583 (E)	593 (D)	603 (C)	613 (A)	
584 (E)	594 (E)	604 (A)	614 (C)	
585 (B)	595 (C)	605 (D)	615 (A)	
586 (B)	596 (D)	606 (B)	616 (B)	
587 (B)	597 (D)	607 (C)	617 (D)	
588 (A)	598 (C)	608 (C)	618 (B)	

Directions (Questions 622–643): For each numbered item, select

   A if the item is associated with (A) ONLY
   B if the item is associated with (B) ONLY
   C if the item is associated with BOTH (A) AND (B)
   D if the item is associated with NEITHER (A) NOR (B)

622. In order for a graft-versus-host reaction to occur, which of the following is essential?
   (A) The host has at least one transplantation antigen not present in the graft.
   (B) The graft contains immunologically competent cells.
   (C) Both
   (D) Neither

623. HLA antigens are controlled by genes that have which of the following properties?
   (A) They are codominant.
   (B) They have a large number of allelic forms.
   (C) Both
   (D) Neither

624. Which of the following is TRUE of the "minor" histocompatibility antigens in humans?
   (A) They cannot be typed serologically.
   (B) They do not contribute to graft rejection.
   (C) Both
   (D) Neither

625. Which of the following is TRUE of immunlogic tolerance?
   (A) It is more easily induced in T cells than in B cells.
   (B) It is more easily induced with large doses of antigen than with small doses.
   (C) Both
   (D) Neither

Questions 626–628
   (A) Class I MHC glycoproteins
   (B) Class II MHC glycoproteins
   (C) Both
   (D) Neither

626. They are involved in antibody responses to T cell-dependent antigens.
627. They are involved in target cell recognition by cytotoxic T cells.
628. They are important in graft rejection.

Questions 629–632
   (A) Fab
   (B) Fc
   (C) Both
   (D) Neither

629. It contains a heavy-chain domain.
630. It contains a complement-binding site.
631. It contains an antigen-combining site.
632. It contains hypervariable regions.

Questions 633–638

633. The immunoglobulins secreted by myelomas and hybridomas are typically
   (A) Homogeneous
   (B) IgA

(C) Both
(D) Neither

634. Immunoglobulin serves as antigen receptor on the surface of which of the following?
(A) T cells
(B) B cells
(C) Both
(D) Neither

635. Injection of BCG organisms into a tumor can result in which of the following?
(A) Intensify the immune response against tumor antigens
(B) Stimulate macrophages, which then damage tumor cells
(C) Both
(D) Neither

636. Which of the following is due to cytotoxic (type II) hypersensitivity?
(A) Poison oak hypersensitivity
(B) Erythroblastosis fetalis due to Rh incompatibility
(C) Both
(D) Neither

637. Desensitization to atopic allergies by parenteral injections of the allergen may be brought about by which of the following?
(A) Production of ''blocking'' antibody
(B) Generation of suppressor T cells
(C) Both
(D) Neither

638. In anaphylactic hypersensitivity to penicillin and in poison ivy allergy, which of the following is TRUE?
(A) The 2 reactions are mediated by sensitized T cells.
(B) The 2 allergens are haptens.
(C) Both
(D) Neither

Questions 639–643
(A) L chain
(B) H chain
(C) Both
(D) Neither

639. Encoded in part by a J segment gene
640. Encoded in part by a D segment gene
641. Contains amino acids that form the binding site for antigen
642. May be kappa or lambda type
643. Primary RNA transcript requires no processing of introns to generate mRNA

Answers (Questions 622–643)

622 (C)	627 (A)	632 (A)	637 (C)	642 (A)
623 (C)	628 (C)	633 (A)	638 (B)	643 (D)
624 (A)	629 (C)	634 (B)	639 (C)	
625 (C)	630 (B)	635 (C)	640 (B)	
626 (B)	631 (A)	636 (B)	641 (C)	

Directions (Questions 644–654): For each question ONE or MORE of the numbered options is correct. Select
A if only 1, 2, AND 3 are correct
B if only 1 AND 3 are correct
C if only 2 AND 4 are correct
D if only 4 is correct
E if ALL are correct

644. Major histocompatibility class I antigens are
(1) cell surface proteins on virtually all cells
(2) key recognition elements for cytotoxic T cells

(3) codominantly expressed

(4) important in the skin test response to *Mycobacterium tuberculosis*

645. Graft-versus-host disease can be avoided or treated by

(1) MHC matching of donor and recipient

(2) alpha interferon

(3) removing mature T cells from the graft

(4) removing B cells from the graft

646. Which of these immunologic abnormalities is the consequence of the loss of helper T (CD4) cells?

(1) decreased in vitro lymphocyte proliferation responses to alloantigens

(2) decreased ability to mount an antibody response to a T cell-dependent antigen

(3) decreased or absent skin tests (delayed hypersensitivity)

(4) decreased anaphylaxis

647. The variable regions of heavy chains and the variable regions of light chains in a given antibody molecule

(1) are different from each other

(2) define the specificity

(3) are encoded by more than one gene segment

(4) contain the hypervariable regions

648. Which of the following are T cell products capable of enhancing certain T cell activities?

(1) interleukin-2

(2) bradykinin

(3) gamma interferon

(4) endotoxin

649. Both class I and class II MHC antigens

(1) are found on the surfaces of all cells

(2) have a high degree of polymorphism

(3) are involved in anaphylaxis

(4) have immunoglobulinlike domains

650. CORRECT statements concerning immunoglobulins include the following:

(1) The ratio of IgA to IgG in saliva is much higher than in serum.

(2) IgA and IgE cannot cross the placenta.

(3) There is IgE on the surface of basophils.

(4) The structure of IgA in saliva and in serum is the same.

651. Factors that play a role in the origin of antibody diversity include

(1) the large number of V genes

(2) association of heavy and light chains

(3) somatic mutation

(4) recombination of V, D, and J gene segments

652. Phagocytosis of bacteria by neutrophils is enhanced if the bacteria are coated with

(1) IgG

(2) IgE

(3) C3b

(4) C9

653. Immunoglobulin allotypes are

(1) found only on heavy chains

(2) determined by class I MHC genes

(3) confined to the variable regions

(4) due to genetic polymorphism with a species

654. CORRECT statements concerning carcinoembryonic antigen include the following:

(1) The level is high in normal fetal serum.

(2) The level is very low in normal adult serum.

(3) The level is elevated in some people with colon carcinoma.

(4) The level in serum rises after a tumor has been excised.

Answers (Questions 644–654)

644 (A)	647 (E)	650 (A)	653 (D)
645 (B)	648 (B)	651 (E)	654 (A)
646 (A)	649 (C)	652 (B)	

Index

NOTE: Page numbers in bold face type indicate a major discussion. A *t* following a page number indicates tabular material; an *i* following a page number indicates an illustration; and an *s* following a page number refers to the summaries of medically important organisms in Part VIII. Drugs are listed under their generic names. When a drug trade name is listed, the reader is referred to the generic drug name.